Complications of Pediatric and Adult Spinal Surgery

Complications of Pediatric and Adult Spinal Surgery

Edited by

Alexander R. Vaccaro

John J. Regan

Alvin H. Crawford

Edward C. Benzel

D. Greg Anderson

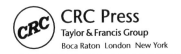

CRC Press
Taylor & Francis Group
Boca Raton London New York

CRC Press is an imprint of the
Taylor & Francis Group, an **informa** business

CRC Press
Taylor & Francis Group
6000 Broken Sound Parkway NW, Suite 300
Boca Raton, FL 33487-2742

First issued in paperback 2019

© 2004 by Taylor and Francis Group, LLC
CRC Press is an imprint of Taylor & Francis Group, an Informa business

No claim to original U.S. Government works

ISBN-13: 978-0-8247-5421-1 (hbk)
ISBN-13: 978-0-367-39387-8 (pbk)

Library of Congress Cataloging-in-Publication Data
A catalog record for this book is available from the Library of Congress.

Visit the Taylor & Francis Web site at
http://www.taylorandfrancis.com

and the CRC Press Web site at
http://www.crcpress.com

Preface

Over the past two decades the field of spinal surgery has expanded and evolved into a complex and technical surgical subspecialty. Fellowship training programs have produced a new breed of spinal specialists, often with practice interests distinct from their counterparts in general orthopedic, neurosurgery, or rehabilitation medicine. As the field of spinal care has evolved, vast changes have occurred in the techniques used for patient diagnosis, nonoperative management, and surgical treatment of spinal conditions. Along with sweeping advances in medical technology have come new challenges and potential complications associated with their applications. Each new technology brings with it a learning curve and a new set of potential pitfalls. To successfully navigate the waters of modern spinal care, the spine physician must be aware of the possibility of specific complications and be prepared to aggressively diagnose and successfully treat these situations. To date, no text or resource exists that comprehensively identifies and offers treatment advice for the myriad of complications experienced in contemporary spinal care.

The goal of this book is to provide an up-to-date and comprehensive overview of potential complications associated with nonoperative and operative management of various spinal pathologies. To achieve this goal, the book contains over 40 chapters written and edited by experienced nationally (and internationally) recognized experts in the field of spinal care. The book is divided into four parts, beginning with complication identification, prevention, and management. This section serves to lay the framework for understanding, diagnosing, and managing complications related to spinal intervention. The second part of the book addresses general complications, that may arise in all areas of spinal care. This section covers specific and challenging scenarios that are familiar to spinal specialists but are not often written about in the format of a book. The third part addresses specific complications that present within a well-defined area of spinal treatment. To improve organization and flow, this section is subdivided by spinal region, starting with occipital-cervical issues and ending with issues involving the lumbosacral region. In these subparts, modern nonoperative and operative interventions including surgical techniques and implant applications, are discussed to clarify the limitations, risks, and appropriate use of the described technologies. Two more subparts, discussing the complications of minimally invasive spinal procedures and pediatric spinal surgery complications, round out the specific complications section.

The section related to minimally invasive techniques is of particular interest, as this aspect of spinal surgery is changing rapidly, often with no good reference to which the spinal specialist can turn for advice on how to manage the frequent setbacks experienced with new and technically challenging innovations. It is paramount for the spine surgeon to be able to accurately compare emerging, less invasive techniques with their traditional open counterparts and thus understand the appropriate role of this new field of spinal surgery. This part not only identifies the benefits of less invasive techniques but also points out the limitations of each technology and the unique risks that may be encountered.

The section on pediatric spinal surgery addresses pathological conditions unique to the pediatric patient, including rare and often difficult-to-manage genetic conditions affecting the spine.

The fourth and final part of the book deals specifically with complication avoidance and addresses unique and important issues such as the involvement of house staff (i.e., residents and fellows) in the care of spinal patients and the legal and ethical aspects of contemporary spinal care. The book's division into subparts enables the reader to quickly reference a topic of interest.

This text provides practical, "in the trenches" information that will be useful to all physicians treating patients with spinal disorders. It fills a void in the available spinal literature, providing a "one-stop" reference for spinal care physicians on preventing and managing the unexpected complications arising in the management of these often-difficult patients. Consequently, it is an indispensable manual for those who care for spinal disorders at all stages of their career.

We thank Michael A. Pahl, M.D., for his assistance with the editing and production of the book.

Alexander R. Vaccaro
John J. Regan
Alvin H. Crawford
Edward C. Benzel
D. Greg Anderson

Contents

Simple Complications

Complication Prevention

Contributors

Kuniyoshi Abumi, M.D., D.M.Sc. Professor, Department of Orthopaedic Surgery, Hokkaido University, Health Administration Center, Sapporo, Japan

Michael C. Ain, M.D. Assistant Professor, Department of Orthopaedic Surgery, Assistant Professor, Department of Neurosurgery, and Director of Orthopaedic Residents, Johns Hopkins Hospital, Baltimore, Maryland, U.S.A.

Todd J. Albert, M.D. Professor and Vice Chairman, Department of Orthopaedic Surgery, Thomas Jefferson University and the Rothman Institute, Philadelphia, Pennsylvania, U.S.A.

Neel Anand, M.D. Director, Spine Trauma, Cedars-Sinai Institute for Spinal Disorders, Los Angeles, California, U.S.A.

D. Greg Anderson, M.D. Assistant Professor, Department of Orthopaedic Surgery, University of Virginia School of Medicine, Charlottesville, Virginia, U.S.A.

Ronald I. Apfelbaum, M.D. Professor, Department of Neurosurgery, University of Utah School of Medicine, Salt Lake City, Utah, U.S.A.

Paul M. Arnold, M.D. Associate Professor, Department of Neurosurgery, University of Kansas School of Medicine, Kansas City, Kansas, U.S.A.

John M. Beiner, M.D. Fellow, Spine Surgery, Department of Orthopaedic Surgery, Thomas Jefferson University and the Rothman Institute, Philadelphia, Pennsylvania, U.S.A.

Gordon R. Bell, M.D. Vice Chairman, Department of Orthopaedic Surgery, and Head, Section of Spinal Surgery, Cleveland Clinic Foundation, Cleveland, Ohio, U.S.A.

Edward C. Benzel, M.D. Director of Spinal Disorders, Department of Neurosurgery, Cleveland Clinic Foundation, Cleveland, Ohio, U.S.A.

Sigurd Berven, M.D. Assistant Professor, Department of Orthopaedic Surgery, University of California, San Francisco, San Francisco, California, U.S.A.

Michael J. Bolesta, M.D. Associate Professor, Department of Orthopaedic Surgery, The University of Texas Southwestern Medical Center, Dallas, Texas, U.S.A.

David S. Bradford, M.D. Professor and Chairman, Department of Orthopaedic Surgery, University of California, San Francisco, San Francisco, California, U.S.A.

Keith H. Bridwell, M.D. Asa C. and Dorothy W. Jones Professor of Orthopaedic Surgery, and Chief, Adult/Pediatric Spine Surgery, Department of Orthopaedic Surgery Barnes-Jewish Hospital and Washington University in St. Louis School of Medicine, St. Louis, Missouri, U.S.A.

Darrel S. Brodke, M.D. Associate Professor, Department of Orthopaedic Surgery, University of Utah, Salt Lake City, Utah, U.S.A.

Zach Broyer, M.D. Clinical Instructor of Physical Medicine and Rehabilitation, Thomas Jefferson University and the Rothman Institute, Philadelphia, Pennsylvania, U.S.A.

Rocco R. Calderone, M.D. Department of Surgery, St. John's Regional Medical Center, Oxnard, California, U.S.A.

Brett M. Cascio, M.D. Resident, Department of Orthopaedic Surgery, Johns Hopkins Hospital, Baltimore, Maryland, U.S.A.

Kanit Chamroontaneskul, M.D. Fellow, Spine Surgery, Department of Orthopaedic Surgery, University of Virginia School of Medicine, Charlottesville, Virginia, U.S.A.

Alvin H. Crawford, M.D. Director, Pediatric Orthopaedics, Cincinnati Children's Hospital Medical Center, Cincinnati, Ohio, U.S.A.

Aaron S. Dumont, M.D. Resident, Department of Neurological Surgery, University of Virginia School of Medicine, Charlottesville, Virginia, U.S.A.

John C. France, M.D. Associate Professor of Orthopaedic Surgery and Neurosurgery, and Chief, Section of Spine Surgery, Department of Orthopaedic Surgery, West Virginia University Health Science Center, Morgantown, West Virginia, U.S.A.

Mitchell K. Freedman, D.O. Clinical Instructor and Director, Department of Physical Medicine and Rehabilitation, Thomas Jefferson University and the Rothman Institute, Philadelphia, Pennsylvania, U.S.A.

Frank Fumich, M.D. Department of Orthopaedic Surgery, West Virginia University Health Science Center, Morgantown, West Virginia, U.S.A.

Peter G. Gabos, M.D. Assistant Professor of Orthopaedic Surgery, Jefferson Medical College, Philadelphia, Pennsylvania, and Pediatric Orthopaedic Surgeon, Alfred I. DuPont Hospital for Children, Wilmington, Delaware, U.S.A.

Steven R. Garfin, M.D. Professor and Chairman, Department of Orthopaedic Surgery, University of California, San Diego, San Diego, California, U.S.A.

Romergryko Geocadin, M.D. Assistant Professor and Director of Neuroscience, Critical Care Unit, Johns Hopkins Bayview Medical Center, Baltimore, Maryland, U.S.A.

Peter C. Gerszten, M.D., M.P.H. Director of Minimally Invasive and Spinal Oncology Programs, and Assistant Professor, Neurological Surgery and Radiation Oncology, University of Pittsburgh School of Medicine, Pittsburgh, Pennsylvania, U.S.A.

Jonathan N. Grauer, M.D. Fellow, Spine Surgery, Department of Orthopaedic Surgery, Thomas Jefferson University and the Rothman Institute, Philadelphia, Pennsylvania, U.S.A.

John J. Gross, Esq. O'Brien & Ryan, LLP, Plymouth Meeting, Pennsylvania, U.S.A.

Heather E. Hansen, Esq. O'Brien & Ryan, LLP, Plymouth Meeting, Pennsylvania, U.S.A.

James S. Harrop, M.D. Assistant Professor, Department of Neurosurgery, Thomas Jefferson University Hospital, Philadelphia, Pennsylvania, U.S.A.

Victor M. Hayes, M.D. Resident, Department of Orthopaedic Surgery, Long Island Jewish Medical Center, New Hyde Park, New York, U.S.A.

Gregory A. Helm, M.D. Associate Professor, Department of Neurosurgery, University of Virginia, School of Medicine, Charlottesville, Virginia, U.S.A.

Harry N. Herkowitz, M.D. Chairman, Department of Orthopaedic Surgery, William Beaumont Hospital, Royal Oak, Michigan, U.S.A.

Alan S. Hilibrand, M.D. Associate Professor of Orthopaedic Surgery and Director of Medical Education, Thomas Jefferson University and the Rothman Institute, Philadelphia, Pennsylvania, U.S.A.

Jeffery Hogg, M.D. Professor of Radiology, Neurology, and Neurosurgery, Department of Radiology, Ruby Memorial Hospital, West Virginia University, Morgantown, West Virginia, U.S.A.

Denise T. Ibrahim, D.O. Clinical Fellow, Division of Pediatric Orthopaedic Surgery, Northwestern University Feinberg School of Medicine Children's Memorial Hospital, Chicago, Illinois, U.S.A.

Manabu Ito, M.D., D.M.Sc. Assistant Professor, Department of Orthopaedic Surgery, Hokkaido University Hospital, Sapporo, Japan

John A. Jane, Jr., M.D. Chief Resident, Department of Neurological Surgery, University of Virginia School of Medicine, Charlottesville, Virginia, U.S.A.

John A. Jane, Sr., M.D., Ph.D. David D. Weaver Professor of Neurosurgery and Chairman, Department of Neurological Surgery, University of Virginia School of Medicine, Charlottesville, Virginia, U.S.A.

Iain H. Kalfas, M.D., F.A.C.S. Head, Section of Spinal Surgery, Department of Neurosurgery, Cleveland Clinic Foundation, Cleveland, Ohio, U.S.A.

Peter Kan, M.D. Resident, Department of Neurosurgery, University of Utah School of Medicine, Salt Lake City, Utah, U.S.A.

Larry T. Khoo, M.D. Assistant Professor, Neurologic and Orthopaedic Surgery, and Co-Director, Comprehensive Spine Center, UCLA Medical Center, Los Angeles, California, U.S.A.

Shyam Kishan, M.D. Resident, Department of Orthopaedic Surgery, New Jersey Medical School, University of Medicine and Dentistry of New Jersey, Newark, New Jersey, U.S.A.

Ira Kornbluth, M.D. Chief Resident, Department of Physical Medicine and Rehabilitation, Thomas Jefferson University Hospital, Philadelphia, Pennsylvania, U.S.A.

John P. Kostuik, M.D. Chief and Professor of Spinal Disorders, Department of Orthopaedic Surgery, Johns Hopkins University School of Medicine, Baltimore, Maryland, U.S.A.

Yoshihisa Kotani, M.D., D.M.Sc. Spine Surgeon, Department of Orthopaedic Surgery, Hokkaido University Hospital, Sapporo, Japan

Brian K. Kwon, M.D.* Fellow, Spine Surgery, Department of Orthopaedic Surgery, Thomas Jefferson University and the Rothman Institute, Philadelphia, Pennsylvania, U.S.A.

Sang-Min Lee, M.D., Ph.D. Assistant Professor, Seoul Spine Institute, Inje University, Sanggye-Paik Hospital, Seoul, Korea

Joan M. Lewis, J.D. Superior Court Judge, San Diego, California, U.S.A.

James K. Liu, M.D. Resident, Department of Neurosurgery, University of Utah School of Medicine, Salt Lake City, Utah, U.S.A.

Steven C. Ludwig, M.D. Assistant Professor, Department of Orthopaedic Surgery, University of Maryland, Baltimore, Maryland, U.S.A.

**Current affiliation*: Combined Neurosurgery and Orthopaedic Spine Program, Vancouver General Hospital, Vancouver, British Columbia, Canada

Robert A. McGuire, M.D. Professor, Department of Orthopaedics, University of Mississippi Medical Center, Jackson, Mississippi, U.S.A.

Joan K. McMahon, M.S.A., B.S.N., C.R.R.N. Spinal Cord Program Coordinator, Department of Nursing, University of Kansas Hospital, Kansas City, Kansas, U.S.A.

Christopher C. Meredith, M.D. Resident, Department of Neurosurgery, University of Kansas Schoool of Medicine, Kansas City, Kansas, U.S.A.

Arthur P. Nestler, R.N. Neurosurgical Nurse Coordinator, University of Pittsburgh School of Medicine, Pittsburgh, Pennsylvania, U.S.A.

Michael A. Pahl, M.D. Jefferson Medical College, Philadelphia, Pennsylvania, U.S.A.

Frank M. Phillips, M.D. Associate Professor of Surgery, Medical Director, Rush University Medical Center, Chicago, Illinois, U.S.A.

Ben B. Pradhan, M.D., M.S.E.* Chief Resident, Department of Orthopaedic Surgery, UCLA School of Medicine, Los Angeles, California, U.S.A.

Louis G. Quartararo, M.D. Assistant Professor, Department of Orthopaedic Surgery, Thomas Jefferson University and the Rothman Institute, Philadelphia, Pennsylvania, U.S.A.

Gannon B. Randolph, M.D. Resident, Department of Orthopaedic Surgery, University of Utah, Salt Lake City, Utah, U.S.A.

John J. Regan, M.D. Director, Cedars-Sinai Institute for Spinal Disorders, Los Angeles, California, U.S.A.

John M. Rhee, M.D. Assistant Professor, Department of Orthopaedic Surgery, The Emory Spine Center, Emory University School of Medicine, Atlanta, Georgia, U.S.A.

K. Daniel Riew, M.D. Associate Professor and Chief, Cervical Spine Surgery, Department of Orthopaedic Surgery, Barnes-Jewish Hospital and Washington University, School of Medicine, St. Louis, Missouri, U.S.A.

Daniele Rigamonti, M.D., F.A.C.S. Professor of Neurosurgery, Johns Hopkins Hospital Baltimore, Maryland, U.S.A.

Anthony S. Rinella, M.D. Instructor, Department of Orthopaedic Surgery and Rehabilitation, Loyola University Medical Center, Maywood, Illinois, U.S.A.

Matthew Robbins, M.D. Jefferson Medical College, Philadelphia, Pennsylvania, U.S.A.

Current affiliation: Spine Surgery Fellow, The Spine Institute, Saint John's Health Center, Santa Monica, California, U.S.A.

Virginia M. Salas, Ph.D. Research Coordinator, Durango Orthopaedic Associates, Durango, Colorado, U.S.A.

John F. Sarwalk, M.D. Interim Head, Professor of Pediatric Orthopaedic Surgery, Northwestern University Feinberg School of Medicine, Children's Memorial Hospital, Chicago, Illinois, U.S.A.

Rick C. Sasso, M.D. Assistant Professor, Department of Clinical Orthopaedic Surgery, Indiana Spine Group, Indianapolis, Indiana, U.S.A.

Martin H. Savitz, M.D., F.A.C.S., F.I.C.S., F.R.C.S. Professor of Neurosciences, Royal College of Physicians and Surgeons, Dean of Surgical Research, American International University, Executive Director, American Academy of Minimally Invasive Spinal Medicine and Surgery, and Adjunct Professor of Bioethics, Drexel University School of Medicine, Philadelphia, Pennsylvania, U.S.A.

Richard P. Schlenk, M.D. Clinical Spine Fellow, Department of Orthopaedic Surgery, Cleveland Clinic Foundation, Cleveland, Ohio, U.S.A.

Daniel M. Schwartz, Ph.D., D.ABNM President and CEO, Surgical Monitoring Associates, Bala Cynwyd, Pennsylvania, U.S.A.

Dilip K. Sengupta, M.D. Fellow, Spinal Surgery, Department of Orthopaedic Surgery, William Beaumont Hospital, Royal Oak, Michigan, U.S.A.

Anthony K. Sestokas, Ph.D., D.ABNM Director of Clinical Operations, Surgical Monitoring Associates, Bala Cynwyd, Pennsylvania, U.S.A.

Alok D. Sharan, M.D. Resident, Division of Orthopaedic Surgery, Department of Surgery, Albany Medical Center, Albany, New York, U.S.A.

Ashwini D. Sharan, M.D. Assistant Professor, Department of Neurosurgery, Thomas Jefferson University Hospital, Philadelphia, Pennsylvania, U.S.A.

Farhan N. Siddiqi, M.D. Resident, Department of Orthopaedic Surgery, Long Island Jewish Medical Center, New Hyde Park, New York, U.S.A.

Jeff S. Silber, M.D. Assistant Professor, Department of Orthopaedic Surgery, Long Island Jewish Medical Center, New Hyde Park, New York, U.S.A.

Marshall E. Smith, M.D. Associate Professor, Division of Otolaryngology–Head and Neck Surgery, University of Utah School of Medicine, Salt Lake City, Utah, U.S.A.

Paul D. Sponseller, M.D., M.B.A. Professor and Head, Pediatric Orthopaedics, Johns Hopkins University, Baltimore, Maryland, U.S.A.

Se-Il Suk, M.D., Ph.D. Professor and Director, Seoul Spine Institute, Inje University Medical School, Sanggye-Paik Hospital, Seoul, Korea

Louise E. Toutant, MSN Nurse Practitioner, Camarillo, California, U.S.A.

Alexander R. Vaccaro, M.D. Professor and Co-Director, Spine Service, Co-Director, Spine Fellowship Program, and Co-Director of the Delaware Valley Regional Spinal Cord Injury Center, Department of Orthopaedic Surgery, Thomas Jefferson University and the Rothman Institute, Philadelphia, Pennsylvania, U.S.A.

Anthony Virella, M.D. Chief Resident, Neurological Surgery, UCLA Medical Center Los Angeles, California, U.S.A.

Michael J. Vives, M.D. Assistant Professor, Department of Orthopaedic Surgery, New Jersey Medical School, University of Medicine and Dentistry of New Jersey, Newark, New Jersey, U.S.A.

Diane E. VonStein, M.D. Fellow, Pediatric Orthopaedics, Cincinnati Children's Hospital Medical Center, Cincinnati, Ohio, U.S.A.

Jeffrey C. Wang, M.D. Chief, Spine Surgery, Department of Orthopaedic Surgery, UCLA Medical Center, UCLA School of Medicine, Los Angeles, California, U.S.A.

K. Michael Webb, M.D. Resident, Department of Neurosurgery, University of Virginia School of Medicine, Charlottesville, Virginia, U.S.A.

William C. Welch, M.D., F.A.C.S., F.I.C.S. Associate Professor, Departments of Neurological and Orthopaedic Surgery and the School of Rehabilitative Sciences, and Director, Neurosurgical Spinal Services, University of Pittsburgh School of Medicine, Pittsburgh, Pennsylvania, U.S.A.

Kirkham B. Wood, M.D. St. Croix Orthopaedics, Stillwater, Minnesota, U.S.A.

Anthony T. Yeung, M.D. President, American Institute of Minimally Invasive Spinal Medicine and Surgery, Arizona Institute for Minimally Invasive Spine Care, Phoenix, Arizona, U.S.A.

Jim A. Youssef, M.D. Durango Orthopaedic Associates, Durango, Colorado, U.S.A.

Christopher M. Zarro, M.D. Resident, Department of Orthopaedic Surgery, University of Maryland, Baltimore, Maryland, U.S.A.

Seth M. Zeidman, M.D. Rochester Brain and Spine Institute, Rochester, New York, U.S.A.

1

The Foundation of Complication Identification, Prevention, and Management

D. Greg Anderson
University of Virginia School of Medicine, Charlottesville, Virginia, U.S.A.

Alexander R. Vaccaro and Michael A. Pahl
Thomas Jefferson University and the Rothman Institute, Philadelphia, Pennsylvania, U.S.A.

I. INTRODUCTION

Few issues are as important to the success of the practicing spinal surgeon as the appropriate recognition and management of complications in his or her patients. In spite of the best quality of medical care, complications are an inevitable part of medical interventions. It is the goal of physicians to minimize the risk of complications and rapidly identify and treat complications when they occur. In many cases, early recognition and aggressive management following a complication can significantly reduce the risk of long-term sequalae.

Because complications represent a difficult and unpleasant event for both the patient and physician, it may be difficult to thoroughly discuss a complication with a patient or patient's family. However, a lack of discussion or avoidance of repeated contact with the patient or family can significantly increase the patient's fear and anguish and lead to ill feelings towards the treating physician. Generally, an extra measure of involvement with the patient and family is the best way to let the patient and family know that every effort is being taken to limit the negative impact of the particular complication. The time spent interacting with the patient following a complication will not only ensure that they understand their medical situation but will empower them to be a partner in determining the course of their medical care. Often, it is helpful to seek consultations with other specialists who provide not only a different perspective on the work-up and treatment of the particular complication but also act as an additional resource to the patient and family for questions regarding their medical situation. The psychological benefit of active caring and open dialogue with the patient and family following a serious complication cannot be overstated.

II. PREVENTION

The management of complications begins prior to surgery with the informed consent process. During the consent process, it is the physician's opportunity to educate the

1

patient on the nature of their spinal condition and the planned spinal intervention. It is critical to ensure that the patient understands the spectrum of treatment options available to them and why the chosen treatment is thought to be appropriate. Common or serious complications that might be anticipated after a particular type of intervention should be discussed. When discussing potential complications, the goal should be to help the patient understand the meaning of specific complications, the likelihood of occurrence, and the goals of early recognition and treatment of the complications if they should occur. This helps to make the patient a partner in the recognition and management of a complication prior to the planned surgical intervention. If possible, the patient's family should also be involved in the consent process for surgery, allowing family members to benefit from this educational process. Having family members present can help to prevent the impression that something "must have been done wrong" should a complication occur.

Complication prevention often begins with good preoperative planning. This is especially true in the field of spine surgery, where modern techniques often require significant logistical preparations. It is critical to obtain all the necessary imaging studies and review them carefully prior to the planned operation. Arrangements should be made for the necessary equipment to be ready in the operating suite, including the appropriate spine table, necessary radiographic support, image guidance technology, and operative microscopes, if necessary, and the required instruments and implants.

A medical evaluation by a specialist may be advisable prior to surgery depending on the patient's age and medical history and should be sought through appropriate consultation. Preparation should be made for perioperative blood products in cases where significant bleeding is anticipated. Necessary operating room personnel including exposure surgeons, neurophysiological monitoring personnel, cell savor personnel, anesthesia staff, instrumentation representatives, and nursing staff are all valuable members of the operating team, and these members should be informed in advance of the surgical plan. Arrangements for postoperative care should also be considered, especially for patients requiring intensive care in the postoperative period.

Positioning of the patient for surgery is an important step in minimizing the risk of complications. Care should be taken to avoid pressure areas, especially over critical neurovascular structures. Use of a spinal frame that removes pressure from the abdominal region is important for prone procedures. Special attention should be taken to ensure that the eyes and face are free of pressure points. Equally important to good positioning is the need to proceed with surgery in an efficient fashion, as prolonged surgery, even with good padding, can be responsible for pressure-related trauma, wound infections, and metabolic stress to the patient.

Wrong site surgery is a complication that is responsible for a very high proportion of malpractice cases and is avoidable with appropriate measures. The prevention of wrong site surgery begins with a preoperative evaluation of the patients and imaging studies. The site of surgery should be clearly documented. Some surgeons find it useful to mark the site and surgical plan directly on a preoperative radiograph to ensure that the operative plan is immediately available in the operating room. The symptomatic side should be identified immediately prior to surgery by the operative team in patients with radicular symptoms to ensure that wrong side surgery is avoided. During surgery, radiographic identification of the vertebral level is mandatory. It is best to place a metallic instrument as close as possible to the spinal canal to avoid confusion. Permanent marking of the desired site can be achieved with removal of a small fragment of lamina or spinous process at the location of the radiographic marker. It is safest to do this once the radiograph is interpreted in order to avoid any potential for confusion as to the precise location of the previously removed localizer. The importance of a good quality intraoperative radiograph cannot be overstated. Unfortunately, patient obesity, spinal deformity, and previous surgery can obscure or complicate the identification of levels. In some regions of the spine, intraoperative radiographic imaging is difficult or impossible, such as the cervicothoracic junction in prone patients with large shoulders. In some cases, a larger exposure may be required to achieve unequivocal identification of spinal levels.

Prevention of technical complications during surgery begins with good surgical technique and experience with the planned procedure. In open procedures, it is important to have adequate exposure of the anatomy and maintain a dry surgical field to allow adequate visualization during the procedure. Correct placement of implants in the spine should be confirmed by radiographic means prior to completion of the procedure. Surgeon fatigue may become a factor in long cases and should be avoided when feasible.

Complication prevention continues in the postoperative period through early mobilization of the patient, if possible. The metabolic status of the patient should be assessed carefully in the postoperative period, and any metabolic abnormalities should be should be corrected as needed. Analgesic medications should be customized to the patient to promote early mobilization.

Following these general principles, the rate of complications can be minimized.

III. IDENTIFICATION

The first step in treating a complication is recognizing that a complication exists. Recognition requires an understanding of the potential problems that are possible and an active routine surveillance for such complications intraoperatively and during the post-operative course. Vigilance for potential complications requires routine subjective assessment of the patient's symptoms and a focused examination supplemented with selective laboratory studies in the postoperative period. Specific tests or studies should be acquired as early as possible to confirm the presence of a complication. Early detection allows early complication treatment, which in most cases leads to the best ultimate outcome.

Significant changes in neurological status dictate the need for rapid imaging of the affected regions of the spine. If the cause of the neurological deterioration is noted, treatment can be instituted in a timely basis. In cases where an explanation of the neurological deterioration is not apparent, a search for other causes of the neurological deterioration (e.g., stroke) should be sought. The use of advanced imaging modalities such as magnetic resonance imaging (MRI) and computed tomography (CT) myelography can effectively reveal the cause of neurological decline in the presence of spinal cord compression.

Some types of complications may not be obvious. An example might be a low-grade deep wound infection in the setting of a benign-appearing wound. In these cases, a high index of suspicion is needed to diagnose this condition. Maintaining a high index of suspicion when evaluating a patient with unexplained signs or symptoms following surgery is the best way to uncover subtle problems and allow institution of appropriate diagnostic and treatment modalities.

IV. MANAGEMENT

When dealing with a serious complication, seeking medical consultation from other specialists is often wise. Eliciting such guidance can have several important benefits. First, opinions for outside physicians can help to highlight medical issues that may not have been considered. Second, because the consultant has more emotional distance from the case, they can often provide balance to the opinion of the treating surgeon. Third, patients and family members generally appreciate having outside medical opinions when facing a serious complication. Fourth, appropriate medical consultation helps to demonstrate a high quality of care should a malpractice claim arise following a given complication. Finally, and most importantly, requesting consultation enhances the level of care provided and minimizes the risk of a poor outcome.

Spine surgery complications often have medicolegal implications. Although frivolous lawsuits are all too common these days, each malpractice claim begins with a perceived suboptimal outcome of some type. To prove malpractice, the plaintiff, depending on the local law, often must convince the judge and/or jury that the care of the patient was below the community "standard." Legal experts generally agree that physicians with positive relationships with their patients are the least likely to be sued following a complication. Documentation of the consent process and the discussion of expected complications becomes paramount in malpractice cases. Other important features include how rapidly and effectively the physician recognized and instituted treatment following the complication. Therefore, it is important that the thought process of the physician managing an unexpected complication be carefully documented in the medical record. Fortunately, the principles of good quality medical practice and thorough documentation are effective in defending most malpractice claims.

V. CONCLUSION

Although prevention of a complication is always best, perioperative complications will never be eliminated. Therefore, the efforts of the treating physician should be directed towards reducing the risk of complications through careful, deliberate planning and attention to detail. Understanding the potential complications that can occur is critical to the preoperative consent process and to anticipating and successfully managing complications in the postoperative period if they should occur. The contributors to this text have provided significant details of specific complications in all areas of the spine in both pediatric and adult patients. In the technically demanding field of spine surgery, a better understanding of complication recognition and management remains a worthy goal for all spine surgeons.

2

Complications of Anesthesia Administration and Positioning for Spinal Surgery

Dilip K. Sengupta and Harry N. Herkowitz
William Beaumont Hospital, Royal Oak, Michigan, U.S.A.

I. COMPLICATIONS RELATED TO ANESTHESIA

A. Hypotensive Anesthesia

Controlled hypotension helps to reduce blood loss during spinal surgery. The mean arterial pressure needs to be safe and adequate for perfusion of the spinal cord and other vital organs. A moderate degree of induced hypotension, usually a mean arterial pressure of 65 or 20 mmHg below the baseline in normotensive subjects, is considered safe in nonmyelopathic patients. Induced hypotension, however, may contribute to spinal cord ischemia and neurological damage. The risk increases significantly in the presence of preoperative hypertension, hypocapnia, anemia, rapid blood loss, or a sudden drop in the blood pressure. The adverse effects may depend on the degree of hypotension induced and the specific drugs used to produce hypotension.

The two most commonly used hypotensive agents are sodium nitroprusside and trimethaphan. Less commonly used agents include nitroglycerin and volatile anesthetic agents.

Inhalation anesthetics induce hypotension during their administration. Enflurane and isoflurane have fewer myocardial effects, decrease systemic vascular resistance to a greater extent, and cause cardiac arrhythmias less frequently than halothane. However, all volatile anesthetics produce a dose-dependent deterioration of somatosensory evoked potential (SSEP) response. Sodium nitroprusside produces a reliable decrease in blood pressure and, at least initially, increases spinal cord blood flow. It also has a "ceiling effect," i.e., it cannot lower blood pressure beyond a certain point. Side effects of its use include tachyphylaxis, toxicity, and rebound hypertension with reflex tachycardia. This may be prevented by use of a β-blocker or an ACE inhibitor as premedication. Blood pressure should be allowed to recover gradually at the end of the surgery to prevent reactionary hemorrhage.

During controlled hypotension using trimethaphan, the autoregulatory control of spinal cord blood flow may be lost, resulting in a pressure-dependent blood flow, which may not be adequate at a low mean arterial pressure. Similar changes are not observed when hypotension is induced with agents like sodium nitroprusside or nitroglycerin. Therefore trimethaphan is not recommended during spinal operations (1).

Systemic hypotension and local compression of the spinal cord both independently affect spinal cord blood flow in an additive way (2). Experimentally, reduction of spinal

5

cord blood flow has been shown to cause deterioration of motor evoked potentials and resultant spinal cord damage. Hypoperfusion causes a slow loss of evoked potentials (>15 min), while cord compression causes a rapid loss (<5 min) of signals. A spinal cord blood flow of at least 65% of baseline is required to maintain the physiological integrity of the spinal cord, and a decrease in blood flow to 12% of baseline is associated with the potential for paralysis (3).

Nielsen (4) recommended that it may be safe to induce controlled hypotension to a mean arterial blood pressure of 55 mmHg as long as the somatosensory and motor-evoked potentials remain unchanged from normal baseline values during specific spinal procedures.

B. Endotracheal Intubation in the Presence of Cervical Spine Injury

Emergency intubation may be necessary at the accident site before cervical spine injury is excluded. Extension of the neck for intubation may cause or aggravate a spinal cord injury and should be avoided when injury to the cervical spine is a possibiltiy. The patient's head should be stabilized between the hands and forearms of an assistant under mild traction, and the head may be gently extended to facilitate intubation.

In an elective operation, an intubation may be performed safely without moving the neck. An awake nasal intubation, with judiciously applied local anesthetic, is the procedure of choice when neck motion is to be avoided. It is often, however, uncomfortable to the patient. Alternately, use of a fiber-optic bronchoscope may facilitate intubation while the head and neck is supported in the neutral position between the hands and forearms of an assistant. Neck motion may also be lessened by leaving the patient in a stiff-neck collar.

C. Spinal Anesthesia

For short-duration spinal surgery, spinal or epidural anesthesia has certain advantages. In patients with pulmonary disease, it avoids bronchospasm associated with intubation and respiratory depression associated with general anesthesia. Other advantages are post-operative analgesia, a lesser incidence of nausea and vomiting, the potential for sympathetic blockade, and less blood loss.

Spinal and epidural anesthesia, however, have several disadvantages when used in spinal surgery. Disastrous complications like paraplegia are extremely rare but have been reported in the literature (5). Should the surgery last longer than the duration of the regional block, conversion to general anesthesia is difficult for most spinal procedures which are performed in the prone position. When the effect of regional blockage lasts longer than the duration of the surgery, it makes postoperative neurological assessment difficult and may delay the recognition of any neurological deficit. If the patient coughs or moves during surgery, it may result in inadvertant iatrogenic neural injury or nerve root prolapse even through a small dural leak.

II. COMPLICATIONS RELATED TO PATIENT POSITIONING

Most posterior lumbar surgical procedures are performed in the prone or knee-chest position. Anterior approaches to the cervical or lumbar spine are performed in the supine position, and approaches to the thoracic and thoraco-lumbar junction are usually performed in a lateral position.

Proper positioning of patients is one of the most challenging tasks in spinal surgery. Numerous complications are associated with improper positioning. Air embolism, peripheral nerve palsy, blindness, quadriplegia, compartment syndrome, pressure necrosis of the skin, excessive bleeding, and venous thrombosis are only some of the complications that may result from improper positioning.

A. Pressure-Related Injuries

The most frequent complication due to prone positioning during spinal surgery is pressure necrosis of the skin. Adequate padding must be placed under the pressure points to prevent skin breakdown or peripheral nerve compressions. For prone positioning, pressure points of particular importance include the face, iliac crests, breasts, and the anterior aspect of the knee joints. The abdomen must be allowed to hang freely to avoid pressure to the vena cava, which may cause excessive venous bleeding during surgery and, in a prolonged operation, may initiate deep vein thrombosis. Lee et al. (6) has shown in a clinical study that hypotensive anesthesia does not lower the venacaval pressure, but the use of a spinal frame, which allows the abdomen to hang free in a prone position, significantly lowers vena caval pressure compared to the prone position on a conventional pad. Anterior tibial compartment syndrome has been reported following lumbar surgery in the knee-chest position due to prolonged pressure in front of the tibia (7). Systemic anticoagulants are often not used in the perioperative period as a preventive measure against postoperative deep vein thrombosis in spinal surgery because of the risk of hematoma around the spinal cord. Elastic bandages and sequential compression devices should be placed on the lower extremities before the induction of the anesthesia.

In the prone position, particular attention must be given to facial positioning. It is preferable to position the head and neck in a neutral rotation and to support the face over a piece of foam with a cutout for the eyes, nose, and mouth (Fig. 1A). The pressure points vulnerable to skin necrosis are the forehead, chin, and tip of the nose. During posterior surgery of the cervical and cranio-cervical junction, great pressure may be exerted during spinal instrumentation. In these situations the head should preferably be positioned in Mayfield tongs, which allows the face to hang free of pressure from any source. The protective padding over the face may shift during the surgical procedure and requires frequent reevaluation. Use of a mirror may facilitate inspection of the face (Fig. 1B). During prolonged surgical procedures exceeding a few hours, elevation of the head-end of the operating table may prevent edema of the face, eyelids, and lips.

Neurological injury is the most common cause of perioperative morbidity resulting from improper positioning. In one study, neurological injury due to operative positioning was found in 72 out of 50,000 operations (0.14%), the most common of which were brachial plexus injuries (38%) (8). Other major peripheral nerves that are vunerable during positioning are the ulnar nerve around the elbow and the radial nerve around the arm. Elbow extension minimizes the exposure of the ulnar nerve to compression. When the elbow is flexed, foam padding should be applied around the elbow. The radial nerve may be injured if the arm hangs over the edge of the operation table. The common peroneal nerve around the fibular neck is most vulnerable to compression injuries in the lateral decubitus position. In the supine or prone positions, which are more frequently used in spinal surgery, the common peroneal nerve may be injured if the lower extremities roll into abduction with external rotation. The superficial location of the nerve around the neck of the fibula may increase the risk of compression. Patients with a history of diabetes

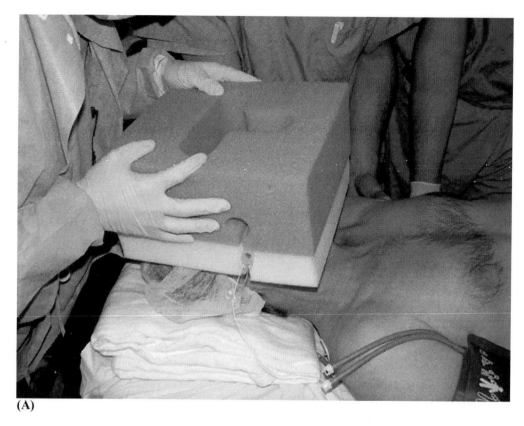

(A)

Figure 1 (A) For prone positioning, the face should be rested over a piece of foam, with cutouts for the mouth, eyeballs, and endotracheal tube to relieve pressure. (B) Use of a mirror permits inspection and reevaluation of the face during surgery, without moving the patient's head.

or alcoholism are particularly prone to develop neurological injury from external pressure and also appear to recover more slowly (9).

In the lateral decubitus position for anterior surgical approaches to the thoracic and thoraco-lumbar spine, the kidney rest should be positioned under the pelvic brim to rotate the iliac crest away from the lower rib margin. If the kidney rest is positioned under the flank or the lower ribs, it may cause pressure to the vena cava and may jeopardize pulmonary function. The head should be supported in the neutral position, as unilateral Horner's syndrome has been reported after anesthesia for patients operated in the lateral position. This is possibly due to extreme lateral flexion of the cervical spine leading to damage of the inferior cervical sympathetic trunk (10).

Moving and turning the patient into and out of the prone position should be performed without hyperextension of the cervical spine or undue manipulation of the peripheral joints. Particular attention is needed in elderly osteoporotic subjects, patients with total joint replacements, and patients with stiff joints such as in ankylosing spondylitis. The endotracheal tube should be properly secured before moving the patient into the prone position. The patient should be properly oxygenated, and then the tube should be disconnected before turning into or out of a prone position to prevent to the tube traction and dislodgement.

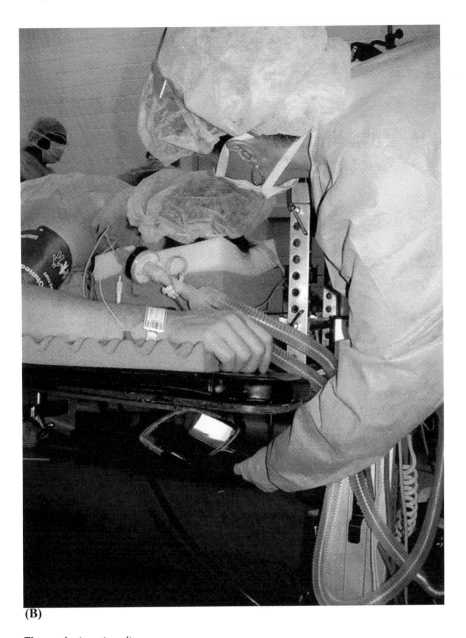

(B)

Figure 1 *(continued)*

The patient may be positioned prone on a normal operating table using chest and pelvic rolls of appropriate sizes. This may not adequately prevent pressure to the abdomen, vena cava, or brachial plexus, and is only suitable for short operative procedures. More desirable bed frames include the four-post frame, Jackson frame, Andrew's frame, or Wilson frame. The key to successful positioning is familiarity with the given table or frame. Sufficient personnel must be present during transfer of the patient to a spinal table for lifting and stabilization, particularly for heavy patients. The Jackson frame (Fig. 2) permits easy access to the whole length of the spine for intraoperative

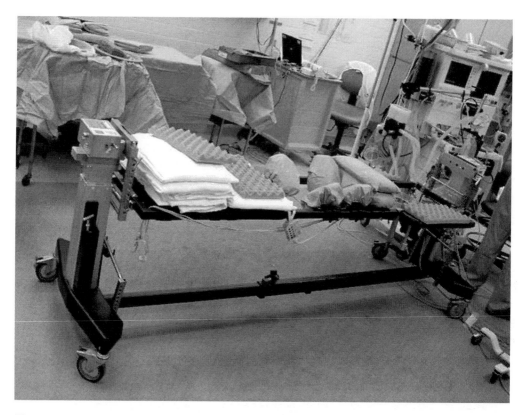

Figure 2 The Jackson frame has legs only at the rostral and caudal ends, leaving the whole length of the spine free for preoperative radiographs. The abdomen may hang freely between the sidebars. The head rests on a transparent headboard (arrow), and the face can be inspected using a mirror, while the patient is positioned prone on the table.

radiographs. Use of a mirror may facilitate inspection of the face, eyes, and tube position, which may shift during patient transfer or during surgery. An Andrews frame (Fig. 3) may permit gradual and controlled transition from a prone position to a knee-chest position, without the need for lifting the patient. However, such a transition must be done under direct vision, and proper attention to all pressure points and tubes connected to the patient must be given during the positioning procedure.

The prone position may affect pulmonary compliance by compressing the abdomen and restricting chest wall movement. Palmon et al. (11) studied the effects of the patient body habitus with the use of three different surgical frames (chest rolls, the Wilson frame, or the Jackson table) with the patient in the prone position. Seventy-seven adult patients took part in this study. Pulmonary compliance decreased when turning the patients from the supine to the prone position in all three body mass groups when using chest rolls or the Wilson frame. However, regardless of body habitus, using the Jackson table for prone positioning was not associated with a significant alteration in pulmonary or hemodynamic functions.

B. Brachial Plexus Injury

The brachial plexus is most vulnerable to injury in the prone position (8,9,12).

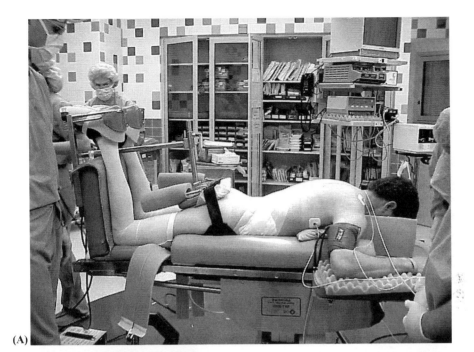

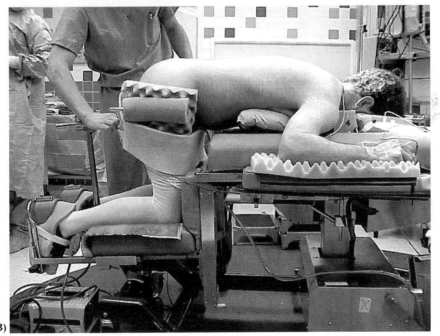

Figure 3 The Andrews frame permits for the conversion of the patient from the prone position (A) to the knees to chest position (B) without moving the patient off of the table.

Neurological injury is believed to occur due to mechanical injury from compression or stretching, or possibly due to ischemia, which may result from moderate compression over a long time period. Typically, neurological injury is associated with long operative procedures, but has been reported with surgical procedures as short as 45 minutes (8). Positions that appear to cause brachial plexus injury, on the basis of both clinical and cadaveric studies, are shoulder abduction with external rotation or shoulder extension or posterior displacement (8,12). The shoulder should not be abducted beyond 90°. The arms should rest at the level of the operating table or slightly lower, and the elbows should be flexed at a right angle allowing the hands to lie alongside the head. Great care should be taken to prevent hyperextension of the shoulders (Fig. 4).

A case reported by Jackson et al. (12) involves the onset of bilateral brachial plexus injury following an operative procedure in the prone position over longitudinal chest rolls with the arms abducted and the elbows flexed. This was felt to be due to unusually large chest rolls and an unsupported head, resulting in posterior shoulder displacement and anterior head displacement. Turning the head may also increase stretch on the contralateral brachial plexus, but this has not been confirmed in cadaveric studies (12,13). General anesthesia increases the risk of neurological injury from malposition because of the loss of muscle tone and the inability of the patient to report any discomfort (9).

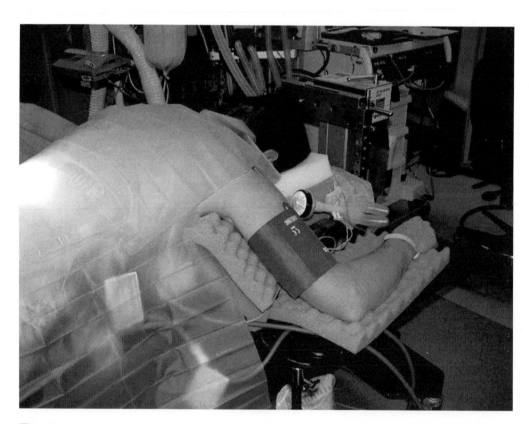

Figure 4 To prevent traction or compression in jury to the brachial plexus, the arm should be placed alongside the head with the elbow flexed at a right angle. It is important to note that the arm should not be abducted beyond a right angle and that the shoulder should not be extended. Padding under the humerus and elbow avoids pressure to the radial and ulnar nerves.

Although brachial plexus injury is more common in spinal surgery in the prone position, supine or lateral positions are not immune to such injuries. In fact, brachial plexus injuries are most frequently reported in the supine position following cardiac surgery with a median sternotomy approach (14,15,16), particularly because of excessive sternal retraction for harvesting the internal mammary artery, which results in traction to the brachial plexus. In a prospective study of 1000 consecutive cardiac surgery patients, brachial plexus injury was reported in 27 patients. The incidence was 10 times higher in cases with harvesting the internal mammary artery for grafting compared to those without (14). Median sternotomy is rarely indicated in spinal surgery, expect where a direct anterior approach to the upper thoracic spine is needed. Infrequently, a traction injury to the brachial plexus may occur during anterior surgery of the cervical spine when the shoulders are strapped down with adhesive tape for better radiological visualization of the lower cervical spine. During surgery in the lateral decubitus position, the brachial plexus of the dependent arm may undergo compression injury. This may be prevented by placing a rolled towel or a bag of fluid under the upper part of the rib cage, immediately distal to the axilla.

Recovery of neurological deficits as a result of patient positioning is observed in over 92% of cases, typically within 6 months (8). Somatosensory evoked potential has been suggested to be a sensitive tool in recognizing an impending brachial plexus injury (16). However, a study in conscious volunteers found no correlation between changes in somatosensory evoked potentials and the development of symptoms (17). Hence, the only reliable method for prevention remains attention to detail while positioning the patient.

C. Ocular Injuries

Postoperative visual loss is one of the most devastating complications reported to occur after spinal surgery in the prone position. Ocular damage may occur due to corneal dryness and abrasion or postoperative visual loss (POVL).

The most common cause of ocular damage is by corneal abrasion (18). The cornea should be protected by closing the eyelids with adhesive tape, preferably after the application of an ophthalmic lubricant. The eyes should then be protected with padding and secured in place. Despite careful preoperative positioning, any movement during surgery may cause the patient to shift, resulting in elevated ocular pressure. The eyes should be frequently reevaluated during surgery. The use of a mirror to view the face of the patient during surgery while in a prone position may be helpful (Fig. 1B).

The etiology of postoperative blindness is incompletely understood and multifactorial (19,20,21,22). This complication is most frequently reported after spinal surgery and cardiopulmonary bypass surgery, but may occur after other nonocular surgeries like liver transplantation, head and neck surgery, and veno-veno bypass. The true incidence is not known, but may vary between 0.05% and 1% for cardiopulmonary bypass or spine surgeries (19). Atheromatous plaque or air emboli, prolonged hypotension and anemia, inadequate venous drainage of the globe, and direct pressure to the eye have all been implicated as causative factors. The most important preventive measure is to avoid direct pressure to the eyeballs. Extreme care must be taken in the prone positioning of a patient. Use of Mayfield tongs allows the head and the face to hang free from pressure, but may not be appropriate for all patients undergoing spinal surgery. Many clinicians prefer foam rubber support with cutouts for the eyes and nose (Fig. 1A). The unexplained intraoperative occurrence of bradyarrhythmia or conduction disturbance may signal increased intraorbital pressure during general anesthesia (7).

The American Society of Anesthesiologists' Committee on Professional Liability has established an International Registry in July 1999 to investigate the mechanism of perioperative Ischemic Optic Neuropathy (ION) (23). The goal of the Registry is to identify potential intraoperative risk factors and patient characteristics, which may predispose to such complications. Although data from a registry cannot determine a definite cause-and-effect relationship, it can be used to find common events or characteristics between patients suffering from the same complications.

According to a recent report based on the registry (24), which collected 47 cases, operations associated with POVL were predominately prone spine procedures ($n = 31$, 67%) followed by cardiopulmonary bypass cases ($n = 8$, 17%), head and neck procedures ($n = 2$, 4%), and liver transplantation with veno-veno bypass ($n = 2$, 4%). Other operations accounted for 4 cases (8%). There is a perception that the incidence of POVL has been increasing recently, particularly in association with prone spine procedures. This may be related to a large increase in the number of complex, long duration, instrumented spine operations occurring over the last decade. Alternatively, this may reflect a reporting bias in which people are more motivated to report cases of POVL associated with the prone position than with other types of cases. Visual loss was predominantly (90%) caused by ischemic optic neuropathy; only 6% of cases were diagnosed as central retinal artery occlusion. The prone position appears to place patients at increased risk of developing POVL. The other important determinant is the number of hours in the prone spine position. The incidence appears to dramatically increase for durations of prone positioning between 5 and 9 hours. The etiology of POVL in prone spine operations may differ from that occurring in operations performed in the supine position.

Ischemic optic neuropathy is divided into anterior and posterior, depending upon the location of the lesion on the optic nerve. The majority of anterior ischemic optic neuropathy cases occur during cardiopulmonary bypass procedures (53%), followed by prone spine cases (12%). Most posterior ischemic optic neuropathy cases have occurred during neck, nose, or sinus operations (48%), followed by prone spine cases (16%) and cardiopulmonary bypass procedures (11%) (18).

Younger age does not appear to be protective. Nearly 50% of POVL occur in patients younger than 50 years of age. Although coexisting diseases may increase the risk of developing this complication, such a high frequency of occurrence in younger, healthier patients suggests that intraoperative physiological variables such as edema formation and venous congestion in the prone position, as well as "normal" physiological variation in ocular hemodynamics, may be important etiological determinants.

D. Air Embolism

Air embolism is one of the most serious complications in spinal surgery. It is predominantly related to operations performed above the level of the heart. The incidence of air embolism is greater in the sitting position than in any other position and may be as high as 25% following neurosurgical procedures (25). However, it has been reported infrequently following surgery in the supine and prone positions (26,27,28).

Prevention of air embolism and its management depends on (a) use of a central venous catheter, and maintaining the central venous pressure above 10 cm to prevent the decline of pressure in the epidural veins, and (b) meticulous monitoring of the patient at risk with ultrasound Doppler and end-tidal PCO_2. If air embolism is detected, air should be sucked out from the left atrium through the central venous catheter. The surgeon should flush the wound with Hartman solution and promptly coagulate any open veins using bipolar cautery. Bleeding bones should be waxed, and the wound should be packed with wet gauze. If the signs of air embolism still persist, the patient should be quickly turned into the right-side-up position to facilitate the removal of air from the right atrium through the central venous catheter.

III. FLUID MANAGEMENT

Safe and adequate perfusion and oxygenation of the vital organs may only be ensured when the patient is maintained normovolemic, with a minimum hematocrit of 0.21% and a mean arterial pressure at or above 55 mmHg.

Controlled hypotension may be easier to induce if the patient is hypovolemic, but this practice is dangerous (4). Fluid requirement may be calculated from the hourly fluid input, urine output, third space loss, and estimated blood loss. Additional fine-tuning may be accomplished by monitoring central venous pressure and pulmonary artery pressure.

When the need for transfusion is anticipated, autologous blood is the safest option for eligible patients. The different methods for obtaining autologous blood for use during or after a planned surgical procedure include preoperative autologous blood donation, perioperative blood salvage, and acute normovolemic hemodilution. Hemodilution with crystalloid infusion to a hematocrit of 0.21 commonly allows 1–2.5 L of blood to be drawn from the patient during induction (4). The right hematocrit and the lowest acceptable hematocrit are controversial issues. The National Blood Resource Education Program Expert Panel recommendation, as circulated to all anesthesiologists in 1989, stated 0.21 to be the minimal value recommended during surgical care (4). In their revised recommendation this value was dropped, while keeping the wording of the document unchanged (29).

IV. INTRAOPERATIVE MONITORING

A. Spinal Cord Monitoring

Nash et al. reported in 1977 on the use of mixed-nerve somatosensory evoked potentials (SSEP) as a method of monitoring spinal cord function during spinal surgery. SSEPs are sensory-based and are highly sensitive to the functional integrity of the dorsal medial tracts, but provide only indirect information regarding the functional integrity of the motor tracts, which lie in the anterior column and are supplied by the anterior spinal artery. Because of this fact, some potential exists for postoperative motor deficit in a patient even without changes in the intraoperative SSEP monitoring signal. Motor-evoked potential has subsequently been developed to directly monitor the functional integrity of the motor tracts in the spinal cord.

Both somatosensory and motor-evoked potentials are affected by various factors besides actual damage to the functional integrity of the spinal cord. These include hypotension, hypoxia, level of anesthesia, and pharmacological effects of the various anesthetic agents. The resulting changes in electrophysiological monitoring signals may be indistinguishable from changes indicating spinal cord damage.

The effect of inhalational anesthetics are dose-related, with increasing doses producing reduced amplitude and increased latency in the monitored signals. A nitrous oxide–narcotic-relaxant combination is commonly used for the maintenance of anesthesia. Supplementation with a low concentration of volatile anesthetics helps to maintain controlled hypotension, reduce narcotic requirements, and at the same time allow for satisfactory interpretation of SSEPs.

MEPs are more frequently affected by the anesthetic agents. Satisfactory monitoring requires obtaining a steady baseline monitoring signal before the surgical procedure can be started. In one study of combined SSEP and MEP motoring in 126 consecutive spinal surgery procedures, MEP motoring had to be abandoned in 18 cases, and SSEP had to be abandoned in 2 cases because of unsatisfactory baseline signal quality (30). In another study isoflurane interfered with the baseline MEP signals more often than propofol, when used in combination with nitrous oxide for the maintenance of anesthesia (31). Muscle relaxants also interfere with MEP signals. Their dose should be titrated to the minimum required for relaxation and should be monitored by recording the compound muscle action potentials (CMAPs).

Availability of spinal cord monitoring and third-generation spinal stabilization implants may motivate the surgeon to achieve a greater correction of deformity. This raises the question, "How sensitive are these monitoring techniques?" In general, MEPs are extremely sensitive, and many centers have experienced no false-negative MEP monitoring. However, although SSEP monitoring is highly sensitive, one center reported 2 cases of false negative monitoring out of 124; one patient awoke with a motor deficit with no SSEP changes, and the other had a sensory deficit despite full recovery of SSEP signals (30). Nuwer et al. (32) reported that SSEPs have a negative predictive value of 99.6% for ruling out motor deficit during surgical correction of scoliosis.

Specificity of these modalities is difficult to determine. Normally, when the monitoring signal is reduced, lost, or delayed, any hemodynamic abnormality like hypotension should be immediately restored to normal. This often returns the monitoring signal back to normal. If not, the spinal instrumentation is loosened or removed, and in many cases the monitoring signal returns. If the patient wakes up without any neurodeficit, it is unreasonable to designate those monitoring changes as false positive, although some of them truly are. In the study previously mentioned, significant monitoring changes occurred in the SSEPs or MEPs or both in 16 out of 124 monitored patients. Ten of the patients were undergoing instrumentation, and six were experiencing hemodynamic changes. After appropriate remedial measures, monitoring signals returned to baseline in 12 cases completely or incompletely, and only 6 cases awoke with a postoperative neurological deficit. In the 10 cases that did not develop a neurological deficit, the transient signal changes may not be false positive, but rather indicate recovery from impending spinal cord ischemia or compression.

B. Wake-Up Test

To date there have been no reports of false-negative wake-up tests; no patient who was neurologically intact intraoperatively at the time of the wake-up test awoke with a neurological deficit at the end of the procedure. If there is loss of monitoring signal during surgery, and the signal fails to return, the wake-up test should be performed immediately before proceeding further with the operative procedure. Ideally the surgeon should notify the anesthesiologist 30–45 minutes in advance of a wake-up test. Long-acting anesthetics and inhalation anesthetics may delay the time to wake-up. Nitrous oxide and propofol are short-acting agents, and muscle relaxants, opioids, and benzodiazepines can be reversed. A continuous narcotic infusion may reduce intraoperative narcotic requirements by 50% and results in a smoother and more rapidly achievable wake-up test. A satisfactory wake-up test consists of satisfactory movement of both hands and feet to command. If there is satisfactory movement of the hands, but not the feet, distraction or rotation on the rod should be reversed and the test must be repeated. If the patient moves neither hands nor feet on command, the most likely explanation is that the patient is still asleep, but of course it may suggest dysfunction of the upper cervical cord or the brainstem. The patient is then asked to open his eyes or mouth. If these tasks are performed flawlessly on command, the compromise must be assumed to be in the spinal cord.

V. SUMMARY

In summary, the complications due to positioning, hypotensive anesthesia, and neurological monitoring are fairly common in spinal surgery and require extra care for prevention. In the prone position, the face and eyes must be protected from pressure in order to prevent the dreadful complication of blindness. Brachial plexus injury may be prevented by avoiding hyperextension of the shoulder and abduction of the arm beyond a right angle. Pressure points over the major superficial nerves like the radial and ulnar nerves in the upper extremity, and the lateral popliteal nerve around the fibular neck must be protected with padding. Abdominal pressure in the prone position may cause venacaval obstruction leading to excessive epidural venous bleeding and venous thrombosis. Postoperative visual loss is a rare but devastating complication, which is reatively more frequent in long spinal operations in prone position, over 6–9 hours. Special attention must be paid to keep the cervical spine immobilized during intubation in the presence of cervical spine injury. Hypotensive anesthesia may prevent blood loss during surgery, but the mean arterial pressure should be controlled above 65 mmHg, or 20 mmHg below the baseline, in order to prevent spinal cord ischaemia. Hypovolemia should be avoided. Neurophysiological monitoring is essential for any deformity surgery, and anesthetics drugs must be appropriately selected to avoid interference with the monitoring signal. Last but not the least, one must remember that, although highly sensitive, a normal spinal cord monitoring signal does not guarantee an absence of neurological injury and should not therefore provoke the surgeon to be overzealous and aggressive in the correction of spinal deformity.

REFERENCES

1. Wilton NC, Tait AR, Kling TF, Jr, Knight PR. The effect of trimethaphan-induced hypotension on canine spinal cord blood flow. Measurement at different cord levels using radiolabelled microspheres. Spine 1988; 13:490–493.
2. Krengel WF, 3rd, Robinson LR, Schneider VA. Combined effects of compression and hypotension on nerve root function. A clinical case. Spine 1993; 18:306–309.
3. Naito M, Owen JH, Bridwell KH, Sugioka Y. Effects of distraction on physiologic integrity of the spinal cord, spinal cord blood flow, and clinical status. Spine 1992; 17:1154–1158.
4. Nielsen CH. Preoperative and postoperative anesthetic considerations for the spinal surgery patient. In: Bridwell KH, DeWald RL, eds. The Text Book of Spinal Surgery. Philadelphia: Lippincott-Raven, 1997:1:31–37.
5. Weinberg L, Harvey WR, Marshall RJ. Post-operative paraplegia following spinal cord infarction. Acta Anaesthesiol Scand 2002; 46:469–472.
6. Lee TC, Yang LC, Chen HJ. Effect of patient position and hypotensive anesthesia on inferior vena caval pressure. Spine 1998; 23:941–948.
7. Geisler FH, Laich DT, Goldflies M, Shepard A. Anterior tibial compartment syndrome as a positioning complication of the prone-sitting position for lumbar surgery. Neurosurgery 1993; 33:1117.

8. Parks BJ. Postoperative peripheral neuropathies. Surgery 1973; 74:348–357.
9. Goettler CE, Pryor JP, Reilly PM. Brachial plexopathy after prone positioning. Crit Care 2002; 6:540–542.
10. Gerber H, Maar K. [Horners syndrome. A complication of the lateral recumbent position (author's transl)]. Anaesthesist 1977; 26:357–358.
11. Palmon SC, Kirsch JR, Depper JA, Toung TJ. The effect of the prone position on pulmonary mechanics is frame-dependent. Anesth Analg 1998; 87:1175–1180.
12. Jackson L, Keats AS. Mechanism of brachial plexus palsy following anesthesia. Anesthesiology 1965; 26:190–194.
13. Bhardwaj D, Peng P. An uncommon mechanism of brachial plexus injury. A case report. Can J Anaesth 1999; 46:173–175.
14. Vahl CF, Carl I, Muller-Vahl H, Struck E. Brachial plexus injury after cardiac surgery. The role of internal mammary artery preparation: a prospective study on 1000 consecutive patients. J Thorac Cardiovasc Surg 1991; 102:724–729.
15. Vander Salm TJ, Cutler BS, Okike ON. Brachial plexus injury following median sternotomy. Part II. J Thorac Cardiovasc Surg 1982; 83:914–917.
16. Jellish WS, Blakeman B, Warf P, Slogoff S. Hands-up positioning during asymmetric sternal retraction for internal mammary artery harvest: a possible method to reduce brachial plexus injury. Anesth Analg 1997; 84:260–265.
17. Lorenzini NA, Poterack KA. Somatosensory evoked potentials are not a sensitive indicator of potential positioning injury in the prone patient. J Clin Monit 1996; 12:171–176.
18. Roth S, Thisted RA, Erickson JP, Black S, Schreider BD. Eye injuries after nonocular surgery. A study of 60,965 anesthetics from 1988 to 1992. Anesthesiology 1996; 85:1020–1027.
19. Williams EL. Postoperative blindness. Anesthesiol Clin North Am 2002; 20:367–384, viii.
20. Cheng MA, Tempelhoff R. Postoperative visual loss, still no answers yet. Anesthesiology 2002; 96:1531–1532.
21. Roth S, Barach P. Postoperative visual loss: still no answers—yet. Anesthesiology 2001; 95:575–577.
22. Lee LA, Lam AM. Unilateral blindness after prone lumbar spine surgery. Anesthesiology 2001; 95:793–795.
23. Anesthesiology ASo. Postoperative Visual Loss Registry, 1999.
24. Lee LA. ASA Postoperative Visual Loss (POVL) Registry. American Society of Anesthesiologists, September 2000.
25. Wilkins RH, Albin MS. An unusual entrance site of venous air embolism during operations in the sitting position. Surg Neurol 1977; 7:71–72.
26. Albin MS. Venous air embolism and lumbar disk surgery. JAMA 1978; 240:1713.
27. Albin MS, Ritter RR, Pruett CE, Kalff K. Venous air embolism during lumbar laminectomy in the prone position: report of three cases. Anesth Analg 1991; 73:346–349.
28. Robinson DA, Albin MS. Venous air embolism and cesarean sections. Anesthesiology 1987; 66:93–94.
29. The use of autologous blood. The National Blood Resource Education Program Expert Panel. JAMA 1990; 263:414–417.
30. Sengupta DK, Grevitt MP, Freeman BJ, Mehdian SMH, Webb JK, Pelosi L. Combined somatosensory (SEP) and motor evoked potentials (MEP) monitoring in orthopaedic spinal surgery (abstr). J Bone Joint Surg [Br] 2002; 84(suppl 3):332.
31. Pelosi L, Stevenson M, Hobbs GJ, Jardine A, Webb JK. Intraoperative motor evoked potentials to transcranial electrical stimulation during two anaesthetic regimens. Clin Neurophysiol 2001; 112:1076–1087.
32. Nuwer MR, Dawson EG, Carlson LG, Kanim LE, Sherman JE. Somatosensory evoked potential spinal cord monitoring reduces neurologic deficits after scoliosis surgery: results of a large multicenter survey. Electroencephalogr Clin Neurophysiol 1995; 96:6–11.

3

Complications of Bone Graft Harvest, Allograft Bone, and Bone Graft Extenders or Alternatives in Spinal Surgery

Jim A. Youssef and Virginia M. Salas
Durango Orthopedic Associates, Durango, Colorado, U.S.A.

I. AUTOGENOUS BONE GRAFTS

A. Properties of Autogenous Bone Grafts

Approximately 500,000 bone-grafting procedures are performed annually in the United States, half of which are associated with spine fusion surgeries. Autogenous bone is the historical gold standard for providing the requisite osteoinductive, osteogenic, and osteoconductive elements for bone graft consolidation. The marrow component of autograft bone is a source of osteoinductive growth factors and osteogenic mesenchymal stem cells (MSCs), a subset of cellular constituents capable of generating new bone. Mineralized bone tissue provides osteoconductive scaffolding and biomechanical integrity. Thus, a relatively high success rate has been achieved with the use of autograft for spinal arthrodesis, and fusion rates range from 60% to over 90%, depending on the surgical approach and the mechanical and biological environment available to the graft (1).

Successful autograft incorporation is influenced by host factors. The relative number of osteogenic cells present in autogenous grafts varies between individuals, and there is potential for progenitor cell numbers and function to vary within the same individual over time or under the influence of disease. Evidence from a number of animal and human studies demonstrates that there is a loss of absolute numbers of stem cell progenitors with aging and that responses to cellular proliferative signals may also change with age (2,3,4). The operative mechanisms contributing to these observations are under investigation. Development of useful models for accurately predicting successful fusions and strategies for mitigating these intrinsic deficits will enhance all approaches to grafting technology.

The relationship between environmental factors and effects on bone healing using autogenous grafts is supported by several studies. Bone marrow cells undergo altered differentiation patterns following environmental exposures to air pollution particulates (5) and cigarette smoke (6). The effects of cigarette smoke on blood forming elements in bone marrow have been observed in molecular studies in vitro (7) and in animal models of posterolateral spinal fusion (8–10), and cigarette smoking has long been appreciated as a predictor of negative outcomes in spine fusion surgeries in humans (11,12). Cigarette smoke contains elements that alter the normal balance of cellular proliferation and programmed cell death, and nicotine specifically has been shown to inhibit expression of important cytokine signaling molecules associated with osteoblast differentiation. Overcoming the inhibitory effects of nicotine on spinal fusion using osteogenic proteins has demonstrated some promise in animal models (9,13). However rigorous studies in humans including long-term risk analysis for the use of osteogenic proteins for this application have not been forthcoming.

Methods for biological manipulation of bone fusion are based on our emerging understanding of the molecular biology of bone growth and repair (14,15). The clinical challenge of achieving high success rates for arthrodesis has been pursued using various techniques for obtaining and delivering osteoinductive agents to the fusion bed, including autologous growth factors and bone marrow and recombinant human proteins. Early human trials using these applications in spinal fusion appear promising (16–20). The efficacy of this approach will undoubtedly depend on our ability to identify, understand, and predict individual risk and capacity to respond to these therapies in the context of aging and disease, genetic makeup, and environmental factors.

B. Common Sources of Autogenous Graft Material: Iliac Crest, Fibula, and Ribs

The most common sources of autogenous bone graft are the iliac crest and the fibula. The preferred source of cancellous graft is the iliac crest with its characteristically high-quality bone marrow content. Cancellous bone contains high proportions of osteoprogenitor cells and its distinctive porosity promotes vascularization and therefore rapid delivery of growth factors and osteogenic proteins. As regeneration progresses, cancellous grafts gain structural integrity through the forces of bone apposition. In biomechanical testing models of bone from the superior iliac spine, specimens from the anterior iliac crest are capable of bearing approximately threefold higher axial loads compared to those from the posterior iliac crest, and the cancellous density is the most important predictor of load to failure in iliac crest grafts (21).

The surgical approach for iliac crest harvest depends on the desired graft composition. Cancellous graft is obtained using currettage and trapdoor or splitting techniques. The subcrest window technique is most commonly used for obtaining bicortical grafts, and tricortical bone is commonly obtained from the anterior ilium posterior to the anterior superior iliac spine. Comparison between the outer table and intracortical methods for harvest from the iliac crest are comparable with regard to postoperative blood loss and severity of donor site pain. However, the intraosseous method requires longer operative time and yields less bone compared to the outer table approach (22).

Alternative approaches for minimally invasive procurement of iliac crest bone graft (ICBG) include motorized trephines for obtaining moderate amounts of graft material (30 cc or less) and corticocancellous acetabular reamers. Morbidity rates reported in patients donating autograft bone with motorized trephines compare favorably to those in patients undergoing anterior iliac crest harvest with traditional open approaches (23). Comparable morbidity has also been reported in studies evaluating the acetabular reamer approach with traditional harvesting techniques (24). Alternative procurement approaches may present options for less invasive grafting procedures, but their clinical utility will depend on the quality and performance of the harvested graft materials.

Complications that have been reported with iliac crest donor-site procedures include chronic pain, neurovascular injury, avulsion fractures of the anterior superior iliac spine, hematoma, infection, herniation of abdominal contents, gait disturbance, cosmetic deformity, violation and instability of the sacroiliac joint, and ureteral injury (25). The neurovascular structures at risk for injuries during iliac bone-graft harvesting include the lateral femoral cutaneous, iliohypogastric, and the ilioinguinal nerves anteriorly and the superior cluneal nerves and superior gluteal neurovascular bundle posteriorly (26,27).

Cortical grafts, while biomechanically superior to cancellous grafts, have the least cross-sectional area of cancellous bone, compared to either the anterior or posterior superior iliac crest. Cortical bone, commonly harvested from the fibula, lacks porous structure and has inferior osteogenic properties compared to cancellous bone graft. Cortical grafts are useful for severe spinal defects or to meet a pressing need for a structurally sound supportive medium. The structural integrity of cortical grafts degrades over time, however, due to osteoclastic resorption.

The use of fibular bone in reconstruction following cervical corpectomy appears to be effective for achieving spinal decompression and stabilization, with fusion rates of 84–86% reported in the literature (28,29). For this application, an allograft source is frequently selected. Complications of autogenous fibula graft harvesting include neurovascular injury, compartment syndrome, extensor hallucis longus weakness, and ankle instability. The neurovascular structures at risk for injury during fibular bone-graft harvesting include the peroneal nerves and their muscular branches in the proximal third of the fibular shaft and the peroneal vessels in the middle third (30).

Compared to the iliac crest and fibula, the use of the rib as a source of autologous graft material is rare, despite its high content of bone morphogenetic protein (31). Vascularized fibular grafts provide an important alternative for achieving arthrodesis in a suboptimal graft bed (32). Vascularized rib strut grafts have found utility in conjunction with other anterior implant techniques in selected patients who have experienced nonunions with avascular grafts or repeated failures using conventional grafting methods (33,34). Autologous rib is also a good source of graft material in staged scoliosis surgical regimens (35). Fusion rates using rib autograft in posterior cervical stabilization constructs compare favorably with iliac crest graft, both exceeding 94%. In a study of 600 patients comparing rib and iliac crest graft sites, the rate of donor site morbidity for rib grafts was approximately sevenfold lower (3.7% vs. 25.3%) than that reported for iliac crest harvest. Complications associated with autologous rib harvest include pneumonia and persistent absorption atelectasis (36).

C. Complications and Morbidity Associated with Iliac Crest Autograft Harvest

Although the literature is replete with references to donor site morbidity associated with ICBG harvest, rigorously controlled, randomized studies quantifying overall donor site morbidity and complication rates associated with its use in spine surgery are lacking (37,38). Prospective studies conclude that the major component of ICBG donor site morbidity is pain, with intensity at 12 months significantly less than that at 3 months, and a trend toward the highest pain scores at 6 months (39,40). The incidence of chronic donor site pain has been reported over a range of 8–36% (41). Major complications associated with ICBG harvest are uncommon, with reported incidence ranging from 0.8 to 25%. Minor complications, however, are more common with reported incidence ranges from 9.4 to over 50% (42).

Patient demographics, surgical approach, surgeon technique, and evaluation tools arguably influence complication and morbidity rates derived from large clinical studies.

In a retrospective independent outcome analysis of 105 patients evaluated 4 years post-operatively, persistent ICBG donor site pain incidence was 34%, with 3% of patients reporting unacceptable pain severity (43). Interestingly, this incidence was significantly greater than previously appreciated by the surgeon (8%). In a 48-month study, morbidity associated with anterior ICBG harvest for single level anterior cervical discectomy and fusion (ACDF) was investigated in a noncontrolled retrospective analysis of 134 patients (44). Acute symptoms in study subjects included difficulty in ambulation in half of the study subjects. Other acute symptoms occurring in less than 10% of the patients included protracted antibiotic usage, persistent drainage at the wound site, and wound dehiscence. Chronic donor site pain occurred in 26.1% of patients with an average score of 3.8 out of 10 on a visual analog scale (VAS). Chronic use of pain medication was reported by 11.2% of patients and 15.7% experienced abnormal sensation at the donor site. Functional disabilities in ambulation, recreational activities, work activities, sexual activity, and activities of daily living were also associated with ICBG donation in 6.5–12.7% of patients, depending on the specific impairment.

A retrospective study in a total of 107 patients specifically compared acute donor site complications between two methods of posterior iliac crest graft harvesting for lumbar fusion (45). In the group of patients who underwent bone graft harvesting from a midline fascia splitting approach, 17.9% reported tenderness at the donor site compared to 54.9% of patients in a similar group that were grafted from a separate incision at the iliac crest. Severity of the tenderness resulting from a second incision was also greater, with 15.7% reporting severe tenderness compared to only 1.8% in the group receiving graft from the midline incision. Furthermore, the incidence of sensory disturbance at the donor site was approximately four times greater in patients undergoing bone graft harvesting from a separate incision (21.6%), compared to a 5.4% incidence in patients who underwent harvesting from a midline approach.

The reported complication rate for ICBG harvest is significantly higher following anterior compared to posterior approaches. A noncontrolled, retrospective, comparative study in 108 patients who underwent surgery for the treatment of chronic osteomyelitis found less morbidity with the harvesting of iliac crest bone graft from the posterior approach (46). The severity and duration of postoperative pain was also greater following anterior harvest.

Surgeons are increasingly challenged to carefully weigh the physical and monetary considerations of selecting among alternative technologies for bone grafting, and many surgeons are unaware of the actual direct and indirect cost incurred by autogenous bone harvesting (47). An appreciation of the morbidities associated with autogenous bone grafts is essential for evaluating utility in terms of clinical, health-related quality of life, and economic outcomes.

II. ALLOGRAFT BONE VERSUS AUTOGRAFT BONE

A. Characteristics of Allograft Materials

Allograft materials obtained from cadaver sources are the most common alternative components to autografts in spinal surgery. Allograft provides an osteoconductive environment, and there is some evidence that it is weakly osteoinductive, but the bone-inductive effects in humans is debated (48). Allografts are devoid of living material and therefore lack the osteogenic elements required for use as a stand-alone bone graft (49). Allograft is available in structural and crushed cancellous form. Structural allograft can be machined as spacers, freeze-dried cancellous croutons, and powder, all to improve the availability of bone graft volume. The major advantages of allograft bone in spine is that it precludes the requirement for autologous bone services and therefore decreases the incidence of bone graft donor site morbidity.

B. Clinical Use of Allograft Bone: Comparison with Autograft

The optimal use of allograft bone must take into account the properties of the source bone and the issues related to its processing for decreased antigenicity, extended shelf life, and sterilization. Freeze-dried material may lose up to 50% of its structural strength upon rehydration (50), and sterilization methods also affect graft properties. Structural cortical allograft is well suited for reconstruction of the anterior column of the spine, particularly if combined with a posterior fusion (51). Corticocancellous allograft offers inferior mechanical support as compared to pure cortical grafts. However, because of its large surface area, it displays more rapid integration compared to cortical bone (52).

Prospective studies in large patient populations conclude that ethylene oxide–sterilized allograft fails to perform as well as autologous bone in combined interbody/posterolateral fusion (53,54). Allograft bone in the form of fresh frozen human femoral head was evaluated against autograft bone in posterolateral lumbar fusions in a randomized clinical trial of 69 patients followed over a period of 6 years. The study concluded that the clinical outcome was comparable between groups receiving either fresh frozen allograft or posterior iliac crest autograft, and the 16% incidence of donor site morbidity associated with spinal fusions at the study site was avoided. Importantly, the authors noted that the source of banked bone was rigorously regulated for harvesting, testing, and storage and located in an area with a low incidence of endemic disease in the typical donor (55). The use of fresh frozen structural allografts is further supported in several studies of single-level anterior interbody arthrodesis in the cervical and lumbar spine demonstrating equivalency in fusion rates between allograft and autograft bone (56,57). However, successful allograft use for multisegmental cervical fusion has not been clearly demonstrated (58).

C. Safety Issues Surrounding the Use of Allograft

Concerns exist regarding the risk of immunogenicity and disease transmission with allograft bone. Allografts must be matched to the recipient for histocompatibility antigen, and fresh frozen allografts are more immunogenic than freeze-dried grafts. Graft immunogenicity is problematic because it contributes to delayed incorporation and increased resorption, which have been observed in allograft remodeling (59). Fresh frozen allografts undergo the least rigorous processing and therefore have increased potential for immugenicity and harboring of pathogens. Viral transmission associated with allograft bone is rare. Four documented cases of HIV seroconversion have been associated with allograft transplant, and bacterial infections have also been reported (60,61). Federal oversight of processing human tissue includes requirements for organizations to validate and monitor procedures for preventing infectious agent contamination. Inconsistent implementation of the U.S. Food and Drug Administration (FDA) screening procedures and processing requirements resulted in over 6800 allograft recalls since 1994 from over 20 different tissue-banking organizations.

The perception of safety associated with allograft use may remain unresolved pending further evidence of improved regulatory enforcement (62). Furthermore, allograft used alone or in combination with autograft for spinal fusions has failed to demonstrate fusion rate equivalency to stand-alone autograft for many applications (63). A variety of synthetic bone substitute materials are currently being developed as bone graft extenders (1). Graft materials, including allograft and allograft composites, are likely to become increasingly specialized for specific clinical applications (64). Evaluation of allograft materials must take into account this potential and the advantages of eliminating donor site complications, procedural costs, and morbidity and the availability of large quantities of graft material.

III. BONE GRAFT EXTENDERS

Bone graft extenders increase the options beyond allograft and autograft bone for enhancing the graft consolidation processes. The osteoconductive properties of bone graft extenders enrich the environment of the graft bed by contributing to a lattice for bone formation aided by the osteogenic properties of endogenous and exogenous graft materials and growth factors. Graft extender technology will likely evolve to incorporate the use of bioactive materials including bone morphogenetic proteins and gene therapy modalities.

A. Demineralized Bone Matrix

Demineralized bone matrix (DBM) was first recognized to induce formation of ectopic bone in laboratory animals as early as 1965 (65). Allograft material is processed and converted into type I collagen and noncollagenous proteins, including BMPs. Various forms of DBM are available including gels, hydrogel carrier products, putties, flexible sheets, pellets, and combination products containing cancellous chips.

Several studies have demonstrated that DBM is primarily osteoconductive and weakly osteoinductive, most likely due to the presence of BMPs whose composition in these preparations is less than 0.01% (1). Commercial preparations of DBM vary with regard to their osteoinductive properties and other biological characteristics. The amount of DBM relative to carrier within a preparation does not necessarily correlate with its efficacy. Improved screening and product testing criteria including bioassays to reliably predict DBM performance will improve the clinical utility of these products (66).

B. Platelet-Derived Growth Factors

Platelet-derived growth factors are commonly prepared intraoperatively as concentrates from autologous blood draws combined in a fibrinogen-thrombin clot matrix. Molded preparations of the platelet gel matrix are applied directly to the graft site. The use of platelet gels is based on the well-documented role of growth factors in several stages of bone healing, including migration, differentiation, and proliferation of osteoprogenitor cells at the graft site (67).

Platelet gels have been utilized in surgical procedures including oral/maxillofacial surgery (68,69) and total knee arthroplasty (70). The use of autologous growth factors in spinal surgery was examined in a retrospective review of 39 patients undergoing lumbar fusions, and there was enough supportive evidence from early radiographic observations to warrant more rigorous clinical studies to definitively support the efficacy of platelet gels as graft extenders for spinal surgery in humans (19).

C. Nonbone Ceramics

Nonbone ceramic materials are valued as bone graft extenders for their osteoconductive properties and are most successfully used to promote bone regeneration in conjunction with osteoinductive agents. Tricalcium phosphate products undergo at least partial conversion to hydroxyapatite over time, and reports of inconsistent biodegradation have compromised their acceptance as mechanically sound graft materials, despite their biocompatibility and osteoconductive properties. Combinations of highly porous beta tricalcium phosphate blocks with bone marrow osteoprogenitor cells have shown osteogenic potential in animal models (71). In other studies, augmentation of tricalcium phosphate formulas with polymeric matrices have resulted in enhanced materials demonstrating improved colonization of bone cells, improved osteoblastic activity, and more robust osteoinduction and osteoconduction activities related to bone remodeling (72). In contrast to the tricalcium phosphates, calcium sulfate products are readily resorbed. The clinical efficacy of calcium sulfate used alone or in combination with bone marrow aspirate, DBM, or autograft bone has been demonstrated in a large multicenter trial for the reconstruction of contained nonstructural bony defects (73). The hydroxyapatites are also characterized by relatively slow resorption rates, resulting in superior mechanical stability. Coralline hydroxyapatite has similar porosity to human trabecular bone and has been used successfully as grafting material for anterior cervical interbody fusions (74).

Synthetic bone graft substitutes are available in unlimited quantities and are easily stored and sterilized. A number of calcium-based bone graft substitutes are marketed in the United States and Europe, yet despite over 15 years of clinical experience with the use of these products, synthetic bone substitutes do not represent a significant market share (75). The use of both allograft and nonallograft synthetic bone graft substitutes will undoubtedly increase as effective combinations with bioactive adjuvants are explored in product-specific applications for spine surgery.

IV. EMERGING BONE MORPHOGENETIC PROTEIN TECHNOLOGIES

A. Osteogenic Properties

Bone morphogenetic proteins (BMPs) are a subgroup of proteins in the transforming growth factor-beta (TGF-β) family. The clinical application of the BMPs in spinal fusion is based on their role in endochondral and intramembranous bone formation during development and promotion of bone healing. Of the numerous growth factors that have been evaluated in preclinical trials, none has demonstrated the potency of the BMP family members for osteogenesis. Bone morphogenetic proteins are the only bioactive molecules capable of inducing in vivo bone formation spontaneously when introduced subcutaneously or intramuscularly (65,76).

Recombinant technologies using mammalian cell expression strategies for producing BMPs result in highly purified homogeneous preparations of single proteins available in reproducible amounts with consistent biological activity. Toxicity and biological efficacy testing, therefore, is relatively straightforward using a recombinant analyte. A second option for obtaining BMPs is through bovine-derived extracts containing a mix of multiple BMPs and other related proteins. Extracts offer the advantage that these protein mixes create a synergistic biological environment for bone regeneration, but mechanistic studies defining the role of each component become more complex. Furthermore, bovine extracts have a potential for harboring elements that may modulate the biological properties of BMPs and its extracts, including immunogens.

Many animal studies have established that fusion rates and biomechanical characteristics of fusion masses obtained with the use of BMPs in spinal fusions are equivalent or
superior to those obtained with autogenous grafts (77–83). The use of BMPs may obviate
the need or compensate for inefficient decortication of the posterior elements normally
required for delivery of growth factors to the site of posterolateral fusion (82). Overcoming
the inhibitory effects on spinal fusion of agents such as nicotine and NSAIDS has also been
attributed to the use of BMPs (9,84). Of the approximately 20 BMPs that have been identified to date, BMP-2 and BMP-7 (also known at osteogenic protein-1, OP-1) are the only
BMPs currently undergoing evaluation in human clinical trials. In addition to establishing
the safety of BMP use in humans, major issues related to clinical efficacy of BMPs for spinal
fusion include optimizing the biological properties of the protein preparations of BMP and
determining the appropriate delivery and quantity of protein to specific graft sites.

B. Safety Issues

The supraphysiological doses of BMPs required to induce biological effects in pre-clinical
and clinical trials is an issue that raises safety concerns. The rhBMP-2 dose-response curve
in humans is steep relative to that reported in animal fusion models, and large doses are
required to achieve arthrodesis reliably. The use of milligram quantities of osteogenic proteins during procedures that involve extensive exposure of raw bone surfaces and other
nonbony tissues that are known to have cellular receptors for BMP has resulted in
untoward effects.

In animal studies, bony overgrowth induced by BMP-2 has been reported to result in
inadvertent bone formation and fusion at adjacent levels (85,86). Carriers that effectively
retain the protein within the fusion bed mitigate the risk of this complication, and combination of rhBMP-2 with different carriers results in different outcomes depending on dose
and inflammatory reactions to the carrier substrate (87). The use of rhBMP-2 in decompressive laminotomy or foraminotomy followed by intertransverse fusion has been associated with bony overgrowth and restenosis (88). There is also evidence to suggest that
rhBMP-2 leads to laminar reconstitution and neuroforaminal narrowing if it is directly
introduced into the laminectomy site, but the degree of neuroforaminal narrowing and
the clinical sequelae were not noted in the animal model cited (89).

Studies in humans undergoing rhBMP-2 augmented PLIF report heterotropic
formation in several patients in the spinal canal adjacent to cages containing collagen carrier and along insertion tracts (85). No clinical sequelae were reported, but these studies
serve to illustrate that the importance of accurate placement and appropriate use of these
potent osteoinductive proteins cannot be overstated.

Bone resorption is also associated with the use of rh-BMP-2. This finding is
consistent with the modulatory role of this growth factor in conjunction with other
proteins in the regulation of bone remodeling. The observed biomechanical superiority
of fusion masses reported with the use of rhBMP-2 suggests that the increased osteoclastic activity is coupled with a greater magnitude of osteoblastic upregulation under the
physiological conditions at these fusion sites (78,82).

In contrast to rhBMP-2, studies with OP-1 have not reported complications related
to bony overgrowth in animal models of posterolateral intertransverse and interbody
fusions (83,90–93). In contrast to BMP-2, bony growth with OP-1 appears to require a
more fastidious biological environment. Ongoing efficacy trials in humans comparing
autograft alone and autograft augmented with OP-1 for posterolateral spinal arthrodesis
are more promising and to date have reported no complications or side effects (20).

Bone formation in the subarachnoid space following deliberate placement of OP-1 over dural tears has been reported in an animal model (94). Despite new bone formation, the animals remained neurologically intact, and there was no evidence of damage to the spinal cord, nor were changes in cerebrospinal fluid (CSF) observed. This study raises awareness that use of these factors in the presence of dural tears must be approached with caution.

Determining the minimal amount of protein required for a specific biological effect and optimizing the delivery and environmental conditions for the use of BMPs will contribute greatly to establishing a reliable safety and efficacy profile for their use in specific spinal applications.

C. Use of BMPs in Spinal Fusions

Bone morphogenetic proteins have undergone extensive testing in over 40 preclinical studies since 1989 and in a number of species including canine, rodent, caprine and non-human primates (95). Bovine BMP extract (bBMPx) in a composite with collagen has demonstrated efficacy in a dose-dependent study design of spinal fusion in a rabbit model (96). The efficacy of bBMPx in nonhuman primates has also demonstrated dose-response efficacy in lumbar spinal fusion and a trend toward an increase in effective dose from rabbit to rhesus to human applications (97).

Prospective randomized trials in human subjects undergoing single-level lumbar spinal fusions corroborate preclinical findings that arthrodesis occurs more reliably in subjects treated with rhBMP-2–filled fusion cages compared to cages filled with autograft bone (98). A similar randomized human trial was conducted using rhBMP-2 in a collagen sponge carrier within cylindrical interbody cages. The use of rhBMP-2 was associated with radiographic evidence of osteoinduction and new bone formation within the disk space outside the cages, with bone density surpassing that observed in autograft control (99). In a study of posterolateral lumbar spine fusions, patients randomized into three groups based on arthrodesis technique were evaluated for fusion status and clinical outcome. At 6 months follow-up, fusion rates in the rhBMP-2–augmented anterior lumbar fusions performed with or without pedicle screw instrumentation were greater compared to instrumented autograft fusions. Patient-reported clinical outcomes were also significantly improved with the use of rhBMP-2 (100).

Safety and efficacy trials using OP-1–augmented posterolateral fusions have recently been reported and are promising. Patient groups randomized to noninstrumented fusions with either autograft and OP-1 or autograft alone were evaluated in a 16-patient study. At 6-month follow-up 75% of patients in the OP-1 group were determined to have achieved solid arthrodesis, compared to 50% of patients in the autograft group. Furthermore, 83% of the OP-1 group reported at least a 20% improvement in Oswestry scores, compared to 50% of the autograft group (101). A similar study in 36 patients with lumbar spinal stenosis and degenerative spondylolisthesis (L3–L5) undergoing a posterolateral spinal fusion following decompression reported a 32% higher clinical success rate in OP-1–treated patients compared to those receiving autograft alone (102). An ongoing Australian study in patients with degenerative spondylolysthesis is currently evaluating uninstrumented posterolateral fusions using autograft on one side and OP-1 putty (OP-1/bovine collagen/CMC mix) on the contralateral side. At 6 month follow-up, fusion masses in the five patients that have been evaluated were noted to be equivalent or greater with OP-1 treatment (103). Many of the ongoing clinical studies with OP-1 are demonstrating promising trends whose statistical significance has yet to be proven in the long term.

The evolution of bone grafting techniques is progressing rapidly. The advancements made during the past 10 years have given rise to new technologies that are less invasive and demonstrate efficacy similar to autogenous bone. The future appears bright as we look to identify alternatives to traditional bone grafting that provide similar clinical results at a reduced cost and with decreased morbidity to our patients.

REFERENCES

1. Wang JC, Hilibrand AS, Youssef JA. Bone graft extenders: biology and options for enhancing graft consolidation. SpineLine 2002; 3(6):6–11.
2. D'Ippolito G, Schiller PC, Ricordi C, Roos BA, Howard GA. Age-related osteogenic potential of mesenchymal stromal stem cells from human vertebral bone marrow. J Bone Miner Res 1999; 14(7):1115–1122.
3. Erdmann J, Kogler C, Diel I, Ziegler R, Pfeilschifter J. Age-associated changes in the stimulatory effect of transforming growth factor beta on human osteogenic colony formation. Mech Ageing Dev 1999; 110(1–2):73–85.
4. Muschler GF, Nitto H, Boehm CA, Easley KA. Age-and gender-related changes in the cellularity of human bone marrow and the prevalence of osteoblastic progenitors. J Orthop Res 2001; 19:117–125.
5. Suwa T, Hogg JC, Vincent R, Mukae H, Fujii T, Van Eeden SF. Ambient air particulates stimulate alveolar macrophages of smokers to promote differentiation of myeloid procursor cells. Exp Lung Res 2002; 28(1):1–18.
6. Liu XD, Zhu YK, Umino T, Spurzem JR, Romberger DJ, Wang H, Reed E, Rennard SI. Cigarette smoke inhibits osteogenic differentiation and proliferation of human osteoprogenitor cells in monolayer and three dimensional collagen gel culture. J Lab Clin Med 2001; 137(3):208–219.
7. Salas VM, Burchiel SW. Apoptosis in Daudi human B cells in response to benzo [a] pyrene and BAP-7,8 dihydrodiol. Toxicol Appl Pharmacol 1998; 151(2):367–376.
8. Daftari TK, Whitesides TE Jr, Heller JG, Goodrich AC, McCarey BE, Hutton WC. The effects of nicotine on the revascularization of bone graft: an experimental study in rabbits. Spine 1994; 19(8):904–911.
9. Silcox DH III, Boden SD, Schimandle JH, Johnson P, Whitesides TE, Hutton WC. Reversing the inhibitory effect of nicotine on spinal fusion using an osteoinductive protein extract. Spine 1998; 23(3):291–296.
10. Theiss SM, Boden SD, Hair G, Titus L, Morone MA, Ugbo J. The effect of nicotine on gene expression during spine fusion. Spine 2000; 25(20):2588–2594.
11. Brown CW, Orme TJ, Richardson HD. The rate of pseudoarthrosis in patients who are smokers and patients who are nonsmokers: a comparison study. Spine 1986; 11(9):942–943.
12. Hadley MN, Reddy SV. Smoking and the human vertebral column: a review of the impact of cigarette use on vertebral bone metabolism and spinal fusion. Neurosurgery 1997; 41(1): 116–124.
13. Patel TC, Erulkar JS, Grauer JN, Troiano NW, Panjabi MM, Friedlaender GE. Osteogenic protein-1 overcomes the inhibitory effect of nicotine on posterolateral lumbar fusion. Spine 2001; 26(15):1656–1661.
14. Ludwig SC, Boden SD. Osteoinductive bone graft substitutes for spinal fusion: a basic science summary. Orthop Clin North Am 1999; 30(4):635–645.
15. Helvering LM, Sharp RL, Ou X, Geiser AG. Regulation of the promoters for the human bone morphogenetic protein-2 and -4 genes. Gene 2000; 256(1–2):123–138.
16. Boden SD, Hair GA, Viggeswarpu M, Liu Y, Titus L. Gene therapy for spine fusion. Clin Orthop 2000; 379S:225–233.
17. Connolly JF. Clinical use of marrow osteoprogenitor cells to stimulate osteogenesis. Clin Orthop 1998; 355S:257–266.

18. Hidaka C, Khan SN, Farmer JC, Sandhu HS. Gene therapy for spinal applications. Orthop Clin North Am 2002; 33(2):439–446.
19. Lowery GL, Kulkarni S, Pennisi AE. Use of autologous growth factors in lumbar spinal fusion. Bone 1999; 25:47–50.
20. Vaccaro AR, Anderson DG, Toth CA. Recombinant human osteogenic protein-1 (bone morphogenetic protein-7) as an osteoinductive agent in spinal fusion. Spine 2002; 27(16S):59–265.
21. Smith MD, Cody DD. Load-bearing capacity of corticocancellous bone grafts in the spine. J Bone Joint Surg Am 1993; 75(8):1206–1213.
22. Mirovsky Y, Neuwirth MG. Comparison between the outer table and intracortical methods of obtaining autogenous bone graft from the iliac crest. Spine 2000; 25(13):1722–1725.
23. Sandor GK, Nish IA, Carmichael RP. Comparison of conventional surgery with motorized trephine in bone harvest from the anterior iliac crest. Oral Surg Oral Med Oral Pathol Oral Radiol Endod 2003; 95(2):150–155.
24. Westrich GH, Geller DS, O'Malley MJ, Deland JT, Helfet DL. Anterior iliac crest bone graft harvesting using the corticocancellous reamer system. J Orthop Trauma 2001; 15(7):500–506.
25. Schnee CL, Freese A, Weil RJ, Marcotte PJ. Analysis of harvest morbidity and radiographic outcome using autograft for anterior cervical fusion. Spine 1997; 22(19):2222–2227.
26. Arrington ED, Smith WJ, Chambers HG, Bucknell AL, Davino NA. Complications of iliac crest bone graft harvesting. Clin Orthop 1996; 329:300–309.
27. Sawin PD, Traynelis VC, Menezes AH. A comparative analysis of fusion rates and donor site morbidity for autogenic rib and iliac crest bone grafts in posterior cervical fusions. J Neurosurg 1998; 88(2):255–265.
28. Mayr MT, Subach BR, Comey CH, Rodts GE, Haid RW Jr. Cervical spinal stenosis: outcome after anterior corpectomy, allograft reconstruction and instrumentation. J Neurosurg 2002; 97(1S):10–16.
29. McKoy BE, Wingate JK, Poletti SC, Johnson DR II, Stanley MD, Glaser JA. Fibular allograft after anterior cervical corpectomy: long-term follow up. Iowa Orthop J 2002; 22:42–46.
30. Pacelli LL, Gillard J, McLoughlin SW, Buehler MJ. A biomechanical analysis of donor site ankle instability following free fibular graft harvest. J Bone Joint Surg Am 2003; 85A(4):597–603.
31. Frenkel SR, Saadeh PB, Mehara BJ, Chin GS, Steinrech DS, Brent B, Gittes GK, Longaker MT. Transforming growth factor beta superfamily members: role in cartilage modeling. Plast Reconstr Surg 2000; 105(3):980–990.
32. Kim CW, Abrams R, Lee G, Hoyt D, Garfin SR. Use of vascularized fibular grafts as a salvage procedure for previously failed spinal arthrodesis. Spine 2001; 26(19):2171–2175.
33. Krishnan KG, Miller A. Reconstruction of the cervical spine using free vascularized bone. Eur Spine J 2002; 11(2):176–183.
34. Deen HG, Zimmerman RS, Lanza LA. Vascular pedicle rib graft in anterior transthoracic fusion procedures. J Neurosurg 1999; 90(1S):155–158.
35. Chugh S, Marks DS, Mangham DC, Thompson AG. Autologous bone grafting in staged scoliosis surgery. The patient as bone bank. Spine 1998; 23(16):1793–1795.
36. Laurie SW, Kaban LB, Mulliken JB, Murray JE. Donor site morbidity after harvesting rib and iliac bone. Plast Reconstr Surg 1984; 73(6):933–938.
37. Gibson JN, Waddel G, Grant IC. Surgery for degenerative lumbar spondylosis. Cochrane Database Syst Rev 2000; 3:CD001352.
38. Turner JA, Ersek M, Herron L, Haselkorn J, Kent D, Ciol MA, Deyo R. Patient outcomes after lumbar spinal fusion. JAMA 1992; 268(7):907–911.
39. Hill NM, Horne JG, Devane PA. Donor site morbidity in the iliac crest bone graft. Aust NZ J Surg 1999; 69(10):726–728.
40. Robertson PA, Wray AC. Natural history of posterior iliac crest bone graft donation for spinal surgery: a prospective analysis of morbidity. Spine 2001; 26(13):1473–1476.

41. Papavero L, Zwonitzer R, Burkard I, Klose K, Hermann H. A composite bone graft substitute for anterior cervical fusion. Spine 2002; 27(10):1037–1043.
42. Banwart JC, Asher MA, Hassanein RS. Iliac crest bone graft harvest donor site morbidity. A statistical evaluation. Spine 1995; 20(9):1055–1060.
43. Heary, RF, Schlenk RP, Sacchieri TA, Barone D, Brotea C. Persistent iliac crest donor site pain: independent outcome assessment. Neurosurgery 2002; 50(3):510–517.
44. Silber JS, Anderson DG, Daffner SD, Brislin BT, Leland JM, Hilibrand AS, Vaccaro AR, Albert TJ. Donor site morbidity after anterior iliac crest bone harvest for single level anterior cervical discectomy and fusion. Spine 2003; 28(2):134–139.
45. David R, Folman Y, Pikarsky I, Leitner Y, Catz A, Gepstein R. Harvesting bone graft from the posterior iliac crest by less traumatic, midline approach. J Spinal Disord Tech 2003; 16(1):27–30.
46. Ahlmann E, Patzakis M, Roidis N, Shepherd L, Holtom P. Comparison of anterior and posterior iliac crest bone grafts in terms of harvest-site morbidity and functional outcomes. J Bone Joint Surg Am 2002; 84A(5):716–720.
47. St. John TA, Vaccaro AR, Sah AP, Schaefer M, Berta SC, Albert T, Hilibrand A. Physical and monetary costs associated with autogenous bone graft harvesting. Am J Orthop 2003; 32(1):18–23.
48. Schwartz Z, Somers A, Mellonig JT. Ability of commercial demineralized freeze-dried bone allograft to induce new bone formation. J Periodontal 1996; 67:918–926.
49. Boden SD. The biology of posterolateral lumbar spinal fusion. Orthop Clin North Am 1998; 29:603–619.
50. Hamer AJ, Strachan JR, Black MM, Ibbotson CJ, Stockley I, Elson RA. Biomechanical properties of cortical allograft bone using a new method of bone strength measurement: a comparison of fresh, fresh-frozen and irradiated bone. J Bone Joint Surg Br 1996; 78:363–368.
51. Ehrler DM, Vaccaro AR. The use of allograft bone in lumbar spine surgery. Clin Orthop 2000; 371:38–45.
52. Whang PG, Wang JC. Bone graft substitutes for spinal fusion. Spine 2003; 3:155–165.
53. Brantigan JW. Pseudarthrosis rate after allograft posterior lumbar interbody fusion with pedicle screw and plate fixation. Spine 1994; 19:1271–1279.
54. Jorgenson SS, Lowe TG, France J. A prospective analysis of autograft vs allograft in posterolateral lumbar fusion in the same patient: a minimum of 1 year follow up in 144 patients. Spine 1994; 19:2048–2053.
55. Gibson S, McLeod I, Wardlaw D, Urbaniak S. Allograft versus autograft in instrumented posterolateral lumbar spinal fusion. Spine 2002; 27(15):1599–1603.
56. Young WF, Rossenwasser RH. An early comparative analysis of the use of fibular allograft versus autogenous iliac crest graft for interbody fusion after anterior cervical discectomy. Spine 1993; 18:1123–1124.
57. Brown MD, Malinin TI, Davis PB. A roentgenographic evaluation of frozen allografts versus autografts in anterior cervical spine fusions. Clin Orthop 1976; 119:231–236.
58. Zdeblick TA, Ducker TB. The use of freeze-dried allograft bone for anterior cervical fusions. Spine 1991; 16:726–729.
59. Tsuang YH, Yang RS, Chen PQ, Liu TK. Experimental allograft in spinal fusion in dogs. Taiwan I Hsueh Hui Tsa Chih 1989; 88:989–994.
60. Simonds, RJ. HIV transmission by organ and tissue transplantation. AIDS 1993; 2S:35–38.
61. Centers for Disease Control. Update: allograft associated bacterial infections, United States 2002. JAMA 2002; 287:1642–1644.
62. Woolf SK, Gross RH. Perceptions of allograft safety and efficacy among spinal deformity surgeons. J Pediatr Orthop 2001; 21:767–771.
63. Floyd T, Ohnmeiss D. A meta-analysis of autograft versus allograft in anterior cervical fusion. Eur Spine J 2000; 9:398–403.

64. Bauer TW, Muschler GF. Bone graft materials. An overview of the basic science. Clin Orthop 2000; 371:10–27.
65. Urist MR. Bone: formation by autoinduction. Science 1965; 150:893–899.
66. Maddox E, Zhan M, Mundy GR, Drohan WN, Burgess WH. Optimizing human demineralized bone matrix for clinical application. Tissue Eng 2000; 6:441–448.
67. Solheim E. Growth factors in bone. Int Orthop 1998; 22:410–416.
68. Witman DH, Berry RL, Grenn DM. Platelet Gel: an autologous alternative to fibrin glue with applications in oral and maxillofacial surgery. J Oral Maxillofac Surg 1997; 55:1294–1299.
69. Anitua E. The use of plasma-rich growth factors (PRGF) in oral surgery. Pract Proced Aesthet Dent 2001; 13:487–493.
70. Mooar PA, Gardner MJ, Klepchik PR, Sherk HH. The efficacy of autologous platelet gel administration in total knee arthroplasty: an analysis of range of motion, hemoglobin, and narcotics requirements. Paper presented at American Academy of Orthopaedic Surgeons 67th Annual Meeting, Orlando, FL, March 15–19, 2000.
71. Dong JU, Shirasaki T, Tateishi T. Promotion of bone formation using highly pure porous beta-TCP combined with bone marrow-derived osteoprogenitor cells. Biomaterials 2002; 23(23):4493–4502.
72. Fini M, Giavaresi G, Aldini NN, Torricelli P, Botter R, Beruto D, Giardino R. A bone substitute composed of polymethymethacrylate and alpha-tricalcium phosphate: results in terms of osteoblast function and bone tissue formation. Biomaterials 2002; 23(23):4523–4531.
73. Kelly CM, Wilkins RM, Gitelis S, Hartjen C, Watson JT Kim PT. The use of a surgical grade calcium sulfate as a bone graft substitute: results of a multicenter trial. Clin Orthop 2001; 382:42–50.
74. Thalgott JS, Fritts K, Giuffre JM, Timlin M. Aterior interbody fusion of the cervical spine with coralline hydroxyapatite. Spine 1999; 24:1295–1299.
75. Bucholz RW. Nolallograft osteoconductive bone graft substitutes. Clin Orthop 2002; 395:44–52.
76. Wozney JM, Rosen V, Celese AJ. Novel regulators of bone formation: molecular clones and activities. Science 1998; 242:1528–1534.
77. Cook SD, Dalton JE, Tan EH, Whitecloud TS, Rueger DC. In vivo evaluation of recombinant human osteogenic protein (rhOP-1) implant as a bone graft substitute for spinal fusions. Spine 1994; 19:1655–1663.
78. Schimandle JH, Boden SD, Hutton WC. Experimental spinal fusion with recombinant human bone morphogenetic protein-2. Spine 1995; 20:1326–1337.
79. Boden SD, Martin GJ, Morone M, Ugbo JL, Titus L, Hutton WC. The use of coalline hydroxyapatite with bone marrow, autogenous bone graft, or osteoinductive bone protein extract for posterolateral lumbar fusion. Spine 1999; 24:320–327.
80. Boden SD, Martin GJ, Morone M, Ugbo JL, Moskovitz PA. Posterolateral lumbar intertransverse process spine arthrodesis with recombinant human bone morphogenetic protein2/hydroxyapatite-tricalcium phosphate after laminectomy in the nonhuman primate. Spine 1999; 24:1179–1185.
81. Muschler GF, Hyodo A, Manning T, Kambic H, Easley K. Evlauation of human bone morphogenetic protein-2 in a canine spinal fusion model. Clin Orthop 1994; 308:229–240.
82. Sandhu HS, Kanim LE, Kabo JM. Evaluation of rhBMP-2 with OPLA carrier in a canine posterolateral (transverse process) spinal fusion model. Spine 1995; 20:2669–2682.
83. Grauer JN, Patel TC, Erulkar JS, Troiano NW, Panjabi MM, Friedlaender GE. Evaluation of OP-1 as a graft substitute for intertransverse process lumbar fusion. Spine 2001; 26: 127–133.
84. Martin GJ, Boden SD, Titus L. Recombinant human bone morphogenetic protein-2 overcomes the inhibitory effect of kitrolak, a nonsteroidal anti-inflammatory drug (NSAID), on posterolateral lumbar intertransverse process spine fusion. Spine 1999; 24:2188–2193.

85. McKay W, Sandhu HS. Rh-BMP-2 use in spinal fusions: focus issue on bone morphogenetic proteins in spinal fusion. Spine 2002; 27(S16):66–85.

86. Poynton, AR, Lane JM. Safety profile for the clinical use of bone morphogenetic proteins in the spine. Spine 2002; 27(16S):40–48.

87. Martin GJ, Boden SD, Morone MA. Posterolateral intertransverse process spinal arthrodesis with rhBMP-2 in a nonhuman primate: important lessons learned regarding dose, carrier and safety. J Spinal Disord 1999; 12:179–189.

88. Postacchini F, Cinotti G. Bone regrowth after surgical decompression for lumbar spinal stenosis. J Bone Joint Surg Br 1992; 74:862–869.

89. Meyer RA, Gruber HE, Howard BA. Safety of recombinant human bone morphogenetic protein-2 after spinal laminectomy in the dog. Spine 1999; 24:747–754.

90. Cunningham BW, Kanayama M, Parker LM. Osteogenic protein versus autologous interbody arthrodesis in sheep thoracic spine. Spine 1999; 24:509–518.

91. Magin MN, Delling G. Improved lumbar vertebral interbody fusion using rhOP-1: a comparison of autogenous bone graft, bovine hydroxyapatite (Bio-Oss), and BMP-7 (rhOP-1) in sheep. Spine 2001; 26:469–478.

92. Laursen M, Hoy K, Hansen ES. Recombinant bone morphogenetic protein-7 as an intracorpal bone growth stimulator in unstable thoracolumbar burst fractures in humans: preliminary results. Eur Spine J 1999; 8:485–490.

93. Jeppsson C, Saveland H, Rydholm U. OP-1 for cervical spine fusion: bridging bone in only 1 of 4 rheumatodi patients. Acta Orthop Scand 1999; 70:559–563.

94. Paramore CG, Lauryssen C, Raussino MJ. The safety of OP-1 for lumbar fusion with decompression-a canine study. Neurosurgery 1999; 44:1151–1155.

95. Sandhu HS, Safdar NK. Animal models for preclinical assessment of bone morphogenetic proteins in the spine. Spine 2002; 27(16S):32–38.

96. Boden SD, Schimandle JH, Hutton WC. The use of an osteoinductive growth factor for lumbar spinal fusion: Part II: Study of dose, carrier and species. Spine 1995; 20:2633–2644.

97. Damien CJ, Grob D, Boden SD, Benedict JJ. Purified bovine BMP extract and collagen for spine arthrodesis. Spine :50–58.

98. Boden SD, Zdeblick TA, Sandhu HS, Heim SE. The use of rhBMP-2 in interbody fusion cages. Definitive evidence of osteoconduction in humans: a preliminary report. Spine 2000; 25:376–381.

99. Burkus JK, Dorchak JD, Sanders DL. Radiographic assessment of interbody fusion using recombinant human bone morphogenetic protein type 2. Spine 2003; 28(4):372–377.

100. Boden SD, Kang J, Sandhu H, Heller JG. Use of recombinant human bone morphogenetic protein-2 to achieve posterolateral lumbar spine fusion in humans: a prospective, randomized clinical pilot trial: 2002 Volvo Award in clinical studies. Spine 2002; 27(3):2662–2673.

101. Patel TC, Vaccaro AR, Truumees E. Safety and efficacy study of OP-1 (rhBMP-7) as an adjunct to posterolateral spinal fusion. Presented at the North American Spine Society 16th Annual Meeting, Seattle, Oct. 31–Nov. 3, 2001.

102. Patel TC, McCullock JA, Vaccaro AR. A pilot safety and efficacy study of OP-1 in posterolateral lumbar fusion as a replacement for iliac crest autograft. Presented at the North American Spine Society 16th Annual Meeting, Seattle, Oct. 31–Nov. 3, 2001.

103. Speck G. Posterolateral fusion using OP-1: a model using degenerative spondylolysthesis. Presented at the International Society for the Lumbar Spine 27th Annual Meeting, Adelaide, Australia, April 9–13, 2000.

4

Intraoperative Injury to the Spinal Cord and Nerve Roots

Paul M. Arnold and Christopher C. Meredith
University of Kansas School of Medicine, Kansas City, Kansas, U.S.A.

Joan K. McMahon
University of Kansas Hospital, Kansas City, Kansas, U.S.A.

I. INTRODUCTION

Intraoperative injury to the spinal cord during spinal surgery, although rare, is a potentially devastating complication of spine surgery. Injury may occur at any stage of the procedure, from patient positioning to wound closure. The increased use of spinal instrumentation in the past decade, while offering patients significant benefit, has also increased the potential risk of intraoperative spinal cord injury. The exact incidence of spinal cord injury is unknown, and most injuries are transient. In this chapter, we will look at the pitfalls and potential ways of preventing iatrogenic spinal cord injury.

II. ROLE OF SPINAL CORD MONITORING

Intraoperative spinal cord monitoring has been increasingly used in the past several years as a means of reducing intraoperative spinal cord injury (4,24,38,41,47,53). Initially used in scoliosis surgery (7,14,15,17,21,35,36,38,39), it has found an expanded role in nonscoliotic pathologies involving the cervical and thoracolumbar spine. In the last few years there has been an increased use of motor-evoked potentials (MEPs), either alone or in combination with somatosensory-evoked potentials (SSEPs) (5,21,29,35,36,38,40,43,51).

The first attempt at intraoperative monitoring was the wake-up test (41). This technique involves waking the patient during the course of surgery and performing a limited neurological exam. While this maneuver provides useful information regarding the neurological status of the patient, it can only be used once during the course of the procedure. It also requires the discontinuation of muscle relaxants around the time of the exam and exposes the patient to the risk of air embolism, inadvertent extubation, and infection.

SSEPs were developed to overcome the problems associated with the wake-up test. SSEPs monitor the sensory pathways located in the posterior white matter of the spinal cord, and thus are most useful in dorsal spinal surgery (14,17,47,51). SSEPs involve stimulating nerves in the upper and lower extremity (such as the peroneal, ulnar, median, or posterior tibial) and then measuring the evoked potentials, usually at cortical sites (17,35). SSEPs have been used in cervical and thoracolumbar cases of tumor, trauma, and infection, but have found their greatest utility in scoliosis surgery (14,29,38,39,47). Through a continuous recording of the amplitude and latency of these potentials, potential injury to the spinal cord can be detected and possibly reversed. SSEPs are used by a majority of surgeons performing scoliosis surgery (14,21,35,36,38,39,47,51).

A significant change in a SSEPs recording involves an amplitude signal decrease by 50% or slowing of the latency by 10% (39). As a rule, ischemic injuries to the spinal cord occur at a slower rate than mechanical insults, which tend to be immediate. Ischemia may occur as a result of systemic or local hypotension or reduced spinal cord perfusion secondary to overdistraction (15). Mechanical injuries may occur secondary to direct compression, derotation, or overdistraction of the spinal cord. In ischemic injuries the amplitude is often significantly reduced, while the latency is unchanged. The latency is significantly prolonged and the amplitude is significantly reduced in mechanical injuries (17).

While SSEP monitoring is a useful tool for intraoperative evaluation of the spinal cord, it has some definite disadvantages (24). It has been reported that there may be a false-positive rate as high as 1.5% and a false-negative rate of 0–13% (4,14,17,24). Anesthetic agents alone may alter the SSEPs, or the leads could become dislodged during the case. Also, because SSEPs are a measure of sensory spinal cord injury function, rather than motor function, there could be injury to the motor tracts without changes in the SSEPs (4).

For this reason, most intraoperative monitoring today involves MEPs (7,40). MEPs can be elicited by stimulating either the spinal cord or the motor strip of the brain. Two types of MEPs are possible: a compound nerve action potential, which measures the action potential of nerves, and the compound muscle action potential, which is recorded on an EMG (electromyogram) (7,29). The compound muscle action potential has several disadvantages: It is extremely difficult to attain reliable recordings during surgery, and there may be wide fluctuations of amplitude during surgery, even though patients may awake with no postoperative deficit. For this reason, compound nerve action potentials have been utilized more and more frequently and are considered highly reliable. A 10% change in latency or an 80% decrease in amplitude has been defined as a significant alteration and correlates with new-onset postoperative neurological deficit (29).

If changes in SSEP or MEP monitoring occur, steps must be taken to ascertain the cause. Alterations may be due to anesthetic changes, technical aspects of the monitoring apparatus, or true neurological injury (7). Consultation with the surgeon, anesthesiologist, and neurophysiologist should take place to determine appropriate action. The test should be performed again, all leads checked, and assessment of whether anesthetic changes (e.g., changes in muscle relaxation) have occurred. Obviously, if some recent manipulation of the spinal cord has taken place immediately before, this should be stopped or reversed, usually in the form of hardware removal, support of blood pressure, or realigning the spinal cord.

III. CERVICAL SPINAL CORD INJURY

Injuries to the cervical spinal cord are among the most feared and potentially dangerous complications in spine surgery. They may occur during patient positioning (15), decompression (5,10,27,33), fusion (5), fixation (1,2,11,28,45,52), or closure and may occur during either dorsal or ventral approaches.

A. Incidence

The incidence of intraoperative injury to the cervical spinal cord is fortunately low (10). However, there have been instances of devastating neurological complications. Smith et al. (45) reported on a patient who died postoperatively following what was thought to be incorrect placement of sublaminar wires. Other patients have suffered quadriparesis and ventilator dependence. Flynn (20) reported on a large series of patients who underwent anterior cervical surgery in a questionnaire of more than 700 surgeons who performed over 80,000 operations. The reported rate of neurological deficit was 0.3%. Kraus and Stauffer (31), as well as Kostuik et al. (30), have reported on spinal injuries occurring during anterior decompression and fusion, as well as those related to instrumentation.

Historically, posterior cervical surgery has been riskier than anterior surgery, with complication rates in the 1–2% range. Some of this increased complication rate may be due to the plethora of hardware available for the posterior cervical spine, including facet, sublaminar (5), and interspinous wiring (45); hooks; Halifax clamps; lateral mass screws (2,11,19,26,28); and, recently, pedicle screws (1). The technically demanding use of transarticular screws has also been introduced in the past few years (54).

Several reports of injury secondary to incorrect placement of clamps or sublaminar wires have been reported (5,45). For these reasons, as well as increased ease of use and superior biomechanics, there has been increased interest in lateral mass screws as a means of posterior cervical fixation (1,2,19,26). The incidence of complications has been reported to be between 0.1–1.8%, mostly related to radiculopathy secondary to nerve root injury during screw placement. Cervical pedicle screws have been used more and more frequently in the past 5 years, with a reported 0.3% complication rate (1,2,19).

B. Spinal Cord Injury During Positioning

Patients may also incur neurological injury during the positioning phase of a case. This may be due to extreme rotation of the neck, spinal cord compression from osteophytic spurs, ischemia secondary to decreased blood flow, and manipulation of the neck in patients with an occult injury.

Operative positioning in patients undergoing cervical spine procedures should be performed in a controlled, deliberate manner. Tong traction may be used in patients undergoing ventral surgery, and the Mayfield head-holder may be used in dorsal surgery to prevent head movement and prevent pressure on the eyes. This will prevent sudden, inadvertent neck movement during the case. Extremes in flexion and extension of the neck should be avoided, particularly in elderly patients. These patients may have spondylotic stenosis, and direct injury to the spinal cord can occur with manipulation of the neck. This potential complication can be avoided, and preoperative plain x-rays should be obtained to assess the degree of spondylosis in these patients.

Vascular compromise can also occur during positioning, particularly during flexion or extension of the neck in patients with carotid or vertebral artery disease. This could cause ischemia and lead to cerebral or spinal cord infarction (15,44).

Patients with a history of trauma should have appropriate imaging before undergoing any type of surgical procedure. Identification of fractures and/or traumatic herniated disks would encourage the use of awake, fiber-optic intubation. These injuries can be identified and prevented with plain x-rays, computed tomography CT scans, or magnetic resonance imaging (MRI) (27,42).

C. Spinal Cord Injury During Decompression

Injury to the cervical spinal can occur during surgical decompression from an anterior or posterior approach (10,48,49). Spinal cord injury during a ventral decompression may be due to direct injury of the spinal cord by inappropriate use of an instrument during bone removal, or indirectly by injury to the carotid or vertebral artery (10,27,33,56). The carotid artery may be torn during exposure: this complication is obvious when encountered and should be repaired with subsequent termination of the procedure (27). The carotid artery may also be occluded due to excessive retraction; this can be prevented by careful observation and meticulous technique (10). Excessive retraction may also lead to dislodgement of a plaque with subsequent intracranial embolus.

Vertebral artery injury can occur if the dissection is taken too far laterally (25,44). This is more frequently seen in re do operations or in patients with unusual anatomy, for example, anomalus foramina transversaria. Bleeding can often be stopped with tamponade, and an arteriogram should be obtained postoperatively to rule out dissection or pseudoaneurysm (49). This complication can be avoided by identifying the midline and landmarks such as the uncovertebral joints (44). An AP x-ray may be useful if these landmarks are obscured.

Direct injury to the spinal cord during anterior decompression is rare, but may occur in patients with particularly significant stenosis (27,48,56). Even a slight increase in spinal cord pressure can cause injury, particularly when removing osteophytes with a Kerrison punch (49). Meticulous technique, adequate illumination and magnification, maintenance of normotension, and attention to hemostasis are all standard means for preventing this problem (33,49,56). Often this complication is not detected until the patient is examined in the recovery room. Direct injury to the spinal cord may also occur with overaggressive or improper use of a drill during decompression (27). Experience, proper technique, and appropriate drill bit selection guard against this complication.

Operative trauma to the spinal cord is also seen in posterior surgery and most often occurs during laminectomy (27,33,48). Again, this may be caused by inadvertent pressure on the spinal cord with the use of rongeurs or punches, particularly in patients with very significant stenosis (31). Some surgeons perform laminectomies by initially using a high-speed drill, making a laminotomy at the most caudad level to be removed, and then inserting the foot plate of a Kerrison punch and proceeding cephalad (27,48). Spinal cord injury can also occur with the direct use of monopolar cautery current on the spinal cord and/or nerve roots.

D. Spinal Cord Injury During Fusion and Fixation

Injury to the spinal cord during the fusion and fixation steps of anterior cervical surgery has become quite rare in the past few years and is easily preventable. Injury to the spinal cord may occur when tapping the bone graft into place following diskectomy (20). This happens when the bone graft is not appropriately shaped and is "hammered" into the spinal cord. This complication is preventable with meticulous bone carpentry (31). Injury to the spinal cord may also occur if there is sudden collapse of the spine following bone graft extrusion. This can also be prevented by appropriate sizing of the bone graft, with particular attention paid to its depth and height (20,31).

Injury during anterior cervical fixation is quite rare, particularly with the advent of screws with unicortical purchase (30). The first anterior cervical screws to be used required bicortical purchase, and intraoperative fluoroscopy was required to assure that the screws did not penetrate the dura. Unicortical fixation was found to be biomechanically equivalent to bicortical purchase, without the risk of neural injury. As long as the plate is centered on the midline and appropriate screw lengths are chosen, spinal injury from this technique should be nonexistent (30).

Neurological deficit may also occur as a result of postoperative epidural hematoma (27,50). This complication has been reported to occur in less than 1% of ventral procedures. Epidural hematomas can be avoided by paying careful attention to hemostasis, particularly right before closure begins. One should spend an extra few minutes making a circumferential search for any occult bleeding, and closure should not begin until the wound is dry. Subfascial drains are used if a large dead space has been created, particularly with a multilevel procedure.

Spinal cord injury during the fusion step of a posterior operation should not occur, since lateral mass screws are placed in a lateral direction within the lateral mass (2,11,19,26,28,52,55), especially if the spinal cord is not exposed with a decompression. As noted above, wires passed in a sublaminar manner may puncture the dura and spinal cord and cause neurological injury. Wiring techniques have largely given way to segmental lateral mass fixation for both biomechanical and safety reasons.

Spinal cord injury is very rare with lateral mass screws, because the screws are aimed laterally (11,19,26,52). However, several studies have reported nerve root injuries or pain secondary to foraminal stenosis. Several techniques (2,28,55) have been described to avoid this pitfall, and the basic principles involve picking the correct drilling point, and aiming the drill laterally in the appropriate three-dimensional trajectory. Several authors stress the use of optimal length screws, generally 14 mm, and of obtaining unicortical purchase (2,28,52). If a problem is detected intraoperatively, either by poor purchase or suboptimal screw location, the screw should be removed and that level skipped if possible.

E. Spinal Cord Injury During Surgery

Injury to the thoracic spinal cord or conus medullaris may occur during dorsal or ventral surgery (3); most of the causes are the same as discussed in the cervical spine section. Spinal cord injury may occur during the decompression, fusion, or fixation phases and may be a result of mechanical or ischemic injury to the thoracic spinal cord. This is especially pertinent when operating ventrally from T4 to T9 (32,46). The major arterial supply to the cord in this region usually enters at T7, and the predominant blood supply to the lower spinal cord, the artery of Adamkiewicz, has a variable appearance, from T9 to L2 (9,46). Thus, there exists a "watershed" region of the spinal cord where blood flow is lowest; diminution of blood supply to this variable area may lead to spinal cord ischemia and infarction (32,46). Therefore, it is important to preserve the artery of Adamkiewicz to prevent injury in the watershed area; preoperative angiography may be useful in identifying this vessel and avoiding injury to it during the procedure (9).

With the advent of adequate rigid anterior thoracolumbar fixation, there has been a parallel increased interest in ventral retroperitoneal surgery that allows decompression, fusion, and fixation in a single stage (18). Most ventral thoracic and thoracolumbar surgery is performed to decompress the anterior spinal cord, whether for tumor, trauma, infection, or disk herniation (22). The spinal cord is therefore compromised when the decompression begins, and any inadvertent pressure during the decompression may injure the spinal cord. This could come in the form of overagressive lesion resection or getting lost in anatomy that is obscured by tumor, bone, or granulation tissue (12). Inadequate decompression may also lead to delayed neurological deficit. Careful attention to preoperative imaging studies, a thorough knowledge of the surgical anatomy, and careful technique may help to avoid those complications (18).

Once decompression is complete, fusion and fixation are performed. Usually at least one vertebral body is resected, and thus a large gap must be bridged (12). Bone from the decompression (in the case of fracture) or from local rib or iliac crest (tumor or infection) is then procured. Injury to the spinal cord may occur if proper sizing and shaping of the graft is not undertaken or if the appropriate-sized cage is not used. These pitfalls can only be avoided with experience and proper technique (18). If methylmethacrylate or another synthetic material is used for grafting, care must be taken to ensure that it does not migrate into the spinal canal.

Injury to the spinal cord may occur during placement of anterior hardware (12). This generally involves misdirection of screws that enter the spinal canal and cause injury to the spinal cord. Proper adherence to technique, familiarity with the instrumentation, knowledge of anatomy and orientation, and intraoperative imaging are all crucial in avoiding instrument-related neurological injury (41).

Postoperative epidural hematoma may also be responsible for lower extremity weakness (Fig. 1). Fractures and tumors in this region may be especially vascular. Achieving adequate hemostasis may be problematic, but it is essential to avoid this complication. Epidural drains and chest tubes are also useful in this regard.

Injury to the spinal cord may also occur from posterior thoracic or thoracolumbar procedures (6,53). Injury may occur during decompression, and this is usually due to poor technique. Extreme care must be taken during laminectomy of the thoracic spine, as there is very little room in the canal for the spinal cord in this region.

Posterior instrumentation of the thoracic and thoracolumbar spine may also be the source of spinal cord complications (6,23,53). Placement of hooks or sublaminar wires particularly at the site of pathology may cause pressure on the spinal cord, and derotation, traction, or other manipulation of the spinal cord may also cause injury. These changes may be detected by intraoperative monitoring and potentially reversed (53). Many surgeons have used all pedicle screw (13,23,24) constructs to avoid having hardware in

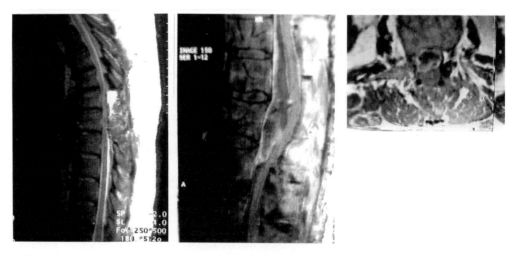

Figure 1 Postoperative epidural hematoma following laminectomy. The patient woke up with paraparesis, and was only minimally improved following reoperation.

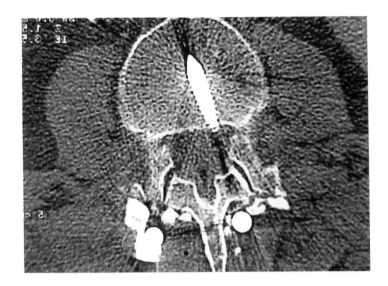

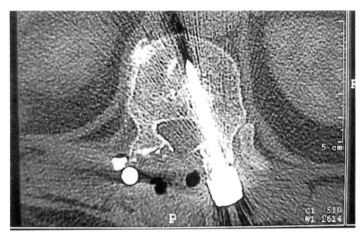

Figure 2   Thoracic pedicle screw placed through the spinal cord. Patient woke up with paraparesis, which did not improve following screw removal.

the canal, and their placement accuracy has been enhanced in recent years with the popularity of frameless stereotaxy (6). Again, epidural hematoma is another avoidable complication of posterior thoracic spine surgery (Fig. 2).

IV. LUMBOSACRAL SPINAL ROOT SURGERY

Many of the same potential complications involved in surgery of the cervical and thoracic spine are potential challenges in the lumbar spine: injury may result during ventral or dorsal decompression, malposition of bone graft, poor hardware placement, and epidural hematoma (43). However, there are some problems that are unique or should be stressed as potential hazards in the lumbar spine. These are pedicle screw injury, nerve root

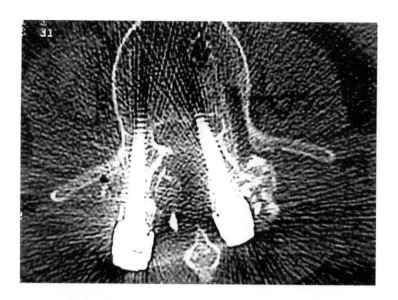

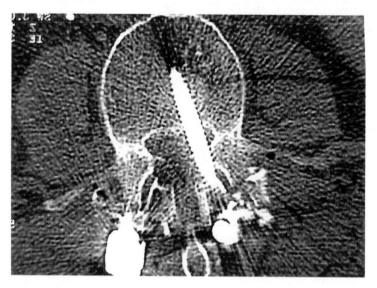

Figure 3   Lumbar pedicle screw, placed too medially. Patient's radiculopathy improved following removal.

retraction, nerve root injury from dural tears, and neural injury due to malplaced interbody devices.

The use of pedicle screw fixation as adjuncts for lumbar degenerative disease has skyrocketed in the past 10 years, and the complication rate in several large studies ranges from 0 to 18% (6,13,34). These complications involve pain and neurological injury and arise out of inappropriate placement of the screws, usually due to technical error (6,13,34). Optimal placement involves a thorough knowledge of pedicular anatomy, with particular attention to the angle of the pedicle. This angle increases as one progresses caudally in the lumbar spine.

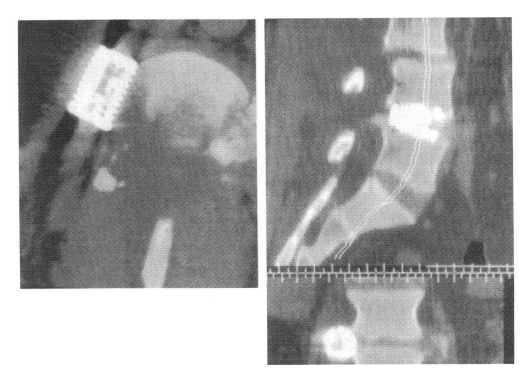

Figure 4 Gross misplacement of interbody cage. Patient woke up with radiculopathy.

Intraoperative fluoroscopy or portable x-rays are useful for confirmation of the pedicle (34). Recent advances in pedicle screw placement are intraoperative frameless navigation, which illustrates the pedicle in three dimensions, and intraoperative EMG, which lets the surgeon know if a nerve root is irritated (43). If standard landmarks are

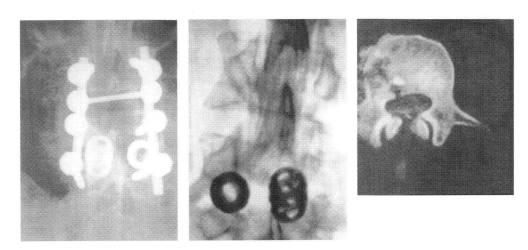

Figure 5 Poor placement of interbody cage. Patient suffered fracture of L4 with severe pain. This resolved with decompression and pedicle screw fixation.

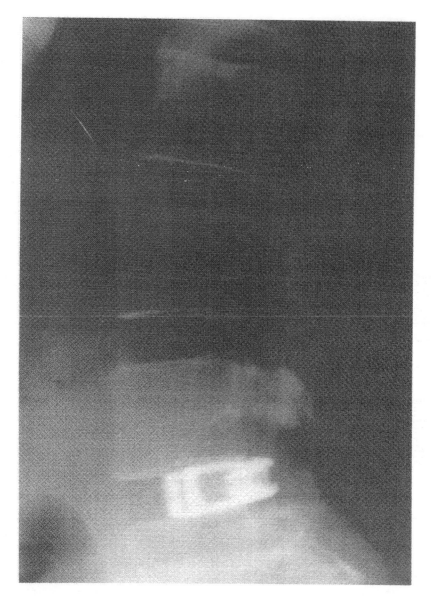

Figure 6 Movement of interbody cage after satisfactory placement. Patient experienced severe back pain, which resolved with removal and placement of a larger cage.

obscured by scar or anomalous anatomy, a laminectomy may be performed and the dorsal aspect of the pedicle directly visualized (Fig. 3).

Nerve root and thecal sac retraction are performed more commonly in the lumbar spine, as there is usually no fear of spinal cord injury at the level of the cauda equiva. However, over-retraction of the nerve roots of the thecal sac may cause neurologic injury, and unfortunately there is no good contemporary intraoperative method of detecting this problem (8). The only means of avoiding this complication is prevention. If there is concern that a nerve root may need to be unduly retracted, it is appropriate to remove more bone or ligament so that less pressure is placed on the nerve.

Nerve roots may also be injured during laminectomy for lumbar stenosis, and few sights are more distressing for the spine surgeon than to see a clump of nerve roots protrude through the dura after removing some stenotic bone (8). This is most likely to occur with particularly tight stenosis, where the dura and ligamentum flavum are adherent, or in a reoperation, where scar tissue prevents development of normal tissue planes. If nerve roots appear outside the dural sac and are still in continuity, they should be meticulously placed back within the sac with a smooth forceps. The durotomy should then be closed, and consideration should be given to the use of synthetic dura and a tissue sealant (8).

Interbody fusion as treatment for low back pain has been described for 50 years, but recently there has been a surge of interest in this procedure (16). Titanium threaded cages have been developed in the last few years to span the intervertebral space while allowing bone to grow through them and produce a fusion (16). Recent enthusiasm for their use has waned in the last 2–3 years, as their initial reports of success have not been sustained. Presized machined allograft has also been used as fusion material. As with any new technology, this procedure involves its own set of pitfalls. These are related to intraoperative injury in the following way: they may migrate and cause nerve root or cauda equina compression. This can be avoided by proper sizing and shaping of the implant and proper placement within the disk space. Use of pedicle screws, with the potential for intraoperative compression of the device (either bone or cage), enhances the stability of the construct. Sufficient bone, up to and including a total facetectomy, should be performed so the nerve roots are not overly stretched when inserting the devices (Figs. 4–6).

Cauda equina or nerve injury may occur when reducing a spondylolisthesis (37). This problem can be avoided by first performing a decompression, as well as using intraoperative neural monitoring to assess neural irritation during the reduction.

V. THE PATIENT WITH A POSTOPERATIVE NEUROLOGICAL DEFICIT

A relevant neurological examination should be performed on postoperative patients as soon as possible. If a patient wakes up with a new deficit, several questions must be answered: Is the deficit partial or complete? Cord or root? What is the cause? Can I fix it? Do I need more information? (20).

If a patient wakes up with a significant injury and has undergone a posterior decompression only (no hardware), the only potentially reversible deficits are an epidural hematoma or a retained disk fragment, both of which may be reversible. We recommend immediate return to the operating room to rule out those causes following appropriate imaging if necessary. If a retained disk fragment is found, it should be removed and the disk space reexplored. If an epidural hematoma is discovered, it should be evaluated and all bleeding sites identified. We also recommend investigating whether the hematoma has spread beyond the confines of the original surgery.

If a patient wakes up with a significant deficit and has undergone bone grafting and/or fixation, x-rays performed in the recovery room are useful for assessing the status of the bone graft and hardware. If there is an obvious problem, the patient should be taken to the OR and the problem corrected. Depending on the type of surgery, further imaging studies may be required, or the patient can return to the OR to rule out a hematoma.

If the patient wakes up with a partial deficit, postoperative x-rays are indicated to evaluate spinal alignment and hardware, followed by an MRI or myelogram/CT to rule out spinal cord pathology. If there is no hematoma or disk, it is likely that the treatment will be nonoperative, such as blood pressure support, corticosteroids, and possibly mannitol.

Finally, if the patient wakes up with a normal neurological exam and then has a progressive neurological deficit, the likely cause is an expanding hematoma, and the patient should be taken back to the OR for immediate evacuation.

The experienced spine surgeon will run into complications from time to time. The best way to treat complications is to avoid them. Proper patient selection, realistic outcome expectations, appropriate preoperative planning, and meticulous surgical technique are all ingredients in complication avoidance. If a complication occurs, the surgeon should do everything in his or her power to correct it, as well as learn from it so as to minimize the potential for occurrence in the future.

REFERENCES

1. Abumi K, Shono Y, Ito M, Taneichi H, Kotani Y, Kaneda K. Complications of pedicle screw fixation in reconstructive surgery of the cervical spine. Spine 2000; 25:962–969.
2. An HS, Gordin R, Renner K. Anatomic considerations for plate-screw fixation of the cervical spine. Spine 1991; 16:5548–5551.
3. Apel DM, Marrero G, King J, Tolo VT, Bassett GS. Avoiding paraplegia during ventral spinal surgery. Spine 1991; 16(suppl):5365–5370.
4. Ben-David B, Haller G, Taylor P. Anterior spinal fusion complicated by paraplegia: a case report of a false-negative somatosensory-evoked potential. Spine 1987; 12:536–539.
5. Blacklock JB. Fracture of a sublaminar stainless steel cable in the upper cervical spine with neurological injury: case report. J Neurosurg 1994; 81:932–933.
6. Brown CA, Lenke LG, Briodwell KH, Geideman WM, Hassan SA, Blanke K. Complications of pediatric thoracolumbar and lumbar pedicle screws. Spine 1998; 23:1566–1571.
7. Calancie BJ, Klose J, Baier S, Green BA. Isoflurane-induced attenuation of motor evoked potentials caused by electrical motor cortex stimulation during surgery. J Neurosurg 1991; 74:897–904.
8. Carrol SE, Wiesel SW. Neurologic complications and lumbar laminectomy. Clin Ortho Rel Res 1992; 284:14–23.
9. Champlin AA, Rael J, Benzel EC, Kesterson L, King JN, Orrison WW, Mirfakhrace M. Preoperative spinal angiography for lateral extracavitary approach to thoracic and lumbar spine. AJNR 1994; 15:73–77.
10. Cloward RB. Complications of ventral cervical disc operation and their treatment. Surgery 1971; 69:175–182.
11. Conant RF, Vaccaro AR, Albert TJ. Complication of posterior occipital and cervical screw placement. Sem Spine Surg 1998; 10:228–236.
12. Cotler JM, Star AM. Complications of spine fusions. In: Cotler JM, Cotler HB, eds. Spinal Fusion: Science and Technique. New York: Springer-Verlag, 1990:361–387.
13. Davne SH, Myers DL. Complications of lumbar spinal fusion with transpedicular instrumentation. Spine 1992; 17:5184–5189.
14. Dawson EG, Sherman JE, Kanim LEA, Nuwer MR. Spinal cord monitoring: results of the Scoliosis Research Society and the European Spinal Deformity Society survey. Spine 1991; 16:5361–5364.
15. Dolan EJ, Transfeldt EE, Tator CH, Tator CH, Simmons EH, Jughes KF. The effect of spinal cord distraction on regional spinal cord blood flow in cats. J Neurosurg 1980; 53: 756–764.
16. Elias WJ, Simmons NE, Kaptain GJ, Chadduck JB, Whitehill R. Complications of posterior lumbar interbody fusion when using a titanium threaded cage device. J Neurosurg 2000; 93(suppl 1):45–52.

17. Epstein NE. Intraoperative evoked potential monitoring. In: Benzel EC, ed. Spine Surgery: Techniques, Complication Avoidance, and Management. New York: Churchill Livingstone, 1999:1249–1257.

18. Fasciszewski T, Winter RB, Lonstein JE, Denis F, Johnson L. The surgical and medical perioperative complications of anterior spinal fusion surgery in the thoracic and lumbar spine in adults: a review of 1223 procedures. Spine 1995; 20:1592–1599.

19. Fehlings MG, Cooper PR, Errico TJ. Posterior plates in the management of cervical instability: long term results in 44 patients. J Neurosurg 1994; 81:341–349.

20. Flynn TB. Neurologic complications of anterior cervical interbody fusion. Spine 1982; 7: 536–539.

21. Forbes HJ, Allen PW, Waller CS, Jones SJ, Edgar MA, Webb PJ, Ransford AO. Spinal cord monitoring in scoliosis surgery: experience with 1168 cases. J Bone Jt Surg 1991; 73B:487–491.

22. Fugita T, Kostuik JP, Huckell CB, Sieber AN. Complications of spinal fusion in adult patients more than 60 years of age. Ortho Clin N Am 1998; 29:669–678.

23. Gertzbein SD, Robbins SE. Accuracy of pedicle screw placement in vivo. Spine 1990; 15:11–14.

24. Ginsburg HH, Shetter AG, Raudzens PA. Postoperative paraplegia with preserved intraoperative somatosensory evoked potentials. J Neurosurg 1985; 63:296–300.

25. Golfinos JG, Dickman CA, Zabramski JM, Sonntag VKH, Spetzler RF. Repair of vertebral artery injury during anterior cervical decompression. Spine 1994; 19:2552–2556.

26. Graham AW, Swank ML, Kinard RE, Lowery GL, Dials BE. Posterior cervical arthrodesis and stabilization with a lateral mass plate: clinical and computed tomographic evaluation of lateral mass screw placement and associated complications. Spine 1996; 21:323–328.

27. Graham JJ. Complications of cervical spine surgery. Spine 1989; 14:1046–1050.

28. Heller JG, Silcox DH, Sutterlin CE. Complications of posterior cervical plating. Spine 1995; 20:2442–2448.

29. Konrad P, Owen JM, Bridwell KH. Magnetic stimulation of the spine to produce lower extremity EMG responses: significance of coil position and the presence of bone. Spine 1994; 19:2812–2818.

30. Kostuik JP, Connolloy PJ, Esses SL, Suh P. Anterior cervical plate fixation with the titanium hollow screw plate system. Spine 1993; 18:1273–1278.

31. Kraus DR, Stauffer ES. Spinal cord injury as a complication of elective anterior cervical fusion. Clin Orthop Rel Res 1975; 112:130–141.

32. Lazorthes G, Gouaze A, Zadeh JO, Santini JJ, Lazorthes Y, Burdin P. Arterial vascularization of the spinal cord: recent studies of the anastomotic substitution pathways. J Neurosurg 1971; 35:253–262.

33. Lesion F, Bovasakao N, Clarisse J, Rousseaux M, Jomin M. Results of surgical treatment of radiculomyelopathy caused by cervical arthrosis based on 1000 operations. Surg Neurol 1985; 23:350–355.

34. Lonstein JE, Denis F, Perra JH, Pinto MR, Smith MD, Winter RB. Complications associated with pedicle screws. J Bone Jt Surg 1999; 81A:1519–1528.

35. MacDonald DB, Alzayed Z, Khoudeir I, Stigsby B. Monitoring scoliosis surgery with combined multiple transcranial electric motor and cortical somatosensory-evoked potentials from the lower and upper extremities. Spine 2003; 28:194–203.

36. MacEwen GD, Bunnell WP, Sriram K. Acute neurologic complications in the treatment of scoliosis: a report of the Scoliosis Research Society. J Bone Jt Surg 1975; 57A:404–408.

37. Maurice HD, Morley TR. Cauda equina lesions following fusion in situ and decompressive laminectomy for severe spondylolisthesis. Four case reports. Spine 1989; 14:214–216.

38. Nuwer MR, Dawson EG, Carlson LG, Kanim LE, Sherman JE. Somatosensory evoked potential spinal cord monitoring reduces neurologic deficits after scoliosis surgery: results of a large multicenter survey. Electroencephalogr Clin Neurophys 1995; 96:6–11.

39. Owen JH. The application of intraoperative monitoring during surgery for spinal deformity. Spine 1999; 24:2649–2662.

40. Owen JH, Tamaki T. Applications of neurophysiological measures during surgery of the spine. In: Frymoyer JW, ed. The Adult Spine: Principles and Practice. Philadelphia: Lippincott-Raven, 1997:673–702.
41. Oxner WM, Kang JD. Management of iatrogenic neurologic loss due to spinal instrumentation. In: Vaccaro AR, Betz RR, Zeidman SM, eds. Principles and Practices of Spine Surgery. Philadelphia: Mosby, 2003:697–710.
42. Robertson HJ, Smith RD. Cervical myelography: survey of modes of practice and major complications. Radiology 1990; 174:79–83.
43. Shields CB, Paloheimo MP, Backman MH, Edmonds HL, Johnson JR, Holt RT. Intraoperative transcranial magnetic motor evoked potentials are difficult to obtain during lumbar disc and spinal tumor operations. Muscle Nerve 1988; 11:993.
44. Smith MD, Emery SE, Dudley A, Murray KJ, Leventhal M. Vertebral artery injury during anterior decompression of the cervical spine: a retrospective review of ten patients. J Bone Jt Surg 1993; 75B:410–415.
45. Smith MD, Phillips WA, Hensinger RN. Complications of fusion of the upper cervical spine. Spine 1991; 16:702–705.
46. Suh TM, Alexander L. Vascular system of the human spinal cord. Arch Neurol Psych 1939; 41:659–677.
47. Tamaki T, Tsuji H, Inove SI, Kobayashi H. The prevention of iatrogenic spinal cord injury utilizing the evoked spinal cord potential. Int Orthop 1981; 4:313–317.
48. Taylor BA, Vaccaro AR, Albert TJ. Complications of anterior and posterior surgical approaches in the treatment of cervical degenerative disc disease. Sem Spine Surg 1999; 11:337–346.
49. Tew JM, Mayfield FH. Complications of surgery of the anterior cervical spine. In: Dunsler SB, ed. Cervical Spondylosis. New York: Raven Press, 1981:191–208.
50. U HS, Wilson CB. Postoperative epidural hematoma as a complication of anterior cervical diskectomy: report of three cases. J Neurosurg 1978; 49:288–291.
51. Vauzelle C, Stagnara P, Jouvinroux P. Functional monitoring of spinal cord activity during spinal surgery. Clin Orthop Rel Res 1973; 93:173–178.
52. Wellman, BJ, Follett KA, Traynelis VC. Complications of posterior articular mass plate fixation of the subaxial cervical spine in 43 consecutive patients. Spine 1998; 23:193–200.
53. Wilber RG, Thompson GH, Shaffer JW, Brown RH, Nash Jr CL. Postoperative neurological deficits in segmental instrumentation: a study using spinal cord monitoring. J Bone Jt Surg 1984; 66A:1178–1187.
54. Wright NM, Lauryssen C. Vertebral artery injury in C1-2 transarticular screw fixation: results of a survey of the AANS/CNS section of disorders of the spine and peripheral nerves. J Neurosurg 1998; 88:634–640.
55. Xu R, Haman SP, Ebraheim NA, Yeasting RA. The anatomic relation of lateral mass screws to the spinal nerves: a comparison of the Magerl, Anderson, and An techniques. Spine 1999; 24:2057–2061.
56. Yonenobu K, Okada K, Fuji T, Fujiwara K, Yamashita K, Ono K. Causes of neurologic deterioration following surgical treatment of cervical myelopathy. Spine 1986; 11:818–823.

5

Intraoperative Injury to the Cauda Equina and Nerve Roots

Michael J. Bolesta
The University of Texas Southwestern Medical Center, Dallas, Texas, U.S.A.

I. MECHANISM OF INJURY

Lumbar surgery is common and in most cases quite safe. Injuries to the cauda equina and nerve roots are an inherent risk, but based on current literature this appears to be relatively uncommon. Nerve roots may be injured in isolation, but cauda equina injuries may be attended by dural injuries. The literature on incidental durotomy indicates that dural disruption occurs relatively frequently (3.5–14% of cases) but can be successfully managed with a low risk of adverse sequelae (1–3). None of these cited studies report associated neurological deficit. If the cauda equina is manipulated during a dural repair, transient neural dysfunction may occur. If dural laceration is attended by root transection, the prognosis would depend on the extent of neural disruption. Combined dural and cauda equina injuries could occur with both manual and power instruments. Misplaced pedicle screws and other types of instrumentation could injure the dura and nerve roots. Cauda equina injury by pedicle screws can occur but is not common in the hands of an experienced spine surgeon unless the anatomy is quite distorted.

Neural injury can occur during attempted decompression. Insertion of Kerrison rongeurs, curettes, and other tools within a stenotic region may contuse the neural elements. Cutting instruments may also lacerate nerves. When there are adhesions, crushing and avulsion injuries may occur; in such cases, rongeurs may inadvertently remove nerve fibers as well as bone and ligamentum flavum.

Power instruments may be used to remove bone without introducing instruments into a stenotic canal but carry the risk of cutting or abrading the underlying nerves and dura. Such instruments may lacerate, contuse, wrap up, and avulse soft tissue, producing severe injury within seconds. High-grade spondylolisthesis is another entity associated with surgically related neurological injury. Even without an attempt at reduction, cauda equina syndrome has been reported (4). Reduction is associated with root palsy, which may occur as often as 25% of cases (5).

Spinal instrumentation has improved our ability to stabilize, to correct deformity, and to achieve improved fusion rates. Some implants depend on hooks for purchase. When inserted into the spinal canal, these may contuse roots during insertion or compress underlying traversing roots. Pedicle screws may fracture the pedicle, compressing or

47

lacerating the adjacent nerve root or dura. Pedicle probes, drills, taps, and screws themselves can have a similar effect if they enter the canal. Of 617 cases discussed by Esses et al. (6) 2.4% of patients experienced transient neuropraxia and 2.3% were noted to have permanent nerve injury. Lonstein et al. (7) noted root irritation after only 9 of 915 operations caused by 11 of 4790 implanted screws; a medially placed screw is the usual cause. Three of their patients had residual neurological weakness despite screw removal. Indirect neural injury can occur when instrumentation systems apply corrective forces. For example, Holland and Kostuik (8) reported a case of L-5 radiculopathy following correction of thoracolumbar scoliosis. Revision surgery is a recognized risk factor for a neural injury, particularly when there has been previous removal of the posterior elements.

Injuries of the cauda equina and nerve roots behave more like peripheral nerve injuries than spinal cord injuries. Thus, the prognosis of blunt injury tends to be more favorable.

II. DETECTION

Some injuries occurring during decompression are self-evident. This is particularly true when attended by leakage of cerebral spinal fluid. Blunt injuries are not always apparent. Bleeding or overlying structures may obscure a macroscopic injury to a root. When the injury occurs from avulsion, the surgeon is painfully aware of the obvious injury. A more difficult situation occurs when the neural elements are not exposed as part of the operation. While normal posterior elements will tend to protect the nerves, correction of deformity or placement of instrumentation can compromise neural function, as noted above.

In some situations electrophysiological monitoring can be quite useful. Somatosensory and more recently motor-evoked potential monitoring are time-honored techniques widely used by scoliosis surgeons. Their primary utility is in thoracic deformity correction. They are very sensitive to ischemia and direct trauma to the spinal cord. The literature is mixed in assessing its utility to monitor cauda equina function. Somatosensory potential monitoring primarily reflects posterior column function, so it may not detect motor paralysis, one of the most feared complications of deformity surgery. Motor-evoked potential monitoring has improved detection of cord injuries, but it is not as useful in presaging impending cauda equina injury. Compound motor action potential monitoring is useful in identifying nerves in pathological altered regions, such as scar. Electromyography has been used in a variety of ways to detect injury or the potential for injury.

Bose (9) studied spontaneous electromyographical activity and compound muscle action potential responses in 61 consecutive cases of instrumented posterior lumbar fusions. Thirteen of the patients exhibited 14 neurophysiological events. Sustained neurotonic electromyographical discharges occurred in 5 of 40 patients during placement of interbody fusion cages, in 2 patients during placement of pedicle screws, and in 1 during rod tightening. These authors also stimulated the pedicle screws after placement and detected six cortical breaches. Only 1 of 61 patients developed a neurological deficit. Temporary paraparesis was presaged by spontaneous electromyographical discharges during thecal sac retraction and disk distraction to place a cage.

Deletis and Vodusek (10) monitored sacral roots using intraoperative recording of the bulbocavernosus reflex in 119 patients using a specific anesthetic technique. Reliable signals were obtained in these 119 individuals who ranged in age from 24 days to 74 years. No dysfunction was noted. Holland and Kostuik (8) reported a case of L5 radiculopathy following scoliosis surgery. Although posterior tibial nerve somatosensory-evoked potentials were normal, there were frequent trains of neurotonic discharges from the left anterior tibial muscle. Persistent postoperative L5 radiculopathy prompted exploration 9 days following the original procedure. They found that the left L5 root was compressed by bony structures. The authors recommended electromyographic monitoring of the lumbosacral myotomes during this type of procedure.

Hormes and Chappuis (11) recommended compound muscle action potential recordings to identify nerve root irritation in the lumbosacral region, particularly when distorted anatomy and scarring precludes visual identification. Continuous electromyography monitoring detects nerve root irritation manifested by spontaneous neurotonic discharges, potentially warning the surgeon of impending or evolving injury before it becomes irreversible.

Jou and Lai (12) used a clip compression model in rabbits to mimic root injury by transpedicular screws. They found spinal somatosensory evoked potential monitoring to be very sensitive to the compromise of a single nerve root using the criteria of more than 20% percent decrease in amplitude and increased latency. Moed (13) studied first sacral root function using stimulus evoked electromyography, continuous electromyography monitoring and continuous somatosensory evoked potential monitoring in a canine model. A 2.0 mm Kirshner wire was inserted under CT guidance to contact the S-1 nerve root. Sixteen of 17 wires compressed or penetrated the nerve root. No spontaneous burst of electromyographical activity was recorded in any specimen. Only 1 of 12 had abnormal somatosensory evoked potential monitoring. The correlation coefficient for the relationship between current thresholds with stimulus evoked electromyography and the distance of the wire from the nerve was 0.801. They concluded that only stimulus evoked electromyography consistently provided reliable information about the proximity of the implant to the nerve root. In a related clinical study, Moed (14) reported on this same technique in 27 patients. They inserted 51 iliosacral screws, using a current threshold of 8 mA or more as safe. Using this criterion, they redirected 4 screws. All 27 patients had normal neurological function after surgery. Postoperative CT showed all screws to be in a safe interosseous position. Owen (15) found that mechanically elicited electromyograms were extremely sensitive to root irritation. They found them to be both sensitive and specific.

The differing results and recommendations among the studies likely represent variations in methods, equipment, and interpretation of the tests. Each surgeon should select monitoring appropriate to his or her own situation. Such monitoring is a adjunct to careful surgical technique.

III. TYPES OF INJURY AND ACUTE MANAGEMENT

The spinal nerves and the rootlets of the cauda equina behave like peripheral nerves, and injuries to them may be classified in a similar fashion. With neuropraxia, nerve function is temporarily suspended, but there is no physical disruption of the axons. This has the best prognosis. In axonotmesis, axon fibers are disrupted on a microscopic level, but the myelin sheaths remain intact. Injured nerves will show Wallerian degeneration, but the nerve sheaths guide subsequent regeneration by the regrowth of axons. Although recovery is more prolonged than with neuropraxia, the prognosis remains good. In neurotmesis both the axons and sheaths are disrupted. The nervous system will attempt to reconnect by axonal sprouting, but the severed ends have to be close and properly aligned. This is not the usual clinical situation with spinal root and cauda equina injury. Hence, neurotmesis carries the worst prognosis.

While conceptually this classification is useful, the clinician may not have sufficient information to accurately diagnose cauda equina or nerve root injuries according to this scheme. A broader classification is complete versus incomplete injury. This is based on the knowledge of nerve roots at risk and their known myotomes and dermatomes. It infers prognosis from the observed deficit. Dense anesthesia and profound motor loss imply complete injury with a guarded prognosis. Partial function gives some hope for spontaneous recovery.

This clinical assessment is affected by numerous factors. Several adjoining roots may innervate a given lower extremity muscle, so that complete paralysis after injury to a single root is unlikely. There is also overlap in sensory function such that complete anesthesia is uncommon. The clinical presentation will determine the type, sequence, and timing of diagnostic testing. Anatomical studies such as radiographs, computerized tomography, and magnetic resonance imaging are useful when implants may account for root injury. The more advanced imaging modalities are indicated whenever there is profound or delayed loss of function. Compression by hematoma, seroma, or pseudomeningocele may cause tardy dysfunction.

Gonzalez-Darder (16) evaluated three methods of nerve repair in a rat model. The dorsal L4 roots were cleanly severed and repaired using a microsurgical technique with direct end-to-end suture, use of an arterial sleeve, or interposition of a nerve graft. Regeneration was assessed 7, 10, and 14 days after surgery using light and electron microscopy. Grafted nerves showed neovascularization, which was interpreted as a favorable endoneurial response. Three of 12 direct suture repairs lacked continuity. The arterial sleeve technique was tedious and produced intense fibrosis and arachnoiditis. Based on microscopic analysis, nerve grafting appeared to be the best of the three techniques. Successful clinical repair of spinal roots or the cauda equina has not been adequately described in the literature. Surgical repair is seldom feasible, and Gonzalez-Darder did not report functional results. This is an area for further investigation.

IV. AVOIDING INJURY

A surgeon with a good appreciation of normal anatomy who uses good technique is less likely to injury the cauda equina or nerve roots. Careful review of the preoperative studies will help the surgeon anticipate the abnormal position of the neural elements when a decompression is necessary. For example, with high-grade spondylolisthesis at the L5-S1 level, the L5 roots are particularly vulnerable to injury. This is particularly true during reduction maneuvers. Boachie-Adjei and coworkers (17) used a meticulous technique, which included partial lumbosacral kyphosis reduction, posterior decompression, and pedicle screw fixation at the lumbosacral junction. Their small series of six patients included two dural tears but no neurological deficits.

Preoperative studies should also be assessed for other anomalies such as conjoined nerve roots. There are also normal variations in neural anatomy and connective tissue, which can tether the nerve root and perhaps render it vulnerable to injury. Yaszemski and White (18) described the presence of a fibrovascular membrane that attached to the nerve roots, which they called the "diskectomy membrane." This membrane, dorsal to the anulus fibrosis at the level of disk, connects the dura of the nerve root to the anulus.

Its consistency ranged from nearly transparent to a firm tissue, which tethered the root laterally. Current imaging modalities would not show this, but awareness by the surgeon will allow him or her to recognize the potential for a fixed root, which may make it vulnerable to manipulation.

Revision surgery is often challenging. When there has been a previous laminotomy or laminectomy there may be dense scarring of the dura and nerve roots to the adjoining bone and soft tissues. Careful dissection to carefully expose and mobilize the scar from the edge of bone will allow entry into the canal if needed for decompression near a previous surgical site. The technique involves identifying the residual posterior bone and carefully dissecting to the edge of the previous laminectomy or laminotomy. Sharp curettes are used to carefully peel the scar away from the edge of the bone. The concavity of the curette faces the ventral surface of the bone, and the convexity is toward the dura. Compound motor action potential monitoring has been found useful in identifying the location of the nerve root when scarring is severe. Again, careful review of studies, particularly gadolinium-enhanced MRI, will often give the surgeon information about the aberrant location of the spinal nerves.

Pedicle screw instrumentation has been a useful and powerful tool for the modern spine surgeon. As already noted, various electrophysiological techniques have been advocated in assessing neural integrity. The use of stimulus evoked electromyographical threshold potentials appears to be the most useful technique in evaluating for the presence of neural irritation. Spinal somatosensory evoked potential monitoring may also detect injury before threshold electromyography can be performed. Combined with continuous electromyographical monitoring, somatosensory evoked potential monitoring may signal injury as it is occurring and act as a warning to modify surgical activity. Various radiographic techniques have been advocated to improve the accuracy of pedicle screw placement. Odgers (19) found that simple lateral radiography was sufficiently accurate in assessing pedicle screw placement and exposed the operating room personnel to less radiation than fluoroscopy. Other surgeons still prefer plain fluoroscopy. Frameless stereotactic techniques improve the accuracy of pedicle screw placement but are cumbersome and probably not necessary for routine simple cases. Expense and the tedious registration process limit the use of this technique. A hybrid system using two-dimensional stereotaxy based on fluoroscopic images is an exciting innovation, which combines the acceptable accuracy of fluoroscopy with lower radiation exposure to the patient and operating room personnel.

The proliferation of minimal incision strategies and more complex instrumentation technology may theoretically increase the risk of neurological injury. The technique of posterior lumbar interbody fusion has always involved a certain degree of dural manipulation, with risk of durotomy, neuropraxia, and even more severe neural injury. Some years ago interbody metal cages were embraced with unbridled enthusiasm. Careful review of the experience with one design by Elias (20) disclosed that the titanium cylinder cages inserted posteriorly yielded an unacceptably high complication rate. Of 67 patients, 10 had a dural laceration, 10 suffered a postoperative radiculopathy, and 1 had a permanent motor deficit combined with sexual dysfunction. Two suffered radiculopathy associated with migration of the cages and another had symptoms from graft material extrusion. Although their complication rate was higher than reported by other investigators, this report illustrates that new technology may be risky when adopted by the wider surgical community. The spine surgeon must weigh the potential benefits of newer technologies against potential risks to the cauda equina, the nerve roots, and other vital structures.

SUMMARY

Nerve root injuries in lumbar spine surgery are uncommon. Good knowledge of anatomy with particular attention to anatomical variations in the individual patient and good technique will usually minimize the risk of nerve injury. Intraoperative imaging and electrophysiological monitoring are useful during higher-risk procedures such as pedicle screw insertion and disk instrumentation via a posterior approach.

REFERENCES

1. Cammisa FP, Jr., Girardi FP, Sangani PK, Parvataneni HK, Cadag S, Sandhu HS. Incidental durotomy in spine surgery. Spine 2000; 25:2663–2667.
2. Jones AA, Stambough JL, Balderston RA, Rothman RH, Booth RE, Jr. Long-term results of lumbar spine surgery complicated by unintended incidental durotomy. Spine 1989; 14: 443–446..
3. Wang JC, Bohlman HH, Riew KD. Dural tears secondary to operations on the lumbar spine. Management and results after a two-year-minimum follow-up of eighty-eight patients. J Bone Joint Surg 1998; 80:1728–1732.
4. Schoenecker PL, Cole HO, Herring JA, Capelli AM, Bradford DS. Cauda equina syndrome after in situ arthrodesis for severe spondylolisthesis at the lumbosacral junction. J Bone Joint Surg 1990; 72:369–377.
5. Hu SS, Bradford DS, Transfeldt EE, Cohen M. Reduction of high-grade spondylolisthesis using Edwards instrumentation. Spine 1996; 21:367–371.
6. Esses SI, Sachs BL, Dreyzin V. Complications associated with the technique of pedicle screw fixation. A selected survey of ABS members. Spine 1993; 18:2231–2238; discussion 2238–2239.
7. Lonstein JE, Denis F, Perra JH, Pinto MR, Smith MD, Winter RB. Complications associated with pedicle screws. J Bone Joint Surg 1999; 81:1519–1528.
8. Holland NR, Kostuik JP. Continuous electromyographic monitoring to detect nerve root injury during thoracolumbar scoliosis surgery. Spine 1997; 22:2547–2550.
9. Bose B, Wierzbowski LR, Sestokas AK. Neurophysiologic monitoring of spinal nerve root function during instrumented posterior lumbar spine surgery. Spine 2002; 27:1444–1450.
10. Deletis V, Vodusek DB. Intraoperative recording of the bulbocavernosus reflex. Neurosurgery 1997; 40:88–93.
11. Hormes JT, Chappuis JL. Monitoring of lumbosacral nerve roots during spinal instrumentation. Spine 1993; 18:2059–2062.
12. Jou IM, Lai KA. Neuromonitoring of an experimental model of clip compression on the spinal nerve root to characterize acute nerve root injury. Spine 1998; 23:932–940.
13. Moed BR, Hartman MJ, Ahmad BK, Cody DD, Craig JG. Evaluation of intraoperative nerve-monitoring during insertion of an iliosacral implant in an animal model. J Bone Joint Surg 1999; 81:1529–1537.
14. Moed BR, Ahmad BK, Craig JG, Jacobson GP, Anders MJ. Intraoperative monitoring with stimulus-evoked electromyography during placement of iliosacral screws. An initial clinical study. J Bone Joint Surg 1998; 80:537–546.
15. Owen JH, Kostuik JP, Gornet M, et al. The use of mechanically elicited electromyograms to protect nerve roots during surgery for spinal degeneration. Spine 1994; 19:1704–1710.
16. Gonzalez-Darder JM. Experimental microsurgical repair of spinal roots. Neurosurgery 1993; 33:1083–1088.
17. Boachie-Adjei O, Do T, Rawlins BA. Partial lumbosacral kyphosis reduction, decompression, and posterior lumbosacral transfixation in high-grade isthmic spondylolisthesis: clinical and radiographic results in six patients. Spine 2002; 27:E161–168.
18. Yaszemski MJ, White AA, 3rd. The discectomy membrane (nerve root fibrovascular membrane): its anatomic description and its surgical importance. J Spinal Disord 1994; 7:230–235.

19. Odgers CJt, Vaccaro AR, Pollack ME, Cotler JM. Accuracy of pedicle screw placement with the assistance of lateral plain radiography. J Spinal Disord 1996; 9:334–338.
20. Elias WJ, Simmons NE, Kaptain GJ, Chadduck JB, Whitehill R. Complications of posterior lumbar interbody fusion when using a titanium threaded cage device. J Neurosurg 2000; 93:45–52.

6

Intraoperative Dural Laceration, Postoperative Cerebrospinal Fluid Fistula, and Postoperative Pseudomeningocele

Seth M. Zeidman
Rochester Brain and Spine Institute, Rochester, New York, U.S.A.

Cerebrospinal fluid (CSF) leaks are relatively uncommon following spinal surgery. Laminectomy, discectomy, and corpectomy can all be complicated by postoperative CSF leak. Postoperative leakage may occur along the suture line following intradural procedures or can result from inadvertent intraoperative durotomy. In the cervical spine, the surgical treatment of ossified posterior longitudinal ligament (OPLL) is associated with pseudomeningocele and CSF fistula, with a reported incidence of 4.5–32% (3,24). Midline posterior dural lacerations are readily repaired primarily. However, far-lateral or ventral dural tears are more difficult to repair.

I. DUROTOMY, CSF LEAK, PSEUDOMENINGOCELE, CSF FISTULA

Cerebrospinal fluid leakage poses a risk of significant morbidity with the potential for development of meningitis, as well as late pseudomeningocele formation. Incidental durotomy is defined as an unintended dural laceration or tear. The risk of only "incidental" durotomy following a laminectomy is 0.3–13%. The risk increases to up to 18% with reoperations. Although infrequent, unintended durotomy is not at all unusual.

Pseudomeningocele is defined as an extradural CSF collection arising from a dural defect. Pseudomeningocele contents are most commonly of cerebrospinal fluid density and may or may not have a demonstrable communication with the subarachnoid space. Iatrogenic pseudomeningoceles are not necessarily associated with an arachnoid tear, but a dural rent is necessary for their formation. If the arachnoid is not violated, the arachnoid membrane may herniate through the dural defect and a CSF-filled arachnoid sac forms. A postsurgical pseudomeningocele is created when cerebrospinal fluid extravasates through a dura-arachnoid tear and becomes encysted within the wound, creating a fluid-filled space with a fibrous capsule lying adjacent to the spinal canal in the laminectomy opening. Because extradural fluid may be contained in either an arachnoid-lined membrane or a fibrous capsule, multiple designations are used to describe this entity. Most authors prefer the term "pseudomeningocele" because, at least initially, the lesion is not

55

arachnoid lined, and therefore does not represent a true meningocele. Pseudomeningoceles have, at various times, been referred to as spurious meningoceles, false cysts, or pseudocysts. Rinaldi and Peach (20) found arachnoidal cells within the capsular membrane of pseudomeningoceles and advocated terming these lesions "true meningoceles." If the proper milieu exists, the extradural fluid collection is reabsorbed and the communication between the intra- and extradural space becomes obliterated.

CSF fistula may result if the extradural fluid communicates with another area such as the pleural space or is in direct communication with the outside world. Smith et al. (24) reported on 22 patients who had undergone anterior decompression for OPLL with myelopathy. Seven of these participants were found to have absence of the dura adjacent to the ossified ligament. The spinal cord and nerve roots were visible through the defect. Although the arachnoid membrane appeared intact and watertight, postoperative cerebrospinal fluid fistula developed in five, and three required reoperation to repair the defect.

II. PRESENTATION

Incidental durotomy, pseudomeningocele, or CSF fistula can each present in a number of manners. Incidental durotomies are typically asymptomatic but can produce postural headaches, nausea, vomiting, dizziness, photophobia, tinnitus, and vertigo. An exceptional case of cerebellar hemorrhage complicating cervical durotomy has been reported (16). Symptoms resulting from CSF leakage have been postulated to result from intracranial hypotension, i.e., a decrease in CSF pressure, leading to traction on the supporting structures of the brain. CSF leaking from a lumbar puncture leads to egress of CSF from the spine and a loss of buoyancy supporting the brain. When the patient assumes an upright posture, the brain sags, and tension on the meninges and other intracranial structures creates the pain. This explanation is probably simplified and somewhat inaccurate. It is more likely that as the body assumes a vertical posture, the hydrostatic pressure within the thecal sac increases, forcing CSF to exit the puncture site. The intracranial vessels compensate for the volume loss volume with vasodilation. Much of the pain is probably related to vascular distention. This process reverses itself when the patient again assumes a supine posture.

Most pseudomeningoceles remain asymptomatic, but can present with a range of findings, including postural headaches, axial neck pain, radiculopathy, and myelopathy. Patients with pseudomeningoceles may also present with symptoms similar to those seen in those with intracranial hypotension, including photophobia, cranial nerve palsies, and tinnitus. Postural headaches, which are relieved in a recumbent position, may be present. Patients may complain of cervical or occipital pain with or without nausea and vomiting while in a standing position. The time interval between the original surgery to the onset of symptoms ranges from days to years. Some pseudomeningoceles may present as a fluctuant mass that can rapidly enlarge with coughing, sneezing, or any maneuver that increased intracranial or intrathecal pressure. Palpation in the region of the cyst may cause pain, as was seen in 100% of the patients with pseudomeningoceles studied by Aldrete and Ghaly (2).

Depending on the location of the lesion, patients with a pseudomeningocele can present with a spinal cord syndrome. Horowitz et al. reported a patient with both Brown-Séquard and Horner syndromes caused by the development of a cervicothoracic pseudomeningocele following an anterior cervical discectomy (8). Pseudomeningoceles can be problematic for a variety of reasons, but perhaps most significantly because they can function as a mass lesion. Hanakita et al. reported a case of spinal cord compression due to a postoperative cervical pseudomeningocele (5). Helle and Conley reported a case of delayed myelopathy as a result of a postoperative cervical pseudomeningocele (6).

More rarely, a patient may present with progressive or delayed myelopathy following cervical spine surgery due to spinal cord herniation (9). Goodman and Gregorius reported a patient with progressive myelopathy who was ultimately determined to have cord herniation. Intraoperatively, the cord was noted to be bulging into the cyst with each heartbeat and respiration. The authors concluded that myelopathy related to a cervical pseudomeningocele may result from either spinal cord herniation or focal cord compression (4).

Patients with CSF fistula can present with the same constellation of symptoms as incidental durotomy or pseudomeningocele (12). They can also become symptomatic with wound swelling, headache, and radiculopathy. Lastly, patients with unrecognized CSF fistulas may present with signs and symptoms of acute or chronic meningitis (1,21).

III. DIAGNOSIS

Magnetic resonance imaging (MRI) is the diagnostic study of choice. Typically it shows a region of low signal intensity on T_1-weighted images and high signal intensity on T_2-weighted images consistent with CSF. Magnetic resonance imaging can delineate the location, extent, and internal characteristics of the lesion and may demonstrate communication with the thecal sac. It may also elucidate other associated pathological entities such as spinal cord compression or nerve root entrapment, as well as differentiate pseudomeningoceles from syringomyelia, arachnoiditis, or recurrent tumor (25). Findings noted in spontaneous intracranial hypotension, including intracranial meningeal enhancement, subdural fluid collections, and caudal displacement of the cerebellar tonsils, may also be visualized. Although MRI is the imaging modality of choice, computed tomography (CT) myelography and radionuclide myelography may provide useful and complementary information in certain cases.

Cutaneous CSF fistulas are often diagnosed by simple inspection of the wound. If there is a watery discharge that produces a clear halo surrounding a central pink stain, then the fluid is assumed to be CSF until proven otherwise.

Determining the presence or absence of CSF by measuring the glucose level is an unreliable method. Analysis of fluid for β_2-transferrin is highly sensitive in detecting CSF, because β_2-transferrin has only been demonstrated in CSF, perilymph, and aqueous humor.

Transferrin is a polypeptide involved in ferrous ion transport. β_1-Transferrin is present in serum, nasal secretions, tears, and saliva. β_2-Transferrin accounts for 15% of the total transferrin content in CSF. A small sample size of fluid (0.5 mL) is required to detect β_2-transferrin. Proteins in the fluid are separated by polyacrylamide gel electrophoresis and then transferred electrophoretically onto a nitrocellulose sheet. The structural differences between the two forms results in a slower migration of β_2-transferrin towards the cathode. The result is two distinct bands produced during electrophoresis. Serum and other body fluids normally have only one band, represented by β_1. The β_2 isoform arises from β_1-transferrin through the loss of sialic acid by the action of neuraminidase. Because neuraminidase is only found in the central nervous system, CSF fluid will have two bands, one representing β_1 and the other representing β_2. Using an antibody reaction (immunoblot), banding patterns are analyzed. Determination of the presence or absence of β_2-transferrin can typically be performed within 3 hours.

IV. MANAGEMENT

A. Preventive

The vast majority of pseudomeningoceles and CSF fistulas are the result of iatrogenic durotomy. A watertight dural closure is the key to avoiding these late complications. When a pseudomeningocele or CSF fistula is encountered, bed rest, an epidural blood patch procedure, or closed drainage may be attempted (7). If unsuccessful, direct surgical repair may be necessary, and in rare cases placement of a lumbar peritoneal (LP) drain or shunt may be considered.

If a Valsalva maneuver reveals a persistent leak, a fibrin sealant should be placed over the area of the leak. Analysis of the results obtained in animal studies suggests that fibrin sealant alone can withstand high hydrostatic pressures. However, since it remains in situ for only 5–7 days, fibrin glue must be supplemented with a dural, muscle, or fat graft placed over the area of the persistent leak. Simply placing Gelfoam or muscle over the dural leak without also applying fibrin glue is ineffective and has been associated with failure to resolve the leak. Paraspinal muscle and overlying fascia should be closed in at least two layers by using No. 0-gauge monofilament with sutures placed 3–4 mm apart. Surgically placed drains may lead to the persistence of communication between the intra- and extradural space and may serve as a nidus for infection. Therefore, these drains should not be routinely used in the repair of a dural tear or a pseudomeningocele.

Some authors argue that all spinal pseudomeningoceles should be treated surgically, whereas others argue that the overwhelming majority of pseudomeningoceles will resolve with time (10). Horowitz et al. reported a case of an anterior cervical pseudomeningocele that resolved after 3 weeks of expectant observation (8). In contrast to lumbar defects, patients with repaired cervical defects may ambulate immediately (7).

Additional recommendations to prevent formation of CSF fistula when the dura is found to be absent adjacent to an ossified portion of the posterior longitudinal ligament in the cervical spine include use of autogenous muscle or fascial dural patches, immediate lumbar subarachnoid shunting, and modification of the usual postoperative regimen, such as limitation of mechanical pulmonary ventilation to the shortest time that is safely possible and use of antiemetic and antitussive medications to protect the remaining coverings of the spinal cord.

The role of a LP shunt in the management of pseudomeningocele and CSF fistulas is incompletely defined. There are reports of successful management of CSF fistulas and pseudomeningocele with a LP shunt. However, the placement of permanent hardware should be avoided whenever possible, and other therapies, including surgical repair, should first be attempted. A LP shunt, in general, should be applied only in those in whom surgical repair has failed or in whom surgical repair was not possible due to the location of the defect.

B. Nonoperative

The majority of patients with incidental durotomy can be treated effectively with watertight dural closure and fibrin glue. Patients can be permitted to ambulate immediately after surgery but should be cautioned to lie flat if they become symptomatic. This will reduce the costs related to the hospital stay and missed work. The role of antibiotic therapy in the management of spinal fistulas and pseudomeningocele remains incompletely defined. Traditional management includes bedrest for up to 7 days to eliminate traction and reduce hydrostatic pressure during the healing process. However, use of antibiotics for CSF fistulas and pseudomeningoceles suggests that they do not decrease the short- or long-term incidence of meningitis and are actually associated with development of multidrug resistance.

Epidural blood patches have been applied successfully to treat patients with postlaminectomy CSF fistulas and pseudomeningoceles. Maycock et al. described a patient who underwent surgical exploration for a CSF fistula following a laminectomy; the site of CSF fistula was not found, and the CSF leak continued postoperatively (13). The CSF fistula was subsequently successfully treated using an epidural blood patch. Clot formation and clot strength are known to increase in the presence of CSF. The injection of blood stops CSF leakage by promoting clot formation over the dural tear and raises extradural tissue pressure relative to subarachnoid pressure, thus decreasing the gradient for CSF efflux. Because only a few case reports exist in the literature, the success rate of the epidural blood patch in the treatment of CSF fistulas and pseudomeningoceles is unclear.

The first investigators who treated pseudomeningoceles with closed lumbar subarachnoid catheters used Teflon or polyethylene catheters. These catheters, initially designed for epidural use, were complicated by frequent blockage and kinking and were therefore somewhat difficult to use. In 1992, Shapiro and Scully (23) reported the use of silicone lumbar subarachnoid catheters in 39 patients with spinal CSF fistulas and pseudomeningoceles. They reported a 92% success rate after 7 days of drainage alone. Complications included a 24% incidence of temporary nerve root irritation that resolved after the drain was removed and a 63% incidence of transient headaches, nausea, and vomiting. There was a 10% incidence of infection (1 wound, 2 discitis, 1 meningitis). In an earlier report Kitchel et al. noted a similar success rate of 90% in 17 patients treated with 4 days of drainage, but the recurrence rate was higher (18%) when compared with that reported by Shapiro and Scully (8%). The complication rate reported by Kitchel et al. (11) was similar to that reported by Shapiro and Scully, with a 58% incidence of headaches, nausea, and vomiting. All patients were successfully treated with adjustment in the rate of CSF drainage, intravenous hydration, and analgesic medication (23). In each study the authors reported one case of meningitis associated with lumbar subarachnoid drainage, and both cases were successfully treated with antibiotic therapy. McCormack et al. reported using an epidural blood patch combined with a brief course of subarachnoid drainage in one patient with spinal implants (15). They speculated that CSF diversion alone in patients with spinal implants may not eliminate the pseudomeningocele because the hardware prevents reapproximation of paraspinal tissues. The blood patch procedure obliterates extradural dead space and provides a substrate for clot formation. Dural healing may thus be optimized because CSF diversion and percutaneous blood patch are complementary in decreasing the CSF pressure differences across the dural breech. Closed subarachnoid drainage, when properly performed and monitored, is a reasonably effective and safe method for treating duralcutaneous CSF leaks after a spinal operation. It may be considered as a nonoperative alternative to the standard procedure of reoperation and direct repair of the dura. A good result is still possible in patients in whom this technique fails and who eventually need surgical management.

C. Operative

Management often consists of insertion of a diverting spinal fluid drain and administration of prophylactic or therapeutic antibiotics. In cases of persistent CSF leakage, surgical reexploration is sometimes necessary. It is the usual practice to treat postoperative cerebrospinal fluid leaks after operations on the spine nonoperatively. If conservative treatment fails, surgical intervention usually entails the suturing of the opening in the dura with or without leaving a fat or muscle graft over the suture line.

The definitive treatment for CSF fistulas and pseudomeningoceles is reoperation and dural repair. Surgical indications include failure of nonoperative measures, progressive radiculopathy, and development of myelopathy. For those with a neurological deficit, a delay in surgery may put the patient at risk for further neurological injury. One method of repairing postsurgical pseudomeningoceles includes separation of the dura from the arachnoid, watertight dural repair utilizing the operative microscope, and the use of overlapping local muscle flaps to reinforce the dura and obliterate the pseudomeningocele cavity.

The surgery should begin with adequate lighting, and the skin incision should be generous enough to completely encompass the leak. Once the pseudomeningocele is visualized, it must be followed deep into the durotomy site. Often the pseudomeningocele may need to be resected to identify the region of interest. The durotomy site is protected with a cottonoid, and any necessary bone resection is performed prior to attempting dural closure to provide adequate room for suturing. Under microscopic magnification, the durotomy site is explored to ensure that nerve root or spinal cord strangulation is not present. In most cases the dura can be closed primarily, without need of a graft, by using No. 4–0 to 7–0 nonabsorbable sutures on a taper or reverse cutting, half-circle needle. For a large defect, a local fascial graft or artificial dura may be used to avoid compressing neural elements. For durotomies that occur in surgically inaccessible areas, such as far lateral durotomies, a small plug of muscle or fat may be introduced through an intentional medial durotomy and pulled into the area of the defect.

Fat is an ideal sealant because it is impermeable to water (14). A thin sheet of autologous subcutaneous fat covers dural repair as well as all exposed dura and can be gently tucked into the lateral recesses. This procedure prevents CSF from seeping around the fat, which may be tacked to the dura with a few sutures. Fibrin glue is spread over the surface of the fat, which is then further covered with Surgicel or Gelfoam. For ventral dural tears (associated with procedures in which disk material is excised), fat is packed into the disk space to seal off the ventral dural leak. The use of a fat graft is recommended as a rapid, effective means of prevention and repair of CSF leaks following cervical spinal surgery.

In recent years, fibrin glue has enjoyed increasing popularity as a dural sealant (18,19). Fibrin glue is solely suited for dural closure augmentation and is not a substitute for surgical techniques, i.e., it should be added to other modalities. The establishment of the definite site of CSF leakage is also of great importance and significantly improves the success rate. Muscle graft in combination with fibrin glue (presumably due to its adhesive sealing properties) is superior to either muscle packing alone or fibrin glue in isolation.

Shaffrey et al. reported 93% effectiveness for those with no preoperative CSF leakage (prophylactic use) and 67% effectiveness in preestablished CSF fistula (therapeutic use) with the application of fibrin glue. They treated 15 patients with CSF leakage with fibrin glue and were successful in 10 cases (22). Milde reported an anaphylactic reaction to fibrin glue (17), and Wilson et al. detected one HIV-1 transmission following the use of nonautologous cryoprecipitate (26).

However, far-lateral tears pose a technically difficult problem for placement of sutures because these sites are inaccessible. In addition, far-lateral tears that are close to a nerve root are potentially dangerous because the suture may impale neural fascicles or cause traction or scarring of the nerve root.

On the basis of these findings, the use of autologous fat transplants is recommended as a rapid, effective means for repair of dural tears or defects that are inaccessible or unsuitable for standard suture technique. Mayfield demonstrated that autologous fat transplants serve as an excellent water sealant, prevent scar formation, and do not adhere to the neural elements; the fat survives for a long time and becomes revascularized.

V. SUMMARY

Close evaluation of preoperative neuroimaging studies, meticulous surgical technique, and liberal use of microscopic magnification will decrease the potential for iatrogenic pseudomeningocele and CSF fistula. All available preoperative neurodiagnostic images should be evaluated for evidence of bone defects caused by possible occult spina bifida or previous surgeries. Each Kerrison rongeur bite should be preceded by the necessary precaution to ensure that the dura mater does not become entrapped between the footplate and bone. The movement of the drill is directed laterally so that even with a slip a dural tear may be avoided. A cottonoid should cover the exposed dura during the drilling. However, when a dural tear does occur, every attempt should be made to achieve a water-tight primary closure. This includes extending the laminectomy, if necessary, to gain better exposure to repair the dura and using loupe magnification or the operating microscope. Failure to close the rent may produce a pseudomeningocele and recurrence of symptoms. Primary closure of the dural rent at the end of discectomy is preferable. To determine if the repair is sound, Valsalva maneuvers should be attempted prior to initiating closure. Failure to provide an adequate closure may result in a CSF fistula that needs to be repaired.

Treatment modalities for CSF fistula and pseudomeningoceles include non-operative management, placement of an epidural blood patch, lumbar subarachnoid drainage, and surgery.

REFERENCES

1. Aarabi B, Alibaii E, Taghipur M, et al. Comparative study of functional recovery for surgically explored and conservatively managed spinal cord missile injuries. Neurosurgery 1996; 39: 1133–1140.
2. Aldrete JA, Ghaly R. Postlaminectomy pseudomeningocele. An unsuspected cause of low back pain. Reg Anesth 1995; 20(1):75–79.
3. Epstein NE, Hollingsworth R. Anterior cervical micro-dural repair of cerebrospinal fluid fistula after surgery for ossification of the posterior longitudinal ligament: technical note. Surg Neurol 1999; 52:511–514.
4. Goodman SJ, Gregorius FK. Cervical pseudomeningocele after laminectomy as a cause of progressive myelopathy. Bull Los Angeles Neurol Soc. 1974; 39(3):121–127.
5. Hanakita J, Kinuta Y, Suzuki T. Spinal cord compression due to postoperative cervical pseudomeningocele. Neurosurgery 1985; 17(2):317–319.
6. Helle TL, Conley FK. Postoperative cervical pseudomeningocele as a cause of delayed myelopathy. Neurosurgery 1981; 9(3):314–316.

7. Hodges SD, Humphreys SC, Eck JC, Covington LA. Management of incidental durotomy without mandatory bed rest. A retrospective review of 20 cases. Spine 1999; 24(19):2062–2064.

8. Horowitz SW, Azar-Kia B, Fine M. Post-operative cervical pseudomeningocele. Am J Neurorad 1990; 11(4):784.

9. Hosono N, Yonenobu K, Ono K. Postoperative cervical pseudomeningocele with herniation of the spinal cord. Spine 1995; 20(19):2147–2150.

10. Kaar GF, Briggs M, Bashir SH. Thecal repair in post-surgical pseudomeningocoele. Br J Neurosurg 1994; 8(6):703–707.

11. Kitchel SH, Eismont FJ, Green BA. Closed subarachnoid drainage for management of cerebrospinal fluid leakage after an operation on the spine. J Bone Joint Surg 1989; 71:984–987.

12. Magliulo G, Sepe C, Varacalli S, et al. Cerebrospinal fluid leak management following cerebellopontine angle surgery. J Otolaryngol 1998; 27:258–262.

13. Maycock NF, van Essen J, Pfitzner J. Post-laminectomy cerebrospinal fluid fistula treated with epidural blood patch. Spine 1994; 19(19):2223–2225.

14. Mayfield FH. Autologous fat transplants for the protection and repair of the spinal dura. Clin Neurosurg 1980; 27:349–361.

15. McCormack BM, Taylor SL, Heath S, Scanlon J. Pseudomeningocele/CSF fistula in a patient with lumbar spinal implants treated with epidural blood patch and a brief course of closed subarachnoid drainage. A case report. Spine 1996; 21(19):2273–2276.

16. Mikawa Y, Watanabe R, Hino Y, Ishii R, Hirano K. Cerebellar hemorrhage complicating cervical durotomy and revision C1-C2 fusion. Spine 1994; 19(10):1169–1171.

17. Milde LN. An anaphylactic reaction to fibrin glue. Anesth Analg 1989; 69:684–686.

18. Nishihira S, McCaffrey TV. The use of fibrin glue for the repair of experimental CSF rhinorrhea. Laryngoscope 1988; 98:625–627.

19. Pomeranz S, Constantini S, Umansky F. The use of fibrin sealant in cerebrospinal fluid leakage. Neurochirurgia 1991; 34:166–169.

20. Rinaldi I, Peach WF Jr. Postoperative lumbar meningocele. Report of two cases. J Neurosurg 1969; 30(4):504–507.

21. Romanick PC, Smith TK, Kopaniky DR, et al. Infection about the spine associated with low-velocity missile injury to the abdomen. J Bone Joint Surg (Am) 1985; 67:1195–1201.

22. Shaffrey CI, Spotnitz WD, Shaffrey ME, et al. Neurosurgical applications of fibrin glue: Augmentation of dural closure in 134 patients, Neurosurgery 1990; 26:207–210.

23. Shapiro SA, Scully T. Closed continuous drainage of cerebrospinal fluid via a lumbar subarachnoid catheter for treatment or prevention of cranial/spinal cerebrospinal fluid fistula. Neurosurgery. 1992 Feb; 30(2): 241–245.

24. Smith MD, Bolesta MJ, Leventhal M, Bohlman HH. Postoperative cerebrospinal-fluid fistula associated with erosion of the dura. Findings after anterior resection of ossification of the posterior longitudinal ligament in the cervical spine . J Bone Joint Surg (Am) 1992; 74(2):270–277.

25. Teplick JG, Peyster RG, Teplick SK, Goodman LR, Haskin ME. CT identification of postlaminectomy pseudomeningocele. Am J Roentgenol 1983; 140(6):1203–1206.

26. Wilson SM, Pell P, Donegan EA. HIV-1 transmission following the use of cryoprecipitated fibrinogen as gel adhesive. Transfusion 1991; 31:51.

7

Postarthrodesis Adjacent Segment Degeneration

Matthew Robbins and Alan S. Hilibrand
Thomas Jefferson University and the Rothman Institute, Philadelphia, Pennsylvania, U.S.A.

I. INTRODUCTION

Throughout the twentieth century, orthopedic surgeons and neurosurgeons have developed techniques to eliminate motion or fuse vertebral bodies in order to eliminate the painful stimuli leading to spinal pain. During the 1980s there was a marked increase in the performance of spinal fusion procedures of both the cervical and the lumbar spine within the United States, for which data have been published (1). The results of fusion, in terms of both radiographic and clinical outcomes, are beyond the scope of this chapter. However, one important sequela of spinal fusion is the alteration in biomechanics caused by eliminating motion at one or more segments in the spinal column and the implications of this motion being accommodated elsewhere in the spinal column. The biomechanical, radiographic, and clinical implications of this "postarthrodesis adjacent segment degeneration" will be the topic of this chapter.

Data regarding adjacent segment degeneration are most plentiful for lumbar spinal fusions, in part because of the longer history of fusion in the treatment of lumbar spinal disorders, as well as the greater number of lumbar spinal fusions performed in the United States. Long-term follow-up of greater than 30 years has been published in the literature (26), and many shorter-term follow-up studies have described the outcomes of surgical treatment of postarthrodesis adjacent segment degeneration of the lumbar spine (33,34). For the cervical spine, less information is available. Most reports are anecdotal, relating to the incidence of repeat surgery among larger groups of patients followed in longer-term follow-up studies of anterior cervical discectomy and fusion (ACDF) for cervical radiculopathy and myelopathy. However, it does appear that there are some fundamental differences between this pathology in the lumbar spine and the cervical spine, primarily owing to biomechanical differences in the functions of those spinal segments. The problem of postarthrodesis adjacent segment degeneration within the thoracic spine itself has not been separately addressed, although many of the reports of lumbar spine adjacent segment degeneration include patients who previously had fusions in the thoracic spine for scoliosis, and there are recent reports of problems within the thoracic spine after thoracolumbar fusion, primarily relating to osteoporotic compression fractures (33). For the purpose of this review, we will include thoracic level pathology within our discussion of post-arthrodesis adjacent segment degeneration in the lumbar spine.

II. CERVICAL SPINE

A. Scope of the Problem

Anterior cervical discectomy and fusion has a long history of use in the treatment of cervical spondylosis with radiculopathy and myelopathy (2). It has been demonstrated in the hands of many surgeons to be a successful procedure with relatively high rates of fusion and successful clinical outcomes (5,6,7,12). The posterior approach to cervical radiculopathy has also proven to be successful in the hands of several authors (3,4,9). However, with both approaches there is the potential for patients to develop new clinical disease referable to adjacent segments. This has been termed "adjacent segment disease" of the cervical spine (19). This term will be used throughout this chapter to differentiate degenerative changes on radiographs without clinical sequelae (referred to as "adjacent segment degeneration") from the development of new symptoms referable to an adjacent segment at which there are also radiographic degenerative changes termed "adjacent segment disease." This problem is less well studied in the cervical than in the lumbar spine. Most clinical data regarding this entity have been noted anecdotally within reports from long-term follow-up studies of anterior cervical fusion and posterolateral foraminotomy procedures (Table 1). Furthermore, the biomechanical effects of anterior cervical fusion upon adjacent segments are less well understood, and to date no studies have been published that assess the impact of anterior cervical fusion upon adjacent segments in the lower and the upper cervical spine in the same cadaveric model.

B. Evidence from Long-Term Follow-Up Studies of Anterior Cervical Discectomy and Fusion

Bohlman et al. conducted a follow-up study to assess the success of the Robinson technique of anterior cervical discectomy and arthrodesis for patients with cervical radiculopathy (5). In this study, 122 patients were followed for an average of 6 years. At follow-up, 11 of these patients had symptoms that were related to either an adjacent segment above or below the level of fusion. Nine of the 11 symptomatic patients went on to have another surgical procedure. In another study of the outcomes of cervical fusion, Gore and Sepic followed 133 patients for an average of 5 years (6). Indications for anterior cervical fusion in this study were cervical spondylosis in 75% of the patients, disc herniation in 16%, and spondylosis existing at one level and disc protrusion at another in 9%. These authors evaluated their patients during follow-up by reviewing the office chart, hospital record, pre- and postroentgenograms, and interviewing the patient. Patients reported symptoms referable to adjacent segments with a prevalence of 14% (18 of the 133 patients), with 11 undergoing further surgery.

The long-term results of cervical discectomy and interbody fusion and its association with adjacent segment disease were also discussed in a study by Williams et al. (7). These authors reviewed the charts, roentgenograms and interviewed 60 patients at an average follow-up of 55 months. Of these 60 patients, 42 had single level fusions and 18 had fusions of more than one level. Williams et al. discovered that 15 patients required further surgery, with 10 of these needing surgery at a different level from the original procedure. Therefore, in this follow-up study, adjacent segment disease requiring further surgery was present in one out of six patients at a relatively short follow-up of less than 5 years.

Table 1 Adjacent Segment Disease in the Cervical Spine

Study	Follow-up (y)	Number of patients	Approximate annual incidence	Overall prevalence	Type of procedure	Associations/Risk factors
Biomechanical studies						
Bohlman et al. (5)	6	122	1.5%	9%	Anterior	
Gore and Sepic (6)	5	133	2.8%	14%	Anterior	
Williams et al. (7)	4.6	60	3.6%	16.7%	Anterior	Better outcomes in men (not statistically significant)
Lunsford et al. (8)	3	253	2.2%	6.7%	Anterior	No difference between fusion/nonfusion groups
Henderson et al. (9)	2.8	736	3%	9%	Posterior	
Radiographic studies						
Baba et al. (10)	8.5	106	2.9%	25%	Anterior	⇑ angular motion
Herkowitz et al. (12)	4.2	33		41% anterior vs. 50% posterior	Anterior or Posterior	
Clinical studies						
Hilibrand et al. (19)	Up to 21 years	374 (409 cases)	2.9%	19.2%	Anterior	Single level ACDF C5-6 / C6-7 ACDF Advanced spondylosis

Lunsford et al. followed 334 patients who had anterior discectomies for either hard or soft disc compression of nerve root(s) or the spinal cord itself (8). The results of patients with and without fusion were compared, and no significant differences were discovered. Additionally, there were no differences between the soft and hard disc compression cases. The development of adjacent segment disease requiring surgery was noted in 6.7%, although no data were provided regarding the overall incidence of new symptoms from an adjacent level, and follow-up was short (less than 3 years average). Furthermore, no differences existed in the incidence of adjacent segment disease whether the initial operation was a discectomy or a discectomy with a fusion.

C. Evidence from Long-Term Follow-Up Studies of Posterior Decompression by Posterolateral Foraminotomy for Cervical Radiculopathy

In addition to following patients who had undergone surgery via an anterior approach for cervical disease, studies have also assessed the efficacy and complications of decompression via the posterior surgical approach. Henderson et al. (9) analyzed 846 patients who had posterior-lateral foraminotomy for cervical radiculopathy. While the previous studies discussed involved fusion, it is important to note that these patients underwent a decompression without fusion. In this study patients were followed for a mean length of 2.8 years. Investigators reported no significant differences in outcome for this approach based on the indication for surgery (i.e., patients with hard or soft disc protrusions vs. those with spondylotic radiculopathy). Of the 736 patients followed, 103 (13.9%) needed an additional procedure. Specifically 24 of these patients (3.3%) required another surgery at the same level for a recurrence of previous radiculopathy. Therefore, new onset of radiculopathy not referable to the initial operative site was present in 79 of the patients, for an overall prevalence of adjacent segment disease of 9% and an annual incidence of over 3%.

D. Limitations of the Previous Studies

These studies were conceived and performed to assess the long-term outcomes of treating the patient's presenting symptoms. Many of them note patients requiring additional surgery at adjacent levels. However, the studies mostly record additional procedures and not new symptoms. This presents a problem in accounting for the prevalence of adjacent segment disease, since not all patients who have symptoms will need or opt for further surgical intervention. In addition, the studies did not describe the temporal onset of adjacent segment disease. Moreover, they did not report risk factors associated with onset of disease in adjacent segments.

E. Radiographic Studies of Postarthodesis Adjacent Segment Degeneration in the Cervical Spine

Baba et al. (10) studied adjacent segment degeneration among patients who had undergone anterior cervical fusion for spondylotic myeloradiculopathy. The authors evaluated radiographs of 106 patients with an average follow-up length of 8.5 years. The new development of spinal canal stenosis in upper adjacent segments occurred in 26 patients (25%) postoperatively. Another finding was increased angular motion in each of the adjacent segments. Furthermore, when vertebral slip in the sagittal plane was assessed, researchers found both anterior and posterior slip in the adjacent segments above and below the level of fusion. In upper adjacent segments, anterior slip occurred in 16 patients (15%) and 12 (11%) patients had evidence of posterior slip. The lower adjacent segments demonstrated anterior slip in 2 patients (2%) and posterior slip in 10 patients (11%). Although these authors report adjacent segment degeneration to be more common than the others, this study only assessed radiographic changes. It is unknown how many of these patients actually had symptomatic adjacent segment disease.

Iseda et al. (11) investigated the occurrence of adjacent segment degeneration in patients with anterior interbody fusion compared with those treated with laminoplasty. The study consisted of 14 patients, with 7 having anterior interbody fusion and the other 7 receiving laminoplasty. Magnetic resonance imaging (MRI) was done at 6 and 12 months postoperatively to assess the adjacent discs. A significant decrease in intensity of the adjacent discs on T2-weighted images in the anterior interbody fusion group was found at both 6 and 12 months. These changes were not found with laminoplasty. The authors suggest that laminoplasty may be less likely to cause adjacent segment degeneration than anterior interbody fusion. There were several limitations of this study, however; first, patients were only followed over a short period of time, during which few, if any, would be expected to develop symptomatic adjacent segment disease. Second, a decrease in water content of the discs, as evidenced by the decreased intensity of T2 images, does not necessarily represent progressive adjacent segment degeneration. Moreover, when comparing laminoplasty with ACDF, the adjacent levels differ. With laminoplasty the adjacent levels are C2-C3 and C7-T1, which have been found to be much less likely to develop degenerative changes than the levels adjacent to the anterior fusions, which were C4-C5, C5-C6, and C6-C7 (19).

Several other studies have reported radiographic findings of adjacent segment degeneration. In the study previously described by Gore and Sepic (6), roentgenograms were reviewed before and after patients received operative treatment. In this study 31 of 121 patients developed spondylosis at levels other than those fused. The authors also noted an increase in preexisting spondylosis in 30 patients, suggesting that over half of the patients had evidence of radiographic adjacent segment disease. Herkowitz et al. (12) also did imaging studies of the patients in their study comparing anterior and posterior procedures for treating cervical radiculopathy. Results supported a natural history of progressive degeneration, with 41% (7/17) of patients with anterior fusion having degenerative changes in the adjacent level, compared to 50% (8/16) of patients in the laminotomy-foraminotomy group. In another radiographic study of adjacent segment degeneration, Hunter et al. (13) found degenerative radiographic changes in eight of nine patients who had anterior cervical fusions and had been followed for 7–15 years postoperatively. However, these changes did not correlate with clinical symptoms. While the studies presented previously assessed the changes in adjacent segments after fusion, Cherubino et al. (14) compared the findings in patients with cervical fusions to a control group. These researchers found a decreased height among in the interspaces between C3-C4 and C6-C7 of 16.7% and 15.9%, respectively, when compared to the age-matched control group.

The results of these studies suggest that radiographic adjacent segment degeneration is much more common than symptomatic adjacent segment disease. Overall, radiographic studies demonstrate a 25–89% incidence of radiographic degeneration adjacent to the fusion (6,10,12,15,16,17,19). However, none of these have been able to correlate radiographic degeneration and long-term clinical outcomes (13,14,17,18).

F. Clinical Studies of Adjacent Segment Degeneration of the Cervical Spine

In a clinical study of symptomatic adjacent segment disease, Hilibrand et al. (19) analyzed 409 procedures in 374 patients who were followed for up to 21 years. Investigators in this study performed an extensive chart review in order to specifically document any new symptoms referable to an adjacent level. Symptoms of radiculopathy or myelopathy were required to be present on two or more office visits. To more accurately predict the true prevalence of adjacent segment disease, a survivorship analysis was constructed. This study also assessed the most likely levels for adjacent segment disease, associations with the length of fusion, and any association with preexisting radiographic degeneration at adjacent levels.

The most striking result of this study was a 13.6% prevalence of symptomatic adjacent segment disease at 5 years and 25.6% at 10 years follow-up, based on the Kaplan-Meier survivorship analysis. These results suggested a relatively constant incidence of 3% of patients per year developing new disease at an adjacent level. The most likely levels to develop adjacent segment disease were C5-C6 and C6-C7, (see Fig. 1). Less commonly affected levels were C3-C4, C2-C3, and C7-T1. Contrary to the authors' hypothesis, adjacent segment disease was more likely with single- rather than multilevel fusions: single level fusions had 18% incidence of adjacent segment degeneration compared with 12% in the multilevel group.

This study also examined the temporal onset of adjacent segment disease. A more rapid onset of adjacent segment degeneration was found among patients with significant preexisting spondylosis at an adjacent level. Patients with canal stenosis or a herniated nucleus pulposus causing nerve root or spinal cord compression at the adjacent level at the time of the initial procedure usually developed adjacent segment disease within 2 years of the procedure.

The authors emphasized that this pathology affects a significant number of patients. They also considered whether this pathology is secondary to the biomechanical effects of the fusion itself or due to the natural history of cervical spondylosis (i.e., that they are more severely affected). The authors cited the studies by Henderson et al. (9) and Lunsford, et al. (8) (mentioned earlier) to suggest that adjacent segment degeneration is just as likely in anterior cervical discectomy without fusion and cases of posterior foraminotomy without fusion. They also discussed the paradoxical finding of an increased incidence of adjacent segment disease after a single-level fusion than following a multilevel fusion. This is opposite of what might be expected biomechanically, since an increasingly long rigid segment would be expected to increase the transfer of motion to the adjacent, unoperated segments. The authors consider this a reflection of the inclusion of the most commonly affected levels (C5-C6 and C6-C7) in most multilevel fusions, leaving the adjacent levels, such as C7-T1, as lower risk levels for new disease. Another possibility is that the motion from the fused segments may be accommodated in the upper cervical spine, which is much more mobile than the adjacent segments of the lower cervical spine.

G. Conclusions

There does appear to be a definite incidence of the development of adjacent segment disease of the cervical spine, often leading to reoperation. This has been described in several studies and appears to be on the order of approximately 3% of patients per year who undergo a cervical spine procedure. No clear association has been established between the development of adjacent segment disease and longer, multilevel fusions, nor with anterior cervical plating. In fact, some data suggest that adjacent segment disease of the cervical spine may be less likely with longer fusions. This apparent paradox points up the need for good biomechanical studies which can determine "where the motion goes,"

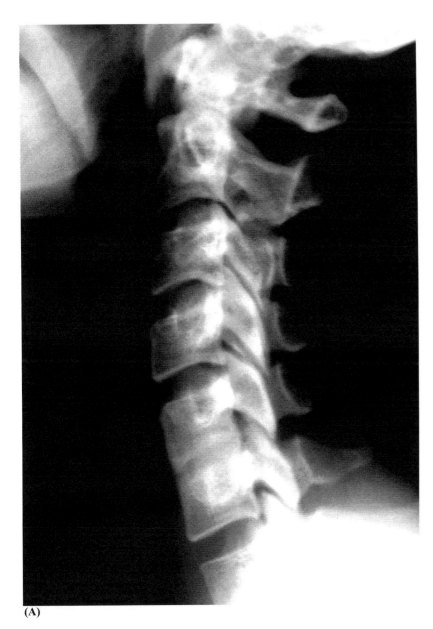

(A)

Figure 1 (A) Lateral radiograph of the cervical spine of a 35-year-old woman one year following C5-6 ACDF for soft disc herniation, now complaining of new left shoulder pain. (B) Sagittal T2-weighted MR images demonstrating an extruded disc fragment left of the spinal cord at the C4-5 level. This patient subsequently underwent C4-5 ACDF with the application of an anterior cervical plate. (C) Lateral radiograph of the same patient 2 years later, who was now complaining of new-onset left forearm pain with paresthesias into the middle and ring fingers. (D) Sagittal T2-weighted MR images obtained at the time of the lateral radiograph in (c). There is a large fragment of disc material extruded from the C6-7 disc space behind the body of C6. (E) Lateral radiograph one year later, following C6-7 ACDF with a separate anterior cervical plate.

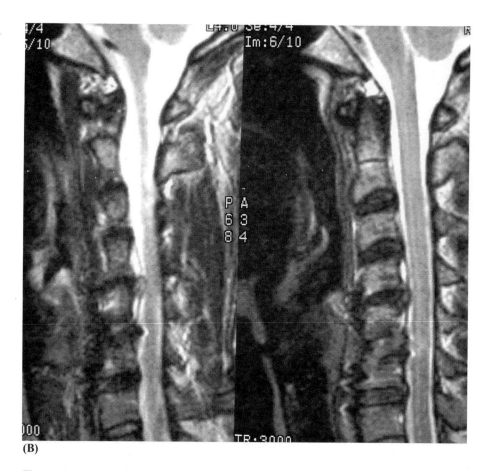

(B)

Figure 1 (*continued*)

whether this be to the adjacent motion segments, to the upper cervical spine, or perhaps just a reduction in overall range of motion following anterior cervical fusion. Furthermore, natural history studies are needed in which the progress of cervical spondylosis in patients with radiculopathy and myelopathy who are candidates for ACDF but do not undergo surgical treatment is followed over longer periods of time.

III. THORACOLUMBAR SPINE

A. Introduction

Postarthrodesis adjacent segment degeneration of the lumbar spine has been given many names, including "adding-on syndrome," "transitional syndrome," and "adjacent segment failure." Longer-term follow-up studies have suggested that at least 50% of patients develop radiographically significant spinal stenosis and/or instability above previous fusion, although there is greater variability in the reported rates of clinical disease requiring further operative treatment. Several forms of postarthrodesis adjacent segment degeneration in the lumbar spine have been described. These include instability above a lumbosacral fusion as well as below a thoracolumbar fusion for scoliosis. This can include

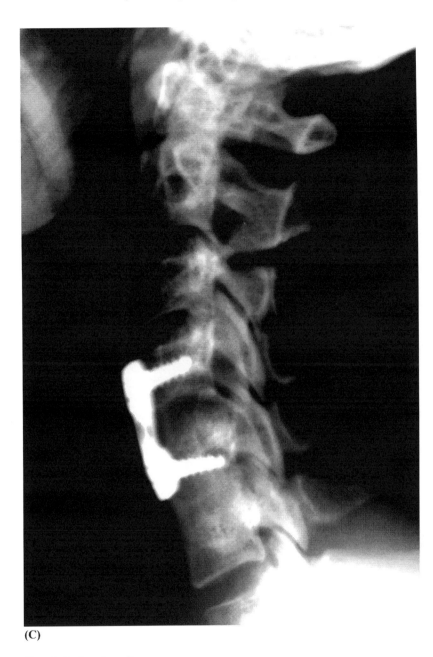

(C)

Figure 1 (*continued*)

anterolisthesis or retrolisthesis and is often associated with spinal stenosis and adjacent facet joint hypertrophy (see Fig. 2). In addition, adjacent vertebral fractures have been described in older patients with fusions from the pelvis into the thoracolumbar region. The larger number of clinical studies of this disorder have provided a set of factors associated with the development of adjacent segment degeneration in the lumbar spine. These will be described in this section and are summarized in Table 2. Once again, the

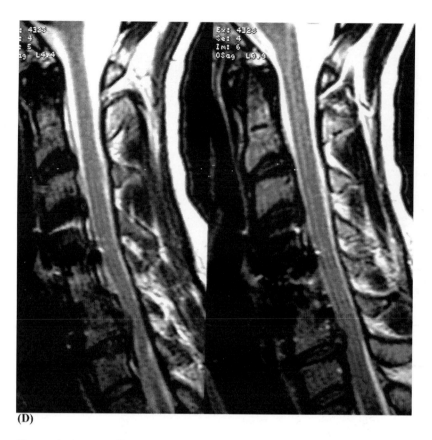

(D)

Figure 1 (*continued*)

problem of postarthrodesis adjacent segment degeneration in the lumbar spine has been studied through biomechanical, radiographic, and clinical means. These are summarized below.

B. Biomechanical Studies

Nagata et al. (20) studied the biomechanical effect of immobilization on the lumbar spine and the adjacent segments. In this study, four canine specimens were tested for the effect of lumbar fusion on the lumbosarcal junction. Researchers discovered that fusions caused increased facet loads and increased total lumbosacral junction motion. Furthermore, these variables increased more as the number of levels fusion increased.

Several other studies have used canine specimens as models to study the biological and biochemical effects of fusions on adjacent segments (21–23). Many of these studies found changes in the composition of the intervertebral discs adjacent to fused levels. In addition, several of the studies found irreversible biochemical changes in the adjacent discs and changes in proteoglycan composition of the discs.

Another biomechanical study that assessed the effects of fusion on adjacent segments in the lumbar spine was performed by Weinhoffer et al. (24). In this study, researchers evaluated cadaveric specimens for the effect of a lumbosacral fusion on intradiscal pressures. The intradiscal pressures were measured at the adjacent L4-L5 and L3-L4 levels.

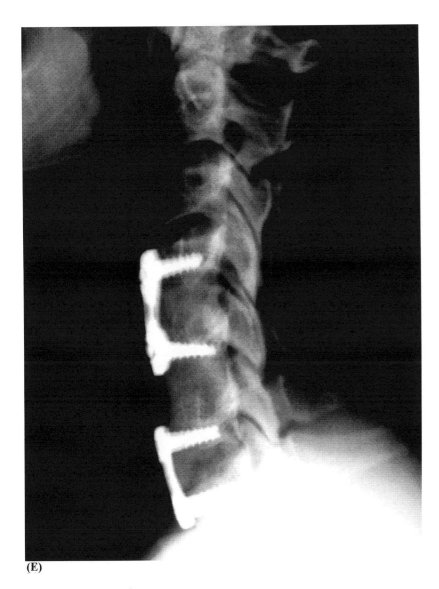

(E)

Figure 1 (*continued*)

Investigators found that as the number of fused levels increased, intradiscal pressures were greater. Moreover, increases in intradiscal pressures were also associated with posterior instrumentation.

Lee and Langrana (25) evaluated the stress placed on adjacent segments as a function of different stabilization techniques of the fused segment. In this study, 16 cadaveric specimens were analyzed for posterior interspinous, bilateral intertransverse, and anterior interbody fusions. These three different fusion techniques were assessed at three levels: L3-L4, L4-L5, and L5-S1. Overall, results of the study were that both bending and stiffness were increased at adjacent segments with all fusion techniques. More specifically, researchers found that the bilateral intertransverse fusion group yielded the best results with the least amount of stress transfer to adjacent levels. The posterior interspi-

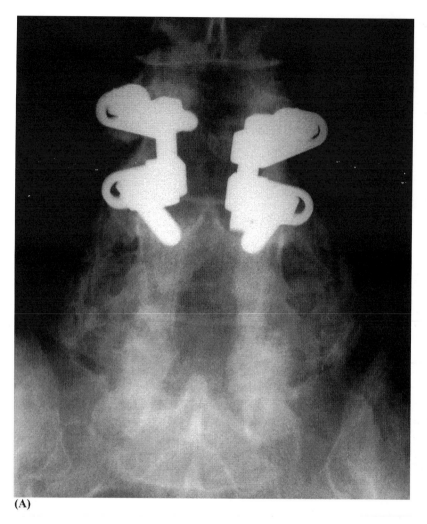

(A)

Figure 2 A 54-year-old woman who had undergone an L4-S1 posterolateral fusion with instrumentation for an isthmic spondylolisthesis. She presented with postarthrodesis adjacent segment degeneration with spondylolisthesis at L3-4 and symptoms of neurogenic claudication and L4 radiculopathy. (A,B) AP and lateral radiographs following removal of hardware and revision L3-4 decompression and posterolateral fusion with segmental internal fixation. (C,D) CT myelography at L2-3 of the same patient 3 years later demonstrating facet and ligamentum flavum hypertrophy and spinal stenosis above the previous L3-4 revision surgical site. The patient presented with progressive gait disturbance and recurrent neurogenic claudication as well as three episodes of urinary incontinence. (E) The patient also complained of postural difficulties and was noted to have significant sagittal imbalance across the previously fused segments L3-S1. (F,G) Post-operative AP and lateral radiographs of the lumbar spine following removal of hardware, laminectomy of L2, transpedicular pedicle subtraction osteotomy of L3, and posterolateral instrumented fusion from T10 to L5.

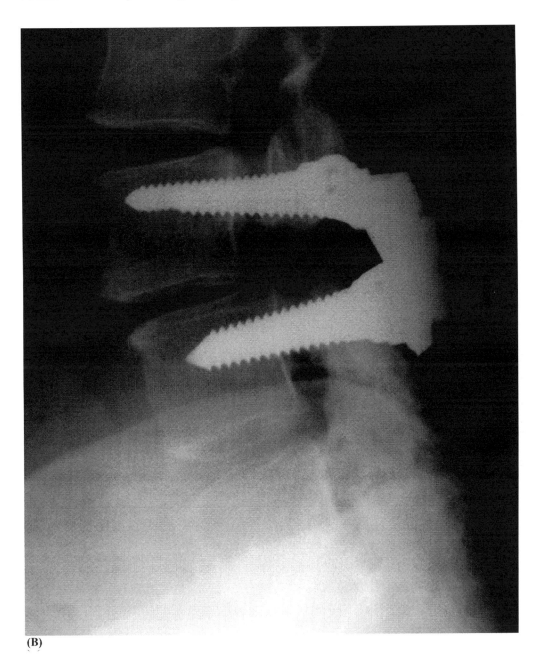

(B)

Figure 2 (*continued*)

nous fusion method resulted in the largest amount of stress placed on the adjacent segments. Data from the study demonstrated that with a loss of motion from fusion of L5-S1, motion was increased in L4-L5 and L3-L4 in all types of fusion. Also in each method of fusion, these authors found greater stress on the adjacent segments, noting that the facet joints received a significant amount of the additional force.

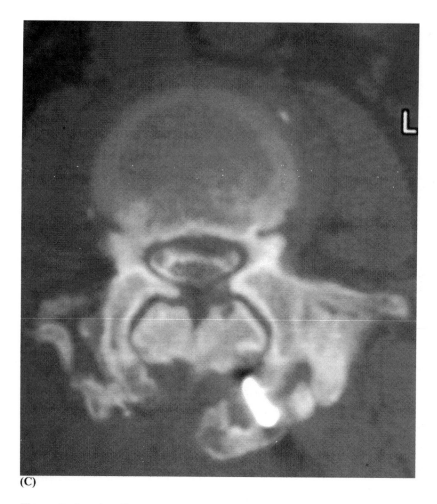

(C)

Figure 2 *(continued)*

C. Radiographic Studies of Lumbar Fusion with Evidence of Adjacent Segment Disease

Lehmann et al. (26) assessed the long-term results of lumbar fusion radiographically. Thirty-three patients with lumbar fusions at or below L3 were followed for an average of 33 years. Radiographic evaluation consisted of flexion-extension lumbar spine films and limited computerized axial tomography (CAT) scans. Adjacent segment degeneration, defined by segmental instability above the fused level, occurred in 45% (15/33) of subjects. The rates of stenotic changes in adjacent segments were 30% in the first level above, 12% in the second level above, and 15% in the level below fusion. When interpreting the results of the study, the authors cautioned that while the radiographic changes suggested a relatively poor outcome of lumbar fusions, the radiographic changes were not correlated with clinical symptoms.

Luk et al. (27) assessed adjacent segment degeneration radiographically in patients with lumbosacral fusions. This study included 22 patients who were followed for an average of 12.8 years. Results of the study revealed that adjacent segments became hypermobile in extension with longer-term follow-up. Investigators interpreted

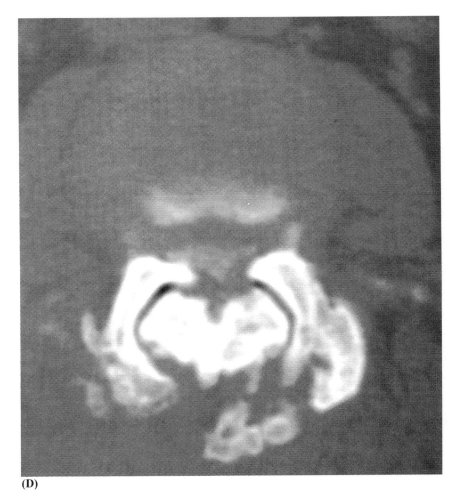

(D)

Figure 2 (*continued*)

hypermobility as evidence of early disc degeneration. Similar to Lehmann et al.'s study, these researchers found a lack of correlation between symptoms and radiographic findings.

In a study by Lee (28), adjacent segment degenerative changes were described. This study followed 18 patients following lumbar fusion for average of 8.5 years with radiographic studies. Findings of adjacent segment degeneration included hypertrophic degenerative arthritis of the facet joints, spinal stenosis, disc degeneration, degenerative spondylolisthesis, and spondylolysis. Of all of these changes, hypertrophic degenerative arthritis of the facet joints was the most common. Moreover, when considering symptoms related to adjacent segments, this study reported that 11 of the 18 patients reported symptoms referable to the adjacent segment within 5 years. As a result of this research, the author believes that lumbar fusions may accelerate degenerative changes in adjacent segments.

Penta et al. (29) evaluated patients with lumbar fusion for adjacent segment degeneration using radiographs and magnetic resonance imaging. This study not only looked at data from patients postoperatively but also preoperative imaging of discs above the level of fusion. Only patients with normal discs preoperatively in the adjacent space to

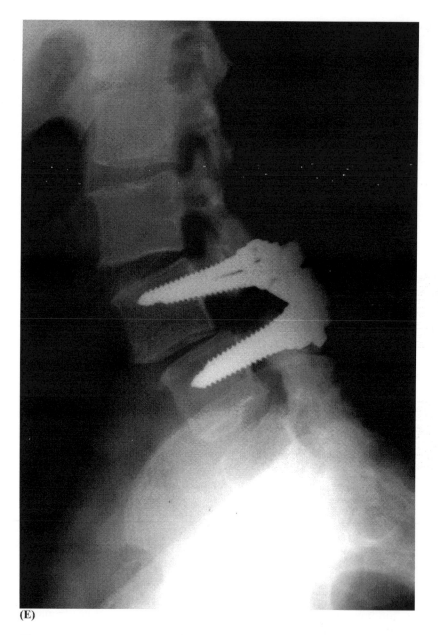

(E)

Figure 2 (*continued*)

the intended fusion were included in the study. Fifty-two patients were followed for a minimum of 10 years. Data from the study showed a 32% prevalence of disc degeneration at the level above the fusion. In nonoperative cases, the investigators reported a 30.7% prevalence of degeneration. Additionally, the length of fusion did not demonstrate a significant effect on adjacent degeneration. Therefore, the overall conclusion reached by these authors was that there is a lack of evidence to support the view that anterior lumbar interbody fusions increase the rate of adjacent segment degeneration.

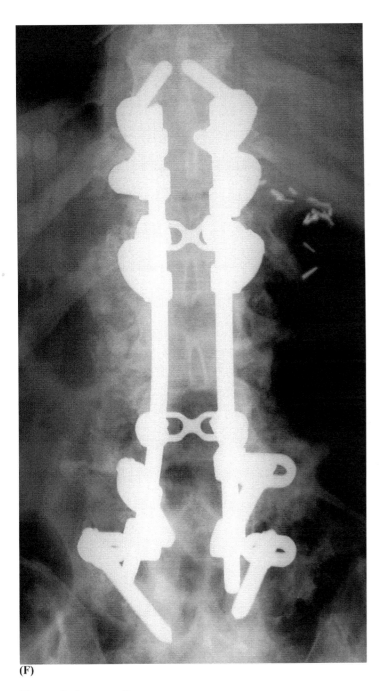

(F)

Figure 2 *(continued)*

Aota et al. (30), found radiographic changes consistent with adjacent segment degeneration in their study of 65 patients with lumbar fusion. The patients were followed for an average of 39 months postoperatively. In 24.6% of the patients postfusion instability was present, with levels above the fusion being affected more than those below.

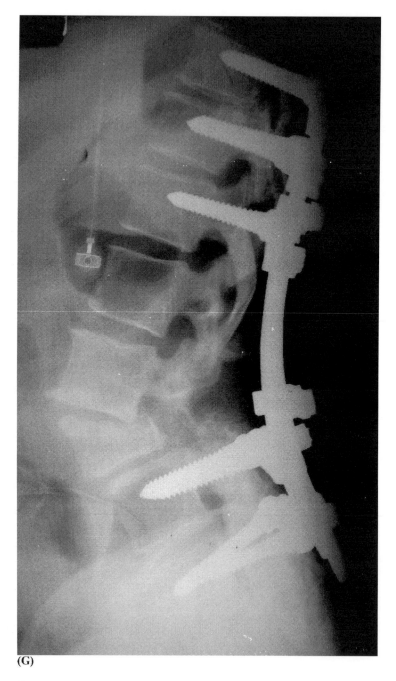

(G)

Figure 2 *(continued)*

The most common type of instability was retrolisthesis. Furthermore, greater instability was correlated with increasing patient age. Therefore, these authors suggest that the surgeon should pay close attention to adjacent segments above the level of fusion and consider the patient's age in determining the appropriate surgical plan.

Table 2 Adjacent Segment Disease in the Lumbar Spine

Study	Follow-up (y)	Number of patients	Approximate annual incidence	Overall prevalence	Type of procedure	Associations/ Risk factors
Biomechanical studies						
Nagata et al. (20)	N/A	4 (canine)				Fusion causes: ⇑ facet loads and lumbosacral motion ⇑ with number of levels fused
Weinhoffer et al. (24)	N/A	6 (cadaveric)			Posterior	Posterior instrumentation
Lee & Langrana (25)	N/A	16 (cadaveric)			Anterior, bilateral-lateral, posterior	Stress on facet joint: greatest with posterior, least with bilateral-lateral
Radiographic studies						
Lehman et al. (26)	33	33	1.4%	45%	Posterior Harrington rod method	
Luk et al. (27)	12.8	22				Hypermobility
Ck Lee (28)	8.5	18	12.2%	61%	Anterior, posterior, bilateral-lateral	
Penta (29)	10 (minimum)	52		32%	Anterior	30.7% prevalence in control vs 32% in surgical group, No effect for length of fusion
Aota (30)	3.25	65	7.6%	24.6%		⇑ age, ⇑ rate for segment above fusion vs. below
Axelsson (31)	1	6	33.3%	33.3%	Postero lateral	
Rahm & Hall (32)	5	49	3.4%	17%	Postero lateral	⇑ age, interbody fusion
Clinical studies						
Etebar & Cahill (33)	3.7	125	3.9%	14.4%		Postmenopausal women Sagittal/coronal imbalance ? Distal hook purchase
Schlegel et al. (34)	13.1	58				
Cochran et al. (35)	9.75	95	1.2% overall / 4.7%	11.6% total 46% distal hook group		

In another study, Axelsson et al. (31) assessed the mobility of segments adjacent to a lumbar fusion. This study evaluated six patients who underwent fusion including implantation of tantalum markers for spinal roentgen stereophotogrammetric analysis. Data was collected at 3, 6, and 12 months postoperatively. Researchers found hypermobility in the adjacent segment of two of the six patients studied, which they suggest may lead to progressive degeneration.

Further evidence of postarthrodesis adjacent segment degeneration was described by Rahm and Hall(32). In their study of 49 patients with lumbar fusion, adjacent segment degeneration occurred in 35% of the patients with an average follow-up of approximately 5 years. Associations of increased rates of adjacent segment degeneration were found with increasing patient age, use of posterior interbody fusion, and worsening of clinical results over time. These authors suggest the limited use of posterior interbody fusion and recommend circumferential fusion when possible based on the increased prevalence of adjacent segment disease in patients with posterior lumbar interbody fusion.

D. Clinical Studies of Lumbar Adjacent Segment Disease

Etebar and Cahill (33) investigated the effects of lumbar fusion on adjacent segments from a clinical perspective. These researchers analyzed the outcomes of 125 patients with instrumented lumbar fusions. The average follow-up was 44.8 months. It was discovered that 18 out of the 125 patients developed symptomatic adjacent segment disease. The authors also correlated adjacent segment symptoms with risk factors, including female sex, postmenopausal status, osteopenia, and a suggested increase in adjacent segment disease with instrumentation, based upon comparison with historical controls. Authors concluded that in the subcategory of postmenopausal women with degenerative disease of the lumbar spine, instrumentation might cause unnecessary morbidity.

A clinical study of the outcome of lumbar fusion performed for adjacent segment disease was published by Schlegel et al. (34). While most of the studies presented focused on the development of adjacent segment disease, the study by Schlegel et al. examined patients being treated for known adjacent segment disease. Fifty-eight patients who required surgery for adjacent segment disease had been symptom-free for an average of 13.1 years after their initial lumbar fusion procedure. Researchers noted that adjacent segment disease occurred at both the adjacent segments and the segments next to the adjacent segment degeneration. The authors suggested that sagittal and coronal imbalance appeared to be risk factors for adjacent segment disease, although the associations were not statistically significant.

Cochran et al. (35) assessed the outcome of bilateral posterior lumbar fusions in patients with adolescent idiopathic scoliosis. Ninety-five patients with a Harrington rod fusion were followed for an average of 9.75 years postoperatively. Degenerative facet changes and disc space narrowing were found in 11 patients. All of these patients were from a group of 24 patients in the study with a distal hook purchase in L4 or L5. Therefore, in this group degenerative changes occurred with a prevalence of 45.8%.

E. Conclusions

It is likely that the true incidence of clinically relevant adjacent segment disease following lumbar and lumbosacral fusion as well as thoracolumbar fusion is much lower than the incidence of radiographic degeneration. Once again, controversy persists between whether this represents new disease caused by the fusion itself or natural progression of the patient's spondylotic process and propensity for instability at the adjacent levels. In the lumbar spine, however, there appear to be more data available, including more biomechanical studies to suggest that there is a biomechanical cause of adjacent segment degeneration, suggesting that in the lumbar spine adjacent segment disease may be more a function of the fusion itself than how it is performed (i.e., anterior, posterior, or combined) as opposed to natural history of the spondylotic disease. On the basis of biomechanical, radiographic, and clinical studies, there appear to be strategies that can help avoid adjacent segment degeneration with current technology, including incorporation of all unstable segments in the fusion, preservation of the adjacent facet joints above lumbosacral and lumbar fusions, avoidance of rigid instrumentation in elderly females with osteoporosis, and perhaps cement augmentation of adjacent vertebral bodies above long fusions of the sacrum. In addition, newer technologies now being developed may further assist in the prevention of adjacent segment degeneration of the lumbar spine. These include the use of bioabsorbable implants, which can stabilize a motion segment immediately following grafting procedures and subsequently resorb and increase the load on the graft, thereby reducing the direct posterior rigidity, which may be associated with adjacent degeneration. In addition, the development of intervertebral disc replacements and prostheses may soon allow preservation of normal lumbar spine mobility while treating painful disc degeneration. In addition, these new implants may be ultimately used to transition from a rigid motion segment to the remaining native segments of the lumbar and thoracic lumbar spine.

REFERENCES

1. Davis H. Increasing rates of cervical and lumbar spine surgery in the United States, 1979–1990. Spine 1994; 19(10):1117–1124.
2. Riley LH Jr, Robinson RA, Johnson KA, Walker AE. The results of anterior interbody fusion of the cervical spine. Review of ninety-three consecutive cases. J Neurosurg 1969; 30(2): 127–133.
3. Silveri CP, Simpson JM, Simeone FA, Balderston RA. Cervical disk disease and the keyhole foraminotomy: proven efficacy at extended long-term follow up. Orthopedics 1997; 20(8):687–692.
4. Scoville WB, Dohrmann GJ, Corkill G. Late results of cervical disc surgery. J Neurosurg 1976; 45:203–210.
5. Bohlman HH, Emery SE, Goodfellow DB, Jones PK. Robinson anterior cervical discectomy and arthrodesis for cervical radiculopathy. Long-term follow-up of one hundred and twenty-two patients. J Bone Joint Surg 1993; 75-A:1298–1307.
6. Gore DR, Sepic SB. Anterior cervical fusion for degenerated or protruded discs: a review of one hundred forty-six patients. Spine 1984; 9(7):667–671.
7. Williams JL, Allen MB, Harkess JW. Late results of cervical discectomy and interbody fusion: some factors influencing the results. J Bone Joint Surg 1968; 50-A:277–286.
8. Lunsford LD, Bissonette DJ, Jannetta PJ, Sheptak PE, Zorub DS. Anterior surgery for cervical disc disease, part 1: treatment of lateral cervical disc herniation in 253 cases. J Neurosurg 1980; 53:1–11.
9. Henderson CM, Hennessy RG, Shuey HM, Shackelford EG. Posterior-lateral foraminotomy as an exclusive operative technique for cervical radiculopathy: a review of 846 consecutively operated cases. Neurosurgery 1983; 13(5):504–512.

10. Baba H, Furusawa N, Imura S, Kawahara N, Tsuchiya H, Tomita K. Late radiographic findings after anterior cervical fusion for spondylotic myeloradiculopathy. Spine 1993; 18(15):2167–2173.

11. Iseda T, Goya T, Nakano S, Kodama T, Moriyama T, Wakisaka S. Serial changes in signal intensities of the adjacent discs on T2-weighted sagittal images after surgical treatment of cervical spondylosis: anterior interbody fusion versus expansive laminoplasty. Acta Neurochir (Wien) 2001; 143:707–710.

12. Herkowitz HN, Kurz LT, Overholt DP. Surgical management of cervical soft disc herniation: a comparison between the anterior and posterior approach. Spine 1990; 15(10):1026–1030.

13. Hunter LY, Braunstein EM, Bailey RW. Radiographic changes following anterior cervical fusion. Spine 1980; 5(5):399–401.

14. Cherubino P, Benazzo F, Borromeo U, Perle S. Degenerative arthritis of the adjacent spinal joints following anterior cervical spinal fusion: clinicoradiologic and statistical correlations. Itali J Orthop Traumatol 1990; 16(4):533–543.

15. Clements DH, O'Leary PF. Anterior cervical discectomy and fusion. Spine 1990; 15:1023–1025.

16. Goffin J, van Loon J, Van Calenbergh F, Plets C. Long-term results after anterior cervical fusion and osteosynthetic stabilization for fractures and /or dislocations of the cervical spine. J Spinal Disord 1995; 8:500–508.

17. McGrory BJ, Klassen RA. Arthrodesis of the cervical spine for fractures and dislocations in children and adolescents. A long-term follow-up study. J Bone Joint Surg 1994; 76-A: 1606–1616.

18. Dohler JR, Kahn MR, Hughes SP. Instability of the cervical spine after anterior interbody fusion. A study on its incidence and clinical significance in 21 patients. Arch Orthop Traumatic Surg 1985; 104:247–250.

19. Hilibrand AS, Carlson GD, Palumbo MA, Jones PK, Bohlman HH. Radiculopathy and myelopathy at segments adjacent to the site of a previous anterior cervical arthrodesis. J Bone Joint Surg 1999; 81-A(4):519–528.

20. Nagata H, Schendel MJ, Transfeldt EE, Lewis JL. The effects of immobilization of long segments of the spine on the adjacent and distal facet force and lumbosacral motion. Spine 1993; 18(16):2471–2479.

21. Bushell GR, Ghosh P, Taylor TF, Sutherland JM, Braund KG. The effect of spinal fusion on the collagen and proteoglycans of the canine intervertebral disc. J Surg Res 1978; 25:61–69.

22. Cole TC, Burkhardt D, Ghosh P, Ryan M, Taylor, T. Effects of spinal fusion on the proteoglycans of the canine intervertebral disc. J Orthop Res 1985; 3(3):277–291.

23. Cole TC, Ghosh P, Hannan NJ, Taylor TK, Bellenger CR. The response of the canine intervertebral disc to immobilization produced by spinal arthrodesis is dependent on constitutional factors. J Orthop Res 1987; 5(3):337–347.

24. Weinhoffer SL, Guyer RD, Herbert M, Griffith SL. Intradiscal pressure measurements above an instrumented fusion. Spine 1995; 20(5):526–531.

25. Lee CK, Langrana NA. Lumbosacral spinal fusion: a biomechanical study. Spine 1984; 9(6):574–581.

26. Lehmann TR, Spratt KF, Tozzi JE, Weinstein JN, Reinarz SJ, El-Khoury GY, Colby H. Long-term follow-up of lower lumbar fusion patients. Spine 1987; 12(2):97–104.

27. Luk KD, Lee FB, Leong JC, Hsu LC. The effect on the lumbosacral spine of long spinal fusion for idiopathic scoliosis: a minimum 10-year follow-up. Spine 1987; 12(10):996–1000.

28. Lee, CK. Accelerated degeneration of the segment adjacent to a lumbar fusion. Spine 1988; 13(3):375–377.

29. Penta M, Sandhu A, Fraser RD. Magnetic resonance imaging assessment of disc degeneration 10 years after anterior lumbar interbody fusion. Spine 1995; 20(6):743–747.

30. Aota Y, Kumano K, Hirabayashi S. Postfusion instability at the adjacent segments after rigid pedicle screw fixation for degenerative lumbar spinal disorders. J Spinal Disord 1995; 8(6): 464–473.

31. Axelsson P, Johnsson R, Stromqvist B. The spondylolytic vertebra and its adjacent segment: mobility measured before and after posterolateral fusion. Spine 1997; 22(4):414–417.

32. Rahm MD, Hall BB. Adjacent-segment degeneration after lumbar fusion with instrumentation: a retrospective study. J Spinal Disord 1996; 9(5):392–400.

33. Etebar S, Cahill DW. Risk factors for adjacent-segment failure following lumbar fixation with rigid instrumentation for degenerative instability. J Neurosurg 1999; 90:163–169.

34. Schlegel JD, Smith JA, Schleusener RL. Lumbar motion segment pathology adjacent to thoracolumbar, lumbar, and lumbosacral fusions. Spine 1996; 21(8):970–981.

35. Cochran T, Irstam L, Nachemson A. Long-term anatomic and functional changes in patients with adolescent idiopathic scoliosis treated by Harrington rod fusion. Spine 1983; 8(6):576–583.

8

Cervical, Thoracic, and Lumbar Pseudarthrosis: Diagnosis and Management

William C. Welch, Art Nestler, and Peter C. Gerszten
University of Pittsburgh School of Medicine, University of Pittsburgh Medical Center, Presbyterian University Hospital, Pittsburgh, Pennsylvania, U.S.A.

I. OVERVIEW

The diagnosis and management of bone nonunion or pseudarthrosis ("false joint") following attempted surgical fusion in the spine can be troublesome. Labeling a patient as having a failed surgical fusion attempt is painful for both the operating surgeon and the patient, as this diagnosis carries with it the understanding that further therapies may be in order. The patient is often confused about the diagnosis and may doubt the surgeon's skills. Patients want to know what went wrong, and extra efforts are required on the part of the surgeon to explain the possible causative factors and subsequent treatment options.

The diagnosis of pseudarthrosis may be an initiating or precipitating factor in stimulating the patient to seek other surgical treatments or legal remedies. Confounding this is the difficulty with confirmation of the diagnosis. The purpose of this chapter is to provide the reader with a greater understanding as to the potential causes of pseudarthrosis, the diagnosis, and both surgical and non-surgical treatment options.

II. INCIDENCE AND CAUSATIVE FACTORS

The incidence of cervical pseudarthrosis varies from 0% to more than 50% (1–7). The incidence of lumbar pseudarthrosis also varies considerably, from 0% to over 50% (1,8,9). Over the last 20 years, pseudoarthrosis rates have varied as much as 5–86%. Steffe reported on a series of 12 patients who underwent an uninstrumented posterior lumbar interbody fusion and found a failure rate of 100% due to the continued instability of the surgical construct (10).

A number of known, common risk factors exist for the development of pseudarthrosis in both the cervical and lumbar spine. The major risk factor for the development of pseudarthrosis is patient use of nicotine products. These include chewing tobacco, cigarette smoking, and, probably, cigar smoking. A number of clinical and animal trials support the fact that nicotine reduces vascularity and may contribute to nonunion by other means as well (11,12). Many clinical trials exclude nicotine users because of these facts.

Another significant influence on the development of pseudarthrosis is the location and number of segments fused. For example, fusion along the posterior para-axial spine has a relatively high rate of pseudarthrosis, especially when compared to fusion in the anterior axial spine (1). Factors include the presence of osteoporosis, number of levels fused, surgical technique, use of nicotine products, use of antimetabolic agents, use of nonsteroidal anti-inflammatory agents, presence of collagen disorders, and location of the fusion. Studies also suggest that patients undergoing fusion surgery for treatment of degenerative disk disease have the highest rate of pseudarthrosis (13,14). Other factors that influence the rate of reported pseudoarthrosis include age, litigation, and worker's compensation involvement.

III. DIAGNOSIS OF PSEUDARTHROSIS

Most diagnostic evaluations begin with the suspicion that the postoperative patient may have a symptomatic pseudarthrosis. Pain is the factor that drives this evaluation. Surgeons and care-takers, for the most part, will not treat asymptomatic psuedarthrosis unless the surgeon feels that nontreatment poses a risk for implant failure or continued significant discomfort for the patient. Furthermore, even when a relatively definitive diagnosis of pseudarthrosis is made, intervention is not always required.

The typical history of a patient who has developed a pseudarthrosis usually shows initial improvement followed by progressive pain. The initial improvement is felt to be due to the neurological decompression with subsequent stabilization if instrumentation was used. Over time, as a pseudarthrosis develops, pain may become a prominent complaint due to residual instability. The etiology of the localized pain is not fully understood. Possible causative factors include cytokine production from metal wear debris, chronic localized inflammation, or microfracture of bone in various stages of healing (15). There has been no identification of nervous innervation of the fibrotic material within a bony defect, although nervous innervation has been identified adjacent to such defects (16). The histological evaluation of areas of pseudarthrosis demonstrates fibrous tissue between bone segments. There may also be small, nonviable fragments of bone imbedded in the fibrous tissue (16).

Physical findings do not necessarily help to make the diagnosis of pseudarthrosis. Localized pain may occur at the site of lumbar psedarthrosis, but this is not a specific or sensitive finding. Occasionally, migrated instrumentation is palpable beneath the skin. This is most often seen in the thoracic region in cases where sublaminar hooks have become free from the lamina. Instrumentation rarely erodes through the skin. This may occur in cases of infection or progressive kyphotic deformity related to pseudarthrosis (14).

Whereas eroded or infected instrumentation usually requires further surgical treatment, broken instrumentation generally does not require removal, especially in the thoracic and lumbar. The identification of broken instrumentation does not necessarily confirm that a pseudarthrosis is present. In many instances the fusion is solid and the instrumentation failed during the healing process due to repeated stresses or micromotion causing metal fatigue (Fig. 1). The instances where surgical extraction of extruded instrumentation or interbody fusion devices should be considered are those where the extruded instrumentation may cause injury to vascular or other structures.

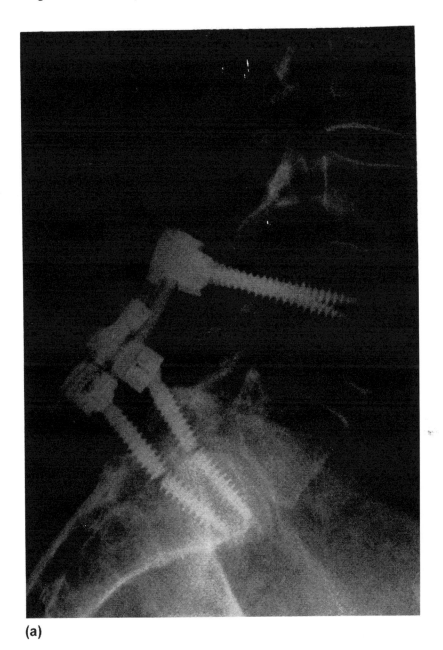

(a)

Figure 1 Lateral (a) and antero-posterior (b) radiographs view of an L4-S1 instrumented fusion demonstrating broken S1 pedicle screw and solid fusion.

When a patient has not had a successful outcome following a fusion procedure, one of the many components of the differential diagnosis includes the diagnosis of pseudarthrosis. When considering the diagnosis, radiographic evaluation is in order. It is important to note, however, that the most definitive test for pseudarthrosis is operative reexploration (13,17–19).

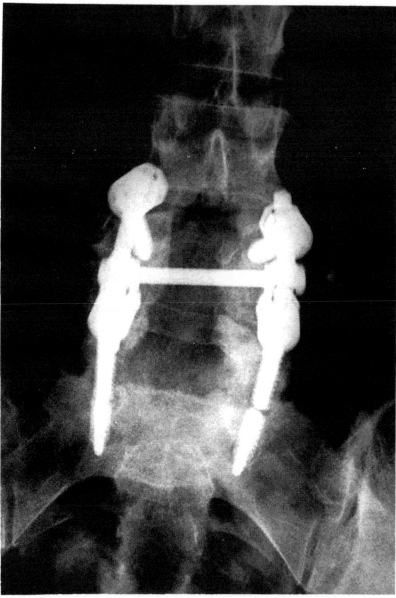

(b)

Figure 1 (*continued*)

A classification scheme has been developed to describe types of spinal pseudarthrosis in the lumbar spine. Resorption of the bone graft and gross atrophy of the fusion mass is described as an "atrophic-type" pseudarthrosis. The presence of bone with nonunion in the frontal plane is described as a "transverse-type" pseudarthrosis. Presence of large quantities of solid bone that is not connected to the vertebral segments is deemed "shingle-type" pseudarthrosis. Finally, more than one defect may be present in the fusion mass. This type of pseudarthrosis is termed "complex" (20).

A. Cervical Pseudarthrosis

Cervical pseudarthrosis is a fairly rare occurrence in the subaxial spine, but it occurs with relative frequency in the posterior para-axial spine (Fig. 2) (1). The diagnosis can be difficult to make on plain radiographs alone. In general, the diagnosis of a radiographically solid fusion is made in the cervical spine when there is bridging trabecular bone between an anterior interbody graft and the vertebral bodies (21–26).

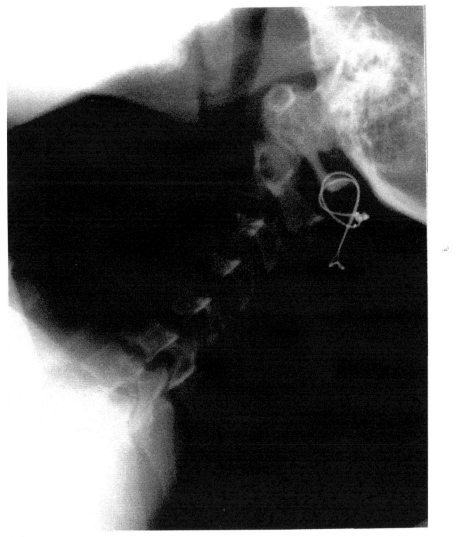

(a)

Figure 2   Lateral (a) radiograph of a failed posterior C1-2 fusion showing lucency between the ring of C1 and C2. Lateral radiograph (b) of the revised posterior C1-2 fusion utilizing transarticular screws, sublaminar wiring, and an implanted bone growth stimulator. Note solid fusion of the ring of C1 to the lamina of C2.

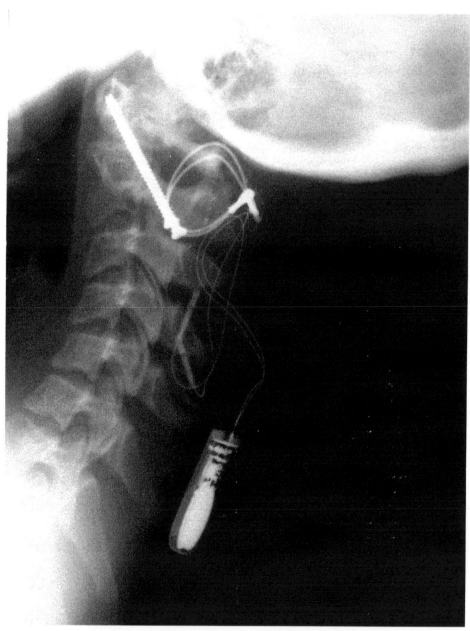

(b)

Figure 2 (*continued*)

Extrusion of the instrumentation, lucencies across the interbody endplate or interbody fusion cage endplate, lucencies around posterior lateral mass screws, instrumentation failure such as broken screws or rods, or gross movement across the fused segment suggests pseudarthrosis (Figs. 3, 4).

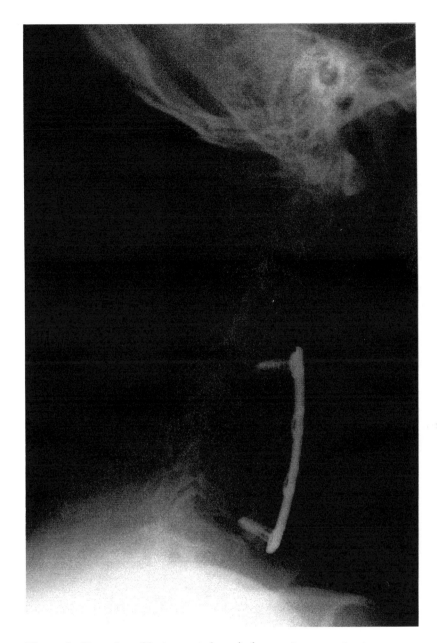

Figure 3   Extrusion of instrumented cervical corpectomy construct.

Indications of pseudarthrosis include evidence of a translucent line across the fracture site or fusion site, lack of osteosynthetic incorporation of graft, or translational movement across the involved segment (Figs. 5, 6). Other suggestive radiographic features include instrumentation failure and extrusion of the bone graft. The radiographic diagnosis may be made by measuring the distance between the tips of the posterior spinous processes on flexion and extension lateral radiographs. A change in distance of 2 mm or more was highly suggestive of pseudarthrosis in one study (27).

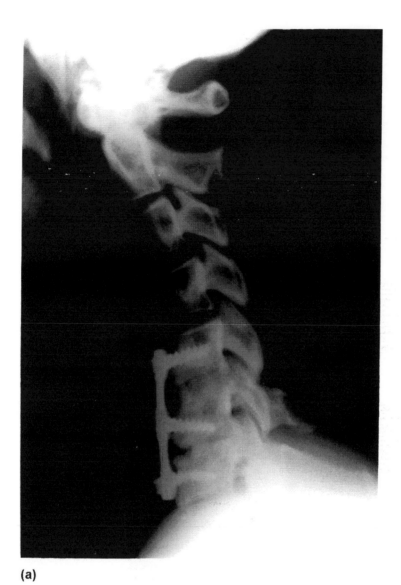

(a)

Figure 4 Neutral (a), extension (b), and flexion (c) lateral radiographic studies demonstrating C5-6–7 instrumented fusion with pseudarthrosis at C6-7 and associated screw failure.

B. Thoracic and Lumbar Pseudarthrosis

The incidence of pure thoracic pseudarthrosis appears low, but this may be related to the relative infrequency of thoracic fusions without the inclusion of the lumbar spine. The diagnosis of thoracic pseudarthrosis is made in a fashion similar to the cervical spine. Anterior constructs may show evidence of "pistoning" of the strut graft without osteosynthetic incorporation of the strut graft. Extrusion of the graft and progressive bone cut-out of the instrumentation are strong suggestions of pseudarthrosis. The diagnosis of lumbar pseudarthrosis is suggested when there is little or no bone along the posterior transverse processes and no evidence of fusion in the facet joints.

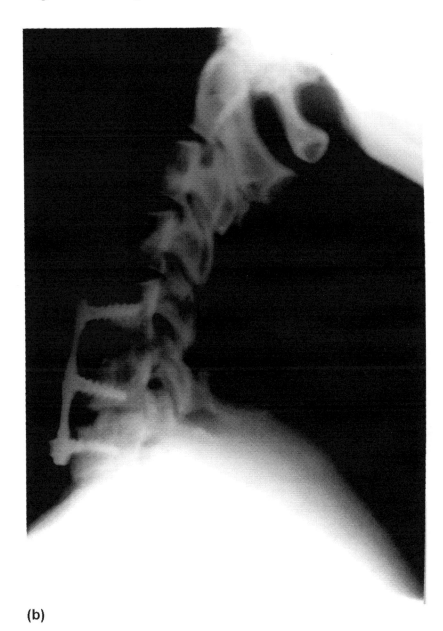

(b)

Figure 4 *(continued)*

Posterior thoracic constructs may exhibit evidence of fusion failure when progressive kyphosis occurs. Progressive dislodgement of posterior thoracic constructs may also indicate pseudarthrosis. Since osteosynthetic bony incorporation may be more difficult to identify in the thoracic region, the absence of this finding may not necessarily indicate pseudarthrosis.

The lumbar spine has been well studied with regards to the diagnosis of pseudarthrosis because of the frequency of lumbar operations and the relatively high rate of nonunion. In the lumbar spine, solid fusion is believed to have occurred when bridging bone is

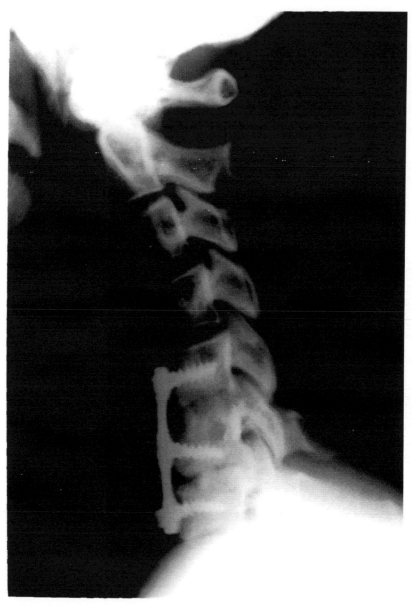

(c)

Figure 4 (*continued*)

identified between transverse processes in the lumbar spine and there is little or no motion on dynamic studies. In the lumbar spine, studies evaluating for the presence of pseudo-arthrosis have allowed up to 5° of motion to be measured across the vertebral endplates and still be consistent with a solid fusion (28). Other criteria include not only the presence of bone along the lateral gutters, but also incorporation of the bone graft into the transverse processes and lateral bony elements.

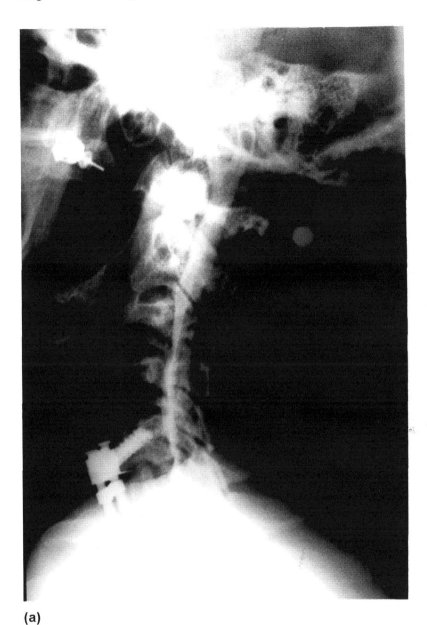

(a)

Figure 5 Lateral (a) view of a cervical myelogram with dynamic plate fixation from C5 to C7. The strut graft has not incorporated into the C5 vertebral body. This is confirmed on the CT scan (b), which shows luciencies around the graft.

The presence of movement on dynamic studies may suggest that nonunion has occurred (Fig. 7). Standard antero-posterior and lateral radiographs accurately diagnose pseudarthrosis in less than 50% of patients (29). There is debate as to the amount of flexion-extension movement that is allowable across the endplates to determine the presence of a nonunion. In studies that incorporated interbody fusion cages, up to 5° of movement was allowed before the diagnosis of pseudarthrosis was made (28).

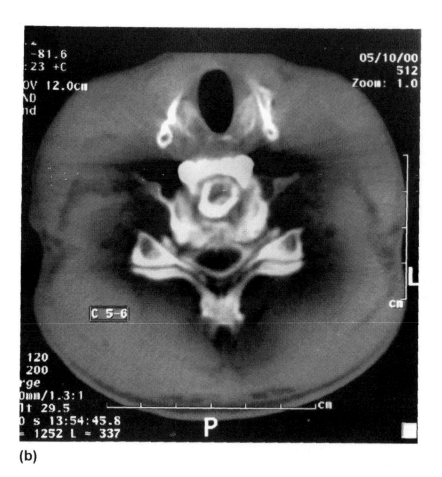

(b)

Figure 5 (*continued*)

When lumbar instrumentation is present, one may identify lucency at the bone/screw interface in the presence of pseudarthrosis. These bone "halos" may indicate nonunion (Fig. 8). The diagnosis of instrumentation failure does not necessarily indicate the presence of a nonunion as the screws may have failed during the healing process after being subjected to repeated cyclic stresses.

Radionucleide studies are neither sensitive nor specific in the diagnosis of pseudarthrosis (29,30). One study reported a sensitivity (true positive/true positive + false negative) of 0.5 and specificity (true negative/true negative + false positive) of 0.58 using this imaging technique and comparing the independent assessment to surgical findings (31). As such, the predictive value of this test for the accurate diagnosis is little better than chance alone.

Standard axial computed tomography (CT) scanning through the area of question may show evidence of bony pseudarthrosis such as bony resorption or halo formation around instrumentation. The sensitivity of the studies may be increased if sagittal and coronal reformation or three-dimensional (3-D) segmentation studies are obtained (32). The reviewing physician must take into account that volume averaging may alter the specificity in the diagnosis of pseudarthrosis. For example, volume averaging may increase the false-negative rate by making small bony clefts appear as solid masses.

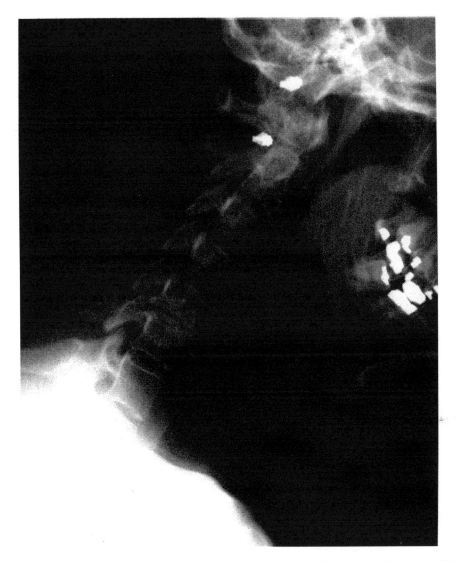

Figure 6 C5-6 pseudarthrosis following anterior cervical discectomy with autograft fusion. Note the collapse of the graft with associated radiographic luciencies.

One must keep in mind that radiation spray from metal implants may render the study uninterpretable. Also, it is important to note that the CT-obtained studies describe only bony structures. The CT does not determine motion. As such, a stable fibrous union may be interpreted as a bone pseudarthrosis but may not cause symptoms or require surgical treatment.

The diagnosis of pseudarthrosis may be particularily difficult to make in patients with interbody fusion cages. The identification of bone resorption around a cage certainly leads one to believe that nonunion is present (Fig. 9). The lack of bone resorption, however, does not necessarily indicate that a solid fusion has occurred. Even with the use of CT scanning, pseudarthrosis may not be accurately diagnosed in interbody fusion cage constructs (33). Another potential method of evaluation of fusion in and around

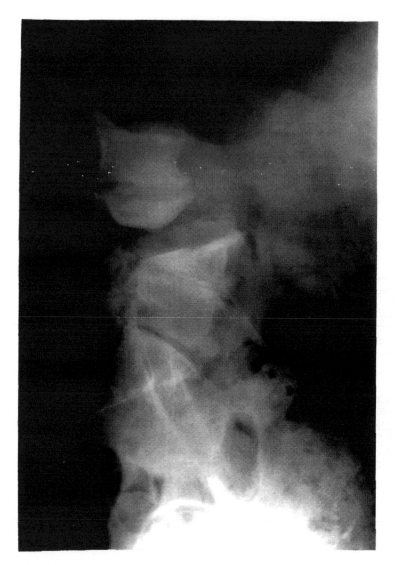

Figure 7   Gross pseudarthrosis at L4-5 following spinal infection.

interbody fusion cages is to inject contrast material around the cage. The presence of contrast material surrounding the cage suggests bony resorption and pseudarthrosis. The development of solid anterior bridging bone across the fused segment may be the best indicator of solid fusion.

Perhaps the single best summary regarding the difficulties and inaccuracies of relying on radiographic evaluations to evaluate for pseudarthrosis is that by Brodsky and colleagues (34). This study examined the results of surgical exploration in over 200 patients and correlated intraoperative findings with preoperative radiographs including stress films, polytomograms, and CT scans. The intraoperative findings were not accurately reflected by plain film studies in 36% of patients. The correlation was even less accurate for polytomograms, stress films, and CT scans.

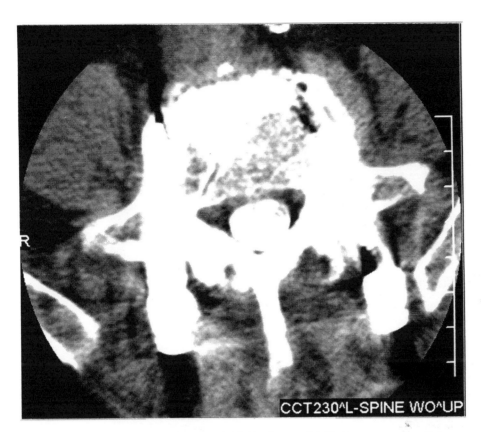

Figure 8 CT scan at S1 level 9 months following an L4-S1 instrumented pedicle screw fusion construct. There is a "halo" around the right S1 screw tip suggesting bone-screw failure and associated movement.

IV. TREATMENT

In general, treatment modalities for pseudarthrosis include correction, when possible, of underlying causative factors of pseudarthrosis. As noted by many authors, fusion can and will only occur in an environment that restricts motion, allows the ingrowth and differentiation of cells, and favors bone deposition over bone resorption. The bone-development side of this equation is positively influenced by the presence of material(s) that promote cellular differentiation into bone-forming cells (osteoinduction). The development or attraction of bone-forming cells to the site of fusion (osteogenesis) also promotes fusion (35). The presence of a bone lattice or scaffold or matrix (osteoconduction) can also induce bone fusion as well. Adequate bone immobility, through either the use of an external brace or internal bracing with instrumentation, also reduces bone absorption.

The fusion environment is negatively affected by osteoporosis, obesity, and anti-metabolic medicines. Nicotine administration has been shown to have an extremely negative impact on fusion success in an animal model (12). Clinical trials also support this animal trial. Brown and colleagues showed that pseudarthrosis rates were higher in patients who used tobacco products (11). Improvement of the local host environment may occur

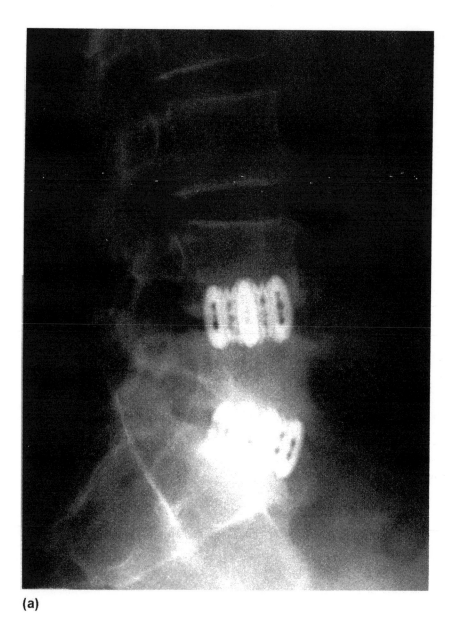

(a)

Figure 9 Lateral (a) and antero-posterior (b) radiographs demonstrating potential lucency around the single L4-5 interbody fusion cage.

as a result of discontinuation of tobacco use and maintenance of an ideal body habitus. The discontinuation of certain medications such as anti-metabolic medicines and phenytoin may also be appropriate in certain instances. Many surgeons will avoid prescription of anti-inflammatory medicines, steroidal or nonsteroidal, for at least 10 weeks following the fusion.

Nonsteroidal and steroidal anti-inflammatory medicines may reduce osteoblastic activity and should be avoided in the early postfusion period.

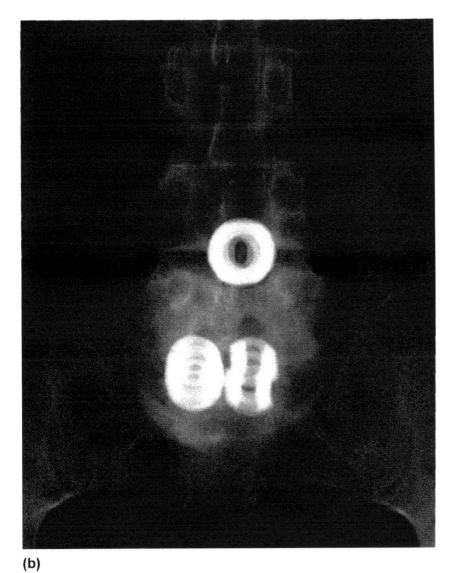

(b)

Figure 9 (*continued*)

Another general treatment that can be considered is the use of internal bone growth stimulators. The application of an external bone growth stimulator may also be considered. Pulsed electromagnetic field (PEMF) external bone growth stimulators have been shown to stimulate bone growth, even in the presence of pseudarthrosis (36).

Implanted bone growth stimulators are based on the concept that stress generates electrical potentials in long bone fractures. Further investigation demonstrated that electronegativity was present on the side of the bone under compression and electropositivity was present on the side of bone under tension (37). Other studies have demonstrated that electrical potentials in vitro influence bone development and new bone is formed at the site of electrical current (38).

The mechanism of action of electrical stimulation may be its ability to trigger cellular mitosis, cause a recruitment of osteogenic cells, or generate chemical signals such as hydroxyl radicals, which may improve the fusion environment. Other responses to electrical stimulation that may stimulate osteogenesis include triggering of a secondary messenger system, release of growth factors, and modulation of calcium.

Implanted stimulators have a significant track record of clinical success in lumbar and thoracolumbar fusion applications. A large study examining the results of direct current stimulation in circumferential fusion utilizing allograft was performed. This study had a comparison control arm of patients who received similar surgeries without stimulation. The study showed a statistically significant improvement in fusion results in patients receiving stimulation compared to those who did not receive stimulation (39). Other studies have shown similar results. Kane noted, in a prospective, randomized, multicenter trial, a statistically significant improvement in fusion success with electrical stimulation (40). In two separate studies, both Rogozinski and Kucharzyk noted similar statistically significant improvement in fusion rates in patients undergoing instrumented fusion (41,42). Tejano et al. (43) reported a 91.5% fusion rate in "difficult" patients in noninstrumented fusions, and Pettine et al. (44) showed a 96% fusion rate in high-risk patients.

There are certain general principles of surgical repair of pseudarthroses. One should consider exploration of the entire fusion mass to be certain that multiple areas of pseudarthrosis are not present. Fibrotic material must be removed in its entirety, and bleeding bone must be identified.

Autologous bone has generally been considered to be the optimal matrix for fusion for use in the cervical, thoracic, and lumbar spine (45). This concept is evolving as studies demonstrating that bone substitutes can have equal and perhaps superior fusion rates (46). Bone morphogenic proteins (BMPs) may also significantly change the way in which pseudarthrosis is treated (47). Specifically, one could propose the use of a human recombinant BMP if it were shown to have fusion rates superior to other modalities of treatment despite the expected cost differential.

A. Cervical Pseudarthrosis

A large number of patients undergo single-level anterior cervical discectomy with or without fusion. These procedures are generally very successful, and the incidence of pseudarthrosis is low (45). However, surgical nonunion following anterior cervical discectomy and fusion has the greatest prevalance of cervical pseudarthrosis. The treatment of cervical pseudarthrosis will depend on patient symptoms. Tolerable neck pain with evidence of radiographic pseudarthrosis does not necessarily require further treatment (45). Persistent neck pain may require intervention. Intervention may be nonsurgical or surgical, depending on the severity of symptoms, host factors, status of instrumentation (if present), location of the surgical site, and the time course of the nonunion.

Initial nonsurgical treatments may include external bracing with the use of a rigid cervical collar, pain medicines, facet or epidural steroid injections, facet rhizotomies or other modalities such as the use of an external electrical stimulator. Anti-inflammatory medicines may also be considered.

Before deciding to perform surgery for the correction of cervical nonunion, several factors must be taken into consideration, including the patient's level of function and employment status, the ability to correct the underlying etiological factors for nonhealing, and the patient's willingness to undergo further surgery. Fortunately, the results of surgical correction for pseudarthrosis in the cervical spine often yield good clinical and radiographic outcomes.

Repair of a symptomatic anterior cervical pseudarthrosis can be effected using an anterior, posterior, or combined approach. Studies indicate that repair of symptomatic cervical spine pseudarthrosis is usually very successful regardless of the surgical approach (24,48). One earlier randomized study examined the surgical correction of pseudarthrosis following anterior cervical discectomy with fusion (49). Patients underwent either resection of the failed graft followed by interbody fusion with tricortical iliac crest autograft bone placement or posterior cervical wiring with autograft bone placement. Sixteen out of 17 patients who underwent posterior revision surgery had evidence of a solid fusion. Thirteen out of 17 patients who underwent an anterior revision had evidence of solid bone union. Fifteen out of 17 patients in the posterior group and 10 out of 17 patients in the anterior group had "excellent" or "good" clinical outcomes. The results of this study have been supported by other studies (50).

Posterior approaches for pseudarthrosis have met with excellent success for the correction of symptomatic cervical pseudarthrosis following anterior surgery. In one study, 19 patients were treated with a posterior decompression and triple wire fusion technique (21). Solid arthrodesis was obtained in all patients. A similar trial was reported in nine patients, all of whom had undergone unsuccessful anterior cervical arthrodesis. In this study, the patients underwent posterior Rogers wiring without the use of bone grafting (51). Seven out of nine patients showed subsequent evidence of solid fusion, which developed across the prior failed anterior arthrodesis.

Advocates of anterior revision surgery include Coric and colleagues, who examined 19 consecutive patients with cervical pseudarthrosis (52). Each patient underwent anterior revision surgery using allograft bone and anterior cervical plating. All patients developed a solid bony fusion at each operative level. Zdeblick and colleagues performed repeat anterior cervical discectomy or corpectomy without instrumentation in 35 patients (26). Autograft bone was used in all cases. Thirty-four out of 35 patients developed solid bone fusions, and excellent clinical results were noted in 29. Tribus et al. reported similar results in 16 consecutive patients treated for cervical pseudarthrosis following a revision anterior cervical corpectomy, autogenous bone grafting, and anterior cervical instrumentation (25). Radiographic stability (no motion on flexion-extension films) was obtained in all patients, and 11 out of 16 patients reported improvement in pain in the postoperative period.

Circumferential fusion has been reported for the repair of cervical pseudarthrosis. Lowery and colleagues reported a subset of 44 patients who underwent circumferential fusion for cervical pseudarthrosis (53). The 7 patients treated with circumferential fusion all developed a solid fusion.

B. Thoracic and Lumbar Pseudarthrosis

Salvage rates in terms of radiographically healed fusion for failed primary pseudarthrosis are generally in the 50% range (54–57). Reoperation for failed fusion has a high rate of failure itself. Generally, the surgeon must consider the cause of initial failure and decide if these causitive factors can be overcome. The surgery is made even more difficult because of the scar tissue that must be dissected, the higher rate of cerebrospinal fluid leak, the difficulty in removing previous pseudarthrosis material, and the potential increased difficulty in placing instrumentation.

It is generally accepted that, in revision cases, instrumentation is beneficial (1,9,14). The instrumentation should provide as rigid a construct as possible. This usually requires pedicle screw fixation but may also include sublaminar wiring and other supplements.

In light of the high failure rates for revision surgery, surgeons should consider circumferential fusion for revision purposes. Circumferential fusions have an extremely high rate of solid arthrodesis in both primary and revision settings (8,58,59). They offer the advantages of increased bony surface area for fusion and direct support of the anterior spinal column. The increased bony surface area for fusion will help to increase the rate of fusion, while support of the anterior column may reduce cyclic fatigue of the posterior applied instrumentation. It is important to note, however, that even with successful bony fusion following a circumferential fusion, the overall clinical and return to work outcomes may remain poor (60,61).

Circumferential fusion may be accomplished through either a posterior approach alone, a combined lateral and posterior approach, or a combined anterior and posterior approach. Circumferential fusion via a posterior approach generally requires a unilateral or bilateral hemilaminectomy (10,62–64). As stated by Albert and colleagues, "The use of a combined anteroposterior fusion for pseudarthrosis repair is practical and intuitive" (65). Furthermore, the anterior column in most instances has not been compromised by prior surgical attempts.

V. CONCLUSIONS

Pseudarthrosis is problematic in all regards. Patients with pseudarthrosis may report the presence of significant pain, which is usually the reason that they were willing to undergo the initial surgical intervention. In the patient's mind, the initial surgical intervention, which may have significantly improved their extremity discomfort, has failed. Unfortunately, the patient in whom a pseudarthrosis has occurred is again at high risk, and maybe higher, for a subsequent nonunion with revision surgery.

The ability to obtain an accurate diagnosis is difficult. Patients are frequently referred for invasive diagnostic testing, including myelography, diskography, and other injection-associated tests. No single test, including surgical reexploration, is completely specific or sensitive.

Treatment is fraught with risk. More traditional reoperative procedures are frequently unsuccessful, and many patients remain symptomatic. More advanced surgical procedures, such as combined anterior and posterior approaches, are time consuming, expensive, and carry with them associated surgical morbidity. Furthermore, advanced treatment modalities may be very expensive, especially if biologics such as bone morphogenic proteins are used.

Compounding these issues is the fact that even if a solid fusion is obtained, many patients treated for pseudarthrosis will remain symptomatic (60). Furthermore, worker's compensation and other socioeconomic issues may cloud the overall outcome of patients treated for this disease.

Ultimately, the best treatment for pseudarthrosis may be its avoidance through patient selection, modulation of underlying systemic risk factors, when possible, and application of appropriate surgical techniques.

REFERENCES

1. Lauerman WC, Bradford DS, Transfeldt EE, Ogilvie JW. Management of pseudarthrosis after arthrodesis of the spine for idiopathic scoliosis. J Bone Joint Surg 1991; 73-A(2):222–236.
2. Bohlman HH, Emery SE, Goodfellow DB, Jones PK. Robinson anterior cervical discectomy and arthrodesis for cervical radiculopathy. J Bone Joint Surg 1993; 75-A(9):1298–1307.
3. Emery SE, Bolesta MJ, Banks MA, Jones PK. Robinson anterior cervical fusion: comparison of the standard and modified techniques. Spine 1994; 19(6):660–663.
4. Riley LH, Robinson RA, Johnson KA, Walker AE. The results of anterior interbody fusion of the cervical spine: review of ninety-three consecutive cases. J Neurosurgery 1969; 30:127–133.
5. Epstein NE. Anterior cervical diskectomy and fusion without plate instrumentation in 178 patients. J Spinal Disord 2000; 13(1):1–8.
6. Epstein NE. Evaluation and treatment of clinical instability associated with pseudarthrosis after anterior cervical surgery for ossification of the posterior longitudinal ligament. Surg Neurol 1998; 49:246–252.
7. Aronson N, Filtzer D, Bagan M. Anterior cervical fusion by the Smith-Robinson approach. J Neurosurg 1969; 29:397–404.
8. Brantigan JW, Steffee AD, Lewis ML, Quinn LM, Persenaire JM. Lumbar interbody fusion using the Brantigan I/F cage for posterior lumbar interbody fusion and the variable pedicle screw placement system. Spine 2000; 25(11):1437–1446.
9. Lorenz M, Zindrick M, Schwaegler P, Vrbos L, Collatz MA, Behal R, Cram R. A comparison of single level fusions with and without hardware. Spine 1991; 16(8):S455–458.
10. Brantigan JW, Steffee AD. A carbon fiber implant to aid interbody lumbar fusion—two-year clinical results in the first 26 patients. Spine 1993; 18(14):2106–2177.
11. Brown CW, Orme TJ, Richardson HD. The rate of pseudarthrosis (surgical nonunion) in patients who are smokers and patients who are nonsmokers: a comparison study. Spine 1986; 11:942–943.
12. Silcox DH, Daftari T, Boden SD, Schimandle JH, Hutton WC, Whitesides Jr TE. The effect of nicotine on spinal fusion. Spine 1995; 20(14):1549–1553.
13. Rothman RH, Booth R. Failures of spinal fusion. Orthop Clin North Am 1975; 6(1):299–303.
14. Raiszadeh R, Heggeness M, Esses SI. Thoracolumbar pseudarthrosis. Am J Orthop 2000: 513–520.
15. Cunningham B, Orbegoso C, Dmitriev A, Hallab N, Sefter J, Asdourian P, McAfee P. An in-vivo rabbit model and an applied clinical study of retrieved instrumentation cases. Spine 2002.
16. Heggeness MH, Esses SI, Mody DR. A histologic study of lumbar pseudarthrosis. Spine 1993; 18(8):1016–1020.
17. Cleveland M, Bosworth D, Thompson F. Pseudarthrosis of the lumbosacral spine. J Bone Joint Surg 1948; 30A:302–312.
18. DePalma A, Rothman R. The nature of pseudarthrosis. Clin Orthop 1968; 59:113–118.
19. Flatley TJ, Derderian HD. Closed loop instrumentation of the lumbar spine. Clin Orthop 1985; 196:273–278.
20. Heggeness MH, Esses SI. Classification of pseudarthroses of the lumbar spine. Spine 1991; 16(8 suppl):S449–S454.
21. Farey ID, McAfee PC, Davis RF, Long DM. Pseudarthrosis of the cervical spine after anterior arthrodesis. J Bone Joint Surg 1990; 72-A(8):1171–1177.
22. Hilibrand AS, Dina TS. The use of diagnostic imaging to assess spinal arthrodesis. Orthop Clin North Am 1998; 29(4):591–601.
23. Martin GJ, Haid RW, MacMillan M, Rodts GE, Berkman R. Anterior cervical discectomy with freeze-dried fibula allograft: overview of 317 cases and literature review. Spine 1999; 24(9):852–859.
24. Phillips FM, Carlson G, Emery SE, Bohlman HH. Anterior cervical pseudarthrosis: natural history and treatment. Spine 1997; 22(14):1585–1589.

25. Tribus CB, Corteen DP, Zdeblick TA. The efficacy of anterior cervical plating in the management of symptomatic pseudoarthrosis of the cervical spine. Spine 1999; 24(9):860–864.

26. Zdeblick TA, Hughes SS, Riew KD, Bohlman HH. Failed anterior cervical discectomy and arthrodesis: Analysis and treatment of thirty-five patients. J Bone Joint Surg 1997; 79-A(4):523–532.

27. Cannada L, Scherping S, Yoo J, Jones P, Emery S. Pseudarthrosis of the cervical spine: a comparison of radiographic diagnostic measures. Spine 2003; 28:46–50.

28. Alpert S. PMA P950002—summary of safety and effectiveness. BAK interbody fusion system with instrumentation. Washington, DC: PMA Document Main Center (HFZ-401), 1996.

29. Dawson EG, Clader TJ, Bassett LW. A comparison of different methods used to diagnose pseudarthrosis following posterior spinal fusion for scoliosis. J Bone Joint Surg 1985; 67-A(8):1153–1159.

30. McMaster M, Merrick M. The scintigraphic assessment of the scoliotic spine after fusion. J Bone Joint Surg 1976; 58B:305–312.

31. Albert TJ, Pinto M, Smith MD, Balderston RA, Cotler JM, Park CH. Accuracy of SPECT scanning in diagnosing pseudoarthrosis: a prospective study. J Spinal Disord 1998; 11(3):197–199.

32. Lang P, Genant HK, Chafetz N, Steiger P, Morris JM. Three-dimensional computed tomogrpahy and multiplanar reformations in the assessment of pseudarthrosis in posterior lumbar fusion patients. Spine 1988; 13(1):69–75.

33. McAfee PC, Cunningham BW, Lee GA, Orbegoso CM, Haggerty CJ, Fedder IL, Griffith SL. Revision strategies for salvaging or improving failed cylindrical cages. Spine 1999; 24(20): 2147–2153.

34. Brodsky AE, Kovalsky ES, Khalil MA. Correlation of radiologic assessment of lumbar spine fusions with surgical exploration. Spine 1991; 16(6):S261–S265.

35. Lindholm TS, Nilsson OS, Lindholm TC. Extraskeletal and intraskeletal new bone formation induced by demineralized bone matrix combined with bone marrow cells. Clin Orthop 1982:251–255.

36. Simmons JW. Treatment of failed posterior lumbar interbody fusion (PLIF) of the spine with pulsing electromagnetic fields. Clin Orthop 1985; 193:127–132.

37. Fukada E, Yasuda I. On the piezoelectric effects of bone. J Physiol Soc Jpn 1957; 12:1158.

38. Oishi M, ST O. Electrical bone graft stimulation for spinal fusion: a review. Neurosurgery 2000; 47(5):1041–1056.

39. Meril AJ. Direct current stimulation of allograft in anterior and posterior lumbar interbody fusion. Spine 1994; 19(21):2393–2398.

40. Kane WJ. Direct current electrical bone growth stimulation for spinal fusion. Spine 1998; 13(3):363–365.

41. Rogozinski A, Rogozinski C. Efficacy of implanted bone growth stimulation in instrumented lumbosacral spine fusion. Spine 1996; 21:2479–2483.

42. Kucharzyk D. A controlled prospective outcome study of implantable electrical stimulation with spinal instrumentation in a high-risk spinal fusion population. Spine 1999; 24(5):465–469.

43. Tejano N, Puno R, Ignacio J. The use of implantable direct current stimulation in multi-level spinal fusion without instrumentation: a prospective clinical and radiographic evaluation with long-term follow-up. Spine 1996; 21(6):1905–1908.

44. Pettine K, Salib R, Walker S. External electrical stimulation and bracing for treatment of spondylolysis. A case report. Spine 1993; 18(4):436–439.

45. Zdeblick TA, Ducker TB. The use of freeze-dried allograft bone for anterior cervical fusions. Spine 1991; 16:726–729.

46. Welch WC, Gerszten PC, Sherman JD, Ullrich P, Latus G, Macenski M. A prospective randomized study of interbody fusion: bone substitute or autograft. Biotechnologies in Spinal Surgery Congress, Halle, Germany, April 11–13, 2002.

47. Sandhu HS, Boden SD. Biologic enhancement of spinal fusion. Orthop Clin North Am 1998; 29(4):621–631.

48. Newman M. The outcome of pseudarthrosis after cervical anterior fusion. Spine 1993; 18(16):2380–2382.
49. Brodsky AE, Khalil MA, Sassard WR, Newman BP. Repair of symptomatic pseudarthrosis of anterior cervical fusion posterior versus anterior repair. Spine 1992; 17(10):1137–1143.
50. Siambanes D, Miz GS. Treatment of symptomatic anterior cervical nonunion using the Rogers interspinous wiring technique. Am J Orthop 1998:792–796.
51. Fuji T, Yonenobu K, Fujiwara K, Yamashita K, Ono K, Okada K. Interspinous wiring without bone grafting for nonunion or delayed union following anterior spinal fusion of the cervical spine. Spine 1986; 11(10):982–987.
52. Coric D, Brnach Jr CL, Jenkins JD. Revision of anterior cervical pseudarthrosis with anterior allograft fusion and plating. J Neurosurg 1997; 86:969–974.
53. Lowery GL, Swank M, McDonough RF. Surgical revision for failed anterior cervical fusions. Spine 1995; 20(22):2436–2441.
54. Waddell G, Kummel E, Lotto W, Graham J, Hall H, McCulloch J. Failed lumbar disc surgery and repeat surgery following industrial injuries. J Bone Joint Surg 1979; 61-A(2):201–207.
55. Lehman T, LaRocca H. Repeat lumbar surgery: a review of patients with failure from previous lumbar surgery treated by spinal canal exploration and lumbar spinal fusion. Spine 1981; 6:615–619.
56. Frymoyer J, Hanley E, Howe J, et al. Disc excision and spine fusion in the management of lumbar disc disease. Spine 1978; 3:1–11.
57. Finnegan WJ, Fenlin JM, Marvel JP, Nardini RJ, Rothman RH. Results of surgical intervention in the symptomatic multiply-operated back patient. J Bone Joint Surg 1979; 61-A(7): 1077–1082.
58. Enker P, Steffee AD. Interbody fusion and instrumentation. Clin Orthop 1994; 300:90–101.
59. Etminan M, Girardi F, Khan S, Cammisa F. Revision strategies for lumbar pseudarthrosis. Orthop Clin North Am 2002:381–392.
60. Gertzbein SD, Hollopeter MR, Hall S. Pseudarthrosis of the lumbar spine outcome after circumferential fusion. Spine 1998; 23(21):2352–2357.
61. Cohen D, Chotivichit A, Fujita T, et al. Pseudarthrosis repair: autogenous iliac crest versus femoral ring allograft. Clin Orthop 2000; 37:46–55.
62. Patel AK, Welch WC. Posterior lumbar interbody fusion using metallic cages: current techniques. Operat Techn Orthop 2000; 10:311–319.
63. Ray CD. Threaded titanium cages for lumbar interbody fusions. Spine 1997; 22(6):667–680.
64. Kuslich SD, Ulstrom CL, Griffith SL, Ahern JW, Dowdle JD. The Bagby and Kuslich method of lumbar interbody fusion. History, techniques, and 2-year follow-up results of a United States prospective, multicenter trial. Spine 1998; 23(11):1267–1278.
65. Albert TJ, Pinto M, Denis F. Management of symptomatic lumbar pseudarthrosis with anteroposterior fusion—a functional and radiographic outcome study. Spine 2000; 23(1):123–129.

9

Complications and Risks of Blood Products, Hemostatic Agents, Dural Substitutes, and Sealants

K. Michael Webb and Gregory A. Helm
University of Virginia Health Sciences System, Charlottesville, Virginia, U.S.A.

I. INTRODUCTION

The ability to maintain hemodynamic stability, stop intraoperative bleeding, and manage cerebrospinal fluid leakage has long been important to the successful practice of spine surgery. Over the last several years, many advancements have been made in these areas that have improved the morbidity of spinal procedures, particularly complex ones involving extensive dissection, instrumentation, and lengthy operative times. However, each new advance brings its own set of unique iatrogenic risks, of which the spine surgeon must be aware. This chapter will discuss the risks, benefits, and efficacy of intraoperative blood transfusions, topical hemostatic agents, and dural substitutes, allowing the spine surgeon to make informed decisions regarding the use of these adjuncts.

II. RISKS OF AUTOLOGOUS AND BANKED BLOOD

A. Banked Blood

Blood transfusion has significantly improved the ability of physicians to ameliorate the effect of acute surgical blood loss, allowing for more complex and lengthy surgical procedures. The increased awareness of transfusion-related complications has prompted intense scrutiny of indications for transfusion, leading to numerous consensus conferences attempting to standardize guidelines for packed red blood cell transfusion. Nevertheless, concrete indications for perioperative blood transfusion remain controversial, and a wide variety exists in clinical practice. Thus, a discussion of the risks of blood transfusion is necessary so that more informed risk/benefit decisions regarding perioperative blood transfusion can be made.

    The most common transfusion reactions are hypersensitivity reactions, hemolytic reactions, febrile nonhemolytic reactions, transfusion-related acute lung injury (TRALI), and bacterial/viral contamination.

Hypersensitivity reactions range from itching and hives to life-threatening anaphylactic shock. They are caused by immunoglobulin E antibodies in the recipient to donor antigens and have an incidence of 1:150,000 transfusions (1).

Hemolytic reactions occur in approximately 1:250,000–1,000,000 blood transfusions (2). They are caused by preformed recipient antibodies against donor antigens such as Rh, ABO, Kell, Kidd, and Duffy. These reactions are almost always related to clerical error and are preventable.

Febrile nonhemolytic reactions are caused by the release of cytokines from recipient leukocytes activated by recipient antibodies. They occur in less than 2% of transfusions and are more common in patients who have received multiple previous transfusions (1).

TRALI is an incompletely understood phenomenon thought to occur in approximately 1:5000 transfusions, although the true incidence may be underestimated. It is thought to be caused by human leukocyte antigen/granulocyte antibodies in donor plasma, which activate recipient neutrophils, subsequently causing lung injury similar in clinical appearance to adult respiratory distress syndrome (ARDS), although with an 80–90% incidence of recovery (1,2).

Viral and bacterial contamination of blood products has received much attention recently and has been the impetus for the increased scrutiny of indications for intraoperative transfusion and an increase in autologous blood donation. Despite this increased attention, infectious contamination of blood products is quite rare. Viral contamination with hepatitis A is found in approximately 1:1,000,000 units, hepatitis B in between 1:30,000–1:250,000, hepatitis C in 1:30,000–1:150,000 (1). Human immunovirus (HIV) contamination is found in approximately 1:677,000 units (3). Bacterial contamination is also uncommon, occurring in 1:500,000 units; the most commonly involved pathogen is Yersinia enterocolitica, although Salmonella, Pseudomonas, Treponema pallidum, Borrelia burgdorferi, and staphylococcal infections can occur (3).

Other transfusion-related complications are related to phlebotomy, namely vasovagal syncope and volume overload in patients with severe cardiac dysfunction. Allogenic transfusions have also been reported to alter recipient immune responses, potentially causing increased postoperative infections, although this is controversial and conflicting studies exist (3).

B. Autologous Blood

Because of the increased awareness of bloodborne pathogens, preoperative autologous donation has increased by nearly 70%. Autologous donation is a multidisciplinary undertaking which is more time-consuming and costly compared to allogenic donations. However, this is offset by its decreased risk of transfusion reactions and bloodborne infections. There has also been an increase in directed donations, in which blood is donated for the patient by relatives or friends. Interestingly, this has not been shown to decrease the risk of bloodborne infection.

Because of the increased cost associated with autologous donations, they are appropriate for surgeries in which the expected blood loss is large and the likelihood of transfusion high. Thus, autologous donations are not indicated for routine spine surgery such as lumbar or cervical discectomies, laminectomies, or routine one-level fusion procedures with instrumentation. In more complex spinal procedures such as multilevel instrumentation procedures and spinal deformities, autologous donation is a reasonable option.

Donations are typically started 4–6 weeks before surgery and are generally made at one-week intervals. There is no minimum interval for blood donation, although the hemoglobin value should be greater than 11 g/dL. Donations should not be made within 72 hours of the planned procedure to allow restoration of plasma volume. During the donation period, oral iron supplementation is frequently used. Once donated, autogenic blood can be stored for up to 5–6 weeks. Autologous donation is contraindicated in patients with critical left main coronary artery disease, unstable angina, aortic stenosis, hypertrophic cardiomyopathy, ventricular dysrythmias, recent myocardial infarction, and congestive heart failure.

The risks of autologous blood donation are significantly less. With the risk of transfusion reactions and infectious contamination virtually eliminated, the greatest risk of donation is vasovagal reaction, which occurs in 2–5% of patients (3). Additionally, clerical errors can occur; allogenic units have been transfused into patients who have donated autologous blood and autologous donations infused into unintended recipients.

II. HEMOSTATIC AGENTS

A. Efficacy

Hemostasis is of primary importance to the spine surgeon, especially in complex cases with significant fluid shifts and resultant hemodynamic changes. Hemostatic adjuncts are typically either mechanical, such as electrocautery, or chemical, which take advantage of the bodies natural coagulation cascade to promote local thrombosis and hemostasis. Topical adjuncts to hemostasis have been available since the 1940s and continue to be widely used in all types of surgery. Although helpful, topical hemostatic agents require a functioning coagulation system to work properly. Thus, they lose effectiveness in coagulopathies, and appropriate tests of coagulation status such as activated partial thromboplastin and prothrombin time should be checked as indicated. Furthermore, these agents also cause hemostasis by activating platelets and are not effective in platelet dysfunction syndromes or low platelet counts.

Although there are many brands and packaging methods for hemostatic agents, they generally fall into three categories: (a) gelatin sponges (such as Gelfoam®, which may be soaked in bovine thrombin before use), (b) microfibrillar collagen (Avitene®), and (c) oxidized rengenerated cellulose (Surgicel®). Recently, a new hemostatic agent, FloSeal®, has been introduced. It is composed of a dehydrated collagen matrix that is regenerated before use with bovine thrombin. Although most hemostatic adjuncts have been in use for many years, few objective studies exist evaluating their efficacy and complication rates. The body of anecdotal evidence suggests that these agents are roughly equivalent, and the decision to use one versus another is largely made based on ease of use and personal experience.

Some reports have studied hemostatic agents both in vivo and in vitro. A recent in vitro study looking at platelet activation and clotting times found that collagen-based hemostatic agents were more effective in both platelet activation and clotting time than gelatin sponges, which were in turn more effective than oxidized regenerated cellulose. However, these differences were not apparent when all agents were presoaked with bovine thrombin (4), which is a common clinical practice. In vivo animal models have failed to show a statistically significant difference between hemostatic agents (5). However, a recent cardiovascular surgery study found FloSeal to be more effective than thrombin-soaked gelatin sponges in decreasing operative blood loss in humans (6), a finding confirmed by subsequent investigators (7). Thus, it appears that very little difference in efficacy exists between Gelfoam, Avitene, and Surgicel. Floseal may be more effective than these previous agents, although this will likely require further confirmation in studies involving spine surgery.

B. Risks and Complications

Hemostatic agents are foreign bodies, and theoretical potential exists for increased infection rates and complications related to mass effect on neurological structures. The use of hemostatic adjuncts has not been associated with increased infection rates in clinical studies. In an experimental model, oxidized cellulose (Surgicel) has been shown to be less prone to superinfection than gelatin sponge (Gelfoam) and microfibrillar collagen (Avitene) after wound inoculation with Staphylococcus aureus, particularly when less than 20 mg of Surgicel was used (8).

Since hemostatic agents act both by activating the clotting cascade and by absorbing blood, creating a tamponade effect, there is a possibility of causing neurological compromise via mass effect. Many case reports exist regarding neurological compression with hemostatic agents, spanning all surgical locations and hemostatic agents (9–14). The common theme throughout these case reports is that hemostatic agents are an adjunct, not a substitute, to proper surgical technique and should not be overused. When possible, they should be removed after hemostasis has been achieved. Additionally, gelatin sponges can have a significant amount of air contained within them, which increases the size and mass effect of the sponge after moistening. Therefore, gelatin sponges should be presoaked in either thrombin or saline and squeezed to remove any remaining air bubbles before use.

III. DURAL SUBSTITUTES, SEALANTS, AND FIBRIN GLUE

A. Efficacy

The first reported use of a dural substitute was in 1895, and since that time surgeons have been searching for the ideal material for duraplasty. Clinical interest in synthetic dural substitutes remains high, and new materials are introduced with great frequency. When evaluating these studies, the important concepts are:

1. Is it easy to use?
2. Does it cause adhesions to the underlying leptomeninges and neural tissue with and without trauma?
3. Does it increase the rate of CSF leakage?
4. Does it increase the rate of infection?

Several dural substitutes are currently in use. The most commonly used are lyophilized bovine pericardium, expanded polytetrafluoroethylene (PTFE or GoreTex®), and bioresorbable collagen-matrix sheets.

Lyophilized bovine pericardium is prepared by freeze-drying bovine pericardial tissue, which is then gamma-irradiated for sterilization. The use of lyophilized bovine pericardium increased in response to reports of Creutzfeld-Jakob disease transmission associated with previously popular cadaveric dural substitutes. There has been concern, particularly in England, regarding the potential transmission of bovine spongiform encephalopathy with the use of bovine pericardium. However, no such occurrence has been reported.

Lyophilized bovine pericardium is easy to use, inexpensive, and can be closed in a water-tight fashion with sutures. A recent clinical study in which the major indication for use was closure of lumbosacral myelocoeles revealed excellent results with no CSF leakage, neural compression, or adhesion (15).

PTFE is associated with the least amount of adhesions and inflammatory reaction in several clinical studies (16–18). However, concern over CSF leakage through suture holes and difficult handling characteristics have diminished enthusiasm for its use among surgeons.

Collagen matrices have long been used as dural substitutes. In the natural state they are somewhat porous, and previous attempts to make collagen sponges watertight and able to hold stitches resulted in intense inflammatory reactions, sometimes leading to the formation of dense adhesions to the underlying neural tissue or hemorrhagic neomembrane formation causing neural compression. These complications were not related to the collagen itself, rather to the materials used to alter it. With the increased realization that overt cerebrospinal fluid (CSF) leakage is related more to inadequate multilayer closure than to strict watertightness, interest has revived in collagen-matrix onlay grafts, Duragen® being a recent addition to this market. A recent study using collagen matrix sponges for duraplasty in both cranial and spinal operations showed no incidence of CSF leakage or neural adhesions in the patients who had undergone spinal surgery (19).

B. Risks

1. Neural Compression

Neural compression has been reported with dural substitutes, almost always as a result of hemorrhage from a neovascular membrane formation surrounding the dural graft. Most reports of hemorrhage involve the use of silastic, a silicone-based polymer no longer available (19–22), occurring up to 20 years after its implantation (23). Newer, less reactive substitutes are currently used, and neural compression from duraplasty has been reported in only two other dural substitutes, both of which involve materials no longer in use (24,25).

2. Infection

Similar to hemostatic agents, dural substitutes are foreign bodies that can theoretically predispose to infection. Clinical studies, however, have not borne this out, and dural substitution has not been shown to increase infection rates (19,26).

C. Fibrin Glue

Fibrin glue has been investigated as a hemostatic adjunct in cardiovascular surgery and as a method to prevent CSF leakage, either prophylactically or in conjunction with dural repair for persistent leakage. Fibrin glue mimics the coagulation cascade, whereby fibrinogen is cleaved by thrombin to fibrin strands, which are then crosslinked by Factor XIII to form a stable fibrin clot. Fibrin glue is a useful adjunct in preventing CSF leakage and prevented CSF leakage in approximately 90% of patients in one clinical study. In patients with a preexisting CSF fistula, adjunctive fibrin glue was successful in 67% (27).

Because fibrin glue is made from human blood products, there is a slight risk of infection from fibrin glue. However, clinical studies have confirmed the safety of its use (28), and new single donor sources will likely reduce the theoretical risk of infection even further.

IV. CONCLUSION

Blood transfusions, topical hemostatic agents, dural substitutes, and fibrin glue are all useful adjuncts to the spinal surgeon. However, these products are no substitute for proper and meticulous surgical technique and are associated with unique risks and benefits, of which spine surgeons should be aware.

REFERENCES

1. Wall MH, Prielipp RC. Transfusion in the operating room and the intensive care unit: current practice and future directions. Int Anesthesiol Clin 2000; 38(4):149–169.
2. Goodnough LT, Brecher ME, Kanter MH, AuBuchon JP. Transfusion medicine. First of two parts—blood transfusion. N Engl J Med 1999; 340(6):438–447.
3. Velez-Pestana LI, Yawn D, Fitch JC. Transfusion medicine in the preoperative period. Int Anesthesiol Clin 2002; 40(2):159–166.
4. Wagner WR, Pachence JM, Ristich J, Johnson PC. Comparative in vitro analysis of topical hemostatic agents. J Surg Res 1996; 66(2):100–108.
5. Kheirabadi BS, Field-Ridley A, Pearson R, MacPhee M, Drohan W, Tuthill D. Comparative study of the efficacy of the common topical hemostatic agents with fibrin sealant in a rabbit aortic anastomosis model. J Surg Res 2002; 106(1):99–107.
6. Oz MC, Cosgrove DM, III, Badduke BR, Hill JD, Flannery MR, Palumbo R, et al. Controlled clinical trial of a novel hemostatic agent in cardiac surgery. The Fusion Matrix Study Group. Ann Thorac Surg 2000; 69(5):1376–1382.
7. Weaver FA, Hood DB, Zatina M, Messina L, Badduke B. Gelatin-thrombin-based hemostatic sealant for intraoperative bleeding in vascular surgery. Ann Vasc Surg 2002; 16(3):286–293.
8. Scher KS, Coil JA, Jr. Effects of oxidized cellulose and microfibrillar collagen on infection. Surgery 1982; 91(3):301–304.
9. Alander DH, Stauffer ES. Gelfoam-induced acute quadriparesis after cervical decompression and fusion. Spine 1995; 20(8):970–971.
10. Awwad EE, Smith KR, Jr. MRI of marked dural sac compression by Surgicel in the immediately postoperative period after uncomplicated lumbar laminectomy. J Comput Assist Tomogr 1999; 23(6):969–975.
11. Banerjee T, Goldschmidt K. 'Surgiceloma' manifested as cauda equina syndrome. South Med J 1998; 91(5):481–483.
12. Brodbelt AR, Miles JB, Foy PM, Broome JC. Intraspinal oxidised cellulose (Surgicel) causing delayed paraplegia after thoracotomy—a report of three cases. Ann R Coll Surg Engl 2002; 84(2):97–99.
13. Friedman J, Whitecloud TS, III. Lumbar cauda equina syndrome associated with the use of gelfoam: case report. Spine 2001; 26(20):E485–E487.
14. Herndon JH, Grillo HC, Riseborough EJ, Rich JC, Jr. Compression of the brain and spinal cord following use of gelfoam. Arch Surg 1972; 104(1):107.
15. Filippi R, Schwarz M, Voth D, Reisch R, Grunert P, Perneczky A. Bovine pericardium for duraplasty: clinical results in 32 patients. Neurosurg Rev 2001; 24(2–3):103–107.
16. Barbolt TA, Odin M, Leger M, Kangas L, Hoiste J, Liu SH. Biocompatibility evaluation of dura mater substitutes in an animal model. Neurol Res 2001; 23(8):813–820.

17. Park YK, Tator CH. Prevention of arachnoiditis and postoperative tethering of the spinal cord with Gore-Tex surgical membrane: an experimental study with rats. Neurosurgery 1998; 42(4):813–823.

18. Yamagata S, Goto K, Oda Y, Kikuchi H. Clinical experience with expanded polytetrafluoro-ethylene sheet used as an artificial dura mater. Neurol Med Chir (Tokyo) 1993; 33(8):582–585.

19. Narotam PK, van Dellen JR, Bhoola KD. A clinicopathological study of collagen sponge as a dural graft in neurosurgery. J Neurosurg 1995; 82(3):406–412.

20. Banerjee T, Meagher JN, Hunt WE. Unusual complications with use of silastic dural substitute. Am Surg 1974; 40(7):434–437.

21. Fontana R, Talamonti G, D'Angelo V, Arena O, Monte V, Collice M. Spontaneous haema-toma as unusual complication of silastic dural substitute. Report of 2 cases. Acta Neurochir (Wien) 1992; 115(1–2):64–66.

22. Ng TH, Chan KH, Leung SY, Mann KS. An unusual complication of silastic dural substitute: case report. Neurosurgery 1990; 27(3):491–493.

23. Ohbayashi N, Inagawa T, Katoh Y, Kumano K, Nagasako R, Hada H. Complication of silastic dural substitute 20 years after dural plasty. Surg Neurol 1994; 41(4):338–341.

24. Gudmundsson G, Sogaard I. Complications to the use of vicryl-collagen dural substitute. Acta Neurochir (Wien) 1995; 132(1–3):145–147.

25. Ongkiko CM, Jr., Keller JT, Mayfield FH, Dunsker SB. An unusual complication of Dura Film as a dural substitute. Report of two cases. J Neurosurg 1984; 60(5):1076–1079.

26. Yamada K, Miyamoto S, Takayama M, Nagata I, Hashimoto N, Ikada Y, et al. Clinical application of a new bioabsorbable artificial dura mater. J Neurosurg 2002; 96(4):731–735.

27. Shaffrey CI, Spotnitz WD, Shaffrey ME, Jane JA. Neurosurgical applications of fibrin glue: augmentation of dural closure in 134 patients. Neurosurgery 1990; 26(2):207–210.

28. Greenhalgh DG, Gamelli RL, Lee M, Delavari M, Lynch JB, Hansbrough JF, et al. Multicenter trial to evaluate the safety and potential efficacy of pooled human fibrin sealant for the treatment of burn wounds. J Trauma 1999; 46(3):433–440.

10

Complications Related to Anterior Surgical Exposures of the Thoracic, Lumbar, and Sacral Spine

Rocco R. Calderone
St. John's Regional Medical Center, Oxnard, California, U.S.A.

Louise E. Toutant
Camarillo, California, U.S.A.

I. INTRODUCTION

Anterior surgical exposure of the thoracic, lumbar, and sacral spine is currently used for trauma, deformity, degenerative conditions, and most recently disk replacement surgery. Burns first described an anterior surgical approach for spondylolisthesis in 1933 (1), followed by Ito's description of anterior spine surgery for Pott's disease in 1934 (2). Lane and Moore reported a transperitoneal approach for anterior lumbar interbody fusion in 1948 (3), and Iwahara et al. discussed anterior lumbar fusion via a retroperitoneal approach in 1963 (4). Hodgson reported on anterior spinal fusion for spinal tuberculosis in 1960 and on anterior spinal surgery for deranged intervertebral disks and spondylolisthesis in 1968 (5,6). Dwyer used the anterior spinal approach for scoliosis in 1969 (7). Advances in medical technology continue to increase the utility of anterior surgical approaches to the thoracic, lumbar, and sacral spine for a variety of spinal disorders.

As many of these procedures are undertaken with a thoracic, vascular, or general surgeon, the terms "approach surgeon" and "access surgeon" have entered the medical vocabulary. An approach or access surgeon is a surgeon who has developed and refined his or her skills to meet the needs of a spine surgeon for the exposure of the anterior spine. Along with the access surgeon, the spine surgeon must define the region of exposure and the surrounding workspace. As such, the spine surgeon requires an intimate knowledge of the proximity of vital structures within the path of dissection.

This chapter discusses complications related to exposure of the vital structures anterior to the spine and potential injuries or altered vital functions associated with anterior surgical exposure of the thoracic, lumbar, and sacral spine. A review of the literature was undertaken to identify the most common approach-related complications. Rare or potential complications in vital structures within the path of dissection are discussed from a theoretical perspective. This overview is organized in specific anatomical or systemic categories along with recommendations for complication avoidance or treatment.

119

II. COMPLICATIONS OF INCISION, FASCIA, AND MUSCLE LAYERS

A. Incisional Complications

Technical points are associated with the incision that help prevent complications. The size and location of the incision will depend on the levels of exposure required for the procedure. Use of limited incisions requires the ability to extend the exposure quickly and efficiently if bleeding or other complications are encountered.

A left-sided incision is the most common approach to both the thoracic and lumbar spine, which avoids the vena cava system on the right. The aorta on the left side is more elastic for mobilization. A retroperitoneal approach on the left avoids the liver, which may crowd lumbar exposure from the right.

Access to the thoracic spine begins with an incision along the ribs, one or two segments above the vertebral level of exposure, since the ribs are downsloping as they course anteriorly (8). A common error is to place an incision too low in the thoracic spine, resulting in the intended spinal segment of interest being located underneath an over-hanging rib. Trying to access a vertebral segment with an incision placed too low is cumbersome and adds significant difficulty to the procedure. If more extensive access to the thoracic spine is needed, excision of a rib may be required.

Approach to the thoracolumbar junction requires an incision over the tenth rib, which slopes downward, for a combined flank approach to the retroperitoneum. This long incision is less cosmetic but allows extensive access to the thoracolumbar spine for deformity, trauma, or tumor surgery.

The approach to the lumbar spine allows choice of a flank or hypogastric incision. The hypogastric incision is more cosmetic and may be oriented longitudinally as a paramedian incision, obliquely or horizontally. A paramedian incision allows extensive exposure of the lumbar spine. An oblique incision allows access to two levels. A horizontal hypogastric incision for one-level access will be hidden below the beltline for a lumbo-sacral exposure. The mini-open hypogastric incision is most cosmetic (9).

In contrast to the thoracic spine, incision placement for the lumbar spine more commonly errs in being too high. Because of the lumbar lordosis, visualization of the disk space requires an approach caudal to the vertebral segment of interest (10). Working on a vertebral level straight on adds considerable difficulty if visualization of the posterior disk space is necessary.

B. Seroma and Abscess Formation

Separation of large surface areas in the plane between subcutaneous fat and fascia pro-duces a space at risk for seroma formation. Serous fluids may potentially accumulate within closed areas of lymph-bearing tissues forming pockets that can become infected, secondarily forming an abscess (11). Formation of a seroma in the retroperitoneum is uncommon in anterior lumbar spine surgery, with two retrospective reviews noting one case each, for an incidence of 0.1% (9,12).

If large areas are undermined, placement of closed-suction drains between the subcutaneous fat and fascial layers may be required to prevent seroma formation. Once a seroma has formed, repeat aspiration and pressure dressings are required. Percutaneous placement of a drain is also an option to evacuate fluid until the tissue planes adhere. A retroperitoneal seroma may be drained via computed tomography (CT)–guided needle aspiration (9). A superficial abscess may be evacuated and treated with packing or a drain, while a deep abscess in the retroperitoneum or an emphyema in the chest will require open debridement and parenteral antibiotics.

C. Wound Hematoma

Inadequate hemostasis can lead to formation of a wound hematoma in various potential spaces, including the subcutaneous, fascial, or subfascial layers. The chest wall contains superficial branches of the intercostal artery and veins. The anterior abdominal wall vasculature consists of the superficial epigastric vessels in the subcutaneous layer, the superior and inferior epigastric vessels deep to the rectus abdominus muscle, and laterally the lumbar and circumflex iliac arteries. These vessels are all potential sites for hematoma formation following thoracic and lumbar surgery. Attention to hemostasis of these branches will prevent postoperative hematoma formation

Risk of wound hematoma formation is increased when closure of the incision occurs under the circumstances of hypotension or epinephrine infiltration (11). Both of these instances may lead to an inaccurate assessment of hemostasis. Once the hypotension is eliminated or the epinephrine is metabolized, additional bleeding may occur post-operatively.

As with seromas, wound hematomas serve as a nidus for bacteria, with resultant infection or abscess formation. A wound hematoma interferes with the progression of tissue healing. In the subcutaneous region this may lead to scar formation and a less cosmetic incision. A hematoma in the deeper layers can result in incomplete fascial apposition, delayed healing, wound dehiscence, or hernia formation.

A rectus sheath hematoma can occur with a hypogastric incision following a retro-peritoneal approach to the anterior lumbar spine. The hematoma forms within the closed confines of the anterior and posterior fascial sheaths of the rectus above the arcuate line. Superior or inferior epigastric vessel bleeding within the rectus sheath causes pain that may mimic an acute abdomen. However, bowel sounds are present.

Before the advent of ultrasound and CT, the diagnosis of rectus sheath hematoma was made in less than 30% of cases (11). Sudden, sharp, and progressively severe pain is felt in the side of the abdomen where the bleeding occurs and remains localized. The tender mass does not cross the midline and remains palpable when the patient tenses the rectus muscle (Fothergill's sign). Ecchymosis of the overlying skin appears 3 days after onset.

An incision below the umbilicus and inferior to the arcuate line does not allow for the formation of a rectus sheath hematoma. Here the hematoma can expand by pushing away the peritoneal layer and crossing the midline with less chance of tamponade and "acute abdomen"–type pain.

Once the hematoma forms, treatment depends on the size and time of diagnosis. A rectus sheath hematoma is usually self-limiting, only occasionally requiring evacuation or epigastric vessel ligation. An asymptomatic hematoma diagnosed late during the stage of hematoma organization can be treated with heat to facilitate resolution. A large hema-toma discovered early requires sterile percutaneous or open drainage. Some surgeons advocate ligation of the inferior epigastric artery and vein in every case at the time of the exposure for rectus incisions (13).

D. Wound Dehiscence

In contrast to posterior spine surgery, incisions for anterior spinal surgery must withstand intra-abdominal or intrathoracic pressure during healing. Separation of the fascial layers, or wound dehiscence, is more common with the anterior approach to the lumbar spine. Evisceration indicates dehiscence with extrusion of abdominal contents beyond the confines of the fascial barrier. The incidence of wound dehiscence of abdominal incisions in general surgery is 0.5–3% (11), is more common over the age of 45, and is associated with morbid obesity, diabetes, malnutrition, hypoproteinemia, malignancy, chemotherapy, radiation, uremia, coughing, as well as poor closure technique.

Wound infection or abscess is another factor associated with dehiscence, especially if the infection involves the fascial layer. Wound infection in anterior spinal surgery is not common, as evidenced by two large studies that cited an incidence of 0.4 and 0.6% (9,12). The reported incidence varies considerably depending on diagnosis, procedure, and comorbidities. In deformity surgery of the anterior thoracic and lumbar spine, including neuromuscular disorders, the infection rate has been reported to be 4.8% (14).

Wound dehiscence is distinguished from subcutaneous hematoma by separation of the fascial layers. The diagnostic appearance of a pinkish or salmon-colored fluid draining from the wound is a classic finding in 85% of the cases on the fourth or fifth postoperative day (11). A larger dehiscence will present with obvious evisceration of abdominal contents. Unrecognized, wound dehiscence may present beyond the first postoperative week with wound disruption and evisceration at the time of skin suture removal.

Treatment of wound dehiscence depends upon the timing and presentation. With appropriate and timely treatment overall mortality rates from wound dehiscence are less than 1% (11). Wound dehiscence with evisceration requires urgent intervention. The eviscerated peritoneal contents should be covered with moist sterile towels, while preparation of the operating room is undertaken for exploration and repair of fascia and wound. Perioperative broad-spectrum antibiotics are recommended. Dehiscence without evisceration allows more time for operative planning.

Reclosure of the fascial layer may not always be possible. In these circumstances anterior abdominal retention sutures serve to prevent evisceration with wound healing by secondary intention. In the event that the patient's condition precludes a return to the operating room, dehiscence without evisceration can be treated with a sterile occlusive wound dressing, an abdominal binder to prevent evisceration, and parenteral antibiotics.

Repair of an incisional hernia may be undertaken electively after infection-free wound healing has been achieved and the patient's condition is stable. The incidence of postoperative incisional hernia with wound dehiscence is greater than 30% (11).

E. Abdominal Wall Hernias

An incisional hernia is a late sequaela of wound dehiscence and occurs when there is a deficiency of the fascial layer in the area of incision. The deficiency occurs as a result of dehiscence of the repaired fascial incision postoperatively or as a result of incompetency of the fascial support over time. Postoperative hematoma or infection may contribute to the formation of a hernia. Other associated risk factors include obesity and diabetes. The documented incidence of incisional hernias associated with anterior lumbar spinal surgery using a flank incision is 1% (12) and 0.29% using a mini-open hypogastric incision (9).

Symptoms include abdominal discomfort, which is worse at the end of the day. Incisional hernias generally enlarge over time, and disfigurement may be present. Peritoneal contents can herniate through the defect and become incarcerated or strangulated. Strangulation indicates incarceration with vascular compromise, which is a surgical emergency.

Incisional hernias are among the most difficult to repair. With large abdominal wall hernias, the muscles may lose tone and retract. When atrophy and retraction occur, reapproximation of the fascia is not possible. Edge-to-edge repair of incisional hernias has a 50% recurrence rate, and defects greater than 10 cm have an even higher incidence of recurrence (15). Successful repair of most incisional hernias and all recurrent incisional hernias requires synthetic mesh prostheses. The general surgery literature cites a 10% risk of infection in incisional hernioplasty with prosthetic mesh (15).

F. Muscle Injury

Injury and dysfunction can occur from incision through muscle within the path of approach to the anterior spine. Compromised muscle function results from hematoma formation, dehiscence, and poor technical reapproximation of muscle with wound closure. An incision can cause partial or complete denervation of the muscle.

Although rare, clinically apparent muscle dysfunction has been reported involving the latissimus dorsi muscle and the serratus anterior (16,17). The thoracodorsal nerve arises from the brachial plexus and travels deep to the subscapularis innervating the latissimus dorsi proximally. The long thoracic nerve lying in the midaxillary line innervates the underlying serratus anterior. Documented case reports cite postoperative ipsilateral shoulder elevation and winging of the scapula due to weakness and denervation of the latissimus and serratus anterior muscles (16). Rupture of the latissimus dorsi after thoracotomy or thoracoabdominal incisions has been reported as acute and delayed (17). Acute rupture is generally due to inadequate repair. Delayed rupture is often secondary to debilitating conditions such as chronic renal failure or malignancy. Rupture of the latissimus produces a fusiform soft tissue mass below the scapula. It is associated with weakness of shoulder extension, internal rotation, and adduction. This complication is self-limited and usually does not require repair. Over time the cosmetic deformity improves and the pectoralis major, teres major, deltoid, and subscapularis muscles compensate for the weakness associated with loss of latissimus function. Limited disability from loss of latissimus function has supported sacrifice of this muscle in reconstructive free flap surgery. Likewise, the cosmetic deformity and limited disability of a winged scapula is generally untreated.

Incisional modifications have been proposed in the literature to avoid incision in the latissimus and serratus anterior muscles. A muscle-sparing incision with mobilization of the latissimus dorsi and the serratus anterior allows retraction of the muscle fibers without division (18). A very limited thoracotomy through the auscultatory triangle has also been described (19).

III. LUNG, PLEURAL, AND DIAPHRAGMATIC COMPLICATIONS

A. Injury to the Lung

A significant injury to the lung parenchyma would be unexpected in anterior thoracic spine surgery. The lung parenchyma is, however, at risk for injury during intercostal incision into the pleural cavity and while dissecting around the thoracic spine with the lung packed towards the midline. Potential complications include pneumothorax, pleural effusion, hemothorax, and diaphragm dysfunction or rupture.

The capacity of the lung for healing a small injury is excellent (20). An inadvertent laceration of the lung during incision of the parietal pleura will create an air leak and bleeding. An air leak from the lung risks potential tension pneumothorax postoperatively, which will quickly seal on its own with standard thoracostomy tube treatment. Rarely does bleeding from a small lung laceration require suturing, as the bleeding will clot rapidly, especially with the lung packed.

B. Pneumothorax

During the intercostal approach to the anterior thoracic spine the pleural space is exposed. Evacuation of air postoperatively through a thoracostomy tube prevents pneumothorax. Lung re-expansion and cessation of air leakage occur within a few days. A small residual pneumothorax after chest tube removal is not considered a complication. Residual air within the pleural space will reabsorb over several days. Two separate studies cite the incidence of significant pneumothorax after discontinuation of chest tubes in anterior thoracic surgery for spinal deformity at 1.8 and 4% (12,14). Bronchopleural fistula is a rare complication of anterior approach to the thoracic spine. The one reported case study was treated successfully with a thoracostomy tube (14) and suction.

C. Pleural Effusion and Hemothorax

A significant collection of fluid or blood within the pleural cavity may complicate anterior thoracic spine surgery and requires drainage. A chest radiograph reveals opacification at the lung base and blunting of the costovertebral angle. Fluid will have a meniscus best seen on the lateral view. A phenomenon known as subpulmonary trapping may give the appearance of an elevated hemidiaphragm but no blunting of the costovertebral angle, hiding a large hemothorax (20). A lateral decubitus x-ray will help confirm the diagnosis of a hemothorax.

Postoperative drainage of 500 mLs total or 100 mL per hour over 5 hours raises the index of suspicion of a surgically correctable lesion. Both the rate and character of bleeding is important in deciding upon thoracotomy with exploration. Bleeding from the vena cava, aorta, or intercostal vessels must be considered when drainage is significant. Hemothorax from a dissecting aortic aneurysm or from an avulsed intercostal artery after anterior thoracic spine surgeries have been documented as sources of bleeding (21).

D. Tension Pneumothorax

A tension pneumothorax may occur postoperatively as a result of laceration to the lung or chest tube occlusion or malfunction. Air accumulates in the closed intrathoracic cavity, creating increased pressure, which results in shifting of the mediastinum and displacement of major vessels; this decreases venous return and causes cardiovascular collapse. Dilated neck veins, hyperresonance of the chest field, and mediastinal shift on radiograph are noted. Immediate release of pleural pressure is required with needle decompression and chest tube insertion.

E. Open Pneumothorax

An open pneumothorax might result from a central venous catheter insertion attempt, incompetent closure, or dehiscence of the thoracotomy or air leakage around an existing chest tube. Signs and symptoms include a "sucking sound" on inspiration at the affected site with signs of reduced venous return–neck vein distension and tachycardia.

Immediately apply a sterile occlusive dressing over the site and observe closely for signs and symptoms of the development of a tension pneumothorax. The chest wound closure may need revision.

F. Diaphragm Dysfunction and Rupture

The anterior thoracolumbar spine approach requires incision into the diaphragm for simultaneous exposure of the thoracic and retroperitoneal cavities. The standard incision into the diaphragm lies in its periphery; incision towards the central portion of the diaphragm may disrupt branches of the phrenic nerve, resulting in paralysis of the hemidiaphragm (22). A poor technical repair, postoperative infection, and significant comorbidities can contribute to impairment in the integrity of the diaphragm. Factors that cause disruption of the diaphragm are similar to those that precipitate hernia formation. Adequate technical repair of the diaphragm is required to prevent rupture.

A chest radiograph will illustrate the gastric bubble or nasogastric tube within the region of the pleural space, and bowel sounds may be heard over the lung field. Urgent repair of a massive diaphragmatic rupture is necessary if high-volume herniation of abdominal contents into the chest prevents adequate ventilation (20). Progressive displacement over several days in an acute rupture with increasing gaseous distention of the herniated stomach results in respiratory compromise and requires reduction of the abdominal viscera with repair of the diaphragmatic defect. Exploration, reduction, and repair of the diaphragm can be accomplished early through a retroperitoneal approach.

Late rupture of the diaphragm may lead to gradual herniation through a small defect; respiratory compromise may not manifest. A delayed presentation may require a transthoracic approach to free any adhesions that may have formed in the pleural space with the abdominal viscera prior to the reduction (20). Repair usually can be accomplished by direct suture, but a prosthetic patch of nonabsorbable material occasionally is required (20).

IV. COMPLICATIONS OF ABDOMINAL VISCERA

A. Peritoneal Complications and Bowel Perforation

Peritoneal perforation is common with retroperitoneal approaches and usually is not clinically significant. The peritoneum has the capacity for rapid healing of any defects. An inadvertent breech of the peritoneal layer is generally repaired primarily at the time of injury. Adhesion formation from peritoneal repair alone is not common. Adhesions and scarring occur with osteomyelitis of the vertebral body, retroperitoneal sarcoma, and prior radiation treatment (10).

Ileus after retroperitoneal surgery usually resolves within 3 days. The incidence of an ileus that required nasogastric decompression beyond 3 days varied from 0.6% in one review to 6% in another (9,14). Adhesion formation and ileus are more common with a transperitoneal approach to the lumbar spine than a retroperitoneal approach (23). Intraperitoneal adhesions form secondary to inflammation and hypoxemia associated with traumatic handling and retraction of the abdominal viscera; infection also contributes to adhesion formation. Adhesions appear around the 10th postoperative day and become maximal at around 3–4 weeks. Over time attenuation of adhesions occurs. Reoperation of an intraperitoneal approach becomes very difficult around the 3rd or 4th week secondary to postoperative adhesions (23).

Although bowel injury is uncommon, the sigmoid colon is the section of bowel most at risk during anterior retroperitoneal approach to the lower lumbar and sacral spine. Anterior to the sacral spine the colon transitions from an intraperitoneal to a retroperitoneal location. A single report of bowel injury during retroperitoneal approach to the lumbosacral spine involved the sigmoid colon (24).

The duodenum is also located in the retroperitoneum anterior to the spine around the level of T12-L1. There is potential for bowel injury here during anterior thoracolumbar surgery, although there were no reports of duodenal injury in the case series reviewed.

Bowel perforation during anterior spinal surgery requires immediate evacuation of contaminant through lavage and intravenous antibiotics. Injured bowel must be isolated and appropriately repaired or colostomy performed (23). The spinal procedure may need to be abandoned in the presence of significant contamination. Peritonitis may result from an injury to the bowel. Postoperative peritonitis raises the suspicion of unrecognized bowel perforation. Delayed diagnosis of bowel injury carries a high mortality rate.

B. Pancreas

The pancreas along with the duodenum is located deep within the retroperitoneal space. The glandular tissue of the pancreas is arched over the abdominal aorta at the level of the superior mesenteric artery and left renal artery and vein. It lies at the second lumbar vertebral body. The pancreas is reflected toward the midline along with peritoneum and the kidney with exposure of the upper lumbar spine.

Pancreatitis secondary to anterior spinal surgery is very rare. Two reports of pancreatitis following anterior spine surgery appear in the literature (24,25). No significant trauma to the pancreas was identified and the cause was determined by exclusion. Direct injury to the pancreas due to surgical trauma or retraction may result in a chemical pancreatitis.

Signs and symptoms of pancreatic injury are nonspecific, and while an elevated amylase correlates with the diagnosis of pancreatitis, a further diagnostic workup is warranted to exclude other more common causes such as biliary calculi. A preoperative history of alcohol use is a predisposing factor and use of narcotics has been noted to cause spasm of the sphincter of Oddi.

C. Spleen and Liver

The spleen lies within the peritoneum on the left side below the diaphragm at the upper lumbar spine. Injury during exposure of the spine is rare. There is a solitary case report of injury to the spleen as a complication of anterior spine surgery (26). Careful handling of the spleen during reflection of the peritoneum and retractor placement will avoid contusion or hematoma during anterior exposure of the upper lumbar spine and thoraco-lumbar region.

There are no reports of injury to the liver in the spine literature. Approach to the anterior spine is almost exclusively left-sided, avoiding any potential risk to the liver. A right-sided approach with injury to the liver may result in laceration to the liver par-enchyma. Treatment of approach-related injury to the spleen or liver parenchyma consists of control of bleeding and observation with rare clinical consequence.

V. GENITOURINARY COMPLICATIONS

A. Injury to the Ureter

Of all urological structures, the ureter is at greatest risk of injury during retroperitoneal dissection. Despite its proximity to the lumber spine, the incidence of ureteral injury is low and may go unrecognized at the time of surgery. Several large retrospective reviews reported no cases of ureteral injury. One case of ureteral injury in a series representing an incidence of 0.1% involved a same-side revision retroperitoneal exposure (12). Failure of identification of the ureter may result in partial or complete ureter laceration, inadvertent suture ligation, vascular clipping or crush injury from clamping or faulty retractor blade placement. This can occur especially during urgent repair of a vascular injury through limited retroperitoneal exposure (27). Preoperative stent placement is a useful adjunct in identification and protection of the ureter in morbidly obese patients or those with suspected retroperitoneal scarring undergoing a retroperitoneal approach to the spine.

The ureter lies lateral to the aorta on the left and lateral to the vena cava on the right. In the retroperitoneal space it rests atop the psoas muscle and just lateral to the tips of the transverse processes of the lower lumbar vertebra. It has been noted in lean persons to lie directly on the anterior longitudinal ligament in the groove between the psoas muscle and vertebral body (27). The ureter may be adherent to the peritoneal layer causing it to be elevated from the psoas muscle as the peritoneum is mobilized and retracted medially. The ureter crosses anterior to the common iliac arteries just proximal to the point of bifurcation into the internal and external iliac arteries. It is enveloped in fatty tissue and is distinguished from artery or nerve by observation of peristaltic contractions in its muscular wall (27).

During retroperitoneal approach to the lumbar spine some surgeons advocate reflection of the ipsilateral ureter medially and anteriorly with the peritoneal sac (10). Alternatively, the ureter may also be preserved and protected in its position overlying the psoas muscle during the retroperitoneal approach (9). In the transperitoneal approach the ureter is often not visualized or exposed unless it is lying close to the midline.

Injury to the ureter most commonly results in flank pain, fever, and ileus. Hematuria is present in only 11% of ureteral injuries (28). Leakage of urine into the retroperitoneal space without significant obstruction is generally subtle. Five percent of patients with ureteral injury may be asymptomatic, with diagnosis of hydronephrosis and nonfunctioning kidney reported years later (29). The diagnosis of ureteral injury is established by demonstration and localization of urinary extravasation or high-grade obstruction on imaging studies. Analysis of aspirated retroperitoneal fluid can distinguish a urinoma from a seroma or lymphocele.

An injury to the ureter suspected at the time of surgery can be confirmed or localized with the administration of intravenous indigo carmine dye. Diagnosed postoperatively, a ureteral injury is treated with an indwelling ureteral stent or open repair.

B. Sterility and Impotence

Retrograde ejaculation is a potential complication that results in sterility in male patients undergoing anterior spinal surgery at the lumbosacral region. Retrograde ejaculation occurs from lack of sympathetic innervation to the internal vesicle sphincter at the bladder neck with semen propelled backwards into the bladder at the time of ejaculation. Although of low incidence, male patients planning to have children need to consider the risk of sterility. This complication is of even greater concern in pediatric or adolescent patients undergoing anterior lumbosacral surgery. The sympathetic nerve fibers known as the superior hypogastric plexus that control the internal bladder sphincter are located in the retroperitoneum anterior to the L5-S1 region between the bifurcation of the iliac vessels.

The incidence of retrograde ejaculation after anterior spinal surgery has been debated in numerous studies and has been reported to be as high as 6% (30) and as low as 0% (31). Rajaraman et al. reported an incidence of 3%. Recently, Sasso et al. reported a 10-fold increase in retrograde ejaculation with a transperitoneal approach to the lumbosacral spine compared to the retroperitoneal exposure with an incidence of 10% versus 0.86%, respectively (32). Faciszewski et al. reported an incidence of 0.5% of all cases with retroperitoneal exposure (12). Brau noted a 0.3% incidence with one case of retrograde ejaculation out of 345 male patients with retroperitoneal exposure (9).

Avoidance of this complication by gentle blunt dissection without use of electrocautery of the soft tissues anterior to the L5-S1 disk space is recommended. Access to the L5-S1 interspace without injury to sympathetic function of the superior hypogastric plexus will thus be achieved without trauma to these fine nerve fibers. Treatment consists of observation, as many patients will recover antegrade ejaculation. Flynn et al. reported recovery in one third of the patients within 6 months (33). Rajaraman et al. reported recovery in one of two cases by 15 months (24). Preoperatively, sperm donation can be considered in male patients planning to father children after surgery.

Erection is controlled by the parasympathetic nerves of the second, third, and fourth sacral segments. The parasympathetic nerves regulate blood flow in the venous plexus at the base of the penis. Impotence or inability to obtain or maintain erection may occur if there is injury to these parasympathetic nerves. This complication is independent and unrelated to retrograde ejaculation. Impotence after approach to the anterior lumbosacral spine is unrelated to the surgery, as the second, third, and fourth sacral nerves are well beyond the field of exposure.

In an anectodal retrospective survey of worldwide spine surgeons by Flynn and Price, the rate of impotence after spinal surgery was 0.44% (33). They also noted that the rate of impotence after anterior spinal surgery was higher among Frenchmen compared to other nationalities (33). The survey concluded, however, that impotence was found to be no more common in anterior versus posterior spinal surgery and that the cause was nonorganic (31,33). Faciszewski et al. reported a 0.8% incidence of impotence, which was higher than the reported rate of retrograde ejaculation (12). Overall, there is no supporting physiological evidence that impotence after anterior lumbosacral surgery is secondary to neurological injury and in general is psychogenic.

C. Injury to Kidney

Injury to the kidney during anterior approach to the spine is unexpected and not reported in the literature. Surgery in the region of the upper lumbar and thoracolumbar junction of the spine requires dissection around the kidney. The kidney is mobilized toward the midline along with the peritoneum. Injury in the form of blunt trauma from retraction or a minor cortical laceration may result in a Grade I or II injury to the kidney. Grades III through V injuries generally result from significant trauma or severe penetrating injury (34). Grade I and II injuries are generally managed with control of bleeding through tamponade and without need for operative repair. Late injury to the kidney after anterior spinal surgery in the form of hydronephrosis may result as a sequelae of ureteral injury as noted above.

D. Bladder and Urinary Complications

The bladder lies deep in the pelvis behind the pubic symphysis. This location renders it unlikely to be injured during an anterior approach to the lumbosacral spine. Spinal surgery rarely extends beyond the pelvic brim. There are no reports of clinically significant direct bladder injury due to the surgical approach to the spine in the literature. Direct trauma from retractor placement may cause minimal bladder contusion. Complications involving micturition, however, do occur.

Normal micturition is not possible without functioning of the nervi erigentes. Innervation to the bladder consists of efferent parasympathetic nerves from sacral segments two, three, and four to the detrusor muscle for contraction and sphincter vesicae for inhibition. Excessive traction on these nerves may result from retraction or packing the bladder downwards during exposure of anterior sacrum (35).

Urinary retention is common following spine surgery and may or may not be related to the approach. In most cases this resolves within the first week postoperatively and may not be considered a complication unless it persists. Treatment for urinary retention secondary to neuropraxia of the parasympathetic nerves requires a self-catheterization program pending recovery of bladder control. The incidence of urinary tract infection and need for antibiotics is increased with urinary retention and need for prolonged or repeated catheterization.

Urinary incontinence as a complication is unrelated to an anterior spine approach and noted in only a single case of neurogenic spine deformity surgery (14). Imaging studies of the spinal canal may be indicated to exclude other causes.

VI. LYMPHATIC COMPLICATIONS

A. Chylothorax

Thoracic duct injury is an uncommon complication to anterior thoracic spine surgery (37). The thoracic duct, azygos, and hemiazygos venous systems lie within the posterior mediastinum. The thoracic duct and azygous veins lie to the right side of the aorta, which provides protection during the left-sided approach. The hemiazygos vein lies along the left and has a more varied pattern. The thoracic duct proceeds cephalad, crosses over the midline from right to left in the upper thorax, and empties into the venous system at the junction of the left internal jugular and subclavian veins. Complications related to a profuse venous bleed from the azygous system can be difficult to control. The thoracic duct is most at risk in the upper thoracic spine; inadvertent injury may occur during dissection and attempts at hemostasis. Repair of the thoracic duct can be undertaken at the time of surgery, but ligation may be necessary to prevent leakage of this thin-walled structure. A delay in diagnosis may result in chronic duct leakage into the pleural cavity with formation of a chylothorax.

B. Chyloretroperitoneum

A significant amount of lymphatic tissue exists within the retroperitoneal space. Lymphatic drainage of the retroperitoneum moves in a cephalad direction towards the cisterna chyli. From the cisterna chyli lymph drains into the thoracic duct, which passes under the median arcuate ligament of the diaphragm and into the posterior mediastinum to the right of the aorta. This process may be disrupted in the retroperitoneum as well as in the chest.

The rare complication of chyloretroperitoneum can result from disruption of these lymphatic channels during extensive dissection within the retroperitoneum. The discovery of clear drainage warrants further investigation and a fluid analysis to rule out urinoma or seroma.

In a review of 1123 patients who underwent anterior spinal surgery, one patient (0.1%) presented with clear drainage 4 months after anterior fusion from L2 to S1. Two thousand seven hundred milliliters of lymphatic fluid was drained percutaneously with CT guidance. The patient was successfully treated with sclerosing therapy using tetracycline and half-strength Betadine. The retroperitoneaum was also drained for 4 months for complete resolution of the lymphocele (12).

VII. PERIPHERAL, AUTONOMIC, AND CENTRAL NEUROLOGICAL COMPLICATIONS

A. Intercostal Nerve Injury

A common approach-related complication of thoracotomy is severe radicular intercostal pain. When described as postthoracotomy pain syndrome it connotes moderate or severe pain, persisting beyond the usual course of postoperative pain, in the distribution of the intercostal nerves. Injury to the intercostal nerve may occur from blunt trauma or retraction, laceration, coagulation and ligation of bleeding intercostal vessels, or inadvertent suture ligation during wound closure.

Pain persisting for longer than 6 months occurred in as many as 9% of patients after thoracotomy for anterior spine surgery (12). Treatment consists of analgesics or an intercostal nerve block injection. Injection of a long-acting local anesthetic applied posteriorly along the inferior edge of the rib may be repeated daily for several days.

B. Stellate Ganglion Injury

The stellate ganglion is at risk of injury during approach to the upper thoracic spine. The sympathetic trunk and ganglia lie lateral to the spine with the stellate ganglion at the level of the T1 vertebra. Injury to the stellate ganglion and sympathetic nerves results in an ipsilateral facial anhydrosis, ptosis, and meiosis (Horner's syndrome). Of 42 thoracotomies extending to the T1 or T2 levels, there was a 7% occurrence rate of Horner's syndrome; of these 3 cases none resolved (12). Dissection lateral to the upper thoracic spine and T1 level and use of electrocautery in this area is to be avoided. Meiosis may be treated intermittently with use of ophthalmological drops.

C. Subcostal, Iliohypogastric, and Ilioinguinal Nerves

Nerves of the anterior abdominal wall include the anterior and lateral branches of the intercostals (T7–T11), subcostal (T12), iliohypogastric (L1), and ilioinguinal (L1). These nerves radiate around to the anterior abdomen angling in a caudal direction. Flank incisions for the retroperitoneal approach to the lumbar spine may cross one of these branches. Postoperatively a patient may experience numbness, paresthesia, or dysesthesia in the anterior abdomen, hypogastric, inguinal, or anterior medial thigh regions innervated by these nerves. The ilioinguinal nerve lies above the iliac crest and has been affected by incisions for iliac crest bone harvesting, as is the case for the lateral femoral cutaneous nerve (38). Treatment is generally conservative and in the majority of cases symptoms resolve within 6 months (24). Nerve blocks or neurectomy may be employed in rare cases of unremitting neuralgia.

D. Genitofemoral and Femoral Nerve Injury

Neuropraxia of the genitofemoral or femoral nerve may occur from anterior exposure of the lumbar spine. The genitofemoral nerve lies on top of the psoas muscle, lateral to the lumbar spine. The femoral nerve is deep to the psoas. Although uncommon, neuropraxia may result during retroperitoneal exposure by retraction or compression on the psoas. The genitofemoral nerve by location is more susceptible to direct pressure, and thus it appears that any neuropraxia of the femoral nerve by direct pressure would also involve genitofemoral injury.

Neuropraxia or injury to the genitofemoral nerve produces numbness along the ipsilateral inguinal, proximal anterior thigh, and groin regions. Femoral nerve palsy results in postoperative numbness in the anterior thigh, absence of patellar reflex, and quadriceps weakness. Femoral nerve palsy has been reported in two cases of retroperitoneal exposure of the lumbar spine (39). Neuropraxic injury to the genitofemoral or femoral nerves is expected to resolve within 3–6 months. Physical rehabiliation will avoid muscle atrophy during recovery.

Papastefanou et al. illustrated through cadaver dissection that the most likely cause of femoral nerve palsy during anterior spinal surgery occurs as a result of tight constriction of the nerve by the psoas muscle when the lumbar spine is immobile and the hip is positioned in extension for long periods of time as opposed to direct pressure or hematoma (39).

Hematoma within the iliacus is another cause of femoral nerve neuropraxia. Hematoma location affecting the femoral nerve has been documented between the periosteum and the iliacus muscle, in the iliopsoas muscle, between the psoas muscle and the fascia of the iliacus and in the groove between the psoas and the iliacus muscles before they join to form a common tendon (39). These are all locations that are generally not involved in exposure of the anterior lumbosacral spine.

E. Injury to the Sympathetic Chain, Obturator Nerve, and Lumbar Plexus

The lumbar sympathetic chain is located lateral to the vertebral body. Sympathetic chain injury is generally self-limiting with resolution of symptoms within 4–6 months. Post-sympathectomy neuralgia is a syndrome defined as a burning or deep aching pain in the proximal part of the leg, groin, and anterior thigh persisting for greater than 6 months. Uncommonly long-term symptoms of dysesthesias and paresthesias to the ipsilateral lower extremity may result (24). As a complication to anterior spine surgery the reported incidence of symptoms in one large series was 0.43% (12).

More commonly, an injury to the sympathetic chain produces the postoperative phenomenon of a contralateral cold foot. A lack of vasoconstriction to the leg in which the sympathetic nerves were injured produces a warm leg on the ipsilateral side that gives the impression that the opposite foot has become cold. Intact pulses in the contralateral "cold" foot are important to confirm that the symptoms are not of vascular thrombotic origin (10).

The obturator nerve innervates the adductor muscles of the medial thigh. It arises from L2, 3, and 4 and lies lateral to the vertebral body in the groove between the vertebral body and psoas muscle. Injury to the obturator nerve is manifested by weakness of hip adduction. Both the obturator nerve and sympathetic chain are at risk of injury during dissection lateral to the left common iliac vein for exposure of anterior L4-L5 disc space. The obturator nerve passes anterior to the iliolumbar and ascending lumbar veins. The sympathetic chain passes posterior to these veins. There may also be an accessory obturator nerve lateral to the main obturator nerve. Distinguishing the obturator and sympathetic nerves from the vascular branches is necessary for their protection. The L4-L5 region is an area of potential massive bleeding during exposure, and difficult visualization during hemostasis may risk injury to these nerves from ligatures, vascular clips, or electrocautery (40). Obturator nerve injury may require focused physical rehabilitation. Hip adductor weakness may not be apparent with intact accessory obturator innervation.

The lumbar plexus, composed of nerve roots L2 through L5, passes deep to the psoas muscle. This is beyond the field of exposure in anterior lumbar spine surgery cases. Straying lateral to the pedicle or retracting the psoas risks injury to the plexus and significant paresis to the lower extremity (10). The psoas may require some retraction in the upper lumbar spine especially if it is hypertrophic and obscures the lateral verebral body (10). Care must be taken to avoid dissection beyond the lateral margin of the disk and pedicle and to avoid excessive pressure on the psoas.

There is one documented report of lumbar plexus injury with ipsilateral quadricep and hamstring weakness as a complication of exposure lateral to the vertebral body and deep to the psoas muscle (12). Isolated nerve root injuries have also been noted due to lateral graft impingement (12). Recovery of strength depends upon the extent of injury. Extensive physical rehabilitation may be required.

F. Spinal Cord and Cauda Equina Injury

Complications of direct trauma or vascular insult to the spinal cord are of major concern in anterior approaches to the thoracic spine. Paraplegia after anterior thoracic spine surgery in patients without preoperative paralysis generally occurs from spinal cord impingement. One large series cited an incidence of 0.2%, both cases from cord impingement by bone graft migration or kyphotic instability (12). Anterior lumbar spinal exposure alone presents little risk to the dura and cauda equina. Three large series of anterior lumbar spine surgery had no dural or cauda equina injuries (9,12,14).

Vascular insult to the spinal cord is theorized from ligation of the posterior intercostal arteries near the thoracic spine during anterior exposure. This concern is greatest in the T9-T10 region where the artery of Adamkiewicz is considered to be the major anterior radicular artery to the spinal cord. One prominent study noted no neurological injuries from spinal cord infarction (41); Winter et al. reviewed 1197 cases of anterior spinal surgery in the region of T1 through L3 with no resultant paraplegias as a result of segmental vessel ligation despite an earlier study by Apel et al. noting three cases of paraplegia from anterior spinal surgery for congenital kyphoscoliosis (42). Westfall et al. also reported no cases of spinal cord ischemia as a result of ligation of multiple segmental arteries on one side of the vertebral column in 85 cases of anterior spinal deformity surgery (14).

Segmental artery ligation in anterior exposure of the spine is recommended unilaterally at the midvertebral body level, in the convexity of a scoliotic curve, and with the avoidance of hypotensive anesthesia to prevent the possibility of spinal cord ischemia (41). The segmental vessels on the convex side of a scoliosis are generally smaller and more attenuated. Radicular branches to the spinal cord enter through the intervertebral foramen, and thus ligation and electrocautery should be avoided in proximity to the neuroforamen. Collateral circulation from the contralateral segmental artery may thus remain in continuity with the dorsal branch of the ipsilateral intercostal artery entering the neuroforamen.

Some surgeons have advocated clamping of segmental arteries with spinal cord monitoring prior to ligation. This has not been universally adopted as necessary in most cases. Patients at greatest risk include those with significant deformity or kyphosis, multiple surgeries, need for corpectomy, spinal cord compression, or preoperative neurological deficit (41). Preoperative angiography has not been shown to be definitive in predicting risk of neurological compromise from segmental vessel ligation (41,42).

VIII. VASCULAR COMPLICATIONS

A. Incidence and Type of Vascular Complication

Anterior spine surgery requires mobilization and retraction of major vascular structures. As such, vascular injuries in anterior thoracic and lumbar spine surgery are among the most common approach-related complications. The commonly used left-sided approach to the spine places the aorta in closer proximity to the field of dissection. However, the aorta is more elastic and less susceptible to injury from mobilization than the vena cava.

Factors contributing to difficulties during exposure include adhesion to the major vessels anterior to the spine associated with vertebral osteomyelitis, inflammatory disk disease and osteophytic ridging, old fractures, and revision surgery (10). Vascular disease and aging cause the aorta to become tortuous and calcified rendering it less elastic and less resistant to injury from retraction. Vessel injury can occur from direct laceration or trauma from retraction and pressure. Injury may be acute with profuse bleeding or delayed as with intimal injuries; examples include vessel injury from the edge of a retrator blade and injury during insertion of a pin retractor.

The reported incidence of vascular injury ranges from 0.8 to 18.4% (9,12,21,24,43,44). Pertinent findings within these studies are reviewed in detail.

A large retrospective review of 1223 cases by Facizewski et al. (12) noted three injuries: one to the aorta and two to the ascending lumbar vein. The incidence of vascular injury was lower than in other studies, but also represented the only instance of a direct laceration to the aorta.

In contrast, Brau reported on 686 cases of retroperitoneal exposure of the lumbar spine via a hypogastric approach through the rectus sheath with 12 cases of vascular injury (9). Half of the vascular complications were arterial and half venous. The six arterial injuries were all thrombotic: four left common iliac artery thromboses, two common femoral thromboses. The cases of thrombosis of the iliac artery were discovered intra-operatively and treated with arteriotomy and thrombectomy. An intimal tear was noted on one of these. The two femoral arterial injuries manifested postoperatively as a pulseless, cold left leg, both undergoing left femoral thrombectomy and left leg fasciotomies. Of the six venous injuries, all involved injury to the left common iliac vein. Intraoperative repair of the left common iliac vein was performed in all six cases with related blood loss ranging from 300 to 900 cc. The venous complications presented intraoperatively with profuse bleeding, whereas arterial injuries were thrombotic in nature, sometimes presenting late. The left common iliac artery and vein represented the main vessels at risk in anterior lumbar surgery especially in the region of L4 to S1, which encompassed 82% of patients within the study. It is also of note that thrombotic complications to the iliac artery were all discovered intraoperatively by direct inspection.

Similarly, Harmon (43) reported eight vascular injuries, and Rajaraman et al. (24) reported four in their retrospective reviews of anterior lumbar spinal surgery. All vascular injuries in both studies were venous.

A review of anterior thoracic and lumbar spine surgery by Oskouian and Johnson noted five thrombotic vascular complications and seven direct vascular injuries (21). The five thrombotic complications involved deep venous thromboses of the common iliac. Of the seven direct vascular injuries, five were venous injuries presenting acutely: three to the common iliac vein in patients with retroperitoneal scarring from previous surgery and two to the inferior vena cava in patients with osteomyelitis. The other two vascular injuries were arterial, and both presented in a delayed fashion. Both of these patients had undergone anterior thoracotomy. One patient sustained an avulsed intercostal artery, which bled 2 days postoperatively, requiring reoperation and ligation. The second arterial complication involved a dissecting thoracic aortic aneurysm that ruptured and was fatal. On postmortem the aneurysm was found to correspond to an area of aorta wall calcification, which was retracted during anterior spine surgery.

The direct venous injuries within this study all involved the inferior vena cava or common iliac vein in the region of L3 through L5. In addition, the five cases of deep venous thrombosis all involved the common iliac vein after L4-L5 surgery. The arterial injuries both presented in a delayed fashion, and both occurred in the thoracic region. This study highlights retroperitoneal scarring from previous surgery and osteomyelitis as risk factors to venous injuries as well as age-related vascular disease with wall calcification as a risk factor for aortic injury in approaches to the anterior spine (21).

A review by Baker et al. compared retroperitoneal approach by hypogastric incision to retroperitoneal approach by flank incision in anterior lumbar spine surgery (44). They found a higher incidence of vascular injury, 18.4%, associated with hypogastric incision as compared to 7.7% in flank incision approaches. Of the 16 vascular injuries, 12 occurred during the exposure of the spine. Vascular injuries requiring repair consisted of 11 tears to the common iliac vein, 4 tears to the inferior vena cava, and one avulsion of the iliolumbar vein. No arterial injuries occurred. The flank incision consisted of an anterolateral approach to the retroperitoneum through the external oblique, internal oblique, and transversus abdominis muscles. The hypogastric incision consisted of approach to the retroperitoneum with a paramedian incision through the rectus sheath and around the rectus abdominis muscle. Twenty-six cases were approached through the flank and 76 through the hypogastric incision. Although many more patients underwent hypogastric incision, the percentage of vascular injury was more than twice that with the anterolateral incision. The authors attributed this to a smaller incision and more limited operative field when using a hypogastric incision. The study also noted that the exposure of the spine was the most hazardous part of the operation with regard to vascular complications (44).

The region of the fourth lumbar vertebra is an area where the vena cava and left common iliac vein are most at risk for injury. A left-sided approach with exposure of the L4-L5 interspace requires mobilization of the aorta, iliac artery, vena cava, and left common iliac vein with retraction to the right side of L4. Tethering this are the iliolumbar vessels and ascending lumbar branches, which renders these vessels relatively immobile.

The left common iliac vein is at risk of injury during exposure of the L5-S1 disk space. Exposing the area within the bifurcation of the vena cava into the iliac vessels requires mobilization and retraction of the left common iliac vein superior and laterally as it is commonly draped across the L5-S1 disk. Injury to the left common iliac requires proximal and distal control and repair of the perforation.

B. Intercostal, Lumbar, and Middle Sacral Vessel Complications

Mobilization of the aorta and vena cava requires ligation and division of segmental arteries and veins. Intercostal vessels in the thorax and lumbar vessels within the retroperitoneum represent potential sources of bleeding. Intercostal and lumbar arteries are high-pressure conduits in direct communication with the descending aorta. Laceration or injury from the trauma of retraction can occur with arterial wall spasm. Delayed bleeding may result when spasm is relieved postoperatively resulting in significant bleeding (21). Segmental vessels should be handled carefully. Those that have been divided or placed under tension of retraction should be ligated even if not currently bleeding.

The middle sacral artery and vein are also located within the bifurcation of the iliac vessels overlying the L5-S1 level. These vessels are generally smaller than lumbar segmental vessels, are often easily accessible, and less susceptible to injury. They have not been identified as major sources of vascular complication. However, there may be more than one tributary, and occasionally they are larger than average. Ligation and division of all branches is necessary for safe access to the anterior L5-S1 region.

C. Iliolumbar Vein and Ascending Lumbar Vein Complications

Consistently problematic vessels during the approach to the L4-L5 disk are the iliolumbar and ascending lumbar veins. The iliolumbar vein is a segmental vein at the level of the fifth lumbar vertebra. The iliolumbar vein can be a source of massive hemorrhage as it directly communicates with the common iliac vein. These veins act as tethers for retraction of the left common iliac vein toward the midline and are prone to avulsion and sidewall injury of the common iliac vein. Control of these veins is necessary to mobilize and retract the inferior vena cava and left iliac vein toward the midline.

Variations of the iliolumbar vein have been documented in cadaver dissections (40). The obturator nerve crossed superficial to the iliolumbar vein in all dissections. The lumbar sympathetic trunk passed deep to the iliolumbar vein in all specimens except one, in which it was superficial. Eleven of the 16 specimens demonstrated one main stem iliolumbar vein with the ascending lumbar vein arising off of the iliolumbar. Five of the 16 dissections contained two iliolumbar veins; a proximal and distal accessory vein approximately 3 cm apart draining into the left common iliac vein. In two specimens the ascending lumbar vein drained directly into the left common iliac vein separate from and proximal to the iliolumbar vein.

Ligating the iliolumbar vein can be difficult. The main stem of the iliolumbar vein in some patients is as short as 0.5 cm and as wide as 1 cm between the common iliac vein and tributaries of the iliolumbar. In addition, the proximity of the obturator nerve and lumbar sympathetic chain adds difficulty in this crowded space. As such, electrocautery is not recommended for control of these veins. All tributaries may need to be ligated or clipped prior to division of the iliolumbar vein.

In the case of iliolumbar vein avulsion, the bleeding may be massive and sudden. The iliolumbar vein is a direct conduit from the valveless area of the common iliac vein and vena cava. Direct pressure on the vena cava and common iliac vein is necessary to control bleeding and identify the site for repair.

D. Anatomical Variations in Retroperitoneal Vasculature

The retroperitoneal vasculature anterior to the lumbosacral junction has been the subject of numerous anatomical studies. In a venous anatomy of 440 surgical cases, Harmon (45) noted that the bifurcation of the vena cava into the right and left common iliac veins occurred atop the middle of L4-L5 disk space in the majority of cases. High bifurcation of the vena cava occurring above the L4-L5 disk space occurred in only 9% of cases, whereas low bifurcation below the mid L5-S1 disk space occurred in 4%. The bifurcation into the right and left common iliac arteries was one vertebral segment above the bifurcation of the iliac veins. In only 1% of cases was the L4-L5 disk accessible between the bifurcations of the iliac vessels in the midline, due to a high bifurcation of the common iliac vein at the L3 vertebra. Conversely, reflection of the left iliac vessels to the right for approach to the L5-S1 disk space was necessary in only 5% of the cases. Elasticity of the arterial walls permitted a greater degree of safe retraction as compared to veins. Other anatomical variations included the vena cava and iliacs lying to the left of the vertebra at the lumbosacral junction, extremely large left common iliac veins, large middle sacral veins, or left iliolumbar tributaries.

Recent studies of vascular anatomy anterior to the lumbosacral region on arteriograms and venograms provided documentation that approximately 14% of patients had bifurcation of the aorta at the L-3 level, 48% at the L-4 level, and 38% at the L-5 level. The inferior vena cava bifurcation was found with the left iliac vein overlying the L-5 vertebra in 86% of patients and overlying the L-4 vertebra in the remainder (46). A review of MRI films demonstrated the left common iliac vein overlying the L5-S1 intervertebral disk in approximately 18% of patients (47). There is a high incidence of vascular injury in the region from L4-S1. A working knowledge of the variations within this region is important to safe exposure.

D. Thrombotic Complications

Thrombosis of both the venous and arterial systems in anterior spinal surgery has been documented in the literature in retrospective reviews as well as individual case reports more frequently in anterior lumbar spine surgery than anterior thoracic spine surgery. Thrombosis has been noted postoperatively after intimal injury from retraction and after wall injury as postrepair thrombosis.

1. Arterial Thrombosis

Risk factors for arterial thrombosis include atherosclerosis, hypercoagulable states, morbid obesity, hypertension, diabetes, hormone replacement therapy, and tobacco use. Atherosclerotic plaques can rupture and result in a vessel occlusion. There are four case reports of documented arterial thrombosis: three involving the left common iliac artery and one involving the distal aorta and bilateral common iliac arteries (48–51). The potential for intimal injury during retraction of vessels is stressed as an initiating cause of arterial thrombosis. A delay in diagnosis with resultant ischemia to the lower extremities carries a high morbidity and mortality rate.

The left common iliac artery is most at risk of injury during access to the L4-L5 disk, which requires the left iliac artery along with the left iliac vein to be retracted to the contralateral side (10). Again, intimal injury or vessel occlusion may occur during sustained retraction predisposing to postoperative thrombosis particularly for spine exposure in this region.

Diagnosis of arterial thrombosis requires careful assessment of neurological status and peripheral pulses. Arterial pulses should be checked intraoperatively after removing vessel retractors; arterial spasm may be present as a result of sustained retraction. Absence of pulsation at this time may require intraoperative arteriogram or thrombectomy.

Postoperative leg paralysis and numbness may appear to be a neurological injury when in fact it is secondary to arterial thrombosis.

2. Venous Thrombosis

Two large reviews of retroperitoneal approaches to the anterior spine cited an approximate incidence of deep venous thrombosis (DVT) of approximately 1%. Neither study used prophylactic anticoagulation in their patients. Baker et al. noted one case in a series of 102 patients, which occurred postrepair of the left iliac vein (44). There were 11 total vein repairs in the series. Brau noted 7 cases in 686 patients despite intraoperative and postoperative compression stockings (9).

Venous injuries postrepair require close follow-up for potential DVT. Symptoms of calf pain and leg swelling signal the need for further evaluation. A Doppler study or venogram is usually diagnostic. Prophylactic measures to prevent DVT include compressive stockings or sequential compression foot or leg pumps and early mobilization. Anticoagulation may be needed for prevention and treatment.

Tachycardia, shortness of breath, cough, chest pain, decreased PAO_2, and hemoptysis are diagnostic clues to pulmonary embolism (PE). A ventilation and perfusion scan, pulmonary angiogram, or CT scan may be indicated. The incidence of fatal PE in a review of 1223 anterior spine surgery cases using only compression boots and stockings for DVT was 0.16% (12). Inferior vena cava filter placement represents an alternative to anticoagulation for preventing PE.

IX. COMPLICATIONS OF ANTERIOR EXPOSURE IN REVISION SPINE SURGERY

The literature concerning revision anterior spine surgery identifies two common complications: vascular and ureteral.

A. Vascular Injuries in Revision Anterior Spine Surgery

Oskouian and Johnson reported on three of the five direct vascular injuries to the common iliac vein in 207 revision anterior spinal cases (21). These three cases had a prior retroperitoneal exposure and surgery at the L4-L5 interspace. Dense scarring in the retroperitoneum was encountered during revision surgery, resulting in common iliac vein injury that required direct vascular repair.

Rajaraman et al. reported a complication of major venous injury during reexploration of an anterior lumbar interbody fusion (24). Dense adhesions had formed between the posterior vessel wall and the intrumentation; the procedure was abandoned due to significant blood loss.

Harmon also reported an iliac vein injury during revision anterior surgery that required extensive dissection for control of bleeding and vein repair (45). Incidentally, this case and another revision retroperitoneal case in the same series both resulted in a complication of retrograde ejaculation. Retroperitoneal scarring obscured the anatomy and the identification of veins and the ureter. He proposed a transperitoneal approach for revision cases.

Raskas and Delamarter documented vascular complications after revision retroperitoneal lumbar spine surgery (49). This vascular complication involved a left iliac artery thrombosis.

In revision anterior surgery, venous injuries were more common than arterial. However, no series contained enough revision cases to draw definitive conclusions. Nonetheless, the predilection of vascular injuries within revision surgeries illustrates the risks created by retroperitoneal scarring.

B. Ureteral Injuries in revision anterior spine surgery

Retroperitoneal scarring encountered in revision anterior spine surgery risks injury to the ureter as well as the retroperitoneal vessels. Faciszewski et al. documented one ureteral injury in 1223 cases, which occurred in a revision surgery (12). The ureter was found to be tortuous and encased in scar tissue. A recommendation to avoid ureteral injury included use of a retroperitoneal approach on the opposite side to the previous surgery. Identification of the ureter within the field of retroperitoneal scarring is difficult, and preoperative stent placement is recommended if revision retroperitoneal surgery is performed on the same side.

X. CONCLUSION

Anterior access to the thoracic, lumbar, and sacral spine offers direct access to the vertebral body and disk spaces in degenerative, deformity, and trauma surgery, but numerous vital structures lie in close proximity. Approach-related complications encompass iatrogenic injury to these vital structures within the path of dissection or in the adjacent zones under pressure of retraction. Complications include injury to the fascial and muscular layers, vessels, visceral structures of the chest and abdomen, diaphragm, peripheral or autonomic nerves, thoracic duct, ureter, dura, and spinal cord. Many of these complications are immediately apparent and remedied at the time of injury without further clinical sequelae. Other structural injuries may not become apparent until the postoperative period.

A greater number of exposure-related risks were reported for the anterior lumbar spine than for the anterior thoracic spine. In addition, a larger number of studies and cases existed for lumbar surgery. The lower lumbar, and sacral region presented the most vascular complications. Risks of anterior spinal surgery were also increased in patients with comorbidities and in patients over the age of 60 (12). Overall, safe navigation during anterior exposure of the spine is critical.

REFERENCES

1. Burns BH. An operation for spondylolisthesis. Lancet 1933; 224:1233.
2. Ito H, Tsuchiya J, Asami G. A new radical operation for Pott's disease. J Bone Joint Surg 1934; 16:499–515.
3. Lane LD, Moore SE. Transperitoneal approach to the intervertebral disc in the lumbar area. Ann Surg 1948; 127:537–551.
4. Iwahara T, et al. Results of anterior spine fusion by extraperitoneal approach for spondylolisthesis. J Jpn Orthop Assoc 1963; 36:1094.
5. Hodgson AR, Stock FE. Anterior spine fusion for the treatment of tuberculosis of the spine. J Bone Joint Surg 1960; 42A:295–309.
6. Hodgson AR, Wong SK. A description of a technique and evaluation of results in anterior spinal fusion for deranged intervertebral disk and spondylolisthesis. Clin Orthop 1968; 56:133–162.

7. Dwyer AF, Newton NC, Sherwood AA. An anterior approach to scoliosis: a preliminary report. Clin Orthop 1969; 62:192–202.

8. Calderone RR. Anterior thoracolumbar techniques: surgical approaches. Vaccaro AR, ed. Fractures of the Cervical, Thoracic, and Lumbar Spine. New York: Marcel Dekker, 2003:543–568.

9. Brau SA. Mini-open approach to the spine for anterior lumbar interbody fusion: description of the procedure, results and complications. Spine J 2002; 2(3):216–223.

10. Watkins R. Anterior lumbar interbody fusion surgical complications. Clinical Orthop Rel Res 1992; 284:47–53.

11. Fischer JE, Fegelman E, Johannigman J. Surgical complications. In: Schwartz SI, ed. Principles of Surgery. 7th ed. New York: McGraw-Hill, 1999:441–484.

12. Faciszewski T, Winter RB, Lonstein JE, Denis, F, Johnson L. The surgical and medical perioperative complications of anterior spinal fusion surgery in the thoracic and lumbar spine in adults; a review of 1223 procedures. Spine 1995; 20(14):1592–1599.

13. Daly JM, Adams JT, Fantini GA, Fischer JE. Abdominal wall, omentum, mesentery, and retroperitoneum. In: Schwartz SI, ed. Principles of Surgery. 7th ed. New York: McGraw-Hill, 1999:1551–1584.

14. Westfall SH, Akbarnia BA, Merenda JT, Naunheim KS, Connors RH, Kaminski DL, Weber, TR. Exposure of the anterior spine. Technique, complications, and results in 85 patients. Am J Surg 1987; 154:700–704.

15. Wantz G. Abdominal wall hernias. In: Schwartz SI, ed. Principles of Surgery. 7th ed. New York: McGraw-Hill, 1999:1585–1612.

16. Jodoin A, Gillet P, Dupuis PR, Maurais G. Surgical treatment of post traumatic kyphosis: a report of 16 cases. Can J Surg 1989; 32:36–42.

17. Lazio BE, Staab M, Stambough JL, Hurst JM. Latissimus dorsi rupture: an unusual complication of anterior spine surgery. Spinal Disord 6(1):83–86.

18. Hazelrigg SR, Landrenau RJ, Boley TM, Priesmeyer M, Schmaltz A, Nawarawong W. The effect of muscle-sparing versus standard posterolateral thoracotomy on pulmonary function, muscle strength, and postoperative pain. J Thorac Cardiovasc Surg 1991; 101:34–40.

19. Horowitz MD, Ancalmo N, Ochnsner JL. Thoracotomy through the auscultoatory triangle. Ann Thorac Surg 1989; 47:782–783.

20. Rusch VW, Ginsberg RJ. Chest wall, pleura, lung and mediastinum. In: Schwartz SI, ed. Principles of Surgery. 7th ed. New York: McGraw-Hill, 1999:667–790.

21. Oskouian RJ, Johnson JP. Vascular complications in anterior thoracolumbar spinal reconstruction. J Neurosurg Spine 2002; 96:1–5.

22. Calderone RR. Spine anatomy and surgical approaches. In: Capen DA, Haye W, eds. Management of Spine Trauma. Philadelphia: Mosby, 1998:6–32.

23. Solomin JS, Wittman DW, West MA, Barie PS. Intraabdominal infections. In: Schwartz SI, ed. Principles of Surgery. 7th ed. New York: McGraw-Hill, 1999:1515–1550.

24. Rajaraman V, Vingan R, Roth P, Heary R, Conklin L, Jacobs, GJ. Visceral and vascular complications resulting from anterior lumbar interbody fusion. Neurosurg Spine 1999; 91:60–64.

25. Korovessis PG, Stamatakis M, Baikousis A. Relapsing pancreatitis after combined anterior and posterior instrumentation for neuropathic scoliosis. J Spinal Disord 9(4):347–350.

26. Hodge WA, Dewald RL. Splenic injury complicating the anterior thoracoabdominal approach for scoliosis. J Bone Joint Surg 1983; 65:396–397.

27. Isiklar UZ, Lindsey RW, Coburn M. Ureteral injury after anterior lumbar interbody fusion. Spine 1996; 21(20):2379–2382.

28. Sagalowsky AI, Peters PC. Genitourinary trauma. In: Walsh PC, Retik AB, Vaughan ED, Wein AJ, eds. Cambell's Urology. 7th ed. Philadelphia: WB Saunders, 1998:3085–3120.

29. Franke JJ, Smith JA Jr. Surgery of the ureter. In: Walsh PC, Retik AB, Vaughan ED, Wein AJ, eds. Cambell's Urology. 7th ed. Philadelphia: WB Saunders, 1998:3062–3084.

30. Cohn EB, Ignatoff JM, Keeler TC, Shapiro DE, Blum MD. Anterior spine: technique and experience with 66 patients. J Urol 2000; 164:416–418.

31. Flynn JC, Hoque MA. Anterior fusion of the lumbar spine. J Bone Joint Surg 1979; 61-A(8).
32. Sasso R, Burkus K, Lehuec JC. Retrograde Ejaculation after lumbar interbody fusion: transperitoneal versus retroperitoneal. Spine J 2002; 2(5S):55S.
33. Flynn JC, Price CT. Sexual complications of anterior fusion of the lumbar spine. Spine 1984; 9(5):489–492.
34. Pearle MS, McConnell, Peters PC. Urology. In: Schwartz SI, ed. Principles of Surgery. 7th ed. New York: McGraw-Hill, 1999:1755–1832.
35. Faraj AA, Webb JK, Lemberger RJ. Urinary bladder dysfunction following anterior lumbosacral spine fusion: case report and review of the literature. Eur Spine J 1996; 5:121–124.
36. Regan JJ, Yuan H, MCAfee PC. Laproscopic fusion of the lumbar spine: minimally invasive spine surgery. Spine; 24(4):402–411.
37. Nakai S, Zielke K. Chylothorax; A rare complication after anterior and posterior spinal correction, report on six cases. Spine 1986; 11:830–833.
38. Bents RT. Ilioinguinal neuralgia following anterior iliac crest bone harvesting. Orthopedics 2002; 12:1389–1390.
39. Papastefanou SL, Stevens K, Mulholland RC. Femoral nerve palsy, an unusual complication of anterior lumbar interbody fusion. Spine 1994; 19(24):2842–2844.
40. Jasani V, Jaffray D. The anatomy of the iliolumbar vein. A cadaver study. J Bone Joint Surg 2002; 84-B(7):1046–1049.
41. Winter RB, Lonstein JE, Denis F, Leonard AS, Garamella JJ. Paraplegia resulting from vessel ligation. Spine 1996; 21(10):1232–1234.
42. Apel D, Marrero G, King J, Tolo V, Bassett G. Avoiding paraplegia during anterior spinal surgery: the role of SSEP monitoring with temporary occlusion of segmental spinal arteries. Spine 1991; 16S:S365–S370.
43. Harmon PH. A simplified surgical technique for anterior lumbar discectomy and fusion: avoidance of complications; anatomy of retroperitoneal veins. Clin Orthop 1964; 37:130–144.
44. Baker JK, Reardon PR, Reardon MJ, Heggeness MH. Vascular injury in anterior lumbar surgery. Spine 1993; 18(15):2227–2230.
45. Harmon PH. Anterior extraperitoneal lumbar disc excision and vertebral body fusion; a study of long term results, operative technique, including observations upon variations in the left common iliac veins and their connections. Clin Orthop 1960; 18:169–182.
46. Vraney RT, Phillips FM, Wetzel T, Brustein M. Peridiscal vascular anatomy of the lower lumbar spine. Spine 1999; 24(21):2183–2187.
47. Capellades J, Pellise F, Rovira A, Grive E, Pedraza S, Villanueva C. Magnetic resonance anatomic study of iliocava junction and left iliac vein positions related to L5-S1 disc. Spine 2000; 25(3):1695–1700.
48. Marsicano J, Mirovsky Y, Remer S, Bloom N, Neuwirth M. Thrombotic occlusion of the left common iliac artery after anterior retroperitoneal approach to the lumbar spine. Spine 1994; 19:357–359.
49. Raskas DS, Delamarter RB. Occlusion of the left iliac artery after retroperitoneal exposure of the spine. Clini Orthop Rel Res 1997; 338:86–89.
50. Khazim R, Boos N, Webb JK. Progressive thrombotic occlusion of the left common iliac artery after anterior lumbar interbody fusion. Eur J Spine 1998; 7:239–241.
51. Castro FP Jr, Hartz RS, Frigon V, Whitecloud TS III. Aortic thrombosis after lumbar spine surgery: a case report. J Spin Disord 2000; 13(6):538–540.

11

Postoperative Spinal Wound Infections and Postprocedural Diskitis

Michael J. Vives and Shyam Kishan
University of Medicine and Dentistry of New Jersey, Newark, New Jersey, U.S.A.

I. INTRODUCTION

The number of invasive spinal procedures continues to increase. Performed for a variety of indications, spinal interventions range from diagnostics, such as diskography, myelography, and lumbar puncture, to minimally invasive therapeutics such as epidural steroid injections and intradiscal electrothermal therapy (IDET), to formal open procedures ranging from discectomy to instrumented fusions. Unfortunately, all invasive procedures are associated with a risk for postprocedural infection. As the complexity of the intervention increases, so does the rate of infection (1). Despite improvements in technique, postoperative care, and the development of broad, powerful antibiotics, infectious complications result in significant morbidity and occasional mortality (2). Rates quoted for infection are related to the type of surgery performed as well as the anatomical site of the procedure and range from < 1% to almost 13% (3–7). The key to the management of this potentially devastating problem lies in early diagnosis and aggressive treatment. This chapter focuses on factors involved in the pathogenesis, the clinical presentation, diagnosis and the treatment of postprocedure infection of the spine.

II. PATHOGENESIS AND PREVENTION

Efforts at prevention require an understanding of the pathogenesis of postoperative infection. The various factors influencing the development of infection may be broadly classified into three main categories: microbiological, patient/host, and surgical (1). All three groups are interrelated, and thus infection can be described as being multifactorial.

A. Microbiological Factors

For a clinical infection to occur, bacteria must be present at the operative/procedural site. The route may be from direct inoculation at the time of the procedure (8–10), soiling of the incision in the immediate postoperative period (11), or hematogenous seeding (12). Most postprocedural infections result from direct inoculation of the wound and thus are operative infections.

The infective agents are fairly consistent in the literature. The culprits in acute infection are usually gram-positive cocci: *Staphylococcus aureus*, *Staphylococcus epidermidis*, and beta-hemolytic streptococci. The organism most commonly identified has been *S. aureus* (2,6,13). *Klebsiella*, *Escherichia coli*, *Pseudomonas*, *Aerobacter*, and *Proteus* are the gram-negative representatives (1). Delayed or chronic infections are usually due to skin flora of low virulence such as *Propionibacterium* (9) and diphtheroids (2). Intravenous drug abusers have a higher incidence of infections with gram-negative rods (1). Infections with nosocomial organisms are more common in patients with prolonged hospital stays (13) and those in intensive care units.

The concept of antiseptic technique is credited to Joseph Lister, who started the routine use of carbolic acid as a prep and as an intraoperative nebulizer to reduce infection. The discovery of sulfonamides, and later that of penicillin, revolutionized treatment of infection and paved the way for the advancement of surgery. However, it was not until the 1970s that the effect of preoperative antibiotics upon infection rates was studied. Keller and Pappas reported a dramatic decrease in infection rates from 2.7 to 0% with the use of preoperative prophylactic antibiotics (3). Infection rates after lumbar discectomy dropped from 9.3 to 1% after the use of preoperative antibiotics in a study in 1975 (14). A placebo-controlled study demonstrated that infection rates were significantly less (4.3%) with preoperative prophylaxis compared to 12.7% in the placebo group in patients undergoing clean lumbar surgery (15). In a laboratory study, Guiboux et al. (16) demonstrated that postoperative disk space infection in a rabbit model was effectively prevented by a single preoperative dose of intravenous cefazolin or vancomycin given within one hour before surgery. No benefit was found in this study to giving postoperative antibiotics. In a later study, the authors (17) found that prophylactic preoperative antibiotics were efficacious in a rabbit spine instrumentation model as well. Thus, most spine surgeons recommend administering a first-generation cephalosporin (or clindamycin/vancomycin in patients with penicillin or cephalosporin allergy) within the hour before surgery. As the antibiotic levels have been shown to decrease with operative time (18,19), some have recommended redosing the patient with the prophylactic antibiotic after 4 hours, of operative time. Clinical studies comparing a single preoperative antibiotic dose to multiple dose (continued postoperatively) prophylaxis have failed to demonstrate statistically significant differences (15,20). Despite these findings, many surgeons continue to favor postoperative anti-biotics for 24–48 hours if any procedure more extensive than a laminotomy/discectomy was performed.

B. Patient/Host Factors

Many patient-related factors have been identified as playing an important role in the pathogenesis of infection. These can be broadly classified as nonmodifiable and modifiable factors.

Higher rates of infection have been observed in older patients (21). Mental retardation was found to be a statistically significant factor in a study on infections after neuromuscular scoliosis surgery (11). Insensate patients with spinal dysraphism under-going neuromuscular scoliosis surgery were found to be at higher risk for postoperative infection (11). Spinal trauma patients with a neurological deficit have a higher risk for infection than elective procedures (12).

Obesity has been quoted as a risk factor by several authors (13,22,23). This may be related to both biophysiological alterations in obesity and technical issues during surgery. Tissue dissection in these patients can be extensive, leading to more surface area for bacterial colonization. The frequent use of electrocautery as well as deep and wide retraction often leads to excessive fat necrosis in the obese patient (22). Furthermore, as the vascularity of the fat is less than that of muscle, oxygen, leukocyte, and antibiotic penetration are compromised, all favorable conditions for bacterial proliferation (1).

Malignancy, chemotherapy, immune suppression, and malnutrition have all been implicated as risk factors for postprocedural infections (2,23–25). Klein and Garfin (24) reported preoperative malnourishment in 25% of 114 elective lumbar fusion patients. Eleven of the 13 reported complications in this series occurred in the malnourished group.

Serum albumin levels less than 3.5 g/dL and a total lymphocyte count less than 1500–2000 cells/mm^3 have been associated with a higher risk for infection (24,25). Malnutrition should be addressed and corrected if possible before elective surgery. In a study of nutrition in orthopedic surgery, Jensen et al. (25) found that a large number of patients (42%) undergoing orthopedic procedures are already malnourished. Surgery was postulated to induce further catabolism and exacerbated the state of malnutrition in these patients. As proteins are used for energy purposes in such a catabolic state, immunoglobulin synthesis is depressed leading to an immunodeficient state. Wound healing may be affected, and patient rehabilitation is often delayed. The authors found a definite correlation between the complication rate and malnutrition. Paradoxically, obesity also can be a risk factor for malnutrition, especially in those patients undergoing rapid weight reduction (1).

Diabetes (2,26–29) is a risk factor for postoperative infection, especially when uncontrolled. White cell function (chemotaxis and phagocytosis) is affected with blood glucose levels higher than 200 mg/dL (30,31). Other causes of immunosuppression, such as rheumatoid arthritis (particularly requiring corticosteroid treatment), cancer patients on chemotherapy, and HIV patients with low CD4 counts, all can increase the potential for postoperative infectious complications. Operating through previously irradiated tissue has also been shown to increase risk for postoperative infection (2), as has revision surgery (13). In a large series (2), 4 of 20 patients with metastatic disease who underwent spine surgery developed wound infection. All 4 patients had been irradiated preoperatively. Radiation affects the vascularity of the tissue as well as the ability to heal. Therefore, consideration should be given to delaying radiation postoperatively to allow wound healing. In a study of 850 spine procedures, Wimmer et al. (13) concluded that revision surgery was a risk factor for postoperative infection, with an 8% risk for infection as compared to a 1.8% risk in primary surgeries.

Modifiable factors include smoking (32), indwelling venous catheters, concurrent infections, and extended preoperative hospitalization (13). Many surgeons will attempt to address modifiable factors preoperatively in order to eliminate unnecessary risk of postoperative complications. Both for the risk of infection, as well as pseudarthrosis, smokers should be counseled to quit preoperatively. Any coexisting infection should be identified and treated prior to elective spine surgery (1,2,26,27,29). Systemic problems such as diabetes and malnutrition should be optimized whenever possible. In patients hospitalized for prolonged periods, consideration may be given to discharging the patient home prior to elective surgery to allow reestablishment of normal skin flora.

Surgical Factors

In addition to patient-related risk factors, there are numerous intraoperative variables that may predispose a patient to an infectious complication. It is difficult to know with certainty the efficacy of any particular operative technique in lowering the infection rate due to the number of confounding variables. Time-tested principles and some available literature do, however, allow for some recommendations.

Most surgeons shave or clip hair from the incision site on the operating table just before the prep to decrease the colonization of the wound with skin flora. A detergent scrub followed by a prep containing an iodophore (povidone-iodine) or chlorhexidine, sometimes combined with alcohol is recommended. The prep should be left in contact with the skin for the minimum recommended time to ensure adequate antisepsis. Authors have recommended a surgical scrub for at least 5–10 minutes in preparation for surgery (1). A povidone-iodine–impregnated bio-occlusive membrane is frequently applied to isolate the skin from the surgical wound. Most infections arise from skin flora, and thus a conscious effort must be made to avoid contact of fingers or instruments with the skin during surgery. Double gloving may prevent wound contamination by unrecognized glove holes, and sterile vests may prevent contamination during an inadvertent turn or lean.

As a generalization, the invasiveness or complexity of the procedure is directly related to the infectious complication rate. Postprocedure diskitis has been reported after a plethora of spinal interventions including less invasive procedures such as diskography (33,34), chemonucleolysis (35,36), myelography (37), paraspinal injections, lumbar punctures, and epidural injections. Discectomy has infection rates ranging from 0.6 to 5%, with paradoxically higher risk for infection with microdiscectomy (1,38). Some authors, however, have reported a lower incidence of postprocedural infection (0.4%) with the operating microscope compared with conventional open discectomy (2.8%) (39). Given these conflicting observations, no consensus exists as to the risk of added infection through use of the microscope by surgeons familiar with the technique (40). Fusion without instrumentation has been associated with infection rates ranging from 0.4 to 4.3%. The use of internal fixation raises the risk significantly (6.6% in one study (27) to 8.7% in another (7)]. Modern modular implants tend to be bulky and can cause soft tissue irritation. The presence of a foreign body implant provides infectious organisms with a surface for bacteria to lay down a glycocalyx, which protects them from antibiotic penetration (1). Also the irritation caused by the implants has been postulated as providing an inflamed area, with potential for seroma formation, which may subsequently become infected (1). Finally, metallosis from micromotion of the instrumentation, with subsequent granuloma formation and the potential for colonization, has been postulated as an additional contributing factor (8).

Anterior cervical surgery generally has a very low infection rate of 0–1% (2,6,41). When infection occurs after an anterior surgical procedure, a high index of suspicion must be maintained to rule out pharyngo-esophageal injury. Recommendations to decrease the risk of injury include the use of blunt retractors, which are intermittently released. Caution should be exercised to place the deep retractors beneath the longus colli (1). Posterior cervical surgery has a higher rate of infection, comparable to posterior lumbar surgery at about 1% for simple decompressions (41) and as high as 4.5% (42) to about 9% for instrumented fusion (5).

Surgical time correlates with the absolute numbers of bacteria found in the wound. More than 10^5 organisms (which is the microbiological definition of most infections) were demonstrated in surgical wounds after 5.7 hours (22). Another study showed an increased risk for infection with operative times greater than 3 hours (13). With this in mind, the surgeon should perform careful preoperative planning and routinely check the OR inventory for the presence of the correct instruments and implants to minimize operative time and improve efficiency.

The time-honored fundamentals of good surgical technique continue to be applicable when minimizing the risk for perioperative infections. Meticulous dissection is recommended, staying in avascular planes, avoiding the creation of large flaps and potential dead spaces. Gentle handling of the tissues and debridement of devitalized material is crucial. Intermittent release of the retractors to allow tissue perfusion and frequent irrigation with bactericidal antibiotics have been suggested as helpful maneuvers. Topical polymixin and bacitracin in solutions used for lavage has been shown to decrease the intraoperative bacterial growth from 64% to 4% (43). In dogs, irrigation of contaminated osseous wounds with bacitracin eliminated clinical evidence of infection and significantly reduced the number of positive cultures and pathological evidence of infection when compared with dogs that received no treatment or irrigation with normal saline solution (44). Careful hemostasis during surgery is recommended, as increased blood loss greater than 1000 cc has also been correlated with an increased risk of infection (13). Additionally, allogeneic blood transfusions have been suggested as a risk for infection (23). The issue of whether to drain the wound or not is controversial. Drainage is often considered if the wound continues to ooze despite attempts at hemostasis. Attention should be paid to a meticulous closure, with careful re-approximation of the tissues in a layered watertight closure that obliterates dead space. Finally, an occlusive dressing and hygienic assistance to prevent soiling of the wound with urine or feces is especially important in posterior lumbar procedures, particularly in the setting of incontinence.

III. CLASSIFICATION

When discussing postoperative wound infections, a commonly mentioned distinction is between superficial and deep infections. Superficial infections are limited to the skin and subcutaneous tissues. Deep infections occur below the lumbodorsal fascia posteriorly or the anterior abdominal fascia anteriorly (the platysma in the neck) and may involve the spinal column including diskitis, osteomyelitis, and epidural abscess. Such complications can be further classified as acute (within the first 3 weeks after the procedure) or chronic/delayed (more than 4 weeks after the procedure) (1). Thalgott and colleagues (32) developed a more detailed classification system for posterior spinal wound infection based on the severity of the infection and the host response. Severity of infection was stratified into three groups on the basis of two factors: location (superficial vs. deep) and the microbiological diagnosis (single organism versus polymicrobial). Host response was divided into three groups based on the patient's systemic defenses, metabolic capabilities, and local vascularity.

IV. CLINICAL PRESENTATION AND DIAGNOSIS

The most common symptom suggestive of postoperative spine infection is worsening pain 1–4 weeks after the procedure, usually following a period of initial relief (45). The patient often complains of the return of their original back pain, thus confusing the diagnosis with a mechanical cause. The back pain is often out of proportion to the physical signs, and may be referred to the buttock, thigh, leg, groin, perineum, or abdomen (38). Fever, chills, and night sweats have all been reported but are less common than pain. Fever, when present, is often mild. Floridly septic presentations with high fevers, chills, and sweats are unusual (38). In the setting of a superficial infection, local wound changes such as erythema or drainage may be the presenting complaint (1). Drainage was the most common presentation of infection in a series of patients reported by Weinstein et al. at a mean of 14–15 days after the index procedure (2), as well as in Glassman et al.'s study on delayed infection (26).

Postoperative infection after anterior cervical procedures may present with painful swallowing as a consequence of a retropharyngeal collection. Frank sepsis is uncommon in this subgroup as well. Pain is again the presenting symptom in delayed infections as well, with occasional drainage. The patients may complain of malaise and night sweats.

The most common physical finding in postprocedural diskitis is significant pain with lumbar range of motion (38). The incision is usually unremarkable, and less than 10% of surgical incisions will show signs of purulent infection with erythema, drainage, or dehiscence (45). The presentation of a patient with a neurological deficit should alert one to the possibility of an epidural abscess. Sixteen percent of epidural abscesses are post-operative complications, accounting for 1 in 10,000 admissions (1). The neurological manifestations in this setting may involve sensorimotor dysfunction or bladder and bowel impairment. Cauda equina syndrome has been reported as a manifestation of lumbar epidural involvement.

V. LABORATORY MARKERS

When an infection is suspected, a thorough workup is recommended. Blood work should include a complete white blood cell (WBC) count with differential, an erythrocyte sedimentation rate (ESR), C-reactive protein (CRP), and blood cultures.

The white cell count may be elevated, but usually is not, and thus is an unreliable marker for infection. Less than half of the cases of infective spondylodiskitis had an elevated WBC count in a recent report (46). Advanced age and immunocompromised states often depresses any significant white cell reaction.

The ESR has been used as a reliable criterion for the diagnosis of postprocedural infection. It is a nonspecific indicator of infection, with sensitivities ranging from 78 to 82% and specificities ranging from 38 to 62% (47,48). Greater than 90% of patients with infective diskitis have an elevated ESR (33,45,47,49–51). Kapp and Sybers were among the first to report on the postoperative changes in the ESR (52). They reported that the ESR was rarely elevated greater than 25 during the first postoperative week, and returned to baseline values or lower by the third week after uncomplicated spine surgery. Jonsson and associates reported higher postoperative peaks (102 vs. 75) in more extensive procedures compared with limited procedures such as discectomies (53). Pre- and post-operative ESR values were obtained at various time points after surgery. The ESR peaked on the fourth postoperative day and returned to baseline after 2 weeks in most patients. They concluded that the ESR is not a reliable indicator of infection in the first week after surgery. Persistent elevation of the ESR for up to 6 weeks postoperatively was shown by Thelander and Larsson in about one third of their patients (54). The prolonged elevation of the ESR in uncomplicated postoperative courses makes it less useful as a definitive marker for infection.

The CRP, an acute phase reactant, is perhaps the most sensitive indicator of post-operative infection (47,48). CRP elevation is more rapid than the ESR as is its return to the baseline after surgery. Studies have shown that the levels usually peak on the second or third postoperative day and normalize about 2 weeks after surgery. Rising values after that timeframe correlate well with the presence of infection (48). Some authors recommend obtaining preoperative ESR and CRP values as a baseline for comparison with postoperative measurements (47,48,50,52–54).

VI. IMAGING

Plain radiographs are generally the first imaging modality obtained when infection is suspected. Negative plain radiographs, however, do not exclude infection. There is usually no change in the first 3 weeks, even as clinical and laboratory findings are emerging (38). In the setting of diskitis, the earliest changes, seen from the fourth to the sixth postoperative week, are a decrease in the disk space height, with blurring of the vertebral endplates (45). Paravertebral soft tissue shadows signifying paravertebral abscesses may be visible on the plain x-rays. X-rays may also show lysis around surgical implants, suggesting loosening. Alignment and implant position should be carefully visualized and inspected. Due to the lag in radiographic changes, more advanced imaging modalities are often needed to establish the diagnosis in a timely fashion.

CT scans show the areas of early bone destruction with better detail, and the sagittal and coronal reconstructions may demonstrate instability (45). Early changes include erosive and destructive lesions of the endplates and disk space narrowing. Soft tissue windows may demonstrate paravertebral abscesses. However, the presence of hardware may create artifact by the scatter. CT-guided biopsy of postoperative diskitis/osteomyelitis or needle aspirate of pus from abscess cavities may provide a microbiological diagnosis in selected cases (55). Ideally, material should be sent for Gram stain and cultures to identify the organism and its susceptibilities to antibiotics, prior to starting the commencement of drug treatment.

Technetium 99 m and gallium 67 have been used in the diagnostic investigation of spinal infections, but usually show nonspecific increased uptake (38) in the majority of cases. Gallium 67 often identifies the presence of a postoperative disk space infection earlier than technetium 99 m scans or plain radiographs (56,57). The results, however, are less accurate and predictive than in extremity infections. A sequential technetium 99 m study followed by a gallium 67 study increases the cumulative accuracy of these nuclear medicine investigations (1). Indium 111–labeled WBC scans may also be useful in establishing the diagnosis of spine infection but are infrequently used, again due to suboptimal specificity (10).

The test of choice for imaging suspected postprocedural spine infection is magnetic resonance imaging (MRI) with gadolinium contrast enhancement. Magnetic resonance scans have been shown to have the highest sensitivity and specificity in the diagnosis of postprocedural diskitis, superior to both technetium 99 as well as gallium 67 scans (58) with a reported sensitivity of 93% and a specificity of 97%. Findings on MRI suggestive of a postprocedure diskitis include a decreased signal on T1 and an increased signal on T2-weighted images in the disk space, secondary to edema from the inflammation and infection (Fig. 1). There may be edema of the adjacent endplates seen as increased signal intensity on T2-weighted images (59). Gadolinium administration may show an area of decreased signal intensity in the bone marrow on T1 images, and this sign is considered a very reliable finding for the presence of edema. Van Goethem et al. reported that the absence of Modic I changes and contrast enhancement of the disk space/paraspinal tissues was suggestive of infection in a study comparing MRI scans in asymptomatic individuals to scans of patients with biopsy-proven diskitis (60). Epidural abscesses are seen as areas isointense with the cord or cauda equina on T1-weighted images that may cause efface-ment of the neural structures. T2-weighted images reveal a high signal expression with this lesion, which enhances with gadolinium. In the absence of findings highly suggestive of postprocedural diskitis or osteomyelitis, MRI may not be able to distinguish between benign postoperative fluid collections (seromas, hematomas) and infections.

Infection after anterior cervical spine surgery may be due to injury to the pharynx or esophagus during the operation (61). Delay in presentation of 2–4 months has been

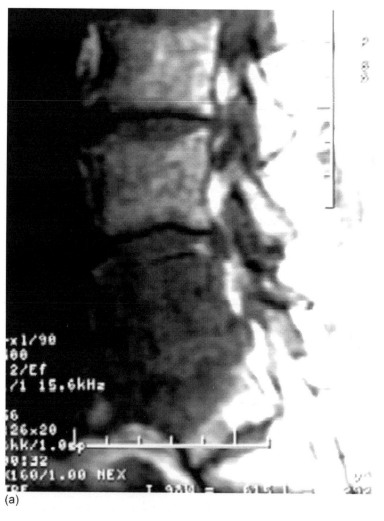

(a)

Figure 1 (a) Sagittal T1-weighted magnetic resonance image of a patient after L5-S1 discectomy. The patient developed a postoperative diskitis involving the L5-S1 interspace with involvement of the vertebral bodies of L5 and S1. (b) Sagittal T2-weighted image demonstrating the increased signal intensity in the involved disk and adjacent vertebral bodies.

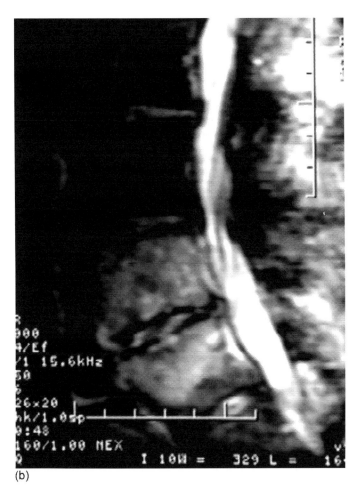

(b)

Figure 1 (*continued*)

reported (62). In addition to the tests described above, an otolaryngology consultation and evaluation should be requested. Contrast esophagogram can demonstrate a leak in 75–100% of these cases (63).

VII. TREATMENT

Once diagnosed, appropriate treatment should be instituted in a timely fashion. Treatment may be nonsurgical or surgical. Common to both is the identification of the organism and administration of the specific antibiotic. In experienced hands, CT-guided biopsy/aspiration may be obtained to direct antibiotic treatment, unless multiple positive blood cultures are obtained. While culture and sensitivity results are pending, the patient may be started on broad-spectrum antibiotics with antistaphylococcal coverage (45).

Indications (38,46) for open surgical management of postprocedural spine infections are as follows: drainage from or dehiscence of the incision, clinical sepsis, neurodeficits due to the presence of a mass effect from a fluid collection, a spinal or epidural abscess, and instability from bone destruction or fixation/hardware failure. Failure of improvement with nonsurgical management (antibiotics and immobilization), especially with negative blood and needle biopsy cultures, is also a surgical indication (38). The goal of surgery is to debride the spine of all necrotic and grossly infected material and then provide sufficient stabilization, when necessary, to prevent deformity or neurological injury.

In cases of refractory diskitis/osteomyelitis following less invasive procedures (diskograms, IDET, etc), minimally invasive techniques utilizing computer- or fluoroscopy-aided percutaneous disk debridement (and even fusion) have been described (64,46,64). Such an approach would be applicable only in cases without significant superficial or deep collections or open, draining wounds. These minimally invasive techniques have the advantages of less postoperative pain, shorter hospital stays, and possibly an accelerated healing response (46,64,65). The success in the lumbar spine is countered by a high complication rate of up to 33% in the thoracic spine. Complications include the need for conversion to open procedures to address vascular injury or to drain an epidural abscess (46).

The principles of open surgical treatment are thorough exploration of the wound to decide if the infection is deep to the fascia and, if so, then opening the entire wound. Necrotic tissue and bone graft should be debrided. There has been debate in the literature about whether the hardware should be left in place or removed. Some recommend removing all bone graft and spinal implants (66). However, there is ample support in the literature for leaving well-fixed posterior instrumentation (particularly titanium) and bone graft in place, even in the face of active infection (3,5,6,29,67). Radical debridement of involved disk and vertebral bodies usually involves anterior surgery with autogenous bone grafting, followed by posterior instrumented fusion (Fig. 2). The procedures may be staged if the patient cannot tolerate a very prolonged operation. Traditionally, anterior instrumentation is recommended after anterior debridement of an infected foci (Fig. 3). However, some recent reports utilizing anterior instrumentation in the cervical spine in the setting of gross infection have cited good results (68–70). Despite these data, postoperative infections following an anterior instrumented fusion are usually managed with removal of all spinal hardware and necrotic and infected tissue with autograft reconstruction of the spinal defect (38). In recent times, allografts have gained favor, as they are easily available. However, a higher incidence of infection has been reported following the use of allograft bone sources (11). This has been theorized to be related to the immune reaction provoked by the graft and the inflammatory changes that result (1). As previously stated, posterior instrumentation may be left in situ if well fixed. Instrumentation should be revised, however, if implants lose fixation, and alternate sites or levels of fixation used. Additional levels may be fused as needed to further stabilize the spine.

Deep tissue specimens should be sent for cultures in the setting of suspected infection due to the high positive culture yield of this tissue (100%) (49). Thorough lavage of the wound with saline is recommended following wound debridement. Addition of an antibiotic to the irrigant has been shown to decrease the bacterial load (44). The wound may be closed over drains (1,6), which are removed when the output decreases to less than 20 cc/12 hours (1). A decision is made at the time of the first washout about the timing of repeat washouts. Heller and Levine recommend reexploration every 48 hours if there is continued drainage (71). Thalgott et al. found that immunocompetent patients who had a single organism needed only one operation with irrigation and debridement and regular suction drains. Those with multiple organisms who were immunocompetent needed up to three surgeries and inflow-outflow irrigation drains, while those with multiple organisms and myonecrosis had wounds that were left open to heal (32). Weinstein et al. (2) left all their deep infections open and packed with gauze until the wound bed appeared

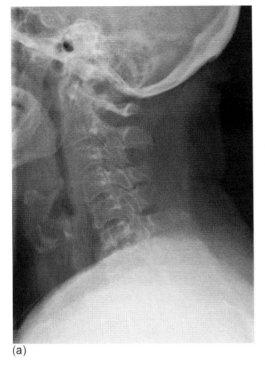

(a)

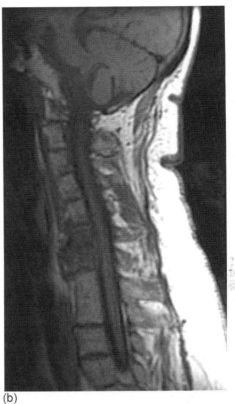

(b)

Figure 2 (a) Plain radiograph of a patient with severe, persistent neck pain after cervical diskography for chronic axial symptoms. Destruction of the endplates about the C6-7 disk space can be seen. (b and c) Sagittal T1-weighted magnetic resonance images before and after intravenous gadolinium administration demonstrate diskitis involving the C6-7 interspace with destruction of the adjacent vertebral bodies and epidural abscess. (d) Postoperative lateral radiograph after anterior debridement with strut reconstruction followed by posterior fusion with segmental instrumentation.

healthy. At this point the wounds were closed over drains in a delayed fashion. Glassman et al. (26) studied the use of antibiotic-impregnated cement beads as an adjunct to serial irrigations and debridements. Tobramycin or a combination of tobramycin and vancomycin were used in the beads. They reported no recurrence in 19 of the 22 patients with deep infections at a mean follow-up of 23 months. Recorded local levels of antibiotics are high and have been shown to be effective in the infected spine injury rabbit model (72).

In the setting of an epidural abscess, the surgical approach is decided by the anatomical location of the abscess (1). Anterior abscesses are approached anteriorly, and posterior absesses are approached from a dorsal direction. Anterior approaches are also effective for debriding vertebral osteomyelitis and for reconstruction of the anterior spinal column. In the case of anterior cervical abscesses, an intraoperative evaluation of the pharynx and esophagus by the head and neck surgeons may be indicated. In the case of pharyngoesophageal fistulae, a diversion may be needed, as well as a local muscle flap (1).

In posterior wounds that are left open for delayed closure, a plastic surgical evaluation may be helpful. The objectives of closure include coverage of the wound, obliteration of dead space, padding of exposed structures, and enhancing the local vascularity, thus

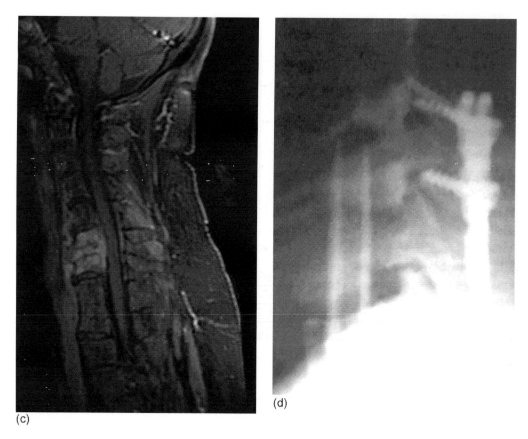

(c)

(d)

Figure 2 (*continued*)

improving antibiotic transport and leukocyte function (73). This has usually been achieved using muscle, myocutaneous, or fasciocutaneous flaps. Tissue expanders have also been used to provide the extra tissue needed for wound coverage (74). These procedures are not without complication. Long operative times, blood loss, recurrent infection, dehiscence, flap failure, seroma, and donor site morbidity have all been described (73). A recent paper points to the possible use of a vacuum-assisted closure device (VAC from KCI Medical, San Antonio, TX) to assist in granulating open wounds over hardware and bone grafts in a report of two cases (73). The two postulated mechanisms of action are removal of excess fluid from the interstitium and stimulation of the local cells mechanically. The interstitial pressure decreases, thus allowing increased blood flow. It is also thought that inhibitory factors in the fluid are removed. Bacterial cell counts from the tissues have been shown to decrease compared to control wounds without the vacuum device. The cost of each drain or sponge change is comparable to other methods routinely used in wound management. Contraindications to its use are the presence of fistulae, neoplasms, bleeding diatheses, and anticoagulation.

Nonsurgical management may be carried out if none of the indications described above are found. Intravenous antibiotics are administered for 6 weeks, followed by 6 weeks of oral antibiotics directed to the specific organism (38). Long-term antibiotic treatment is often selected depending on the virulence of the organism and the presence of internal fixation. The exact duration of antibiotics is determined by the clinical,

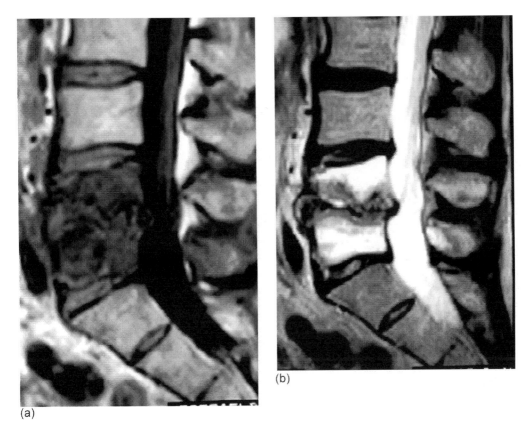

(b)

(a)

Figure 3 (a and b) Sagittal T1- and T2-weighted magnetic resonance images demonstrating L4-5 diskitis/osteomyelitis in a patient who had undergone automated percutaneous discectomy. Progressive destruction of the adjacent vertebral bodies occurred despite antibiotic therapy. (c) Sagittal reconstruction of a CT scan after the anterior debridement demonstrating autograft strut reconstruction. This was followed in a staged manner by a posterior instrumented stabilization.

laboratory, and radiological response to the antibiotics. Bracing is also recommended in the setting of diskitis and osteomyelitis (38). The lumbosacral junction cannot be effectively braced without the addition of a thigh extension, and standard lumbar braces may actually exacerbate motion and pain (75). In patients being managed nonoperatively, serial clinical assessment and surveillance testing of the WBC count, ESR, and the CRP helps determine the response to the antibiotics. If there is no response to 6 weeks of antibiotics and bracing, an open biopsy, surgical debridement, and stabilization may be indicated (38).

VIII. COMPLICATIONS

Complications of postoperative spine infection are related to the morbidity of the infection and the treatment administered. Multiple surgeries may be required. Acute complications include neurodeficits, sepsis, multisystem failure, and death (2). Long-term complications are related to pseudarthroses (2,76,77) of the fusion segments, chronic pain, and poor functional outcome (77).

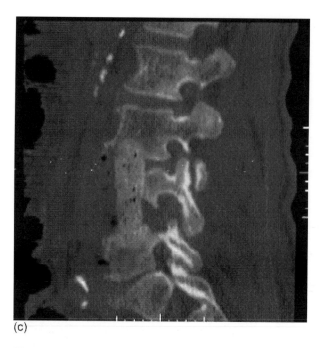

(c)

Figure 3 (*continued*)

IX. OUTCOMES

The long-term prognosis of nonoperatively treated diskitis was reported to be good in one study, with 90% of the patients becoming pain-free and 75% of patients developing a spontaneous bony fusion or stable fibrous union within 2 years of diagnosis of the infection (45). However, a more recent study reported a much higher incidence of back pain (64%) in patients with primary diskitis treated nonoperatively compared to a back pain incidence of 26% in patients who underwent surgery (46). They also reported deterioration among the patients treated nonoperatively, with the development of worsening symptoms, laboratory markers, or spinal deformity, all of which were surgical indications. Przybylski and Sharan (78) reported good outcomes in 17 patients with diskitis and vertebral osteomyelitis treated with debridement, bone grafting, and internal fixation at a mean follow-up of 30 months. Glassman et al. (26) in a study of 22 infected lumbar fusions, reported that 80% of patients felt that they were improved at a final follow-up averaging one year. Thirteen percent of patients reported no change and 5% had worse symptoms. Three patients died from associated medical problems.

Weiss et al. (76) noted in a series of 29 patients with infected lumbar fusions, after a mean follow-up of 37 months, that the overall successful fusion rate was about 62.1% (18 patients). Inclusion of the sacrum in the fusion increased the peudarthrosis rate to 64%. Allograft usage decreased the fusion to 17.2% as compared to 83.3% with autograft. Risk factors identified for poor outcome were the female sex, allograft use, and extension of fusion to the sacrum.

Calderone et al. (77) reviewed several outcome measures comparing functional outcomes in 15 patients with postlumbar fusion infection to a control group of 15 postlumbar fusion patients with no infections. The patients were receiving worker's compensation. There was no statistical difference between the two groups with regard to functional outcome. Fusions were successful in 13 of the 15 control patients as opposed to 6 out of 15 in the infected group. However, only 3 of the uninfected patients and 2 of the infected patients had returned to work at 3-year follow-up. This study showed uniform poor outcomes in the worker's compensation group of patients, but also showed that pseudarthrosis rates were higher after surgeries complicated by postoperative infection.

X. SUMMARY

While uncommon, postprocedural infections are a significant cause of morbidity after spinal interventions. The key to successful management is a high index of clinical suspicion to establish a timely diagnosis and institute treatment. Laboratory markers and advanced imaging modalities may help identify subtle cases of deep infection with benign-appearing wounds. Cases of diskitis/osteomyelitis that occur in the absence of large fluid collections or wound problems can often be treated by CT-guided biopsy and appropriate antibiotic therapy. When operative intervention is necessary, one or more debridements may be required, but well-fixed instrumentation can usually be left in place. Complex wounds may require delayed or vacuum-assisted closure. Occasionally soft tissue reconstructive procedures, such as fasciocutaneous or myocutaneous flaps, may be indicated. Despite eradication of the infection, these complications may be associated with decreased fusion rates and diminished functional outcomes. Ongoing research efforts in this area should, therefore, focus especially on prevention.

REFERENCES

1. Bassewitz HL, Fischgrund JS, Herkowitz HN. Postoperative spine infections. Semin Spine Surg 2000; 12(4):203–211.
2. Weinstein MA, McCabe JP, Cammisa FP, Jr. Postoperative spinal wound infection: a review of 2,391 consecutive index procedures. J Spinal Disord 2000; 13(5):422–426.
3. Keller RB, Pappas AM. Infection after spinal fusion using internal fixation instrumentation. Orthop Clin North Am 1972; 3(1):99–111.
4. Abbey DM, Turner DM, Warson JS, Wirt TC, Scalley RD. Treatment of postoperative wound infections following spinal fusion with instrumentation. J Spinal Disord 1995; 8(4):278–283.
5. Lonstein J, Winter R, Moe J, Gaines D. Wound infection with Harrington instrumentation and spine fusion for scoliosis. Clin Orthop 1973; 96:222–233.
6. Levi AD, Dickman CA, Sonntag VK. Management of postoperative infections after spinal instrumentation. J Neurosurg 1997; 86(6):975–980.
7. Roberts FJ, Walsh A, Wing P, Dvorak M, Schweigel J. The influence of surveillance methods on surgical wound infection rates in a tertiary care spinal surgery service. Spine 1998; 23(3):366–370.
8. Dubousset J, Shufflebarger H, Wenger D. Late "infection" with CD instrumentation. Orthop Trans 1994; 18:121.
9. Richards BS, Herring JA, Johnston CE, Birch JG, Roach JW. Treatment of adolescent idiopathic scoliosis using Texas Scottish Rite Hospital instrumentation. Spine 1994; 19(14): 1598–1605.
10. Viola RW, King HA, Adler SM, Wilson CB. Delayed infection after elective spinal instrumentation and fusion. A retrospective analysis of eight cases. Spine 1997; 22(20):2444–2451.

11. Sponseller PD, LaPorte DM, Hungerford MW, Eck K, Bridwell KH, Lenke LG. Deep wound infections after neuromuscular scoliosis surgery: a multicenter study of risk factors and treatment outcomes. Spine 2000; 25(19):2461–2466.

12. Heggeness MH, Esses SI, Errico T, Yuan HA. Late infection of spinal instrumentation by hematogenous seeding. Spine 1993; 18(4):492–496.

13. Wimmer C, Gluch H, Franzreb M, Ogon M. Predisposing factors for infection in spine surgery: a survey of 850 spinal procedures. J Spinal Disord 1998; 11(2):124–128.

14. Horowitz NH, Curtin JA. Prophylactic antibiotics and wound infections following laminectomy for lumbar disc herniation. J Neurosurg 1975; 43:727–731.

15. Rubinstein E, Findler G, Amit P, Shaked I. Perioperative prophylactic cephazolin in spinal surgery. A double-blind placebo-controlled trial. J Bone Joint Surg Br 1994; 76(1): 99–102.

16. Guiboux JP, Cantor JB, Small SD, Zervos M, Herkowitz HN. The effect of prophylactic antibiotics on iatrogenic intervertebral disc infections. a rabbit model. Spine 1995; 20(6): 685–688.

17. Guiboux JP, Ahlgren B, Patti JE, Bernhard M, Zervos M, Herkowitz HN. The role of prophylactic antibiotics in spinal instrumentation. A rabbit model. Spine 1998; 23(6):653–656.

18. Swoboda SM, Merz C, Kostuik J, Trentler B, Lipsett PA. Does intraoperative blood loss affect antibiotic serum and tissue concentrations? Arch Surg 1996; 131(11):1165–1171.

19. Polly DW, Jr., Meter JJ, Brueckner R, Asplund L, van Dam BE. The effect of intraoperative blood loss on serum cefazolin level in patients undergoing instrumented spinal fusion. A prospective, controlled study. Spine 1996; 21(20):2363–2367.

20. Dobzyniak M, Fischgrund JS, Hankins S. The effect of single versus multiple dose antibiotic prophylaxis on the rate of wound infection in lumbar disc surgery. Annual Meeting of the International Society for Study of the Lumbar Spine. Adelaide, Australia 2000.

21. Swank S, Lonstein JE, Moe JH, Winter RB, Bradford DS. Surgical treatment of adult scoliosis. A review of two hundred and twenty-two cases. J Bone Joint Surg Am 1981; 63(2):268–287.

22. Cruse PJ, Foord R. A five-year prospective study of 23,649 surgical wounds. Arch Surg 1973; 107(2):206–210.

23. Capen DA, Calderone RR, Green A. Perioperative risk factors for wound infections after lower back fusions. Orthop Clin North Am 1996; 27(1):83–86.

24. Klein JD, Garfin SR. Nutritional status in the patient with spinal infection. Orthop Clin North Am 1996; 27(1):33–36.

25. Jensen JE, Jensen TG, Smith TK, Johnston DA, Dudrick SJ. Nutrition in orthopaedic surgery. J Bone Joint Surg Am 1982; 64(9):1263–1272.

26. Glassman SD, Dimar JR, Puno RM, Johnson JR. Salvage of instrumental lumbar fusions complicated by surgical wound infection. Spine 1996; 21(18):2163–2169.

27. Massie JB, Heller JG, Abitbol JJ, McPherson D, Garfin SR. Postoperative posterior spinal wound infections. Clin Orthop 1992; 284:99–108.

28. Simpson JM, Silveri CP, Balderston RA, Simeone FA, An HS. The results of operations on the lumbar spine in patients who have diabetes mellitus. J Bone Joint Surg Am 1993; 75(12): 1823–1829.

29. Stambough JL, Beringer D. Postoperative wound infections complicating adult spine surgery. J Spinal Disord 1992; 5(3):277–285.

30. Nolan CM, Beaty HN, Bagdade JD. Further characterization of the impaired bactericidal function of granulocytes in patients with poorly controlled diabetes. Diabetes 1978; 27(9):889–894.

31. Bagdade JD, Root RK, Bulger RJ. Impaired leukocyte function in patients with poorly controlled diabetes. Diabetes 1974; 23(1):9–15.

32. Thalgott JS, Cotler HB, Sasso RC, LaRocca H, Gardner V. Postoperative infections in spinal implants. Classification and analysis—a multicenter study. Spine 1991; 16(8):981–984.

33. Fraser RD, Osti OL, Vernon-Roberts B. Discitis after discography. J Bone Joint Surg Br 1987; 69(1):26–35.

34. Osti OL, Fraser RD, Vernon-Roberts B. Discitis after discography. The role of prophylactic antibiotics. J Bone Joint Surg Br 1990; 72(2):271–274.

35. Zeiger HE, Jr., Zampella EJ. Intervertebral disc infection after lumbar chemonucleolysis: report of a case. Neurosurgery 1986; 18(5):616–621.

36. Brian JE, Jr., Westerman GR, Chadduck WM. Septic complications of chemonucleolysis. Neurosurgery 1984; 15(5):730–734.

37. Scherbel A, Gardner W. Infections involving the intervertebral disks: diagnosis and management. JAMA 1960; 174:370–374.

38. Silber JS, Anderson G, Vaccaro AR, Anderson PA, McCormick P. Management of post-procedural diskitis. Spine J 2002; 2:279–287.

39. Dauch WA. Infection of the intervertebral space following conventional and microsurgical operation on the herniated lumbar intervertebral disc: a controlled clinical trial. Acta Neurochirurg 1986; 82:43–49.

40. Tronnier V, Schneider R, Kunz U, Albert F, Oldenkott P. Postoperative spondylodiscitis: results of a prospective study about the aetiology of spondylodiscitis after operation for lumbar disc herniation. Acta Neurochir (Wien) 1992; 117(3–4):149–152.

41. Zeidman SM, Ducker TB, Raycroft J. Trends and complications in cervical spine surgery: 1989–1993. J Spinal Disord 1997; 10(6):523–526.

42. Fehlings MG, Cooper PR, Errico TJ. Posterior plates in the management of cervical instability: long-term results in 44 patients. J Neurosurg 1994; 81(3):341–349.

43. Savitz SI, Savitz MH, Goldstein HB, Mouracade CT, Malangone S. Topical irrigation with polymyxin and bacitracin for spinal surgery. Surg Neurol 1998; 50(3):208–212.

44. Rosenstein BD, Wilson FC, Funderburk CH. The use of bacitracin irrigation to prevent infection in postoperative skeletal wounds. An experimental study. J Bone Joint Surg Am 1989; 71(3):427–430.

45. Rawlings CE, 3rd, Wilkins RH, Gallis HA, Goldner JL, Francis R. Postoperative intervertebral disc space infection. Neurosurgery 1983; 13(4):371–376.

46. Hadjipavlou AG, Mader JT, Necessary JT, Muffoletto AJ. Hematogenous pyogenic spinal infections and their surgical management. Spine 2000; 25(13):1668–1679.

47. Fouquet B, Goupille P, Jattiot F, Cotty P, Lapierre F, Valat JP, Amouroux J, Benatre A. Discitis after lumbar disc surgery. Features of "aseptic" and "septic" forms. Spine 1992; 17(3):356–358.

48. Meyer B, Schaller K, Rohde V, Hassler W. The C-reactive protein for detection of early infections after lumbar microdiscectomy. Acta Neurochir (Wien) 1995; 136(3–4):145–150.

49. El-Gindi S, Aref S, Salama M, Andrew J. Infection of intervertebral discs after operation. J Bone Joint Surg Br 1976; 58(1):114–116.

50. Bircher MD, Tasker T, Crawshaw C, Mulholland RC. Discitis following lumbar surgery. Spine 1988; 13(1):98–102.

51. Schulitz KP, Assheuer J. Discitis after procedures on the intervertebral disc. Spine 1994; 19(10):1172–1177.

52. Kapp JP, Sybers WA. Erythrocyte sedimentation rate following uncomplicated lumbar disc operations. Surg Neurol 1979; 12(4):329–330.

53. Jonsson B, Soderholm R, Stromqvist B. Erythrocyte sedimentation rate after lumbar spine surgery. Spine 1991; 16(9):1049–1050.

54. Thelander U, Larsson S. Quantitation of C-reactive protein levels and erythrocyte sedimentation rate after spinal surgery. Spine 1992; 17(4):400–404.

55. Jimenez-Mejias ME, de Dios Colmenero J, Sanchez-Lora FJ, Palomino-Nicas J, Reguera JM, Garcia de la Heras J, Garcia-Ordonez MA, Pachon J. Postoperative spondylodiskitis: etiology, clinical findings, prognosis, and comparison with nonoperative pyogenic spondylodiskitis. Clin Infect Dis 1999; 29(2):339–345.

56. Bruschwein DA, Brown ML, McLeod RA. Gallium scintigraphy in the evaluation of disk-space infections: concise communication. J Nucl Med 1980; 21(10):925–927.

57. Norris S, Ehrlich MG, Keim DE, Guiterman H, McKusick KA. Early diagnosis of disc-space infection using Gallium-67. J Nucl Med 1978; 19(4):384–386.

58. Szypryt EP, Hardy JG, Hinton CE, Worthington BS, Mulholland RC. A comparison between magnetic resonance imaging and scintigraphic bone imaging in the diagnosis of disc space infection in an animal model. Spine 1988; 13(9):1042–1048.

59. Boden SD, Davis DO, Dina TS, Sunner JL, Wiesel SW. Postoperative diskitis: distinguishing early MR imaging findings from normal postoperative disk space changes. Radiology 1992; 184(3):765–771.

60. Van Goethem JW, Parizel PM, van den Hauwe L, Van de Kelft E, Verlooy J, De Schepper AM. The value of MRI in the diagnosis of postoperative spondylodiscitis. Neuroradiology 2000; 42(8):580–585.

61. Anderson PA, Bohlman HH. Anterior decompression and arthrodesis of the cervical spine: long-term motor improvement. Part II—Improvement in complete traumatic quadriplegia. J Bone Joint Surg Am 1992; 74(5):683–692.

62. Kuriloff DB, Blaugrund S, Ryan J, O'Leary P. Delayed neck infection following anterior spine surgery. Laryngoscope 1987; 97(9):1094–1098.

63. Shockley WW, Tate JL, Stucker FJ. Management of perforations of the hypopharynx and cervical esophagus. Laryngoscope 1985; 95(8):939–941.

64. Gebhard JS, Brugman JL. Percutaneous discectomy for the treatment of bacterial diskitis. Spine 1994; 19(7):855–857.

65. Crow WN, Borowski AM, Hadjipavlou AG, Walser EM, Arya S, Calme MB, Amps J, Jensen R, Somisetty S, Alford B, Adesokan A. Percutaneous transpedicular automated nucleotomy for debridement of infected discs. J Vasc Interv Radiol 1998; 9(1 pt 1):161–165.

66. Devlin VJ, Boachie-Adjei O, Bradford DS, Ogilvie JW, Transfeldt EE. Treatment of adult spinal deformity with fusion to the sacrum using CD instrumentation. J Spinal Disord 1991; 4(1):1–14.

67. Moe JH. Complications of scoliosis treatment. Clin Orthop 1967; 53:21–30.

68. Woo H, Rozai A, Cooper P. Modern management of cervical osteomyelitis. 25th Annual Meeting of the Cervical Spine Research Society, Rancho Mirage, December 1997.

69. Vaccaro AR, Harris BM. Presentation and treatment of pyogenic vertebral osteomyelitis. Semin Spine Surg 2000; 12(4):183–191.

70. Hughes J, DiGiancinto G, Sundaresan N. Anterior instrumentation in cervical osteomyelitis. 25th Annual Meeting of the Cervical Spine Research Society, CA, December 1997.

71. Heller JG, Levine MJ. Postoperative infections of the spine. Semin Spine Surg 1996; 8:105–114.

72. Seligson D, Mehta S, Voos K, Henry SL, Johnson JR. The use of antibiotic-impregnated polymethylmethacrylate beads to prevent the evolution of localized infection. J Orthop Trauma 1992; 6(4):401–406.

73. Yuan-Innes MJ, Temple CL, Lacey MS. Vacuum-assisted wound closure: a new approach to spinal wounds with exposed hardware. Spine 2001; 26(3):E30–33.

74. Paonessa KJ, Hostnik WJ, Zide BM. Use of tissue expanders for wound closure of spinal infections or dehiscence. Orthop Clin North Am 1996; 27(1):155–170.

75. Lumsden RM, 2nd, Morris JM. An in vivo study of axial rotation and immoblization at the lumbosacral joint. J Bone Joint Surg Am 1968; 50(8):1591–1602.

76. Weiss LE, Vaccaro AR, Scuderi G, McGuire M, Garfin SR. Pseudarthrosis after postoperative wound infection in the lumbar spine. J Spinal Disord 1997; 10(6):482–487.

77. Calderone RR, Thomas JC, Jr., Haye W, Abeles D. Outcome assessment in spinal infections. Orthop Clin North Am 1996; 27(1):201–205.

78. Przybylski GJ, Sharan AD. Single-stage autogenous bone grafting and internal fixation in the surgical management of pyogenic diskitis and vertebral osteomyelitis. J Neurosurg 2001; 94(1 suppl 1):1–7.

12

The Use of Neuromonitoring for Neurological Injury Detection and Implant Accuracy

Daniel M. Schwartz and Anthony K. Sestokas
Surgical Monitoring Associates, Bala Cynwyd, Pennylvania, U.S.A.

I. INTRODUCTION

Neurological deficit is the most feared complication of spine surgery. It can occur pre-surgically during transfer of the patient to the operating room table, from neck extension for airway management during intubation, during patient positioning for adequate operative exposure, or as a result of surgically induced injury. To be sure, appropriate preoperative preparation, careful surgical planning, precise surgical execution, and constant surgical vigilance can minimize risk for neurological complication. An increasingly important means of injury prevention is continuous intraoperative neurophysiological monitoring (IONM) of spinal cord and spinal nerve root function (1–3). As with any other type of medical test, interpretation of IONM data requires complex clinical decision making, which takes place in the presence of some uncertainty. Decision making is the process of selecting a specific course of action from among a set of alternatives. It begins at the information-gathering stage (e.g., recording a neurophysiological response) and proceeds through the establishment of likelihood estimation (e.g., deciding if the response has changed significantly) until the final act of choosing an action (e.g., alerting the surgeon of evolving spinal cord injury). This chapter discusses the interpretation of IONM data in the context of signal-detection theory (SDT). The goal of this chapter is to reduce the complications associated with misinterpretation of IONM data through careful examination of the intraoperative decision-making process as defined by SDT.

II. SIGNAL DETECTION THEORY

One of the early goals of psychologists was to measure the sensitivity of our sensory systems (vision, hearing, smell, taste, and touch). This led to the concept of a sensitivity threshold defined as the least intense level of sensory stimulation required for a person to detect the presence of the stimulus. What they found was that even though the level of the stimulus remained constant across successive presentations, subjects were inconsistent in their ability to detect the presence of the threshold stimulus. It appeared that factors other than sensory receptor sensitivity influenced the signal detection process. There seemed to be no single fixed value below which a person never detected the stimulus and above which they always identified it. As a result, the accepted definition of threshold was modified as that intensity level at which a person can detect stimulus presence at least 50% of the time.

One approach to resolving the dilemma of sensory threshold measurement is described in SDT, first introduced as a method of applying a statistical decision approach to the study of radar reception (4–6). SDT abandons the concept of a constant threshold in favor of considering stimulus detection as a decision-making process which is governed by the stimulus characteristics, the sensitivity of the person to the stimulus, and cognitive factors. Thus, any given individual will be able to detect an intense sound, light, or smell more easily than a weaker one. Moreover, a more sensitive individual (or one with more training and experience) will require lower stimulus intensity for detection than one who is less sensitive. Finally, and of particular relevance to IONM, an individual who is left to make a decision about the presence or absence of a stimulus (or a neurophysiological change) in the face of uncertainty will do so based on the consequences of any judgment error. That is, the decision will be influenced by what kind of judgment error is worse; stating that no stimulus was present (or that there was no change in the neurophysiological response) when there actually was one, or indicating that there was a stimulus (or a neurophysiological change) when there was none. In simplest form, SDT represents a statistical rule structure for detecting a signal (or change in neurophysiological response) in the presence of uncertainty or "noise". This rule structure forms the very basis for interpreting most medical diagnostic tests, including neurophysiological signals recorded during spine surgery.

To be sure, the ideal would be to have an IONM technique and an interpreter that is always correct. Unfortunately, nothing in medicine is perfect even in the best and most experienced of hands, including neurophysiological monitoring tests and those responsible for interpretation of the data. The goal then is to limit decision error when faced with uncertainty. Moreover, in the case of neurophysiological monitoring, there is a twofold problem: one aspect relates to the sensitivity of the monitoring technique to identifying iatrogenic central nervous system (CNS) injury and the other to the ability of monitoring personnel to detect the change and to alert the surgeon in sufficient time to intervene.

Consider, for example, a surgical neurophysiologist who is monitoring a scoliosis correction. He or she is recording a neurophysiological signal such as a somatosensory-evoked potential (SSEP) throughout surgery. Each recorded potential is compared to some predefined control (baseline) to determine if a significant change has occurred in one or more measurement parameters, namely, amplitude, latency, and morphology. Clearly, this determination is relatively straightforward if the signal is either entirely unchanged relative to its control or completely obliterated and time-locked to a specific surgical maneuver (e.g., rod derotation). The problem arises, however, when the signal lies somewhere between these two extremes. In this situation, the signal change must be interpreted in the presence of uncertainty. Is it secondary to surgical trauma (and therefore significant), or is it associated with natural signal variability due to some external (artifact) and/or internal (physiological) noise factors (and therefore insignificant)? The task of the surgical neurophysiologist is to decide between these two alternatives. SDT describes the process by which the neurophysiologist looks for a particular signal or signal change and attempts to ignore competing noise events in order to make an accurate decision.

III. THE ROLE OF COMPETING "NOISE" IN IONM DECISION MAKING

Interpretation of neurophysiological monitoring data is a complex process. For the most part it is based on determining if certain parameters of the "signal" such as amplitude, latency, and/or morphology (shape) have changed significantly as compared to some control tracing. Regardless of interpreter skill and experience, there is always some level of uncertainty, owing to the contribution of competing internal and external noise sources, which cause the signal of interest to vary from trial to trial in a way that is unrelated to the surgery itself. In other words, evoked potentials, by their very nature, are not stationary.

The human body generates a host of electrical signals from the heart (EKG), brain (EEG), and peripheral muscle (EMG). Once an electrode is attached anywhere on the body, these very large amplitude signals can create a source of "internal noise" that may interact with and mask the neurophysiological signal of interest. To put things into better perspective, EKG electrical voltage is up to 50 times larger than that of intraoperative EMG activity and more than 100 times larger than that of a scalp-recorded cortical SSEP. Generalized EEG activity, which forms the electrical background from which an evoked potential is extracted, ranges in amplitude from 25 to 75 μV in an anesthetized patient, whereas a cortical SSEP may range from 0.1 to 5.0 μV depending on type of anesthesia and presence of preexisting spinal cord compression or disease. Given this, it is easy to understand how evoked potentials are buried in electrophysiological noise. While signal averaging, digital filtering, and other technical manipulations available on neurophysiological recording instruments go a long way toward reducing the contaminating effects of these internal noise sources, they cannot eliminate them completely. Thus, even in the absence of surgical manipulation, and all other things being equal, there will always be some variability in response morphology, amplitude, and latency from trial to trial.

Another source of internal noise comes from the presence of preexisting spinal cord or peripheral nerve disease, which can cause the signal of interest (SSEP) to be degraded before surgery. Owing to neural desynchrony, the response morphology may be poorly resolved and its amplitude markedly reduced, thereby bringing it closer to the physiological "noise floor." Consequently, it will be more difficult to determine when a significant surgically induced change occurs versus one due to moment-to-moment variability because the primary signal voltage (SSEP) might be similar to that of the internal background noise.

Potentially more confounding than internal noise is the effect of external noise or artifact. Examples of such noise sources include but are not limited to (a) high and/or unbalanced recording electrode impedances, (b) contaminating line-frequency (60 Hz and its harmonics) electrical noise (e.g., electronic bed, warming blanket, bad electrical grounding, surgical headlight, surgical microscope, blood warmer), (c) electrostatic interference from contact between two metal surgical instruments, and (d) type and concentration of anesthesia.

Eliminating or limiting the influences of external noise is the responsibility of the surgical neurophysiologist. For example:

1. Careful cleansing and preparation of the skin prior to electrode application will lead to very low and reasonably balanced electrode impedance.
2. Ensuring that the recording electrode cables are braided and not crossing other electrical cables will eliminate the antennae effect of scattered wires and reduce the capacitive inductance effects of other electrical signals.

3. Identifying and eliminating sources of interfering line-frequency noise will "clean up" the neurophysiological signal.
4. Tailoring the anesthesia by replacing potent inhalational agents (e.g., Desflurane, Sevoflurane, Isoflurane) and nitrous oxide (all known to cause significant degradation of the cortical SSEP wave) with a total intravenous anesthetic (TIVA) will boost signal amplitude and improve response consistency.

Each of these proactive steps will foster enhanced signal clarity and act to reduce uncertainty in the detection of significant signal change.

IV. THE ROLE OF COGNITIVE FACTORS IN IONM DECISION MAKING

The interpretation of intraoperative neurophysiological monitoring data can be likened to a sensory stimulus-detection experiment. In both cases there is a constant stream of information, which provides the context within which a decision must be made. This context, commonly known as background "neural noise," can have a marked influence on decision making. In a sensory detection experiment, when a faint stimulus is delivered, a decision about stimulus presence/absence is based on whether ongoing neural activity reflects noise alone or a sensory signal mixed with neural noise. The more intense the signal, of course, the easier it becomes to differentiate the signal from the generalized background neural noise. Hence, cognitive signal-to-noise ratio (CSNR) plays an important role in signal detection.

The surgical neurophysiologist is constantly exposed to streams of information that relate to the quality of the neurophysiological response compared to its control, the surgical manipulation at the moment, the physiological state of the patient (e.g., heart rate, blood pressure, etc), and the consistency of the anesthetic plane. All of this information defines the context (analogous to background neural noise) within which an impression is formed about the significance of neurophysiological response change (analogous to detection of signal presence/absence). If response change occurred only in the presence of CNS injury, then detection would be entirely straightforward. Unfortunately, the influences of external artifact, internal physiological noise, and low CSNR all combine to increase uncertainty about the surgical significance of response change.

V. THE ROLE OF INFORMATION IN IONM DECISION MAKING

It should be clear from the preceding discussion that it is impossible for the surgical neurophysiologist to interpret single-event response changes with perfect accuracy. As a result, a competent surgical neurophysiologist must interpret the data by identifying an array of possible explanations for response change and estimate the relative likelihood of each. This process is not unlike that which underlies differential diagnosis in medicine. One way of managing the effects of uncertainty is to increase the amount of useful clinical information at the disposal of the neurophysiologist (i.e., increase the CSNR). This can be accomplished by monitoring not only one modality such as SSEPs, but by adding other monitoring modalities like transcranial electrical motor–evoked potentials (tceMEPs) together with spontaneous and/or electrically stimulated electromyography (sp/stEMG), thus forming a multimodality IONM battery as we have stressed in previous publications (1–3).

VI. THE ROLE OF CRITERION IN IONM DECISION MAKING

Decision criterion refers to the minimum evidence required by the interpreter of information to say "neurophysiological signal present" or "no significant IONM change" in an
ambiguous situation. The choice of a criterion depends, to a large extent, on perceived
consequences of correct and incorrect outcomes. For example, if the presumed penalty
is greater for saying "no significant IONM change" when there actually was one (false
negative), then the IONM personnel may generally be more willing to state "significant
change." On the other hand, if the consequences are more costly for stating that a change
took place when, in fact, there was none (false alarm), he or she may be more willing to
report "no change." Unquestionably, the penalty for a false-negative IONM report is
potentially devastating neurological compromise; therefore, one would expect the
interpreter's decision criterion to be more biased towards liberal surgical alerts of
significant change. For the same reason, one would also anticipate that the less training
and experience an individual has, the more likely he or she will be to consider any change
significant when the situation is ambiguous.

Figure 1 displays two hypothetical distributions for patients with and without
evolving iatrogenic spinal cord injury, respectively, as a function of intraoperative
neurophysiological signal change. A decision criterion placed in the middle of the signal
change range defines the critical change required before the neurophysiologist alerts the
surgeon. There are four possible outcomes in the decision-making process:

1. **Hit (True Positive)**—there was evolving injury or symptoms, and the IONM data
    were interpreted as having changed significantly from the control (**Yes
    Response**).

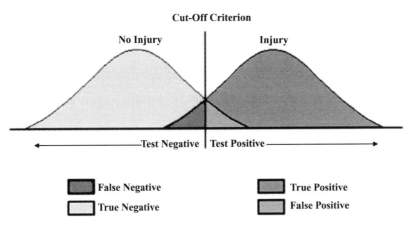

Figure 1 Hypothetical probability distribution curves for patients without intraoperative
iatrogenic injury (left distribution) and those with injury (right distribution) as a function of
intraoperative neurophysiological signal change, ranging from no change on the far left of the
abscissa to extreme change on the right. The vertical line shows a mid-range decision criterion
cut-off point for defining a significant neurophysiological change. Changes falling to the left of
the line do not result in an alert (Test Negative), whereas those falling to the right do (Test Positive).
The four shaded areas indicate possible outcomes in the decision-making process. Note that this
mid-range decision criterion produces an equal number of false-positive and false-negative results.

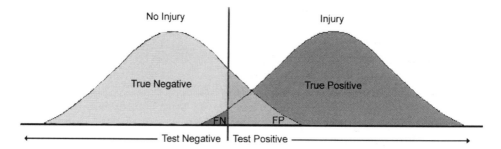

Figure 2 Hypothetical probability distribution curves, as in Figure 1, illustrating the effect of making the decision criterion for significant signal change less stringent by shifting the criterion cut-off point to the left. Note that this decreases the probability of false negatives (FN) and increases the probability of false positives (FP).

3. **Miss (False Negative)**—there was evolving injury or symptoms, but the IONM data were interpreted as not having changed significantly from the control (**No Response**).
4. **False Alarm (False Positive)**—there was not an evolving injury or symptoms, but the IONM data were interpreted as having changed significantly from the control (**Yes Response**).
5. **Correct Rejection (True Negative)**—there was not an evolving spinal cord injury or symptoms, and the IONM data were interpreted as not having changed from the control (**No Response**).

On both hits (true positives) and false alarms (false positives), the interpreter's cognitive state (internal response) exceeds the decision criterion line, resulting in a yes response to the question of significant change.

Suppose, however, that the interpreter's criterion for significant change was set very low so as to call an alert for almost every change, as shown in Figure 2. The interpreter would never miss a neurological compromise when one was developing and thus the hit rate would be incredibly high. Of course the tradeoff for this high hit rate is a higher number of false alarms, which ultimately desensitizes the surgeon and makes him or her less likely to be proactive when informed of a change. Conversely, if the criterion point was set too high, as in Figure 3, such that the interpreter usually reported "no change," the false-positive rate would be markedly lower but at the cost of increasing false negatives.

The point is that there is absolutely no way to adjust the decision criterion cut-off value to achieve all hits with no false positives when the two population distributions illustrated in Figures 1–3 have any overlap, as they do for all neurophysiological tests. It is inevitable, therefore, that errors in IONM interpretation will be made; however, the type of error considered the most costly can be minimized by manipulating the criterion value to achieve the desired result. Ideally, selection of the decision criterion value should be made objectively on the basis of known or estimated prior probabilities of significant events (6); however, this criterion can also be influenced by subjective factors, which may have unintended consequences. For example, a surgeon may suggest that a particular test is "too sensitive" (i.e., after most alerts the patient usually wakes up without a deficit), causing less experienced IONM personnel to raise the decision criterion cut-off for significant response change at the cost of an elevated false-negative rate.

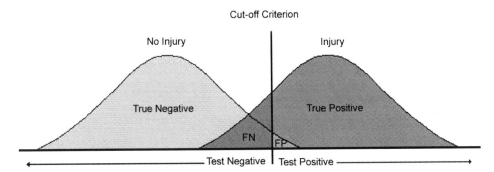

Figure 3 Hypothetical probability distribution curves, as in Figure 1, illustrating the effect of making the decision criterion for significant signal change more stringent by shifting the criterion cut-off point to the right. Note that this increases the probability of false negatives (FN) and decreases the probability of false positives (FP).

VII. THE RECEIVER OPERATING CHARACTERISTIC CURVE

The complete range of an individual's decision options as a function of varying the criterion cut-off can be plotted on a graph known as a receiver operating characteristic (ROC) curve, as illustrated in Figure 4. In application to the study of diagnostic tests, ROC curves consist of plots of true-positive (TP) rates versus false-positive rates, derived experimentally by varying the level of the decision criterion cut-off. The shape of the ROC curve and in particular the depth of its bow characterizes the accuracy of a particular signal-detection system. The deeper the curve bow, the better the system is at detecting the signal in noise. A perfect test would be one with a true-positive rate of 1 and a false-positive rate of 0. The ROC curve for a test that approaches perfection would begin at the origin, rise steeply to a true-positive rate near 1.0, and then flatten out abruptly, creating a deep bow. Conversely, a poor test would be one with a true-positive rate that is close to the false-positive rates thereby producing an ROC curve near the diagonal line, with little or no bow.

As discussed previously, "noise" of all types (i.e., external, internal, and cognitive) can impact greatly on decision making by increasing the level of interpretative ambiguity. Because noise reduces relative signal strength and makes the signal harder to detect, it will affect the contour of the ROC curve, shifting it down and to the right. Conversely, the stronger or more discernable the signal, the more the ROC curve will shift up and to the left. Finally, acquiring more information (such as monitoring more than one modality) has the equivalent effect of increasing signal strength and/or SNR, thereby simplifying decision making. We can see, therefore, that signal detection is governed by the strength of the signal, by the level of the background noise from which the signal must be extracted, and by the amount of complementary information available.

VIII. ACCURACY OF IONM

While it is generally understood that the purpose of IONM tests is to differentiate between normal CNS electrical function and evolving dysfunction, a quantitative appreciation of

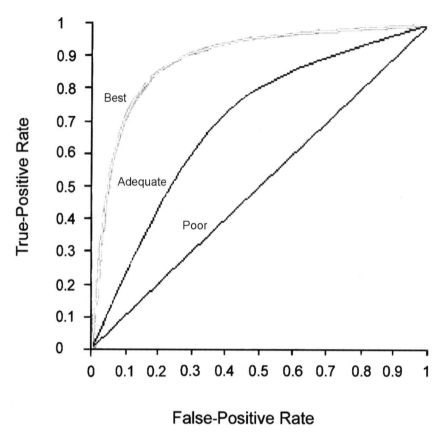

Figure 4 Receiver operating characteristic (ROC) curves showing the tradeoff between true-positive and false-positive rates for three hypothetical tests with different accuracies.

their predictive value is often lacking. Understanding the relationship between the results of these monitoring tests and actual presence or absence of evolving CNS dysfunction serves to (a) increase the likelihood of correct interpretation of each monitoring modality and (b) improve the neurophysiologist's ability to select the best modalities for each specific surgery.

There are several characteristics that describe the utility of any diagnostic test, including IONM procedures. As described above, accuracy can be quantified by the receiver operating characteristics of a test. Sensitivity and specificity are two commonly used measures that can be derived from the ROC curve.

Sensitivity denotes the likelihood that a test result will be positive in the presence of disease or symptom or, in the case of surgical monitoring, that there is a significant neurophysiological response change (e.g., SSEP, tceMEP, EMG) in the presence of evolving CNS dysfunction (i.e., the probability of a true positive or hit). When the sensitivity of a test is high, the false negative rate is by definition low, since the sum of these two probabilities is 1. Highly sensitive tests are best applied when the a priori probability of a specific disease or symptom is low and the purpose of such testing is to rule out the disease. Given that sensitive tests are usually positive in the face of disease, they are the test of choice when the stakes are high for a false-negative result such as spinal cord injury. A simple mnemonic that describes a highly sensitive test is **SnNout**—when a test has high **Sen**sitivity a **N**egative result rules **Out** the disease or dysfunction.

Specificity, on the other hand, refers to the likelihood of a negative or normal test finding in the absence of disease or for IONM that there is no neurophysiological response change in the absence of evolving CNS dysfunction (i.e., the probability of a true negative). When the specificity of a test is high, the false-positive rate is by definition low, since the sum of these two probabilities is 1. Highly specific tests are useful for confirming an existing impression that the disease or dysfunction already exists because they rarely are positive in the absence of the disease. **SpPin** is the mnemonic that describes such tests— when a test has high **Sp**ecificity, a **P**ositive result rules **In** the disease or dysfunction.

The clinical goal then is to select a test or IONM modality that has both high sensitivity (and therefore low false-negative rate) and high specificity (and therefore low false-positive rate). As was highlighted in the previous discussion on SDT and ROC curves, however, it is difficult to achieve one without sacrificing the other. It is critical, therefore, that IONM personnel utilize these concepts both to select the most appropriate monitoring modalities and to optimize the information necessary to make a reliable and valid clinical decision. Accordingly:

Rule 1—When the penalty is great for a false-negative result and you need to rule out the presence of spinal cord or nerve root injury, *the test should be highly sensitive.*

Rule 2—When a test is used to confirm an existing suspicion that the disease or disorder is present and a false-positive finding is harmful, *the test should be highly specific.*

IX. THE FALSE-POSITIVE CONTROVERSY

A complicating factor when attempting to define the operating characteristics of tests used for injury detection is how best to define "injury." From the spine surgeon's perspective, injury refers only to the presence of new-onset neurologic sequalae (e.g., paraplegia, paraparesis, neuropraxia) following emergence from anesthesia. Hence, any intraoperative change in neurophysiological responses that does not result in postoperative deficit may be mistakenly labeled a false positive in the surgeon's view. A competing argument to this view is that if a significant neurophysiological change prompts some type of surgical or nonsurgical intervention (e.g., raising MAP, initiating intraoperative steroid therapy), which in turn causes resolution of the neurophysiological change, then this reflects evidence of evolving CNS dysfunction or at least symptoms that may precede injury if left unattended. From the neurophysiologist's perspective, therefore, such changes are *not* false-positive events. Rather, they are true-positive precursors to an evolving or impending injurious state. Unfortunately, this concept is greatly misunderstood within the spine surgery community. For example, the observation that tceMEP amplitude is sensitive to reduction in blood pressure does not mean that the test is overly sensitive and yields too high a false-positive rate. Rather, it reflects the current hemodynamic state of the spinal cord.

It should be remembered that the underlying goal of IONM is to identify altered CNS electrical function early enough to initiate propitious intervention that will reverse a potentially devastating neurological outcome. For neurophysiological response change to be considered an actual false-positive event, it would be necessary not to intervene upon surgical notification of such change. Then, if the patient awakens without untoward deficit, it can be classified as a false positive. While this certainly represents an interesting topic for discussion, the ethical and medical-legal implications of such a study are obvious. It is our philosophy and practice, therefore, to define a true positive from both a surgical and a neurophysiological perspective, assuming that IONM personnel are adequately trained to rule out inherent response variability, technical reasons, anesthesia, etc., as causes for neurophysiological response change.

The following list suggests some possible reasons for actual false-positive neurophysiological changes.

1. Technical Errors: (a) inadvertently decreasing the level of stimulation used to elicit an evoked potential, thereby producing an apparently significant amplitude change; (b) having unfavorable signal-to-noise ratio for recording an interpretable response; (c) stimulating a pedicle screw at too high a level such that it produces current spread to an adjacent nerve root; (d) interpreting "neurogenic spinal" evoked potential loss following placement of rigid spinal instrumentation as spinal cord injury when it may be a byproduct of current shunting.

2. Anesthesia Influences: (a) misinterpreting amplitude and/or latency change due to variability imposed by changes in anesthesia; (b) mistaking amplitude loss and morphologic change in subcortical SSEPs secondary to the effects of EMG artifact.

3. Interpretation Errors: (a) setting the decision criteria for neurophysiological change too low; (b) attempting to detect an evoked potential change when the initial amplitude is so small that it is within the range of the neurophysiological noise floor; (c) relying on latency (e.g., 10% rule) rather than amplitude as the primary measure for significant response change. This is a common error in spinal cord monitoring and often leads to false-positive results. (In our experience, intraoperative latency change in the absence of significant amplitude decrease is generally unreliable as a predictor of spinal cord injury and therefore should not be used as such). (e) not being able to distinguish between the acoustic and visual signatures of real neurotonic EMG bursts or trains from metallic artifact caused by surgical instruments; (f) mistaking neurotonic discharges across all or most recording channels as being surgically induced when they actually reflect inadequate anesthetic depth.

X. FALSE NEGATIVES IN IONM

A false negative is defined as absence of a neurophysiological change in the presence of neurological injury. Indeed, it is the most feared result for both the surgeon and the neurophysiologist. Recall from Rule 1 that "When the penalty is great for a false-negative result and you need to rule out the presence of spinal cord or nerve root injury, *the test should be highly sensitive.*" The following case study is illustrative.

A patient undergoing a revision decompressive L2-L4 laminectomy and fusion with pedicle screw fixation was monitored by spontaneous and electrically stimulated EMG activity. EMG activity was recorded over adductor, quadriceps, tibialis anterior, gastrocnemius, and anal sphincter muscles innervated by L2 to low sacral nerve roots, respectively. The neuromuscular junction was unblocked for the entire procedure following initial exposure, as evidenced by recording time-locked contractions of foot flexor muscle to train-of-four posterior tibial nerve stimulation. The monitoring results demonstrated absolutely no evidence of any spontaneous neurotonic EMG activity throughout the decompression and during pedicle probing, marking, and placement of pedicle screws. Electrical stimulation of pedicle screws at 12 mA failed to identify a pedicle cortex breach. Postoperatively the patient developed evidence of left L3 nerve root impingement and was taken back to the operating room for pedicle screw exploration. Upon exposure, the left L3 screw was again stimulated at 12 mA without evidence of a recordable compound muscle action potential. Yet, there was visual evidence of a pedicle wall fracture. At that point the left L3 nerve root was exposed and stimulated. Unexpectedly, the root depolarization threshold was found to be 18 mA, elevated more than four times above normal. This false-negative result has led to recommendations that pedicle screw stimulation protocols should include direct nerve root stimulation so that root depolarization threshold can be used to optimize screw stimulation cut-off intensity. This observation of abnormally elevated nerve root depolarization thresholds is rare but does exist, making direct nerve root stimulation a useful procedural adjunct during screw placement. (For a detailed discussion of how to manage pedicle screw testing in such patients see Ref. (2).)

As is the case with false-positive misclassification, there is also some confusion as to what represents an actual false-negative result. All too often, IONM findings are considered false negative, when in reality the test modality used was not suitable for the specific purpose.

Consider, for example, the findings of Minahan et al. (7). They described two cases in which intraoperative monitoring of so-called "neurogenic motor-evoked potentials" (NMEPs) (8–10) failed to identify impending spinal cord injury, which resulted in paraplegia. Minahan and colleagues used the NMEP believing that it represented a motor response as suggested in the early clinical literature, when in fact, other studies have shown that this response is largely mediated by antidromically activitated sensory fibers (11,12). Indeed, we have recorded NMEPs successfully from several paraplegic patients to demonstrate that the response does not depend on functionally intact spinal motor tracts. In light of these findings, should intraoperative preservation of the NMEP in the face of postoperative paraplegia be considered a false-negative result of IONM or rather an inappropriate use of a test not suited for the intended application?

To illustrate further, a patient monitored with SSEPs developed a C5 nerve root palsy in the immediate postoperative period following a cervical laminaplasty. Review of the IONM records demonstrated highly resolved and very stable ulnar and posterior tibial nerve SSEPs throughout the entire surgical course.

As with the NMEP example described above, one should not consider this a false-negative finding because SSEPs do not provide a valid measure of segmental nerve root function. While the outcome was unfortunate, the test was not at fault, nor was the neurophysiologist since he or she was using SSEPs only to monitor the spinal cord. Of course, if the same result occurred now in the presence of direct nerve root monitoring with spEMG and tceMEPs (13), then a false-negative classification would be entirely valid.

Finally, is it a false-negative result of IONM when the immediate postoperative neurological exam is unremarkable and a neurological deficit develops several hours later? It must be remembered that the goal of IONM is to identify emerging neurological injury or symptoms intraoperatively so as to initiate timely intervention. If there is no functional change in the spinal cord intraoperatively, but the cord becomes edematous during the first 12–18 hours following surgery when monitoring has been discontinued, IONM can not be faulted for failing to predict delayed emergence of neurological sequalae.

For the most part, therefore, false-negative IONM results are due either to gross misinterpretation of the neurophysiological data or to inability to observe a response change because the signal is embedded in excessive physical and/or cognitive noise, as discussed earlier.

In cases of avoidable spinal cord injury due to misinterpretation of electrophysiological data, most such mistakes result from recording parameters that are suboptimal, a type and concentration of anesthesia that is highly compromising, or a complete absence of a monitoring plan or strategy as advocated by Schwartz and Sestokas (14).

XI. MEASURES OF IONM PERFORMANCE

Recall that an optimal intraoperative neurophysiological monitoring modality is one that has high sensitivity and carries an acceptably low false-positive rate. The literature is now replete with hundreds of case reports and retrospective studies attesting to the value of SSEP monitoring for reducing the prevalence of spinal cord injury during scoliosis surgery. The largest multicenter survey of 51,263 scoliosis procedures reported sensitivity of SSEP monitoring to be 92% (15). Not surprisingly, the survey also found a relatively high tendency toward false-positive findings. In this survey no attempt was made to control for differences in the definition of significant change among the respondents. For example, of 90 respondents, one fifth considered a minimal 25–40% amplitude decrease to be significant, while nearly one half identified a nominal 5–8% latency shift as representing significant change. Others used a 50% amplitude loss and/or 10% latency increase criterion. As was discussed earlier, it stands to reason that a definition of "significant change" that either is too liberal or encompasses the wide range of normal variability will result a priori in a high false-positive rate, particularly when applied to a population of patients with low likelihood of developing neurological compromise, such as children with idiopathic scoliosis. York and colleagues (16), for example, showed that amplitude losses as great as 50% and latency shift up to 15%, both of which were within a 2.0 s.d. criterion for change, were not associated with postoperative neurological deficit.

Recently we calculated the receiver operating characteristics of SSEP and tceMEP IONM modalities from 427 patients who had undergone cervical spine surgery. Based on a decision criterion cut-off of 60% amplitude change, we reported 25% sensitivity for SSEPs versus 100% for tceMEPs. Specificity, on the other hand, was 100% for both (17). Similarly, we reported 20% sensitivity for SSEPs and 83% for tceMEPs using a 75% criterion for significant amplitude change in a study of IONM during thoracic spine surgery. Here again, specificity was quite high for both modalities (97% for SSEPs and 100% for tceMEPs) (18). The slightly lower sensitivity noted in these thoracic versus cervical spine surgery patients was because one from the former group showed SSEP changes only, which resolved quickly upon raising the MAP.

Given that the penalty for a false-negative is an unrecognized and potentially devastating neurological injury, the available evidence suggests that SSEPs may not be sufficiently sensitive to serve as a primary monitoring modality in spine surgery without lowering the decision criterion cut-off to a level that results in an excessive false-positive rate. When considered in light of SDT theory, therefore, it is clear that tceMEPs should be the preferred primary modality, with SSEPs assuming a secondary role. Since SSEPs tend to have an equivalently high specificity when an appropriate cut-off criterion is selected (e.g., 60–75%), they may serve better to confirm spinal cord functional integrity when tceMEP data are unchanged, rather than act as the main modality for detection of iatrogenic change.

XII. CONCLUSION

In this chapter, intraoperative neurophysiological monitoring during spine surgery has been analyzed as a problem in clinical decision making. The application of signal-detection theory to IONM provides a quantitative tool that can be used to improve decision accuracy. SDT permeates almost every situation that demands a rational clinical decision in the face of uncertainty. Unfortunately, there are significant gaps and shortcomings in the clinical data, which hinder wide-scale investigation of IONM test performance. One problem that we have addressed herein is how best to define a false-positive or false-negative event so as to allow for meaningful quantitative analysis of test accuracy. It is important that spine surgeons and surgical neurophysiologists begin to formulate integrated databases that permit statistical comparison of IONM data and surgical outcomes. Our own research has been directed at that goal. Until such data exist for the myriad permutations of surgical procedures and monitoring modalities, development and improvement of monitoring strategies will be slow.

Understanding the elements that enter into the decision-making process is critical to improved IONM and therefore to improved patient care. Those involved in providing IONM services must be aware of the factors that affect selection of appropriate decision cut-off criteria for neurophysiological change and must have an appreciation for the roles of sensitivity/specificity and the tradeoff between them when selecting monitoring modalities.

IONM is not a perfect technique; however, when performed by professionals that understand the principals of decision-making theory, it can play a vital role in injury prevention.

REFERENCES

1. Schwartz DM, Sestokas AK, Turner LA, et al. Neurophysiological identification of iatrogenic neural injury during complex spine surgery. Semin Spine Surg 1998; 10:242–251.
2. Schwartz D, Wierzbowski L, Fan D, Sestokas A. Intraoperative neurophysiological monitoring during spine surgery. In: Vaccaro A, Betz R, Zeidman S, eds. Principles and Practices of Spine Surgery. Philadelphia: Mosby, 2002:115–126.
3. Schwartz DM. Intraoperative neurophysiological monitoring during post-traumatic spine surgery. In: Vaccaro AR, ed. Fractures of the Cervical, Thoracic and Lumbar Spine. New York: Marcel Dekker, Inc., 2002:373–383.
4. Tanner WP Jr, Swets JA. A clinical decision-making theory of visual detection. Psychol Rev 1954; 61:401–409.
5. Green DM, Swets JA. Signal Detection Theory and Psychophysics. New York: Wiley, 1966.
6. Swets JA. Measuring the accuracy of diagnostic systems. Science 1988; 240:1285–1293.
7. Minahan RE, Sepkuty JP, Lesser RP, Sponseller PD, Kostuik JP. Anterior spinal cord injury with preserved neurogenic 'motor' evoked potentials. Clin Neurophysiol 2001; 112:1442–1450.
8. Owen JH, Bridwell KH, Grubb R, et al. The clinical application of neurogenic motor evoked potentials to monitor spinal cord function during surgery. Spine 1991; 16:S385–S390.
9. Owen JH. Monitoring during surgery for spinal deformities. In: Bridwell K, DeWald RL, eds. Textbook of Spinal Surgery. Philadelphia: Lippincott-Raven, 1997:39–60.

10. Padberg AM, Wilson-Holden TJ, Lenke LG, Bridwell KH. Somatosensory and motor-evoked potential monitoring without a wake-up test during idiopathic scoliosis surgery: an accepted standard of care. Spine 1998; 23:1392–1400.

11. Leppanen R, Madigan R, Sears C, et al. Intraoperative collision studies demonstrate descending spinal cord stimulated evoked potentials and ascending somatosensory evoked potentials are mediated through common pathways. J Clin Neurophysiol 1999; 16:170.

12. Toleikis JR, Skelly JP, Carlvin AO, Burkus JK. Spinally elicited peripheral nerve responses are sensory rather than motor. Clin Neurophysiol 2000; 111:736–742.

13. Fan D, Schwartz DM, Vaccaro AR, Hilibrand AS, et al. Intraoperative neurophysiologic detection of iatrogenic C5 nerve root injury during laminectomy for cervical compression myelopathy. Spine 2002; 27(22):2499–2502.

14. Schwartz DM, Sestokas AK. A systems based algorithmic approach to intraoperative neurophysiological monitoring during spine surgery. Semin Spine Surg 2002; 14(2):136–145.

15. Nuwer MR, Dawson EG, Carlson LG, Kanim LE, Sherman JE. Somatosensory evoked potential spinal cord monitoring reduces neurologic deficits after scoliosis surgery: results of a large multicenter survey. Electroencephalogr Clin Neurophysiol 1995; 96(1):6–11.

16. York DH, Chabot RJ, Gaines RW. Response variability of somatosensory evoked potentials during scoliosis surgery. Spine 1987; 12(9):864–876.

17. Hilibrand AS, Schwartz DM, Sethuraman, V, Vaccaro AR, Albert, TJ. Comparison of transcranial electric motor and somatosensory evoked potential monitoring during cervical spine surgery. J Bone Joint Surg. In Press.

18. Schwartz DM, Vacarro AR, Hilibrand AS, Sestokas A, Albert TJ. Transcranial electric motor evoked potential monitoring as an early indicator of emerging thoracic spinal cord ischemic injury. Presented at the Seventeenth Annual Meeting of the North American Spine Society, Montreal, Canada, November 2, 2002.

13
Complications in Revision Spine Surgery

Louis G. Quartararo
Hackensack University Medical Center, Hackensack, New Jersey, U.S.A.

Alexander R. Vaccaro
Thomas Jefferson University and the Rothman Institute, Philadelphia, Pennsylvania, U.S.A.

John P. Kostuik
Johns Hopkins Outpatient Center, Baltimore, Maryland, U.S.A.

I. INTRODUCTION

Spinal surgery in specific clinical scenarios is extremely beneficial in symptomatic patients who fail to respond to nonoperative measures. A small percentage of patients may not improve or may worsen in terms of their subjective or objective complaints. Kostuik has described the "three W's" of surgical failure: "The wrong patient, the wrong diagnosis and the wrong surgery." In other words, accurate patient assessment and diagnosis, with resultant appropriate surgical intervention, will lessen the potential for surgical and postsurgical complications and decrease the need for revision surgery.

II. DIAGNOSIS

When a patient presents with persistent or recurrent symptoms after surgical intervention, the challenge involves distinguishing between organic pathology that may benefit from further surgical intervention as opposed to nonsurgical therapies. A typical elective surgical candidate in this scenario is one who has an objective mechanical lesion such as a recurrent disk herniation, spinal instability, or spinal stenosis. Nonsurgical candidates include those with systemic illness, psychosocial instability, or symptomatic scar tissue deposition (epidural fibrosis or arachnoiditis) responsible for the majority of the symptomatology.

The most important tool in the evaluation of the failed back patient is the history. This includes the history of the pain, the number of previous operations for similar symptoms, the pain-free interval (if any) after the index surgical procedure, and the present pain pattern. In general, the number of previous operations a patient has undergone is inversely proportional to the success rate of any future surgical revision (25,26,44). More than two previous operations for the same pathology has a less than 50% overall successful reoperation rate. The pain-free interval postsurgery also aids in the diagnosis. No relief suggests either the wrong diagnosis, the wrong patient, failure for unknown reasons, lack of motivation, or an inadequate decompression or reconstruction. Gradual recurrent pain at between 1 and 6 months after surgery suggests symptomatic scarring or arachnoiditis. Recurrent pain after 6 months suggests the possibility of new pathology such as recurrent disk herniation or junctional degeneration.

III. SPINAL IMAGING

Radiological studies are important in the diagnosis and surgical planning for a revision spinal procedure. Standing lateral flexion and extension radiographs and upright coronal and side bending radiographs may reveal obvious mechanical instability. Radiographic evaluation of the previous surgical intervention, i.e., laminectomy defects, aids in surgical planning.

Magnetic resonance imaging (MRI) with gadolinium is the tool of choice in revision procedures, allowing assessment of neural structures and distinguishing between epidural scar formation and recurrent or persistent neural compression. Its usefulness, however, decreases with the presence of spinal internal fixation. Computed tomography (CT) myelogram is useful in these situations; however, it is difficult to distinguish between disk and scar tissue using this modality. CT is very useful in diagnosing arachnoiditis and is the test of choice when this diagnosis is suspected.

Single photon emission computed tomography (SPECT) imaging may be useful in identifying bony lesions such as pseudoarthrosis (19). Discography has also proven useful in the evaluation of a persistent pain generator, especially following a previous posterior fusion (5).

IV. COMPLICATIONS

The overall complication rate of revision spine surgery is variously reported, but is in the realm of approximately 10–30% (9,46,52). Complication rates have been reported to be as high as 80% in some studies (9,44).

Interestingly, Lapp et al. (30) have reported no difference in complication rates comparing a series of anterior-posterior spine surgeries, primary vs. revision. In their series of 44 anterior posterior surgeries (18 primaries, 26 revisions) minor complications were reported in 22% of the primary group and 22% of the revision group. Major complications were seen in 22% of the primary surgeries and 12% of the revision surgeries.

A. Infection

Infection rates in primary spine surgery are approximately 1–2% in uninstrumented spine surgeries and 5–11% in instrumented spine surgeries. Revision spine surgery infection rates are somewhat higher. The highest risk patients for infection are those with a history of previous spine infection, with infection rates reported to be as high as 22%. A history of diabetes or smoking also increases infection rates.

B. Pseudarthrosis

Pseudarthrosis may be caused by many factors, some of which include infection, excessive alcohol intake, systemic illness such as diabetes, smoking, and multiple previous spinal procedures with pseudathrosis (Figure 1). Thus, infection rates in this pathology

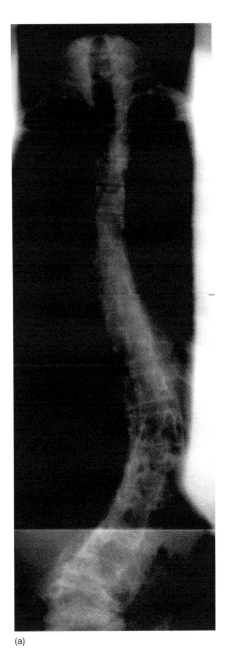

(a)

Figure 1   (a) An AP and (b) lateral x-ray of a 50-year-old male who underwent a stand-alone anterior interbody cage fusion with continuing unrelenting back pain. The patient did well for approximately 10 months but then began to develop unrelenting mechanical back pain with referred leg pain. A diagnosis of continued foraminal stenosis was incorrectly assumed and a posterior multi-level fomaminotomy was performed with worsening back and leg pain. A subsequent diskogram revealed severe concordant pain at the levels of the cage fusion levels as well as the cephalad level, which demonstrated radiographic evidence of junctional degeneration at the L3-4 level. (c) AP and (d) lateral plain radiographs following a posterior stabilization procedure with segmental pedicular fixation and iliac crest autologous bone graft. The patient noted improved low back and referred leg pain at follow-up.

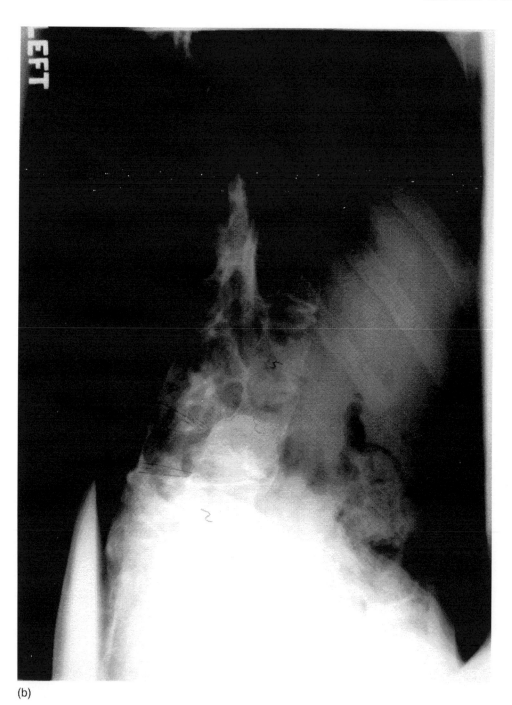

(b)

Figure 1 (*continued*)

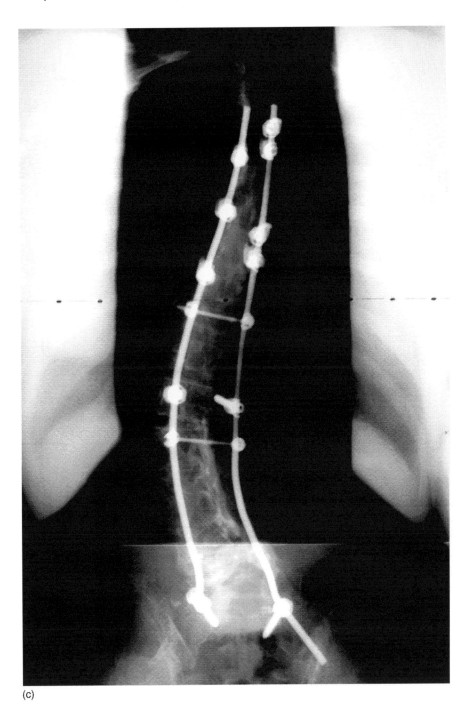

(c)

Figure 1 *(continued)*

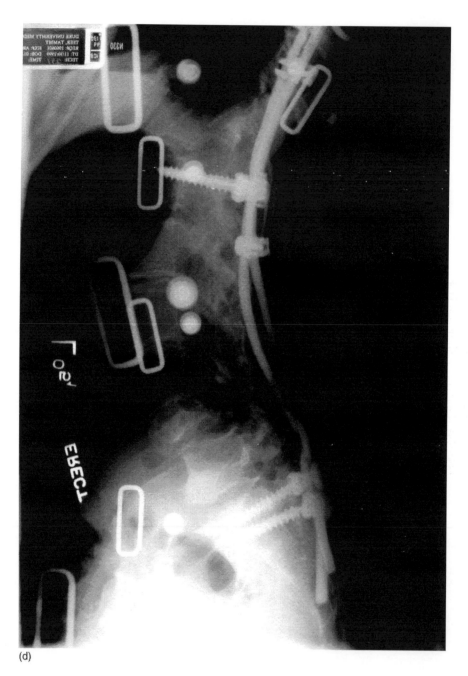

(d)

Figure 1 (*continued*)

(pseudarthrosis) fall somewhere between the rates for a primary surgical procedure and the 22% worst-case scenario.

Infection in the postoperative spine patient has been shown to increase the pseudarthrosis rate. Weiss et al. (50) have shown a 62% fusion rate following a posterior lumbar fusion after a deep infection. The pseudarthrosis rate in the face of infection was also adversely affected by the female sex, use of allograft bone, and fusion to the sacrum. Revisions of these cases are more frequent and are associated with high reinfection rates, as mentioned above.

C. Junctional Degeneration

Adjacent segment failure after rigid internal fixation of the spine has been widely documented and is a common cause of repeat surgery. Patients at highest risk are the elderly, women in the postmenopausal period, patients with a presurgical diagnosis of degenerative instability, and patients demonstrating any anterior translation at adjacent levels on their prefusion films (2,10,15,21,40). Chen et al.'s study (10) on the surgical treatment of junctional degeneration showed a 95% fusion rate and a 77% satisfaction rate. The incidence of another segment undergoing junctional degeneration requiring a third revision fusion was 13%. Revision surgery in this setting requires a thorough understanding of the sagittal and coronal balance of the patient. The goals of surgery are to relieve neurological compression and to stabilize the spine in a way that minimizes the potential for accelerated breakdown above or below the revised decompression and stabilization levels. This may involve extending the fusion to the extremes of the measured Cobb angulation or minimizing the fusion length with circumferential stabilization and avoiding ending the fusion at the apex of a curve or at a compromised vertebral body, i.e., compression fracture.

D. Hardware Complications

1. Screw Malposition

Spinal screw malposition has been reported at rates up to 25% (44). Lonstein et al. reported a screw malposition as low as 5% (33). Painful hardware may occur in up to 24% of cases and is often associated with pseudoarthrosis. Masferrer et al. (37) specifically studied the use of pedicle screws in revision spine cases. In this clinical scenario, the authors demonstrated a very low malposition rate (<5%). The absence of landmarks in the fusion mass leads many surgeons to rely on fluoroscopy for insertion of screws or to use hooks in the fusion mass, depending on its size and quality. Alternative means of improving the accuracy of implant placement includes the use of computer image technology.

2. Hardware Failure

Hardware failure has become less common with advancements in metallurgy, screw and rod design, as well as a better understanding of spinal biomechanics (33). Any hardware failure is suggestive of a potential pseudoarthrosis. Patients with evidence of instrumentation displacement or fatigue failure may fail to improve with nonoperative treatment measures and ultimately may benefit from surgical exploration and refusion. The biggest complication in this setting is the poor potential for refusion due to the local scarred soft tissue environment, lack of bleeding cancellous bony host graft surfaces, and the frequent sparsity of autogenous bone graft donor sites. Preoperative planning is especially important in this setting as the need for soft tissue flaps or harvesting from atypical donor sites should be discussed with the patient prior to surgery. Bone graft alternatives and replacements may also be useful in this setting, i.e., bone morphogenic proteins (BMP)s, which may take time to order and have available.

E. Instability

Postlaminectomy syndrome and instability is a common cause of failed spinal surgery requiring revision surgery. Treatment of this condition with a redecompression and fusion has demonstrated a much higher success rate than a redecompression alone (Figure 2) (17,24). Redecompression alone, however, is effective in situations with no demonstrated instability (21,23). One must keep in mind the potential for iatrogenic instability if further supporting capsular and bony elements are removed in subsequent revision procedures. Epidural scarring, as mentioned below, potentially increases with multiple repeat decompressions.

F. Dural Tear

The rate of dural tears has been variably reported, but can be as high as 5–15%. In a large series of 641 patients, Wang et al. reported a rate of 14%. An analysis by Stolke et al. of 412 primary and 69 reoperations for herniated disk revealed a dural tear prevalence of 1.8% for microdiscectomies, 5.3% for macrodiscectomies, and 17.4% for revision surgical procedures. Thus, the presence of scar adherent to the dura may increase the rate of dural tear. Successful primary repair, followed by short-term bed rest, has not been associated with an increased risk of infection, neural damage, or arachnoiditis (7,49).

G. Epidural Fibrosis and Adhesive Arachnoiditis

After multiple revision spinal surgeries, the rate of epidural fibrosis has been reported to be as high as 60% (17). A poor result may be a result of abundant intracanal scarring, and revision procedures for this diagnosis are often unsatisfactory, with the only viable treatment to date, outside of medication, being an implantable spinal stimulator. The surgical axiom "scar begets scar," should be headed by all surgeons, and scar excision alone for improvement of a patient's symptomatology is not recommended (44).

H. Vascular Injury

Vascular injury in anterior approaches to the spine is a rare injury. Several reports have documented cases of direct vascular injury and/or thrombotic occlusion in anterior spinal procedures (22,29,36,43). Rajaraman et al. (42) specifically examined visceral and vascular complication in a series of 60 anterior lumbar interbody fusions (ALIFs). They noted a 38% incidence of complications (23 of 60 patients). These included 4 vascular injuries, 6 cases of sympathetic dysfunction, 3 neural injuries, 3 instances of sexual dysfunction, and 2 cases of prolonged ileus. They did not find an association between reported complications and the need for revision surgery. Chang et al. (9) recently reported a series of 363 adult deformity surgeries, including 271 revision spine procedures. Five major vascular complications occurred in this group of patients, all in revision anterior procedures.

It is highly recommended that an exposure surgeon with vast experience in approaching the anterior thoracolumbar spine be available in cases of revision surgery due to the potential for injury to the great vessels during the surgical approach. An

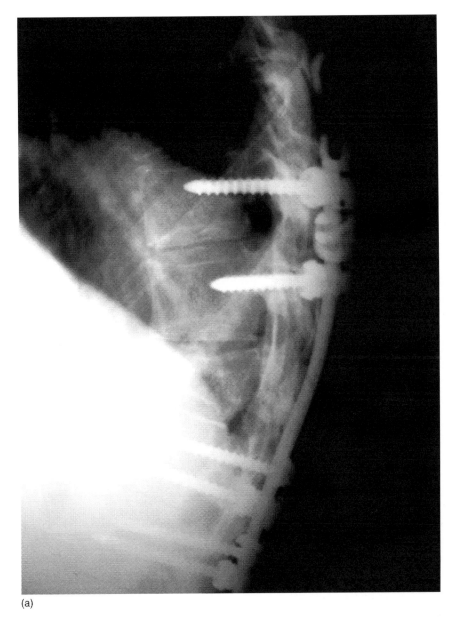

(a)

Figure 2   (a) A lateral plain radiograph of a 33-year-old male who underwent a revision posterior thoracolumbar fusion for a T12 burst fracture. The index procedure initially involved a T12, L1 laminectomy and in situ fusion, which went on to fusion nonhealing and continued back pain. Unfortunately, the patient went on to nonhealing of his revision fusion due to lack of adequate anterior column support with subsequent collapse at the fracture site with progressive kyphosis and unrelenting back pain. (b) An AP plain radiograph at follow-up illustrating a broken rod on the left and a misplaced L1 pedicle screw on the right. (c) AP and (d) lateral plain radiograph following posterior removal of the broken spinal internal fixation, an anterior corpectomy with femoral shaft allograph reconstruction with instrumentation, and then a posterior segmental stabilization procedure. Note the adequate restoration of spinal alignment following the revision stabilization procedure.

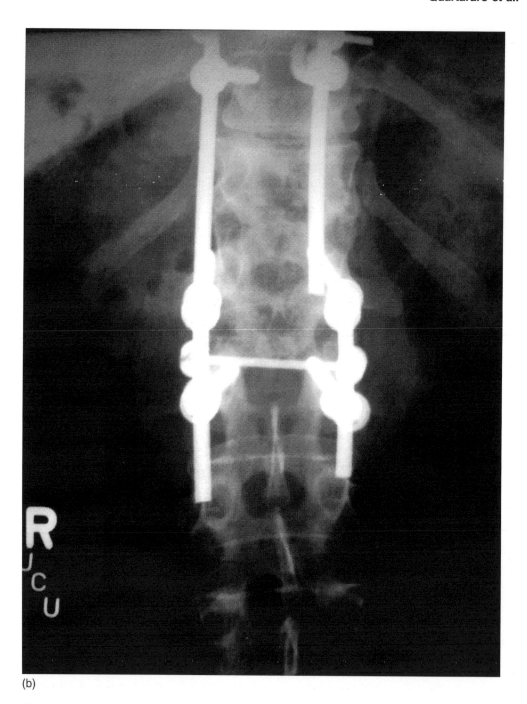

(b)

Figure 2 *(continued)*

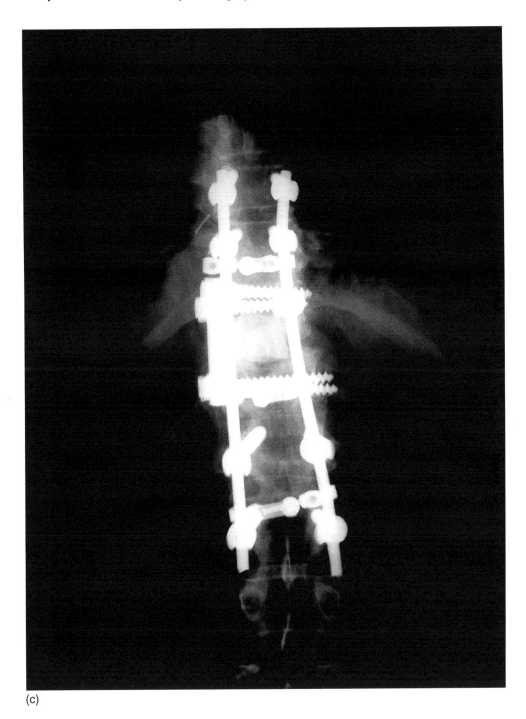

(c)

Figure 2 (*continued*)

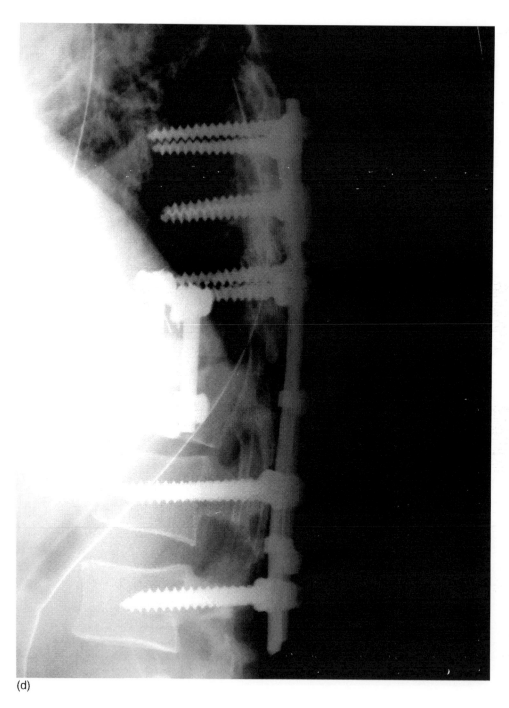

(d)

Figure 2 (*continued*)

additional means of protecting against symptomatic extremity ischemia is through the routine placement of lower extremity pulse oximeters during anterior spinal surgery in case of prolonged vessel traction or manipulation.

I. Lack of Bone Graft Sources

Locating useable bone is extremely difficult in revision spinal surgery due to the finite amount of autogenous bone graft that is available. It is prudent in these circumstances to exploit atypical harvesting sites, i.e., ribs, and have available bone graft extenders and alternatives at the time of surgery.

J. Increased Blood Loss and Operating Room Time

Revision spine surgery is routinely associated with an increased blood loss and operative time due to its complexity as compared to the index procedure. Zheng et al. (53) examined 112 revision posterior spine fusion procedures and noted an average operative time of 280 ± 62 minutes, and a blood loss of 1073 ± 716 mL. Factors predicting operative time were the number of levels fused, increased body weight, and a diagnosis of degenerative scoliosis. Factors responsible for increasing blood loss and transfusions included the number of levels fused and increased age and body weight.

K. Revision Cervical Spine Surgery

Complications associated with cervical revision surgery are primarily related to problems with posterior muscular splaying, i.e., Boutonnière's deformity, and anterior soft tissue trauma resulting in swallowing difficulty and recurrent laryngeal nerve dysfunction. There is a paucity of studies in the literature dedicated specifically to revision cervical spine surgery complications.

1. Esophageal Perforation

Esophageal perforation has been examined in several case reports. Most are related to late perforation by screw migration. Newhouse et al. described 6 intraoperative tears and related them to traumatic injury and the use of spinal internal fixation (38). Van Berge Henegouwen et al. reported on three intraoperative injuries resulting in esophageal perforation (48). Revision procedures, with the presence of scar formation, warrant a much higher degree of diligence with regard to this injury, as a delay in diagnosis can be fatal. A precautionary procedure to guard against missing an occult esophageal tear is the placement of indigo Carmen dye directly into the esophagus through a nasogastric tube at the completion of the cervical spine revision procedure. If the dye is noted in the wound, then a defect in the esophagus is present.

2. Dysphagia

Dysphagia is common after anterior cervical surgery. Primary surgeries report a rate as high as 50% in the first month postsurgery. Revision procedures will have at least as high an incidence, and possibly higher, due to the more extensive nature of these procedures, increased operative time, and the presence of established esophageal dysmotility and scar tissue (4).

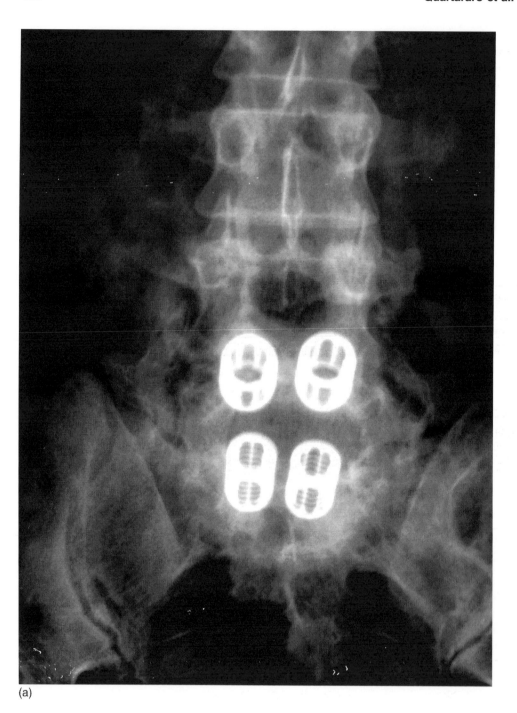

(a)

3. Recurrent Laryngeal Nerve Palsy

In a review of anterior cervical revision surgery, Coric et al. (13) identified only hoarseness as a complication, with 10.5% of patients having transient symptoms. There were no intraoperative complications in this series of 19 patients. Therefore, it is recommended that a careful assessment of vocal cord function be performed prior to a revision cervical procedure. This includes an ENT evaluation of vocal cord motility and placement of the incision in an unadulterated field, if possible. If a vocal cord is noted to be paretic, this should be the side of the surgical approach so as to avoid injury to the intact contralateral recurrent laryngeal nerve.

V. TREATMENT

The surgical treatment of the multiply operated back is as varied as the causes of failure and is dictated by a careful assessment of the aforementioned factors. A review of the literature reveals a wide variation in success rates, ranging from 12 to 84% (52).

A. Repeat Decompression Alone

A repeat decompression without fusion has limited indications in revision lumbar spine surgery (Figure 3). This may be considered in the setting of a recurrent disk herniation in which there is only recurrence of leg pain without back pain and significant bone is not needed to be removed in order to remove the extruded disk fragment. Multiple decompressive surgeries often lead to instability and the development of epidural fibrosis. An adjuvant spinal fusion is often necessary in this clinical situation (17,21,23–25,32,52).

B. Spinal Fusion

Patients with objective mechanical instability and leg or arm pain predominance due to neural compression or a symptomatic pseudoarthrosis often have the best clinical outcomes following a revision surgical fusion procedure. The type of fusion is dictated by the clinical circumstance.

Figure 3 (a) AP and (b) lateral long cassette plain radiographs of a long scoliosis in situ fusion with multiple level symptomatic pseudarthrosis and worsening deformity. (c) AP and (d) lateral long cassette plain radiographs following a revision posterior fusion with instrumentation. There is inadequate restoration of anterior column support at the L4,L5 and L5,S1 levels with minimal spinal anchor support throughout the construct, especially at the L5 level. There is only one point of fixation at the sacral level which may be inadequate in this revision procedure. (e) AP long cassette plain radiographs following partial instrumentation removal for pain. (f) Unfortunately, a pseudarthrosis was missed and the patient developed a progressive flatback syndrome. Clinically the patient developed an obvious flat posture in the side (g) and front (h). (i) AP and (j) lateral long cassette plain radiographs following a revision stabilization procedure again without anterior column support. The patient continue to develop a clinically significant frontal and sagital plane deformity. (k) AP and (l) lateral long cassette plain radiographs following an anterior posterior revision spinal reconstruction procedure. Adequate anterior column reconstruction using instrumentation with lumbar kyphosis resection and segmental stabilization was performed with satisfactory long-term functional results.

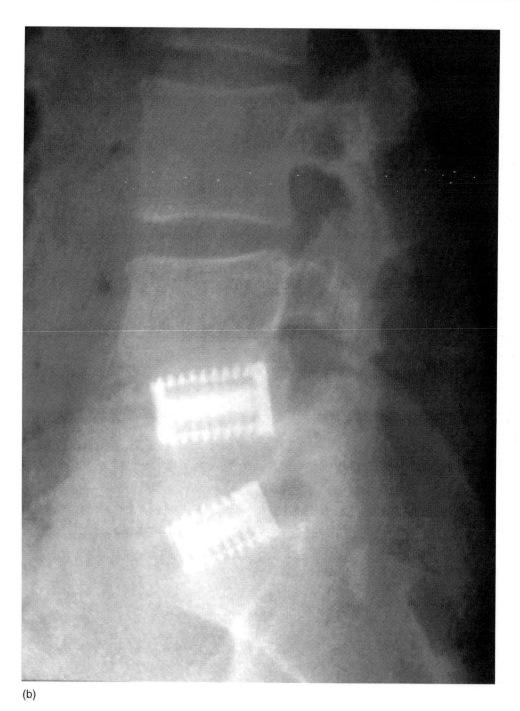

(b)

Figure 3 (*continued*)

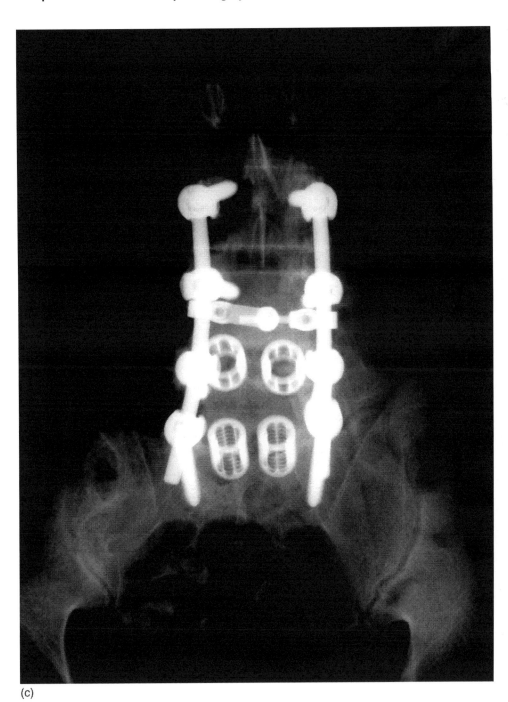

(c)

Figure 3 (*continued*)

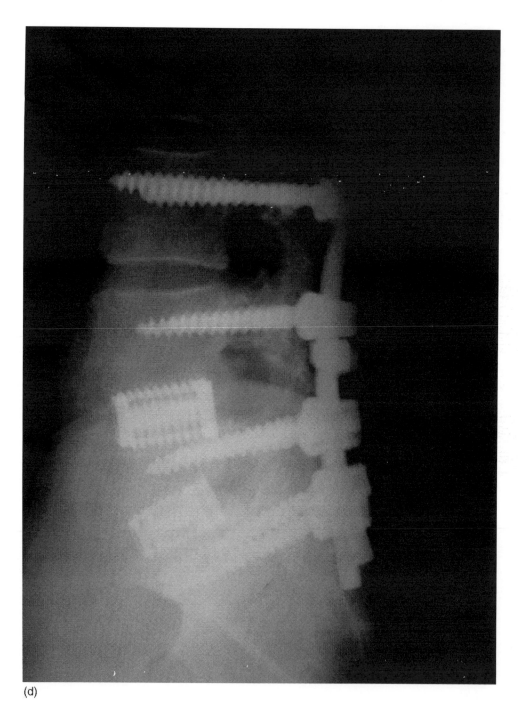

(d)

Figure 3 (*continued*)

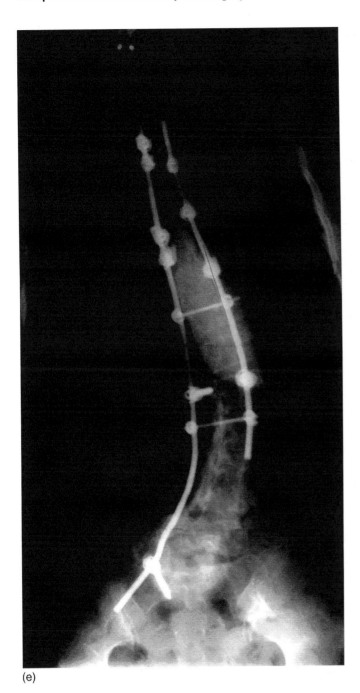

(e)

Figure 3 (*continued*)

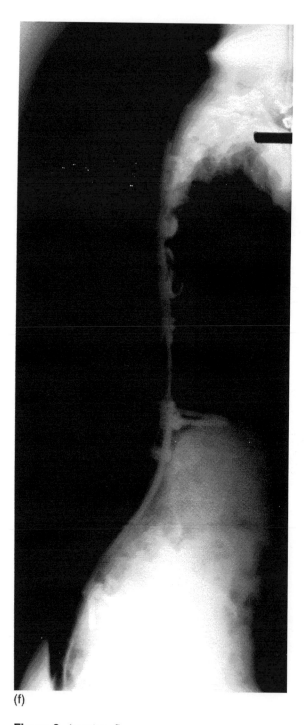

(f)

Figure 3 (*continued*)

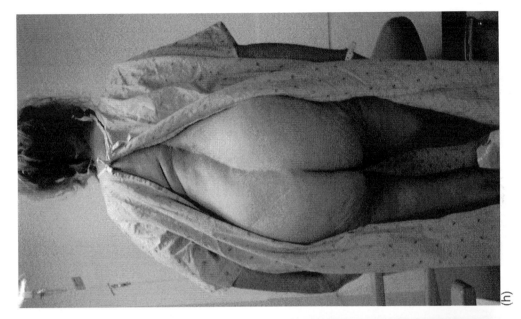

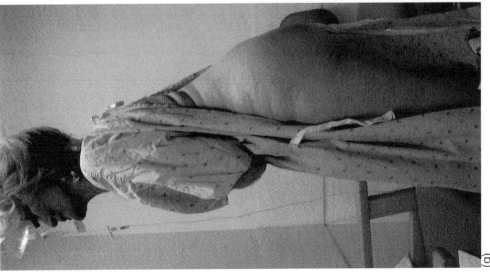

Figure 3 (*continued*)

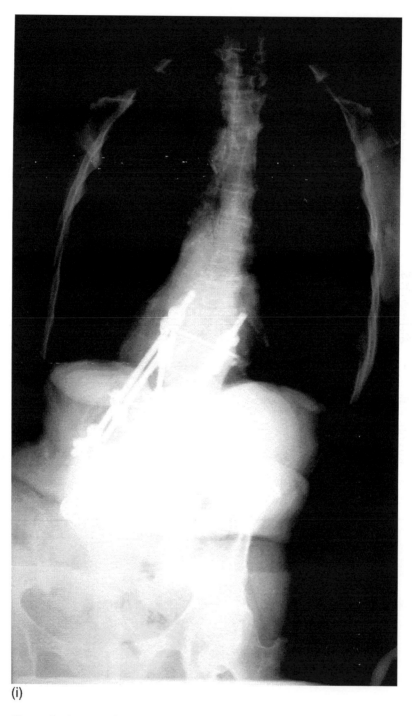

(i)

Figure 3 (*continued*)

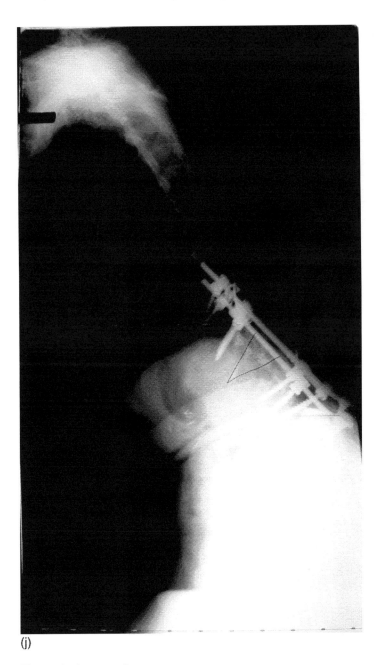

(j)

Figure 3 *(continued)*

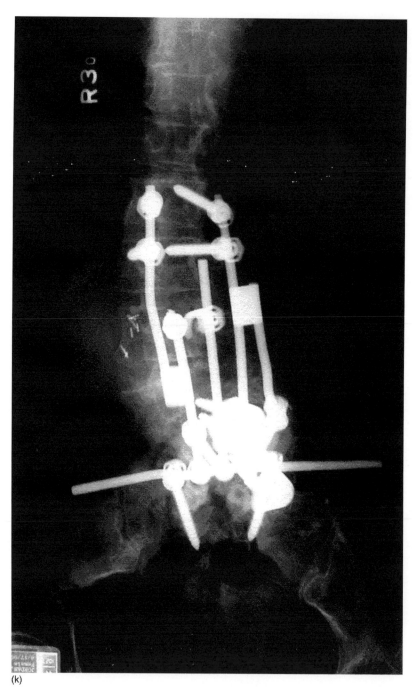

(k)

Figure 3 (*continued*)

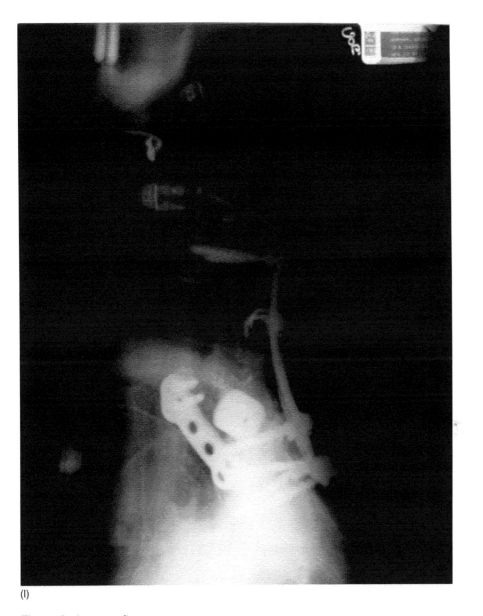

(l)

Figure 3 (*continued*)

1. Posterolateral Fusion

A posterior-lateral instrumented fusion is the most common surgical procedure following a revision decompression for a failed decompressive procedure (32). Success rates are variably reported. Biondi and Greenberg reported a 47% good result rate in their series of 45 patients (6). Kaneda et al. reported a 100% fusion rate and an 87% satisfaction rate following a revision posterior fusion (27). Masferrer et al. reported a 97% fusion rate, an 85% neurological improvement rate, and an 84% satisfaction rate in their series of 95 patients (37). In Saunders and Jacob's series of 50 revision spine patients, an 88% back pain relief rate was reported (45).

Unfortunately a posterior-lateral instrumented fusion alone for pseudarthrosis repair has a high documented failure rate (16,28,31,32). A circumferential fusion should be considered when possible in these cases.

2. Posterior Lumbar Interbody Fusion or Transforaminal Interbody

A posterior revision surgical procedure can provide anterior column support by placing a structural graft past both sides of the dural sleeve into the interbody space following a discectomy. This is ideal when one wishes to avoid the morbidity of an anterior procedure and when objective posterior pathology is present causing radiculopathy or nerve root dysfunction. Chintnavis et al. (11) reported a series of 50 patients who underwent revision disk excision followed by carbon fiber cage insertion, of whom 80% had the interbody cages placed as a stand-alone device (i.e., without pedicle screws). The authors reported a 95% fusion rate, a 92% symptomatic improvement rate, and a 66% patient satisfaction rate.

3. Anterior Interbody Fusion

Direct anterior interbody reconstruction allows the most efficient removal of disk material and optimal disk height restoration with a single-piece, load-sharing interbody device. As previously stated, the anterior disk is often a pain generator, which may remain symptomatic even following a successful posterolateral fusion. Barrick et al. (3) reported on 20 patients who were noted to have a solid posterolateral fusion but with persistent pain thought to be originating from the anterior intervertebral disk. These patients subsequently underwent an anterior interbody fusion, with a 100% fusion rate. The follow-up patient satisfaction rate was 89% (3). This again confirmed that a solid posterolateral fusion may not protect against painful micromotion stimulating a pain generator situated in the anterior intervertebral disk.

4. Anterior-Posterior Circumferential Fusion

Anterior-posterior revision lumbar spine surgery is the optimum procedure for a symptomatic pseudoarthrosis repair. A posterolateral fusion alone has not been consistently effective in the treatment of this problem (16,28,32). Albert et al. (1) reported on a series of 37 pseudoarthrosis patients treated with circumferential fusion. They showed a 90% fusion rate and a 65% functional improvement rate in this patient population. Functional failure was correlated with significant preoperative narcotic use, one or more abnormal neurological findings, and workmen's compensation status. Gertzbein et al. reported on a series of 25 circumferential pseudoarthrosis repairs, demonstrating a 100% fusion rate, but only a 52% significant pain reduction rate. In a large series of adult scoliosis patients, Chang et al. reported a pseudarthrosis repair rate of 94.5% in 132 revision scoliosis cases (9).

Revision cervical fusions for symptomatic anterior pseudarthrosis similarly do well with stabilization of the posterior column. Lowery et al. (34) performed a circumferential fusion for patients with a symptomatic anterior cervical pseudarthrosis, noting a 100% fusion rate in this patient population.

VI. CONCLUSION

The single most important factor in achieving a successful clinical outcome in revision spine surgery is patient selection (16). Although some studies showed that successful pseudarthrosis repair correlated with successful outcomes (5,32), other studies showed that frequently repair of a suspected pseudarthrosis alone did not lead to symptomatic relief (18,20). Factors such as workman's compensation or legal status (1,5,6,31,41), excessive preoperative narcotic use, abnormal pain behavior (1,14), coexisting medical disease or comorbidities (9,25), and preexisting psychological or psychiatric diagnosis (5) all play a potential negative role in the outcomes following a revision spine surgery.

As with most other elective surgical procedures, prevention of the need for a revision procedure is the most successful treatment strategy. Extrapolating from Kostuik's three W's, the three A's of surgical success are appropriate patient selection, appropriate diagnosis, and appropriate surgery. The use of gene therapy and biological implants may make the future of surgical intervention more predictable.

REFERENCES

1. Albert TJ, Pinto M, Denis F. Management of symptomatic lumbar pseudarthrosis with anteroposterior fusion. A functional and radiographic outcome study. Spine 2000; 25(1):123–130.
2. Aota Y, Kumano K, Hirabayashi S. Postfusion instability at the adjacent segments after rigid pedicle screw fixation for degenerative lumbar spinal disorders. J Spinal Disord 1995; 8(6):464–473.
3. Barrick WT, Schofferman JA, Reynolds JB, Goldthwaite ND, McKeehen M, Keaney D, White AH. Anterior lumbar fusion improves discogenic pain at levels of prior posterolateral fusion. Spine 2000; 25(7):853–857.
4. Bazaz R, Lee MJ, Yoo JU. Incidence of dysphasia after anterior cervical spine surgery: a prospective study. Spine 2002; 27(22):2453–2458.
5. Bernard TN Jr. Repeat lumbar spine surgery. Factors influencing outcome. Spine 1993; 18(15):2196–2200.
6. Biondi J, Greenberg BJ. Redecompression and fusion in failed back syndrome patients. J Spinal Disord 1990; 3(4):362–369.
7. Bosacco SJ, Gardner MJ, Guille JT. Evaluation and treatment of dural tears in lumbar spine surgery, a review. COOR 2001; 2001:238–247.
8. Butterman GR, Glazer PA, Hu SS, Bradford DS. Revision of failed lumbar fusions. A comparison of anterior autograft and allograft. Spine 1997; 22(23):2748–2755.
9. Chang JY, Kostuik JP, Sieber AN, Cohen DB. Complications of spinal fusion in treatment of adult spinal deformity. Unpublished manuscript.
10. Chen WJ, Lai PL, Niu CC, Chen LH, Fu TS, Wong CB. Surgical treatment of adjacent instability after lumbar spine fusion. Spine 2001; 26(22):E519–524.
11. Chitnavis B, Barbagallo G, Selway R, Dardis R, Hussain A, Gullan R. Posterior lumbar interbody fusion for revision disc surgery: review of 50 cases in which carbon fiber cages were implanted. J Neurosurg 2001; 95(2 suppl):190–195.
12. Cohen DB, Chotivichit A, Fujita T, Wong TH, Huckell CB, Sieber AN, Kostuik JP, Lawson HC. Pseudarthrosis repair. Autogenous iliac crest versus femoral ring allograft. Clin Orthop 2000; 371:46–55.
13. Coric D, Branch CL Jr, Jenkins JD. Revision of anterior cervical pseudoarthrosis with anterior allograft fusion and plating. J Neurosurg 1997; 86(6):969–974.
14. Dhar S, Porter RW. Failed lumbar spinal surgery. Int Orthop 1992; 16(2):152–156.

15. Etebar S, Cahill DW. Risk factors for adjacent-segment failure following lumbar fixation with rigid instrumentation for degenerative instability. J Neurosurgery 1999; 90(4 suppl):163–169.

16. Etminan M, Girardi FP, Khan SN, Cammisa FP Jr. Revision strategies for lumbar pseudarthrosis. Orthop Clin North Am 2002; 33(2):381–392.

17. Fritsch EW, Heisel J, Rupp S. The failed back surgery syndrome: reasons, intraoperative findings, and long-term results: a report of 182 operative treatments. Spine 1996; 21(5):626–633.

18. Frymoyer JW, Matteri RE, Hanley EN, Kuhlmann D, Howe J. Failed lumbar disc surgery requiring second operation. A long-term follow-up study. Spine 1978; 3(1):7–11.

19. Gates GF, McDonald RJ. Bone SPECT of the back after lumbar surgery. Clin Nucl Med 1999; 24(6):395–403.

20. Gertzbein SD, Hollopeter MR, Hall S. Pseudarthrosis of the lumbar spine. Outcome after circumferential fusion. Spine 1998; 23(21):2352–2357.

21. Guigui P, Ulivieri JM, Lassale B, Deburge A. [Reoperations after surgical treatment of lumbar stenosis] [in French]. Rev Chir Orthop Reparatrice Appar Mot 1995; 81(8):663–371.

22. Hackenberg L, Liljenqvist U, Halm H, Winkelmann W. Occlusion of the left common iliac artery and consecutive thromboembolism of the left popliteal artery following anterior lumbar interbody fusion. J Spinal Disord 2001; 14(4):365–368.

23. Hanley EN Jr. The indications for lumbar spinal fusion with and without instrumentation. Spine. 1995; 20(24 suppl):143S–153S.

24. Hansraj KK, O'Leary PF, Cammisa FP Jr, Hall JC, Fras CI, Cohen MS, Dorey FJ. Decompression, fusion, and instrumentations surgery for complex lumbar spinal stenosis. Clin Orthop 2001; (384):18–25.

25. Herno A, Airaksinen O, Saari T, Sihvonen T. Surgical results of lumbar spinal stenosis. A comparison of patients with or without previous back surgery. Spine 1995; 20(8):964–969.

26. Herno A, Airaksisnen O, Saari T, Sihvonen T, Luukkonen M. The effect of prior back surgery on surgical outcome in patients operated on for lumbar spinal stenosis. A matched-pair study. Acta Neurochir (Wien) 1996; 138(4):357–363.

27. Kaneda K, Higuchi M, Nohara Y, Oguma T, Sato S. Posterolateral fusion with instrumentation in the symptomatic failed back patients. Nippon Seikeigeka Gakki Zasshi 1984; 58(3):323–330.

28. Kim SS, Michelsen CB. Revision surgery for failed back surgery syndrome. Spine 1992; 17(8):957–960.

29. Kulkarni SS, Lowery GL, Ross RE, Ravi Sankar K, Lykomitros V. Arterial complications following anterior lumbar interbody fusion: report of eight cases. Eur Spine J 2003; 12(1):48–54.

30. Lapp MA, Bridwell KH, Lenke LG, Daniel Riew K, Linville DA, Eck KR, Ungacta FF. Long-term complications in adult spinal deformity patients having combined surgery a comparison of primary to revision patients. Spine 2001; 26(8):973–983.

31. Lauerman WC, Bradford DS, Ogilvie JW, Transfeldt EE. Results of lumbar pseudarthrosis repair. J Spinal Disord 1992; 5(2):149–157.

32. Lehmann TR, LaRocca HS. Repeat lumbar surgery. A review of patients with failure from previous lumbar surgery treated by spinal canal exploration and lumbar spinal fusion. Spine 1981; 6(6):615–619.

33. Lonstein JE, Denis F, Perra JH, Pinto MR, Smith MD, Winter RB. Complications associated with pedicle screws. J Bone Joint Surg Am 1999; 81(11):1519–1528.

34. Lowery GL, Swank ML, McDonough RF. Surgical revision for failed anterior cervical fusions. Articular pillar plating or anterior revision? Spine 1995; 20(22):2436–2441.

35. Markwalder TM, Battaglia M. Failed back surgery syndrome, Part I: Analysis of the clinical presentation and results of testing procedures for instability of the lumbar spine in 171 patients. Acta Neurochir (Wien) 1993; 123(1–2):46–51.

36. Marsicano J, Mirovsky Y, Remer S, Bloom N, Neuwirth M. Thrombotic occlusion of the left common iliac artery after an anterior retroperitoneal approach to the lumbar spine. Spine 1994; 19(3):357–359.

37. Masferrer R, Gomez CH, Karahalios DG, Sonntag VK. Efficacy of pedicle screw fixation in the treatment of spinal instability and failed back surgery: a 5-year review. J Neurosurg 1998; 89(3):371–377.

38. Newhouse KE, Lndsey RW, Clark CR, Lieponis J, Murphy MJ. Esophageal perforation following anterior cervical spine surgery. Spine 1989; 14(10):1051–1053.

39. North RB, Campbell JN, James CS, Conover-Walker MK, Wang H, Piantadosi S, Rybock JD, Long DM. Failed back surgery syndrome: 5-year follow-up in 102 patients undergoing repeated operation. Neurosurgery 1991; 28(5):685–691.

40. Phillips FM, Carlson GD, Bohlman HH, Hughes SS. Results of surgery for spinal adjacent to previous lumbar fusion. J Spinal Disord 2000; 13(5):432–437.

41. Quimjian JD, Matrka PJ. Decompression laminectomy and lateral spinal fusion in patients with previously failed lumbar spine surgery. Orthopedics 1988; 11(4):563–569.

42. Rajaraman V, Vingan R, Roth P, Heary RF, Conklin L, Jacobs GB. Visceral and vascular complications resulting form anterior lumbar interbody fusion. J Neurosurg 1999; 91(1 suppl):60–64.

43. Raskas DS, Delamarter RB. Occlusion of the left iliac artery after retroperitoneal exposure of the spine. Clin Orthop 1997; 338:86–89.

44. Rothman-Simeone. The Spine. 4th ed. Philadelphia: WB Saunders Co., 1999.

45. Saunders EA, Jacobs RR. The multiply operated back: fusion of the posterolateral spine with and without nerve root compression. South Med J. 1976; 69(7):868–871.

46. Slosar PJ, Reynolds JB, Schofferman J, Goldthwaite N, White AH, Keaney D. Patient satisfaction after circumferential lumbar fusion. Spine 2000; 25(6):722–726.

47. Stewart G, Sachs BL. Patient outcomes after reoperation on the lumbar spine. J Bone Joint Surg Am 1996; 78(5):706–711.

48. Van Berge Henegouwen DP, Roukema JA, de Nie JC, Vd Werken C. Esophageal perforation during surgery on the cervical spine. Neurosurgery 1991; 29(5):766–768.

49. Wang JC, Bohlman HH, Riew KD. Dural tears secondary to operations on the lumbar spine. Management and results after a two-year-minimum follow-up of eighty-eight patients. J Bone Joint Surg Am 1998; 80(12):1728–1732.

50. Weiss LE, Vaccaro AR, Scuderi G, McGurire M, Garfin SR. Pseudoarthrosis after post-operative wound infection in the lumbar spine. J Spinal Disord 1997; 10(6):482–487.

51. Wetzel FT, La Rocca H. The failed posterior lumbar interbody fusion. Spine 1991; 16(7):839–845.

52. Wong CB, Chen WJ, Chen LH, Niu CC, Lai PL. Clinical outcomes of revision lumbar spinal surgery:124 patients with a minimum of two years of follow-up. Chang Gung Med J 2002; 25(3):175–182.

53. Zheng F, Cammisa FP Jr, Sandhu HS, Girardi FP, Khan SN. Factors predicting hospital stay, operative time, blood loss, and transfusion in patients undergoing revision posterior lumbar spine decompression, fusion, and segmental instrumentation. Spine 2002; 27(8):818–824.

14

Complications Encountered During Surgery for Spinal Trauma

Ashwini D. Sharan and James S. Harrop
Thomas Jefferson University Hospital, Philadelphia, Pennsylvania, U.S.A.

Alok D. Sharan
Albany Medical Center, Albany, New York, U.S.A.

Alexander R. Vaccaro
*Thomas Jefferson University and the Rothman Institute,
Philadelphia, Pennsylvania, U.S.A.*

I. INTRODUCTION

Patients with injuries to the spinal column or cord present a unique challenge for spine surgeons, medical caregivers, and ancillary medical providers. The toll of such injury already poses a significant economic challenge to society, including hospitalization and rehabilitation costs as well as those costs related to lost employment and productivity (18). Despite increasing education and awareness among healthcare workers, certain avoidable and unavoidable complications exist that are unique to this patient population. Starting from the time of injury to definitive nonoperative and operative care, complications may occur that result in neurological deterioration and unfavorable outcomes. This chapter will focus on identifying complications that relate to the surgical management of patients with a spinal column or spinal cord injury.

II. PREOPERATIVE COMPLICATIONS

Prior to the onset of the surgical procedure, the surgeon should carefully decide on all equipment that will be needed (e.g., fluoroscopy machine, image guidance system) during the case and where the specialized equipment will be located to facilitate operating room traffic. For example, the use of a radiolucent operating room table can allow the seamless use of intraoperative imaging technology and avoid the hassle of multiple x-ray attempts when visualization is obscured by extraneous table attachments. All operating room personnel should wear lead aprons prior to scrubbing if fluoroscopy is to be used. This will shorten intraoperative time and decrease the potential for increased blood loss and wound-healing problems. Alternatively, an x-ray cartridge shelf should be placed under an Andrews table if an intraoperative x-ray may be anticipated. Additionally, the shoulders should be taped when working near the cervicothoracic junction or in short-necked patients.

During preoperative planning in spinal trauma, a thorough assessment of all key anatomical features particular to a patient's surgical procedure should be made. This involves an assessment of all intended anchorage sites for spinal fixation to ensure that the appropriate-sized implants are available as well as to determine that an implant can be placed safely without harm to the surrounding soft tissue environment. An example would be the ability to place a C1–2 transarticular screw. A sagittal computed tomography (CT) scan at the level of the C2 isthmus will determine if safe passage of the screw is possible. If the size of this bony passageway is too small, injury to the spinal cord or vertebral artery is possible. Another measurement involves the assessment of the vertebral body and pedicle size (Fig. 1), calvarial thickness for occipital fixation and orientation for screw placement, and the location and distance of the aorta from intended thoracic pedicle screw trajectories as well as anterior spinal implants (35,36). Similarly, measurement of the vertebral body must be made prior to insertion of distractor pins (typically 14 mm) (Fig. 1) during selection of anterior cervical plate screws in the cervical spine and even before selecting the different thoracolumbar plates or anterior column strut implants. (A fibula may suffice in the upper thoracic region, but a humerus allograft may be required in the lower thoracic region.)

In the preoperative phase, the surgeon should develop a plan that will allow stabilization of the spine while avoiding harm to the neural structures. An example would be the need to perform a closed reduction of a dislocated spinal segment. In the presence of an extruded disk fragment in a neurologically intact patient, the immediate surgical goal may be to remove the disk fragment and then perform the reduction (Fig. 2). Many surgeons, however, routinely and safely perform cervical closed reductions emergently in the presence of disk extrusions prior to obtaining a magnetic resonance imaging (MRI) scan (34). Performing the reduction first in patients who cannot be safely monitored neurologically may result in unacceptable pressure on the spinal cord with a worsening of the patients' neurological status.

III. PATIENT POSITIONING

Although oral endotracheal intubation with in-line stabilization of the neck is possible, a useful means of protecting the cervical spinal cord in the setting of cervical spinal instability from harmful manipulation is through the use of an awake fiber optic intubation (1,9,11,12,19,21,32). Once intubation is complete and the patient can voluntarily demonstrate no change in neurological status, final positioning can ensue. Pre- and post-positioning electrophysiological monitoring is helpful to make sure the patient's final resting positioning is not resulting in harmful neural (spinal cord or peripheral nerve) compression that may be reversible if corrected on a timely basis.

Patient positioning in the setting of an unstable fracture may result in further fracture displacement and undesirable neurological deterioration. Protective measures employed by the surgeon may involve awake sedated positioning to allow voluntary patient splinting until final patient positioning is complete or reliance on electrophysiological monitoring during positioning to monitor for any neural embarrassment. Alternatively, utilization of a rotating table such as a Jackson table or via a Stryker frame may allow a more controlled flip from an anterior to a posterior position.

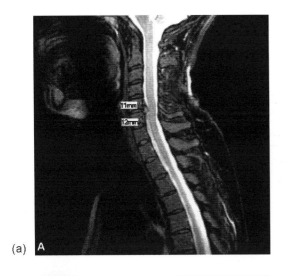

(a)

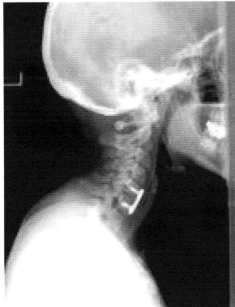

(b)

Figure 1 This patient had an acutely herniated cervical C5-6 disk from a fall resulting in a myelo-radiculopathy. Notice the small caliber of her vertebral body. A 14 mm anterior cervical plate with 10 mm unicortical screws were used. Also note, that the use of 14 mm Caspar distractor pins would likely have resulted in cord injury. (a) Sagittal T2-weighted MRI with measurement of the C5 and the C6 vertebral body showing the acutely herniated disk at C5-6. (b) Postoperative lateral cervical spine x-ray showing the anterior cervical plate and 10 mm screws.

Spinal reconstruction procedures in the setting of trauma have the potential to be lengthy, and therefore careful positioning is an essential aspect of the operation. When the patient is positioned supine, the ulnar nerve at the elbow should be carefully padded (25). Aggressive downward retraction of the shoulders may result in a brachial plexus stretch injury. A common clinical manifestation of this may be a disabling deltoid

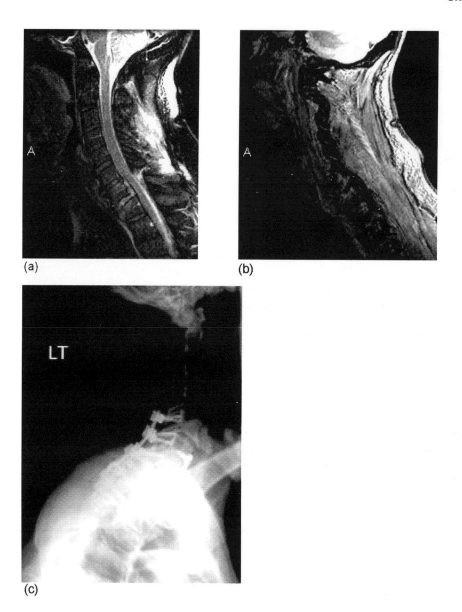

Figure 2 This 53-year-old male developed syncope while driving resulting in a high-speed MVA. He presented with a C7 and T1 left radiculopathies. Plain radiographs identified a C7-T1 subluxation along with bilateral facet dislocations of C6–7 and bilateral C7 pedicle and facet fractures. Due to the unique fracture pattern, a MRI of the cervical spine was obtained and showed a significant hematoma and disc fragment posterior to the C7 vertebral body (a,b). Therefore, an anterior decompression and fusion was performed prior to the posterior procedure. Note maintanence of the overall sagittal balance (c).

palsy. In prone cases, the axilla needs to be carefully padded to again avoid stretch injury to the brachial plexus. In addition, special attention should be made to the wrist, elbows, and heel to avoid any harmful pressure. When the patient is positioned in the lateral decubitus position, the peroneal nerve at the level of the fibular neck must be padded at the knees as protective straps have been seen to irritate the peroneal nerve. Finally, the face, the eyes, the chin, iliac crest, and genitals must be protected when the patient is positioned prone. The eyes should never have pressure on them during any surgical procedure, since this may result in decreased perfusion and potential blindness (16,17,39).

IV. ANESTHESIA

After a traumatic spinal cord injury, the patient may have a contused and swollen spinal cord. Therefore, the maintenance of systemic mean arterial pressure is critical. The induction of anesthesia and resulting blood loss may result in hypotension that is poorly tolerated by a contused spinal cord. It is necessary to have accurate arterial monitoring of blood pressure throughout the surgical procedure, to be aware of the onset of critical hypotension, and to prevent or respond to this problem quickly. Spinal cord monitoring may suggest hypoperfusion of the spinal cord and relative ischemia, although changes detected on monitoring may occur anywhere from 5 to 20 minutes after a potential injury. Communication with the anesthesia team in the setting of severe blood loss is critical. The presence of rapid infuser systems, high-bore intravenous access, and available blood products is necessary to treat acute and rapid bleeding. Additionally, high-volume blood loss should also include replacement of coagulation factors and calcium as well. Thoracolumbar spine injury, a preoperative hematocrit of < 35% and an injury severity score of > 20 has correlated with the need for intraoperative blood transfusion (8). Careful preoperative planning should include routine use of cell saver.

Spinal cord monitoring may play an essential part in the treatment of patients with either an intact spinal injury or incomplete spinal cord injury. Any alteration in the electrophysiological signals should always prompt a search for reversible causes of injury. A typical checklist should begin by investigating the anesthetic agent to determine if any paralytic agents have been employed, assessing mean arterial blood pressure, checking the oxygenation of the patient, and then insuring the absence of a technical problem associated with the monitoring itself (5,6,13,20).

V. INTRAOPERATIVE COMPLICATIONS

A. Proper Instrumentation Use

When planning the surgical levels of stabilization, the trauma surgeon can borrow many of the principles of deformity surgery to lessen the potential for junctional breakdown or iatrogenic spinal deformity in the follow-up period. This involves the avoidance of ending a fusion at the apex of a kyphosis or avoiding distraction in the lower lumbar region in order to prevent the occurrence of a flatback deformity.

Spinal instrumentation has evolved considerably over the last 20 years. The diversity of implants and ease of use have provided the surgeon the ability to safely stabilize complex spinal injuries as well as afford more salvage options in cases in which the primary surgical plan has to be modified. As an example, in high posterior cervical stabilization procedures, the surgeon can now potentially incorporate C1 directly into a C1–2 fusion with a lateral mass screw when placement of a C1–2 transarticular screw or sublaminar wiring is not feasible or desirable (28,29). However, modern instrumentation cannot overcome poor bone quality and sustain stabilization in the setting of certain ligamentous injury (Fig. 3).

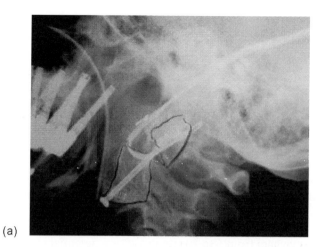

(a)

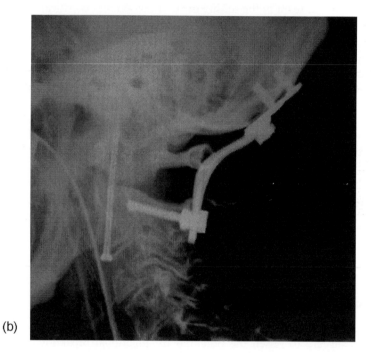

(b)

Figure 3 This 86-year-old male fell, resulting in a type II posterior displaced odontoid fracture, treated initially with anterior odontoid screw after closed reduction. Two weeks after instrumentation, AP cervical radiograph shows posterior displacement with posterior migration of the screw (a). The patient had a posterior instrumentation after reduction with fixation to the occipital bone and C2 pedicle screws (b).

In a similar manner, low posterior cervical fusions may require extension into the upper thoracic spine. This is now less difficult with thoracic pedicle screws designed to fit the pedicle at this level (Fig. 4). Equally, ending a construct at the thoracolumbar junction may not be advisable (Fig. 5). Thus, an important part of the operative planning is to prepare a sterile field in which a salvage construct can be applied. For all cervical

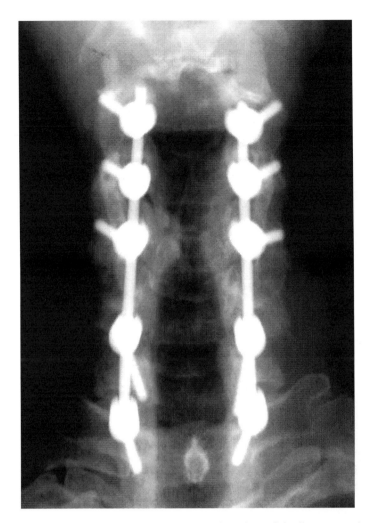

Figure 4 Cervicothoracic fusion in patient that originally presented with rapid cervical myelopathy and severe spinal cord stenosis and straightened cervical curvature. Patient had C3–7 laminectomy followed by posterior instrumented fusion. Note the lateral mass screws are placed at C3–5 and pedicle screws are placed at C7 and T1. Due to the cervical anatomy it is difficult to place C6 lateral mass and C7 pedicle screws. Therefore, the construct was extended one level due the biomechanical disadvantage of the cervicothoracic junction.

cases, the sterile field should include the occiput and cervicothoracic junction. For all other cases, the field may need to include the entire thoracic-lumbar spine.

Accurate identification of intraoperative anatomy may be extremely difficult in particular metabolic disease states such as ankylosing spondylitis and diffuse idiopathic skeletal hyperostosis (DISH). These diseases can make intraoperative anatomical landmarks, especially the midline, difficult to identify for safe cervical decompressive procedures and anterior plate placement (Fig. 6). In these situations the use of myelographic dye placed in the decompression site followed by an antero-posterior x-ray will allow accurate visualization of the midline. Attention to proper patient positioning can also ease the technical challenge of placing anterior instrumentation, especially in the thoracic

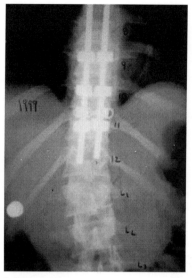

(a)

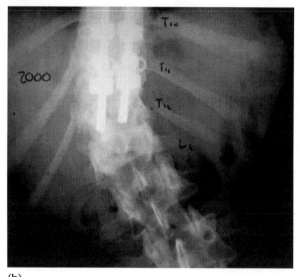

(b)

Figure 5 This 29-year-old male had posterior thoracic fusion after a T6–7 dislocation as a result of a MVA (a). Over the next year we developed severe thoracolumbar junctional breakdown and a scoliotic deformity (b).

spine. A direct lateral decubitus position will make it easier for the surgeon to orient the location of the spinal canal and lessen the potential for inadvertent instrumentation migration into the spinal canal. When performing a posterior stabilization procedure using hooks or wires, the surgeon must be keenly aware of areas of cord edema or swelling. Sublaminar wires or hooks should not be placed in these areas to avoid further cord parenchymal injury (3).

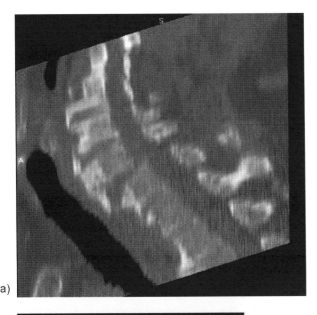

(a)

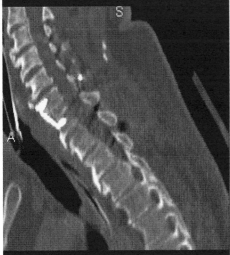

(b)

Figure 6 This 75-year-old male with severe DISH syndrome had a bilateral facet dislocation without a spinal cord injury at C6–7 from a motor vehicle accident. Note the anterior osteophytes, which will make identification of the disk space challenging as well as providing a significant challenge when placing an anterior cervical plate (a). The patient thus underwent an anterior cervical decompression, followed by posterior realignment and reconstruction. (b) Sagittal reconstruction CT revealing realignment of the anterior column and placement of the graft and plate after removing the osteophytes.

B. Biomechanics

Correction of spinal deformity following spinal injury is fraught with many potential pitfalls. The placement of an oversized anterior graft may result in spinal canal lengthening if posterior instability is present. This is hazardous in the setting of a contused spinal cord that poorly tolerates any spinal cord stretching. Distraction in globally unstable thoraco-lumbar injuries may catastrophically result in severe spinal lengthening, especially in the setting of anterior and posterior longitudinal ligament and ligamentum flavum disruption. The surgeon must formulate a surgical strategy that prevents overlengthening of the spinal axis, but allows for correction of an existing spinal deformity and restoration of vertebral body height. An example of this would be the placement of a compression claw hook configuration posteriorly in a flexion distraction injury with loss of anterior vertebral body height. Once the posterior compression claw is fixed, careful graded distraction may now be performed to improve sagittal alignment and restore anterior vertebral body height.

Biomechanical principles must always be respected in the reconstruction of spinal trauma. A popular trend in the late 1980s and early 1990s was the concept of short segment reconstruction of thoracolumbar burst fractures. Unfortunately, a significant number of these reconstructive procedures demonstrated loss of spinal alignment and failure of fixation due to the incompetency of the anterior spinal column. The need to reconstruct the anterior column in this setting became clear in specific injury patterns to avoid this complication. Also, after placing an anterior graft the surgeon can dislocate or decrease the graft-endplate contact with additional posterior compression (Fig. 7). Therefore, care must be taken when placing compression or distraction on posterior tension-band constructs.

C. Dural Tear

Finally, in a small number of cases, cerebrospinal fluid leakage may occur when associated with traumatic dural tears. In general, there is a reported 1–2% incidence of dural tears during elective spine surgery (Fig. 8). A higher incidence of dural laceration has been reported with spinal trauma, although preoperative prediction of dural injury has been poorly correlated. The incidence of traumatically induced dural tears is unclear but should be suspected in the setting of a neurological deficit and obvious lamina fracture on spinal imaging. Primary repair of the dura is typically preferred over patching. However, the majority of the time, an attentive fascial closure with either local drainage through a Jackson-Pratt or a lumbar drain is typically sufficient in cases of trauma, especially when the tear is difficult to locate or an exploration of the source of cerebrospinal fluid (CSF) leakage is undesirable. Others have used fat grafts and fibrin glue and other lumbar drainage to help prevent persistent CSF leakage.

VI. POSTOPERATIVE COMPLICATIONS

A. Visceral Injury

Due to the nature of the injury, spinal trauma patients are at increased risk for certain complications. Many of these patients will have associated closed head injuries, and others will have visceral injuries that delay and complicate their healing. With certain cervical fractures, laryngeal and esophageal injuries have been described. In the setting of thoracic injuries, pulmonary contusions, hemo- or pneumothorax, rib fractures, or aortic dissection may be present. These sometimes require the placement of a chest tube or intubation. Injuries to the lumbar spine can result in abdominal organ injury. Splenic rupture or liver laceration are two common complications with thoracolumbar fractures. Finally, a paralyzed hemi-diaphragm and renal contusions are frequently missed.

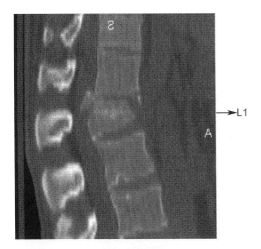

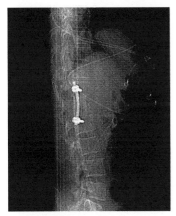

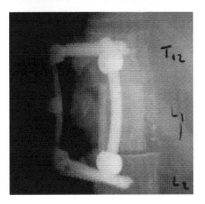

Figure 7 This patient underwent an anterior-posterior thoracic/lumbar reconstruction for a L1 burst fracture. A humerus allograft was packed with autologous cancellous bone from the iliac crest to reconstruct the anterior column and decompress the neural elements. Posterior stabilization was accomplished with pedicle screw fixation. However, compression across the posterior construct although intending to load the anterior column and increase the lordosis resulted in distraction of the anterior elements, making the graft more prone to dislodgement and decreasing the bone graft endplate contact.

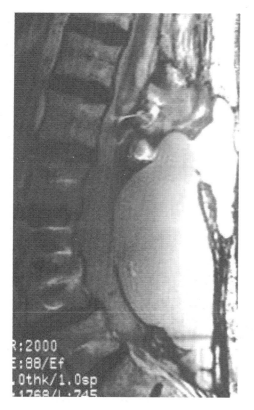

Figure 8 Large pseudomeningocele created by dural tear during previous operation. Patient presented with continued postural headaches after a lumbar fusion.

B. Infection

The rate of perioperative wound infection in the setting of surgically managed trauma has been reported to be greater than 10% (26–27). Risk factors for wound infection include poor nutritional status, obesity, and the use of steroids or other immunosuppressive agents preoperatively. Damage to the soft tissues surrounding the spinal column or cord from the injury can also lead to future infection. Antibiotics are usually all that is necessary for superficial infections, but deep infections typically need irrigation and debridement.

Certain intraoperative risk factors that lead to infection include excessive handling of soft tissue and the placement of retractors for an extended period of time. Periodic release of retractors can ease the soft tissue tension. The use of the bovie to control hemostasis is important, but excessive use can lead to increased infection. Additionally, repeated dosing of antibiotics at scheduled intervals or with excessive bleeding may also be helpful. Finally, attention to post-operative nutritional status to bolster the immune system is essential.

VII. CONCLUSION

Surgery in the setting of spinal trauma is fraught with many potential complications. The spinal surgeon must be attentive to these from the time of admission to the time of surgical stabilization. With meticulous surgical planning and adherence to the principles discussed in this chapter, patient outcomes can be maximized in this unfortunate clinical setting.

REFERENCES

1. Asai T. Fiberoptic tracheal intubation through the laryngeal mask in an awake patient with cervical spine injury [comment]. Anesth Analg 1993; 77:404.
2. Aydinli U, Karaeminogullari O, Tiskaya K, Ozturk C. Dural tears in lumbar burst fractures with greenstick lamina fractures. Spine 2001; 26:E410–E415.
3. Been HD, Kalkman CJ, Traast HS, Ongerboer de Visser BW. Neurologic injury after insertion of laminar hooks during Cotrel-Dubousset instrumentation. Spine 1994; 19:1402–1405.
4. Black P. Cerebrospinal fluid leaks following spinal surgery: use of fat grafts for prevention and repair. Technical note. J Neurosurg 2002; 96:250–252.
5. Bose B, Wierzbowski LR, Sestokas AK. Neurophysiologic monitoring of spinal nerve root function during instrumented posterior lumbar spine surgery. Spine 2002; 27:1444–1450.
6. Calancie B, Harris W, Brindle GF, Green BA, Landy HJ. Threshold-level repetitive transcranial electrical stimulation for intraoperative monitoring of central motor conduction. J Neurosurg 2001; 95:161–168.
7. Carl AL, Matsumoto M, Whalen JT. Anterior dural laceration caused by thoracolumbar and lumbar burst fractures. J Spinal Disord 2000; 13:399–403.
8. Cavallieri S, Riou B, Roche S, Ducart A, Roy-Camille RPV. Intraoperative autologous transfusion in emergency surgery for spine trauma. J Trauma-Injury Infect Crit Care 1994; 36(5):639–643.
9. Crosby E. Airway management after upper cervical spine injury: what have we learned? Can J Anaesth 2002; 49:733–744.
10. De Gelb D, Lenke L, Pond J. Dural tear associated with a flexion distraction subluxation to the cervical spine without neurologic injury. Acta Orthop Belg 1998; 64:224–228.
11. Einav S. Intubation of the trauma patient with a fractured cervical spine: controversies and consensus. Israel J Med Sci 1997; 33:754–756.
12. Fuchs G, Schwarz G, Baumgartner A, Kaltenbock F, Voit-Augustin H, Planinz W. Fiberoptic intubation in 327 neurosurgical patients with lesions of the cervical spine. J Neurosurg Anesthesiol 1999; 11:11–16.
13. Gokaslan ZL, Samudrala S, Deletis V, Wildrick DM, Cooper PR. Intraoperative monitoring of spinal cord function using motor evoked potentials via transcutaneous epidural electrode during anterior cervical spinal surgery. J Spinal Disord 1997; 10:299–303.
14. Kahamba JF, Rath SA, Antoniadis G, Schneider O, Neff U, Richter HP. Laminar and arch fractures with dural tear and nerve root entrapment in patients operated upon for thoracic and lumbar spine injuries. Acta Neurochir 1998; 140:114–119.
15. Keenen TL, Antony J, Benson DR. Dural tears associated with lumbar burst fractures. J Orthop Trauma 1990; 4:243–245.
16. Lee LA, Lam AM. Unilateral blindness after prone lumbar spine surgery [comment]. Anesthesiology 2001; 95:793–795.
17. Manfredini M, Ferrante R, Gildone A, Massari L. Unilateral blindness as a complication of intraoperative positioning for cervical spinal surgery. J Spinal Disord 2000; 13:271–272.
18. Marino RJ. Spinal injury: etiology, demographics, and outcomes. In: Fractures of the Cervical, Thoracic, and Lumbar Spine. New York: Marcel Dekker, 2003:1–8.
19. Meschino A, Devitt JH, Koch JP, Szalai JP, Schwartz ML. The safety of awake tracheal intubation in cervical spine injury [comment]. Can J Anaesth 1992; 39:114–117.
20. Mostegl A, Bauer R, Eichenauer M. Intraoperative somatosensory potential monitoring. A clinical analysis of 127 surgical procedures. Spine 1988; 13:396–400.

21. Muckart DJ, Bhagwanjee S, van der Merwe R. Spinal cord injury as a result of endotracheal intubation in patients with undiagnosed cervical spine fractures [comment]. Anesthesiology 1997; 87:418–420.

22. Nakai S, Yoshizawa H, Kobayashi S, Miyachi M. Esophageal injury secondary to thoracic spinal trauma: the need for early diagnosis and aggressive surgical treatment. J Trauma-Injury Infect Crit Care 1998; 44:1086–1089.

23. Pau A, Silvestro C, Carta F. Can lacerations of the thoraco-lumbar dura be predicted on the basis of radiological patterns of the spinal fractures? Acta Neurochir 1994; 129:186–187.

24. Pollock RA, Purvis JM, Apple DF, Jr., Murray HH Esophageal and hypopharyngeal injuries in patients with cervical spine trauma. Ann Otol Rhinol Laryngol 1981; 90:323–327.

25. Prielipp RC, Morell RC JB. Ulnar nerve injury and perioperative arm positioning. Anesthesiol Clin North Am 2002; 20(3):351–365.

26. Rechtine GR, 2nd, Cahill D, Chrin AM: Treatment of thoracolumbar trauma: comparison of complications of operative versus nonoperative treatment. J Spinal Disord 1999; 12:406–409.

27. Rechtine GR, Bono PL, Cahill D, Bolesta MJ, Chrin AM. Postoperative wound infection after instrumentation of thoracic and lumbar fractures. J Orthop Trauma 2001; 15:566–569.

28. Resnick DK, Benzel EC. C1-C2 pedicle screw fixation with rigid cantilever beam construct: case report and technical note [comment]. Neurosurgery 2002; 50:426–428.

29. Resnick DK, Lapsiwala S, Trost GR. Anatomic suitability of the C1-C2 complex for pedicle screw fixation. Spine 2002; 27:1494–1498.

30. Ryan M, Klein S, Bongard F. Missed injuries associated with spinal cord trauma. Am Surg 1993; 59:371–374.

31. Sar C, Bilen FE. Thoracolumbar flexion-distraction injuries combined with vertebral body fractures. Am J Orthop (Chatham, NI) 2002; 31:147–151.

32. Shatney CH, Brunner RD, Nguyen TQ. The safety of orotracheal intubation in patients with unstable cervical spine fracture or high spinal cord injury. Am J Surg 1995; 70:676–680.

33. Silvestro C, Francaviglia N, Bragazzi R, Piatelli G, Viale GL. On the predictive value of radiological signs for the presence of dural lacerations related to fractures of the lower thoracic or lumbar spine. J Spinal Disord 1991; 4:49–53.

34. Vaccaro AR FS, Flanders AE, Balderston RA, Northrup BE, Cotler JM. Magnetic resonance evaluation of the intervertebral disc, spinal ligaments, and spinal cord before and after closed traction reduction of cervical spine dislocations. Spine 1999; 24:1210–1217.

35. Vaccaro AR, Rizzolo SJ, Allardyce TJ, Ramsey M, Salvo J, Balderston RA, Cotler JM. Placement of pedicle screws in the thoracic spine. Part I: Morphometric analysis of the thoracic vertebrae. J Bone Joint Surg 1995; 77:1193–1199.

36. Vaccaro AR, Rizzolo SJ, Balderston RA, Allardyce TJ, Garfin SR, Dolinskas C, An HS. Placement of pedicle screws in the thoracic spine. Part II: An anatomical and radiographic assessment. J Bone Joint Surg 1995; 77:1200–1206.

37. Venger BH, Simpson RK, Narayan RK. Neurosurgical intervention in penetrating spinal trauma with associated visceral injury. J Neurosurg 1989; 70:514–518.

38. Winton TL, Girotti MJ, Manley PN, Sterns EE. Delayed intestinal perforation after nonpenetrating abdominal trauma. Can J Surg 1985; 28:437–439.

39. Wolfe SW, Lospinuso MF, Burke SW. Unilateral blindness as a complication of patient positioning for spinal surgery. A case report. Spine 1992; 17:600–605.

15

Soft Tissue Complications of Anterior Cervical Surgery: Dysphagia, Dysphonia, and Injuries to the Vital Nonneural Structures of the Neck

James K. Liu, Peter Kan, Marshall E. Smith, and Ronald I. Apfelbaum
University of Utah School of Medicine, Salt Lake City, Utah, U.S.A.

The anterior approach to the cervical spine is one of the most commonly used procedures in spine surgery. It was first introduced in 1958 by Cloward (10), and Smith and Robinson (70). More recently, osteosynthetic plating has been applied to this technique using specialized systems for retraction, distraction, and fixation, which allow for immediate stabilization of the cervical spine. The anterior approach to the cervical spine provides excellent exposure for resection, reconstruction, and stabilization of the cervical spine for traumatic, degenerative, and neoplastic diseases. However, vital structures can be at risk for injury during an anterior approach to the cervical spine. These include the carotid artery, the vertebral artery, the internal jugular vein, the vagus nerve, the sympathetic plexus, the recurrent laryngeal nerve (RLN), the superior laryngeal nerve (SLN), the trachea, and the esophagus. A detailed knowledge of the surgical anatomy is paramount for avoiding complications (47,60–62). Avoidance of complications is mandatory to ensure excellent clinical results (22,30,78,79,82,87,88,91). The authors review the soft tissue complications of anterior cervical spine surgery and discuss the incidence, diagnosis, management, and operative nuances for preventing these complications.

I. DYSPHONIA AND VOCAL CORD PARALYSIS: LARYNGEAL NERVE INJURY

A. Incidence

Vocal cord paralysis is considered the most common neurological complication after anterior cervical spine surgery. In Flynn's review of 82,114 cases, RLN injury comprised 16.7% of all neurological complications and was the single largest complication to result in litigation (22). Symptoms include hoarseness, vocal breathiness or fatigue, weak cough, dysphagia, or aspiration (58). Most cases of vocal cord paralysis are transient, lasting for weeks or months; however, some cases may be permanent. The incidence of RLN injury associated with anterior cervical spine surgery has been reported to be between 0.07% and 11% (3,4,7,11,22,31,34,48,50,66,67,78,82,86,88). Bulger et al. (7) found permanent paralysis rates of 0.98% for both the RLNs and SLNs. Cloward (11) noted 8% transient and 2% permanent paralysis rates. Heeneman et al. (34) found a rate of 11% for vocal motion impairment, with 3.5% of patients having permanent paralysis. In a review by Beutler et al. (4), the incidence of RLN injury was 2.7%, with a significant increase of 9.5% after reoperative anterior fusion. They found no association between the number of disk levels fused or the side of approach with the incidence of RLN injury. In our institutional experience, the overall rates of temporary and permanent vocal cord paralysis were 3% and 0.3%, respectively (1,45). There was an increased incidence of RLN palsy in patients with previous anterior cervical surgery (20%) and in patients who underwent reoperation for failed fusion (10%). In a recent prospective study of 23 patients undergoing anterior cervical surgery, all underwent preoperative and postoperative videolaryngoscopy (24). Postoperatively, two patients had vocal cord paresis: one temporary and one permanent.

Some proposed mechanisms of RLN palsy include direct surgical trauma, nerve division or ligature, pressure or stretch-induced neuropraxia, and postoperative edema (34,58,73,78,83). Although it is widely believed that direct injury to the RLN may occur, there are no data to support such a hypothesis. Direct trauma to the nerve during properly performed anterior cervical spine surgery is unlikely. Although the nerve is not routinely identified, dissection occurs in the fascial plane medial to the sternocleidomastoid muscle and carotid sheath structures, which keeps the approach lateral to the trachea, esophagus, and RLN (Fig. 1). Tew and Mayfield (78) proposed that prolonged

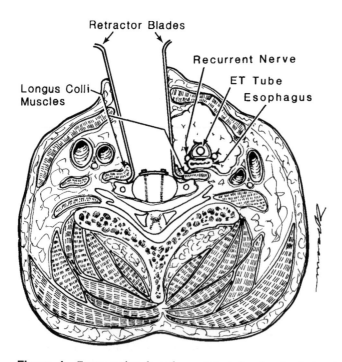

Figure 1 Cross-sectional neck anatomy showing typical retractor placement during anterior cervical surgery. The retractor tips are placed beneath the longus colli muscles with the RLN remaining undissected within interposed soft tissue. (From Ref. 1.)

pressure on the nerve is the most likely cause of vocal cord paralysis in anterior cervical spine surgery. Prolonged pressure decreases mucosal and neuronal capillary blood flow and increases the risk of nerve injury (34,73).

Postoperative vocal cord paralysis has also been reported in patients with intubation who have not undergone neck or thoracic surgery (8,20,32). Studies on vocal cord paralysis after intubation have shown that the endotracheal tube can exert pressure against the RLN in the endolaryngeal portion of the nerve where it passes submucosally before the nerve innervates the vocal cord (Fig. 2). When RLN palsies occur after anterior

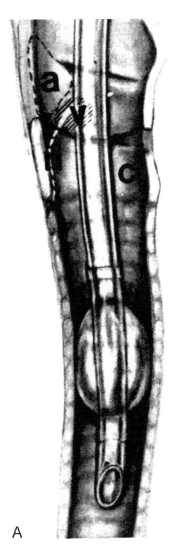

A

Figure 2 (A) Cross-sectional view of endotracheal tube compressing the vulnerable endolaryngeal portion of the RLN. Broken line indicates the course of the RLN (n) where it lies lateral to the cricoid cartilage (c). The nerve is vulnerable to intralaryngeal pressure in the shaded area (v) between the silhouettes of the arytenoids (a) and cricoid cartilages (c). The endotracheal cuff is located well below the point of vulnerability, and the tip is located well above the carina. (B) A sagittally sectioned larynx and trachea with an endotracheal tube in position. (From Ref. 1.)

B

Cricoid Cartilage

Arytenoid Cartilage

Recurrent Laryngeal
Nerve

DIRECTION OF
RETRACTION

Endotracheal
Tube

Thyroid
Cartilage

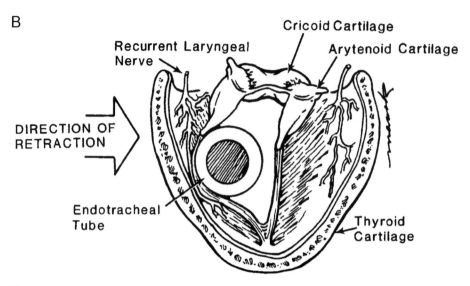

Figure 2 *(continued)*

spinal surgery, it has been postulated that a similar mechanism could occur. This was substantiated by cadaveric studies in which the tracheal mucosa in the region of the vulnerable portion of the RLN was shown to be compressed by the endotracheal shaft after retraction of the larynx (Fig. 3) (1). The anterior ramus of the nerve is the vulnerable segment for compression by the endotracheal tube as the nerve courses submucosally over the thyroid lamina.

The endotracheal tube is fixed at the mouth with tape and distally by the inflated cuff. This makes the system noncompliant so that when the trachea is retracted, the unyielding shaft of the endotracheal tube can compress the wall of the endolarynx. Increases in endotracheal cuff pressure observed after retractor placement during anterior cervical spine surgery have also been implicated in contributing to RLN injury (73). With higher pressures, the endotracheal tube is less able to relocate and center itself in the larynx in response to retraction. This is supported by Jellish et al. (40), who used intraoperative laryngeal electromyography and endotracheal cuff pressure monitoring and found that intraoperative increases in cuff pressure and diminished electromyographic activity occurred in patients with higher rates of postoperative hoarseness. Thus, the most likely sources of RLN palsy during anterior cervical spine surgery are the retractor and/or the endotracheal tube, with clinical evidence favoring the latter as the major source. This supports an endolaryngeal mechanism of injury rather than direct surgical injury.

SLN injury can occur if the dissection is done at higher levels of the cervical spine at or above the larynx (53). This can affect the voice and/or swallowing. The internal branch that provides sensation to the endolarynx crosses the carotid sheath to enter the thyrohyoid membrane. Injury to the SLN may cause dysphagia and aspiration. The external branch courses more inferiorly then follows along the superior thyroid artery, often going between its distal branches above the superior pole of the thyroid gland, to innervate the cricothyroid muscle (54). This muscle controls tension and lengthening of the vocal fold and raises vocal pitch, which is important in singing. Thus, hoarseness and difficulty singing could occur from injury to this nerve. The course these nerves take across the

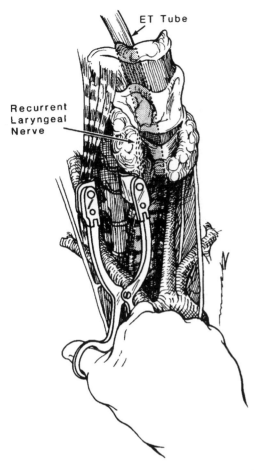

ET Tube

Recurrent
Laryngeal
Nerve

Figure 3 Hypothesized mechanism of RLN injury. Retraction displaces the larynx against the unyielding endotracheal tube shaft with compression on the endolaryngeal segment of the nerve. (From Ref. 1.)

carotid sheath puts them at risk for an injury from anterior cervical spine approach at the level of the larynx or above (levels C4-5 and higher).

B. Diagnosis and Management

Since most laryngeal nerve palsies are transient, most patients can be initially observed. Recovery of function in patients with temporary palsy occurs from 3 weeks to 4 months after surgery. If symptoms of hoarseness persist, or if airway obstruction or aspiration is present, laryngoscopy should be performed to directly assess vocal cord function (7). Even mild changes in the voice, such as vocal fatigue or inability to sing quite as well as preoperatively, can be a significant symptom indicating a laryngeal nerve injury. Vocal cord abduction, adduction, bowing, and elongation with pitch elevation should be evaluated. In RLN palsy there may be impairment of abduction and adduction of the vocal cord, with the cord motionless in the midline to a lateral position. The patient may be at risk of aspiration, especially with thin liquids, if the vocal cords do not approximate well. In SLN palsy, shortening and bowing of the vocal cord and deviation of the posterior larynx to the affected side can be appreciated while having normal abduction and adduction. Hoarseness, vocal fatigue, or reduced pitch range may ensue due to the inability of the cricothyroid muscle to tense the vocal cord during phonation. Patients are also at risk of aspiration due to the loss of sensation in the larynx. Combined SLN and RLN injury may produce a more severe dysphonia.

A useful test in the evaluation of vocal fold paralysis is laryngeal electromyography (EMG) (77). In this procedure, an EMG needle is percutaneously inserted into the cricothyroid muscle or through the cricothyroid membrane into the thyroarytenoid muscle while the patient vocalizes to assess neuromotor function. Patterns of denervation and reinnervation can be identified and prognosis judged for recovery, with an accuracy of 70–90%. This is helpful in determining whether to intervene to improve the voice or to wait for spontaneous improvement. This issue is very important for individuals whose jobs depend on use of their voice. Methods to improve the voice temporarily or permanently can be offered to the patient in an objective manner with information yielded from laryngeal EMG. Injuries to the laryngeal nerves from anterior cervical spine surgery usually occur close to the larynx, so if recovery occurs from a temporary neuropraxia it would be expected within several months after the procedure. The laryngeal EMG can be helpful to determine this. Soon after an injury, presence of normal morphology motor unit potentials on laryngeal EMG is prognostically favorable. Absence of voluntary motor unit activity, fibrillation potentials, and positive sharp waves indicate a poor prognosis, especially when seen more than 3 months after injury. It is, however, important not to equate nerve recovery with phonatory recovery. This is likely due to the phenomenon of misdirected regeneration of abductor and adductor fibers, resulting in synkinetic muscle activity. Individuals with a paralyzed vocal cord may have a normally functioning voice, and those with a mobile but paretic vocal cord can have significant dysphonia.

In cases of permanent vocal cord paralysis, vocal cord medialization can be accomplished by several means for temporary or permanent treatment of dysphonia. For small gaps involving the anterior cord, injection of the paralyzed cord with collagen, fat, gelfoam, acellular dermal matrix (Cimetra®), or Teflon® paste can be done (5,17,19,27,35,55,56,58,63,68). These are widely used rehabilitative techniques and are usually satisfactory in restoring voice and cough and in preventing aspiration. The selected material is injected transorally under topical or general anesthesia between the vocalis muscle and the thyroid cartilage (19,55,68). In the cooperative patient this can be done as an office procedure without sedation using the peroral or percutaneous route and topical local anesthesia (2). The injected mass adducts the anterior membranous cord, producing improved glottic closure with a more effective cough. A disadvantage of these injectable substances is that the result may not be permanent due to resorption. Gelfoam and collagen last for 2–3 months; Cimetra lasts for 6–12 months. Fat has a variable resorption rate. They are all effective for providing temporary improvement in the voice while waiting to see if the nerve recovers. Fine control of the voice is not frequently attained due to loss of ability to tense the cord. An overall improvement in approximately 80% of patients can be expected. Teflon paste, which is permanent, is no longer widely used since a major disadvantage of Teflon injections is delayed formation of granulomas secondary to an inflammatory reaction to the injected Teflon (42). For larger glottal gaps or those involving the posterior larynx, several procedures have been developed that reposition the vocal cord and arytenoid cartilage through external approaches, known as laryngeal framework surgery (37,90). The most widely used are medialization laryngoplasty and arytenoid adduction laryngoplasty (44). These procedures were developed and popularized by Isshiki (38,39) in the 1970s and have become widely used in the United States in the last 15 years. In medialization laryngoplasty (also known as Type I thyroplasty), the larynx is exposed through a skin incision and a window is cut in the thyroid ala at the level of the vocal fold and an implant (usually of silastic or Gore-Tex®) inserted in the paraglottic space to medialize the cord and improve glottal closure (23,51,89). Isshiki's great contribution was to demonstrate that this procedure can be done under local anesthesia so the implant can be placed in optimal position to improve the patient's voice on the operating table (38). Arytenoid adduction, the most effective procedure for closing gaps of the posterior larynx, is also done under local anesthesia and is often combined with a medialization laryngoplasty (44). The procedures can also be revised if needed—an advantage over Teflon injection. Excellent short- and long-term results from these procedures have been reported.

C. Complication Avoidance

Several technical considerations may help prevent vocal cord paralysis. Careful dissection and surgical technique, along with proper retractor placement beneath the bodies of the longus colli muscles away from the tracheoesophageal groove, are critical to preventing direct surgical trauma. The longus colli muscles should be elevated cleanly from the anterior surface of the vertebrae without shredding them to provide a firm anchor point for the retractors. We strongly urge the use of sharp-toothed retractor blades under the longus colli muscles as these will remain in place. Blunt tooth blades do not anchor firmly and can easily slide anteriorly compressing the trachea or esophagus medially and the carotid artery laterally. Intermittent relaxation of the retractors can also be employed and may help prevent injury.

Monitoring of endotracheal cuff pressure and temporarily deflating the cuff after retractor placement may prevent injury to the RLN during anterior cervical spine surgery (1,45,73). The most important factor is deflation of the endotracheal cuff after retractor placement with subsequent reinflation to just-sealed pressures. This should be repeated if the retractor position is changed or elevations in cuff pressure are noted. Significant laryngeal displacement against the endotracheal tube occurs after retractor placement. Since the tube is fixed proximally by tape at the mouth and distally by the inflated balloon, the shaft of the tube can impinge on the lateral wall of the larynx and specifically on the endolaryngeal portion of the recurrent laryngeal nerve as it transverses submucosally to enter the vocal cord musculature. Releasing the cuff pressure by deflating the balloon allows the endotracheal tube to shift away from the inner laryngeal wall (1). The cuff can then be reinflated to just-sealed pressures. This maneuver prevents pressure on the endolaryngeal segment of the RLN. In our experience with a consecutive series of 900 patients, the incidence of temporary RLN palsies dropped from 6.4% (first 250 patients) to 1.7% (subsequent 650 patients) since the introduction of this simple maneuver (1,45). However, there was no significant difference in permanent paralysis rates, which occurred rarely (0.31%).

II. DYSPHAGIA

A. Incidence

Iatrogenic dysphagia has been well documented after anterior cervical spine surgery and has been reported to be transient, with resolution occurring within a few weeks (16).

The incidence of postoperative dysphagia widely ranges from 2 to 80% in several published series (9,10,49,75,84,85). Although the exact etiology has yet to be determined, some have postulated postoperative swelling, hematoma, infection, neurological injury to the pharyngeal plexus, SLN, and/or RLN, and bone graft dislodgement as possible causative factors. Stewart et al. (75) reported a 45% incidence of postoperative dysphagia, with 12% of patients having persistent problems for more than 6 months. Winslow et al. (85) reported an incidence of 60%, with 32% of patients having symptoms greater than 6 months. Buchholz et al. (6) identified impaired pharyngeal contraction near the surgical site, deficient laryngeal closure and laryngeal penetration, and postswallow aspiration in patients with postoperative swallowing deficits. A prospective study of 23 consecutive patients undergoing anterior cervical surgery was conducted in which all subjects underwent preoperative and postoperative videolaryngoscopy and fluoroscopic swallowing studies (24). Eleven patients (48%) exhibited preoperative swallowing abnormalities on the study, though none was symptomatic. Postoperatively, 8 of these 11 had radiographic swallowing abnormalities. There was a tendency for patients undergoing multilevel surgery to demonstrate an increased incidence of swallowing abnormalities on postoperative radiographic studies. In addition, soft tissue swelling was more frequent in patients whose swallowing function was worse postoperatively.

B. Diagnosis and Treatment

In patients with prolonged dysphagia, a videofluoroscopic swallow study (VSS) or endoscopic swallow study (ESS) can be used to determine swallowing integrity and the ability to achieve adequate nutritional intake. It identifies the physiological and anatomical changes of the pharyngolaryngeal swallowing mechanism. Several patterns of swallowing impairments can be identified during VSS, such as reduced pharyngeal wall movement, impaired upper esophageal sphincter opening, incomplete epiglottic deflection, as well as postswallow residue in the vallecula, pyriform sinuses, and posterior pharyngeal wall (49). The pattern of absent pharyngeal swallow is suggestive of neurological injury to the internal branch of the SLN and/or the glossopharyngeal nerve. Deficits in the oral preparatory and/or oral phases of swallowing can also be identified, such as impaired bolus formation, premature spillage of material into the pharynx, hesitancy of the lingual stripping wave, and reduced tongue propulsive action. Any of these deficits suggest the possibility of neurological damage involving the hypoglossal nerve. Additional manometry may reveal elevated pharyngeal pressures in patients with postoperative dysphagia. Based on physiological and anatomical findings of VSS, involvement of the pharyngeal plexus, cranial nerves IX, X, and XII as well as postoperative edema can be implied as possible etiologies of postoperative dysphagia (16). By identifying the physiological and anatomical impairments producing dysphagia, the speech pathologist can implement specific swallowing maneuvers or therapeutic postures to facilitate deglutition.

C. Complication Avoidance

A thorough knowledge of the surgical anatomy may help in identifying and preserving important neurological structures (47,60). Anterior approaches to the C2-C3 level can inadvertently expose the hypoglossal nerve. At the C3-C4 level, both the SLN and hypoglossal nerve are vulnerable to injury. The RLN, as mentioned before, is more commonly damaged from prolonged retraction resulting in an endolayryngeal injury from compression by the endotracheal tube. Careful surgical dissection and proper retractor placement beneath the bodies of the longus colli muscles are important in preventing direct surgical trauma. Deflating and reinflating the endotracheal cuff after retractor placement is critical in preventing endolaryngeal injury to the RLN and has been shown to be very effective in reducing the incidence of RLN palsy, as noted earlier (1).

In performing anterolateral approaches to the upper cervical spine and cranio-vertebral junction, care should be taken to protect the hypoglossal and SLN since both of these nerves are susceptible to injury (52). Although the SLN is usually not seen in this retropharyngeal approach, it is vulnerable to stretch injury from retraction. The key to avoid this complication is to perform wide dissection of the fascial planes, thus allowing less retractive forces required to separate the tissues. If the deep cervical fascia is opened vertically in the lateral exposure to gain access to C4 or higher cervical segments, the SLN must be identified and preserved because this maneuver places the nerve at the most risk for transection.

III. VERTEBRAL ARTERY INJURY

A. Incidence

Injury to the vertebral artery is an uncommon, but serious complication of anterior cervical spine surgery. It is particularly grave because of the difficulty of controlling hemorrhage and the uncertain neurological consequences. The reported incidence of this complication ranges from 0.3 to 0.5% of cases (29,72), although this percentage may be underreported. The incidence of vertebral artery injury is probably higher with more aggressive decompression procedures (29,72,87). Most vertebral artery injuries reported by Smith et al. (72) occurred during vertebrectomies for spinal cord decompression. Vertebral artery injury has been attributed to direct trauma by instruments and high-speed drills during the extended lateral decompression that can be needed to treat some pathological conditions (Fig. 4). Caution, therefore, should be taken when instruments are placed laterally during resection of the uncovertebral joint or performing a foraminotomy (18,64).

B. Diagnosis and Management

Management of vertebral artery injuries requires local hemostasis and prevention of both immediate vertebrobasilar ischemia and vascular embolic complications. When vertebral artery injury occurs during anterior cervical surgery, the status of the collateral circulation is rarely known. The incidence of neurological deficits after sacrificing one vertebral artery is approximately 0.5% (Cervical Spine Research Society, unpublished data). The best management of iatrogenic vertebral artery injury remains controversial. Some surgeons advocate direct exposure of the vessel in the foramen transversarium and microsurgical repair, whereas others recommend simple tamponade with hemostatic packing (14,18,29,64,72).

Golfinos et al. (29) reported three patients who underwent primary microvascular reanastamosis of the vertebral artery at the time of injury. This treatment was recommended as the first-line strategy since it avoids unnecessary sacrifice of the artery and potential ischemic or hemorrhagic complications. Direct microvascular repair restores normal blood flow and minimizes the risk of immediate or delayed ischemic neurological complications. If microvascular anastamosis is not feasible, exposure and ligation of the artery proximally and distally is an alternative option. In patients in whom hemorrhage

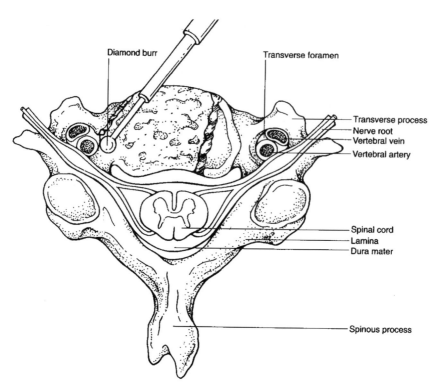

Figure 4 Mechanism of injury to the vertebral artery as a result of excessive lateral drilling or misassessment of the midline. (From Ref. 28.)

can only be controlled by packing or proximal ligation, there remains a risk of delayed pseudoaneurysm formation, vertebrobasilar ischemia, delayed hemorrhage, and fistula formation (14). In such cases, angiography with subsequent endovascular occlusion may be appropriate (18).

C. Complication Avoidance

Avoidance of vertebral artery injuries in anterior cervical spine surgery requires that the surgeon have an understanding of the relationships between the neurovascular anatomy and its surrounding bony landmarks (61). Intraoperative vertebral artery injury can also be avoided by recognizing dilated or tortuous vertebral arteries on preoperative CT and/or MRI scans (80).

The surgeon must keep in mind that the uncinate process serves as an important bony landmark that signifies the lateral border of the spinal canal. The vertebral artery is intimately associated with the lateral border of the uncinate process, which often loses its sharp, bony characteristics with aging (61). Caution should be exercised when the uncinate process is removed in the course of osteophyte removal (Fig. 4). Dissection lateral to the uncinate process needs to be at the level of the posterior aspect of the vertebral body. Dissection in the middle third of the body (from anterior to posterior) may cause damage to the vertebral artery. The longus colli muscles and uncovertebral joints are the key structures for a secure midline dissection during cervical discectomy or corpectomy. Ventral decompression can usually be carried out to a width of 18–20 mm. If wider decompression is needed, careful study of preoperative scans can help the surgeon ascertain the location of the vertebral artery in relationship to the bony anatomy and pathology. Often, dissection to a width of 20–24 mm is possible, if needed.

IV. CAROTID ARTERY AND INTERNAL JUGULAR VEIN INJURY

A. Incidence

Injury to the carotid artery or jugular vein is uncommon, and the incidence is not exactly known (74,78). Vascular complications can be a result of improper and excessive retraction or inadvertent laceration with the scalpel or other surgical instruments. Thrombosis of the carotid artery or cerebral ischemia may occur as a result of prolonged pressure against the carotid artery (30,65,78). Hohf (36) reported four cases of carotid artery injury from anterior spinal fusion—three involving laceration and the other involving a division of the carotid artery.

B. Diagnosis and Management

Diagnosis and treatment of vascular injuries during anterior cervical spine exposure involve recognition, control of bleeding, and repair or ligation when indicated. If the carotid artery is lacerated, primary repair is indicated. Injury to the external jugular vein is of little clinical significance; therefore, it may be sacrificed and ligated safely. Lacerations of the internal jugular vein should be repaired if possible, but may be ligated if necessary (28).

C. Complication Avoidance

To avoid an injury to the carotid artery and internal jugular vein it is necessary to identify the artery before placing the retractor system. Direct palpation and gentle finger dissection helps in avoiding inadvertent injury of this major vessel (74). As emphasized earlier in the chapter, proper placement of retractors requires mobilization of the longus colli muscles along the anterolateral aspect of the vertebral bodies. The blades of the retractor must be placed under the longus colli muscles after elevating them cleanly from their medial side without muscle shredding. Sharp-toothed retractor blades, which hold firmly, will prevent retraction injuries. Although blunt blades may seem safer, they more frequently fail to hold the longus colli muscles. The carotid artery and the jugular vein should be inspected to detect inadvertent injury prior to closure (91).

V. ESOPHAGEAL PERFORATION

A. Incidence

Esophageal perforation after anterior cervical spine surgery and anterior cervical plating is an uncommon but potentially devastating complication. The overall incidence of esophageal perforation after anterior cervical spine surgery has been reported as 0.2–1.15% (26,59,78). Newhouse et al. (59) reported 22 cases of iatrogenic esophageal perforation, four of which were related to hardware. Most complications present in the early postoperative period; however, they may present in a delayed fashion weeks or even months after surgery (43). In a series reported by Newhouse et al. (59), approximately one third of perforations occurred at the time of surgery and were related to sharp or motorized instruments. Delayed perforations recognized after surgery were mostly related to direct erosion of the esophagus by bone, cement, hardware backout, or migration (71). Complications arising from esophageal perforations, such as mediastinitis, esophageal strictures, osteomyelitis, prevertebral or retropharyngeal abscess, and tracheo-esophageal fistulas, can result in high morbidity and extensive hospital stays. Mortality is reported as high as 15–30% and may be greater than 50% if treatment is delayed (26,59).

B. Diagnosis and Treatment

Successful management of esophageal perforations depends on the early recognition of clinical signs and symptoms and immediate treatment. The most frequently occurring symptoms are neck and throat pain, dysphagia, hoarseness, and aspiration. Neck pain and crepitus should alert surgeons to the possibility of an esophageal perforation and possibly a secondary infection. Unexplained fever, leukocytosis, and tachycardia may also indicate an esophageal injury (26,81).

Diagnosis of esophageal perforation traditionally has been by esophagogram, esophagography augmented by CT, and esophagoscopy. However, esophagograms may be difficult to interpret when external and internal devices obscure the esophagus (26,59,81). Lateral cervical radiographs may reveal subcutaneous emphysema and an increased retropharyngeal space. In 50% of patients undergoing endoscopic examination for esophageal perforation, Guadinez et al. (26) found metallic devices, such as cervical plates and screws, inserted for anterior cervical fusion within the lumen of the esophagus. In some cases radiographic examinations may be inconclusive, so clinical suspicion is most important in making a correct and timely diagnosis.

Although minor esophageal injuries have been managed with observation, extraoral feeding, and parenteral antibiotics, nonsurgical management of esophageal perforations are associated with high mortality (46). Most patients require surgical repair and drainage of the esophagus. Perforations detected at the time of surgery should be treated by oversewing the defect, draining the wound, and administering broad coverage antibiotics to cover gram-positive, gram-negative, and anaerobic organisms (59). For extensive and complex esophageal tears, primary closure is not advisable because of the high risk of subsequent esophageal stricture. Alternatively, esophageal advancement or diverting cervical esophagostomy are used. In some cases, interposition of a vascularized sternocleidomastoid myoplasty is recommended for closure of larger defects (81). Postoperatively, extraoral feeding and intravenous antibiotics should be initiated. Follow-up esophagograms within 7–10 days of surgery are recommended to check for anastomotic leaks.

C. Complication Avoidance

Using blunt finger dissection rather than sharp dissection below the superficial cervical fascia can reduce the risk of esophageal perforation. Proper retractor placement should mobilize the esophagus away from the operative field to prevent inadvertent injury from the high-speed drill. During multilevel operations, the medial blades should be released and reset intermittently. It is important that the final cervical internal fixation be smooth so that it does not cause esophageal irritation and subsequent erosion. Careful inspection of the esophagus should be performed prior to wound closure (26,59).

VI. TRACHEAL INJURY

A. Incidence

Although tracheal perforation is a potential complication of anterior cervical spine surgery, it is extremely rare and its true incidence is unknown. In most circumstances it is related to penetration by the sharp blades of a spreading retractor.

B. Diagnosis and Treatment

In most cases direct visualization confirms the diagnosis of intraoperative tracheal injury. Tracheal disruption can be life-threatening and can result in tension pneumothorax, mediastinal emphysema, and esophageal prolapse into the tracheal lumen leading to acute asphyxia, sepsis, and mediastinitis (41). Postoperatively, chest radiographs can assist in the diagnosis.

An absolute indication for surgical repair is a transmural tear with a length exceeding 1 cm that causes pneumothorax and/or pneumomediastinum (25). Short lacerations in the upper third of the trachea, especially if they do not involve the whole thickness of the tracheal wall, can sometimes be treated by antibiotics, intubation with the cuff inflated distal to the tear, and placement of a drain to reduce subcutaneous air accumulation. However, conservative treatment may result in tracheal stenosis. Intubation in these patients must be performed under fiberoptic endoscopic control to ensure correct tube placement.

C. Complication Avoidance

To avoid tracheal injury, Cloward hand-held retractors should be used until the blades of the self-retaining retractor are placed securely beneath the longus colli muscles (78). This maneuver prevents perforation of soft tissue structures by the retractor blades and unnecessary pressure on the trachea.

VII. THORACIC DUCT INJURY

A. Incidence

Stuart (76) compiled the first series of iatrogenic injuries of the thoracic duct during neck surgeries in 1907. Although thoracic duct injury is a well-described complication of neck dissection (12,21), it has rarely been reported after anterior cervical spine surgery. Hart et al. (33) reported one case of thoracic duct injury occurring during cervical discectomy and fusion via an anterior approach. They attributed their complication to an anomalous course of the terminal arch of the thoracic duct that was located more superiorly than its typical position. Nine cases of chylorrhea have been reported in the literature following anterior fusion of the thoracolumbar spine (13,57,69). With left-sided incisions to anterior approaches to the cervicothoracic junction, the thoracic duct may be identified as it enters the dorsal aspect of the subclavian vein. Its small size, inconsistent location, and proximity to the vertebral bodies render the thoracic duct susceptible to injury during left-sided anterior surgical approaches to the spine.

B. Diagnosis and Treatment

Injury to the thoracic duct results in chylorrhea. A prompt search for the source must be made if watery, creamy, or greasy fluid of whitish clotted material is seen during neck surgery. The application of prolonged positive pressure by the anesthesiologist while the patient is in the Trendelenburg position often delineates the location of a leak, as does the use of an operating microscope. The thoracic duct should be ligated with a 3-0 or 4-0 nonabsorbable suture when the site of leakage is identified (15). Chronic loss of chyle can result in serious metabolic derangements secondary to depletion of fluid, electrolytes, and protein as well as decreased immunocompetence caused by peripheral lymphocytopenia. If left untreated, the patient may exhibit progressive weakness, dehydration, and peripheral edema.

Postoperatively, a chylous fistula may present as an elevated skin flap with erythema and edema, which often mimics a seroma or a hematoma. Aspiration of fluid for triglyceride analysis may reveal a cloudy content, depending on the fat content of the patient's diet. Oral feeding should be discontinued and intravenous fluids should be intitiated. If a drain is present, it should be converted from suction to gravity. A pressure dressing is recommended and the patient should be restricted to bed rest in the semi-Fowler position (elevation of head and knee). The fluid and electrolyte balance needs to be maintained (15,33).

C. Complication Avoidance

A thorough knowledge of the neck and lymphatic system anatomy, early recognition, and aggressive management of iatrogenic thoracic duct injury will decrease its incidence and minimize its morbidity. The abundance of thoracic duct branches and variability of their terminations render it susceptible to injury during left-sided surgical neck dissections.

VIII. SYMPATHETIC CHAIN INJURY

A. Incidence

Damage to the cervical sympathetic chain is said to be rare but comprised 4.2% of the neurological complications in Flynn's series (22). Injury to the cervical sympathetic chain is associated with an ipsilateral Horner's syndrome. The sympathetic chain is located between the carotid sheath and the longus colli muscles in the midcervical region. Excessive lateral retraction or extensive dissection of the longus colli muscles from midline can injure the sympathetic chain. This can most likely occur in an anterolateral approach (30), rather than an anterior approach.

B. Diagnosis and Management

Horner's syndrome presents with clinical signs of unilateral ptosis, miosis, and anhydrosis. It is usually temporary or of little clinical significance (30,78).

C. Complication Avoidance

To avoid this complication, one should avoid excessive lateral dissection of the longus colli.

IX. SUMMARY

Soft-tissue complications during anterior cervical spine surgery are rare. RLN injury is the most common neurological complication after anterior cervical spine surgery.

Complications can be minimized by mastering the surgical anatomy, performing careful surgical dissection, placing self-retaining retractor blades properly, and transiently deflating the endotracheal cuff after retractor placement or movement.

REFERENCES

1. Apfelbaum RI, Kriskovich MD, Haller JR. On the incidence, cause, prevention of recurrent laryngeal nerve palsies during anterior cervical spine sugery. Spine 2000; 25:2906–2912.
2. Bastian RW, Delsupehe KG. Indirect larynx and pharynx surgery: a replacement for direct laryngoscopy. Laryngoscope 1996; 106:1280–1286.
3. Bertalanffy H, Eggert H. Complications of anterior cervical discectomy without fusion in 450 consecutive patients. Acta Neurochir (Wien) 1989; 99:41–50.
4. Beutler WJ, Sweeney CA, Connolly PJ. Recurrent laryngeal nerve injury with anterior cervical spine surgery: risk with laterality of surgical approach. Spine 2001; 26:1337–1342.
5. Brandenburg J, Kirkham W, Koshkee D. Vocal cord augmentation with autogenous fat. Laryngoscope 1992; 102:495–500.
6. Buchholz DW, Jones B, Ravich WJ. Dysphagia following anterior cervical fusion. Dysphagia 1993; 8:390.
7. Bulger RF, Rejowski JE, Beatty RA. Vocal cord paralysis associated with anterior cervical fusion. J Neurosurg 1985; 62:657–661.
8. Cavo JW. True vocal cord paralysis following intubation. Laryngoscope 1985; 95:1352–1358.
9. Clements DH, O'Leary PF. Anterior discectomy and fusion. Spine 1990; 15:1023–1025.
10. Cloward RB. The anterior approach for removal of ruptured cervical discs. J. Neurosurg 1958; 15:602–617.
11. Cloward RB. New method of diagnosis and treatment of cervical disc disease. Clin Neurosurg 1962; 8:93–132.
12. Coates HL, DeSanto LW. Bilateral chylothorax as a complication of radial neck dissection. J Laryngol Otol 1976; 90:967–970.
13. Colletta AJ, Mayer PJ. Chylothorax: an unusual complication of anterior thoracic interbody spinal fusion. Spine 1982; 7:46–49.
14. Cosgrove GR, Theron J. Vertebral arteriovenous fistula following anterior cervical spine surgery. J Neurosurg 1987; 66:297–299.
15. Crumley RL, Smith JD. Postoperative chylous fistula prevention and management. Laryngoscope 1976; 86:804–813.
16. Daniels SK, Mahoney MC, Lyons GD. Persistent dysphagia and dysphonia following cervical spine surgery. Ear Nose Throat J 1998; 77:470–475.
17. Dayal VS. Medialization of the vocal cord with fat injection. J Otolaryngol 2002; 31:163–164.
18. de los Reyes RA, Moser FG, Sachs DP, et al. Direct repair of an extracranial vertebral artery pseudoaneurysm: case report and review of the literature. Neurosurgery 1990; 26:528–533.
19. Dedo HH, Urrea RD, Lawson L. Intracordal injection of Teflon in the treatment of 135 patients with dysphonia. Ann Otol Rhinol Laryngol 1973; 82:661–667.
20. Ellis PDM, Pallister WK. Recurrent laryngeal nerve palsy and endotracheal intubation. J Laryngolotol 1975; 89:823–826.
21. Fitz-Hugh GS, Cowgill R. Chylous fistula. Complication of neck dissection. Arch Otolaryngol 1970; 91:543–547.
22. Flynn TB. Neurologic complications of anterior cervical interbody fusion. Spine 1982; 7:536–539.
23. Ford CN. Advances and refinements in phonosurgery. Laryngoscope 1999; 109:1891–1900.
24. Frempong-Boadu A, Houten JK, Osborn B, et al. Swallowing and speech dysfunction in patients undergoing anterior cervical discectomy and fusion: a prospective, objective pre-operative and postoperative assessment. J Spinal Disord Tech 2002; 15:362–368.

25. Gabor S, Renner H, Pinter H, et al. Indications for surgery in tracheobronchial ruptures. Eur J Cardiothorac Surg 2001; 20:399–404.

26. Gaudinez RF, English GM, Gebhard JS, et al. Esophageal perforations after anterior cervical surgery. J Spinal Discord 2000; 13:77–84.

27. Giovanni A, Vallicioni JM, Gras R, et al. Clinical experience with Gore-Tex for vocal cord medialization. Laryngoscope 1999; 109:284–288.

28. Gokaslan ZL, Cooper PR. Ventral and ventrolateral subaxial decompression. In: Benzel EC, ed. Spine Surgery. Philadelphia: Churchill Livingstone, 1999:219–227.

29. Golfinos JG, Dickman CA, Zabramski JM, et al. Repair of vertebral artery injury during anterior cervical decompression. Spine 1994; 19:2552–2556.

30. Graham JJ. Complications of cervical spine surgery: a five year report on the survey of the membership of the Cervical Spine Research Society by the morbidity and mortality committee. Spine 1989; 14:1046–1050.

31. Grisoli F, Graziani N, Fabrizi AP, et al. Anterior discectomy without fusion for treatment of cervical lateral soft disc extrusion: a follow-up of 120 cases. Neurosurgery 1989; 24:853–858.

32. Hahn FW, Martin JT, Lille JC. Vocal cord paralysis with endotracheal intubation. Arch Otolaryngol 1970; 92:226–229.

33. Hart AKE, Greinwald JH Jr, Shaffrey CI et al. Thoracic duct injury during anterior cervical discectomy: a rare complication. J Neurosurg 1998; 88:151–154.

34. Heeneman H. Vocal cord paralysis following approaches to the anterior cervical spine. Laryngoscope 1973; 83:17–21.

35. Hoffmann H, McCabe D, McCulloch T, et al. Laryngeal collagen injection as an adjunct to medialization laryngoplasty. Laryngoscope 2002; 112:1407–1413.

36. Hohf RP. Arterial injuries occurring during orthopedic operations. Clin Orthop 1963; 28: 21–37.

37. Isshiki N. Progress in laryngeal framework surgery. Acta Otolaryngol 2000; 120:120–127.

38. Isshiki N, Morita H, Okamura H, et al. Thyroplasty as a new surgical technique. Acta Otolaryngol 1974; 78:451–457.

39. Isshiki N, Tanabe M, Sawada M. Arytenoid adduction for unilateral vocal cord paralysis. Arch Otolaryngol 1978; 104:555–558.

40. Jellish WS, Jensen RL, Anderson DE, et al. Intraoperative electromyographic assessment of recurrent laryngeal nerve stress and pharyngeal injury during anterior cervical spine surgery with Caspar instrumentation. J Neurosurg 1999; 91:170–174.

41. Kaloud H, Smolle-Juettner FM, Prause G, et al. Iatrogenic ruptures of the tracheobronchial tree. Chest 1997; 112:774–778.

42. Kasperbauer JL, Slavit DH, Maragos NE. Teflon granulomas and overinjection of Teflon: a therapeutic challenge for the otorhinolaryngologist. Ann Otol Rhinol Laryngol 1993; 102:748–751.

43. Kelly MF, Rizzo KA, Spiegel J, et al. Delayed pharyngoesophageal perforation: a complication of anterior spine surgery. Ann Otol Rhinol Laryngol 1991; 100:201–205.

44. Koufman JA, Isaacson G. Laryngoplastic phonosurgery. Otolaryngol Clin North Am 1991; 24:1151–1177.

45. Kriskovich MD, Apfelbaum RI, Haller JR. Vocal fold paralysis after anterior cervical spine surgery: incidence, mechanism, and prevention of injury. Laryngoscope 2000; 110:1467–1473.

46. Loop PD, Groves LK. Collective review, esophageal perforations. Ann Thorac Surg 1970; 10:571–587.

47. Lu J, Ebraheim NA, Nadim Y, et al. Anterior approach to the cervical spine: surgical anatomy. Orthopedics 2000; 23:841–845.

48. Lunsford LD, Bissonette DJ, Jannetta PJ, et al. Anterior surgery for cervical disc disease. J Neurosurg 1980; 53:1–11.

49. Martin RE, Neary MA, Diamant NE. Dysphagia following anterior cervical spine surgery. Dysphagia 1997; 12:2–8.

50. Mayfield FH. Cervical spondylosis: a comparison of the anterior and posterior approaches. Clin Neurosurg 1966; 13:181–187.
51. McCulloch TM, Hoffman HT. Medialization laryngoplasty with expanded polytetrafluoroethylene. Surgical technique and preliminary results. Ann Otol Rhinol Laryngol 1998; 107:427–432.
52. McDonnell DE. Anterolateral cervical approach to the craniovertebral junction. In: Rengachary SS, Wilkins RH, eds. Neurosurgical Operative Atlas. Vol. 1. Park Ridge, IL: American Associations of Neurological Surgeons 1991: 147–164.
53. Melamed H, Harris MB, Awasthi D. Anatomic considerations of superior laryngeal nerve during anterior cervical spine procedures. Spine 2002; 27:E83–E86.
54. Monfared A, Kim D, Jaikumar S, et al. Microsurgical anatomy of the superior and recurrent laryngeal nerves. Neurosurgery 2001; 49:925–933.
55. Montgomery WW. Laryngeal paralysis Teflon injection. Ann Otol Rhinol Laryngol 1979; 88:647–657.
56. Morpeth JF, Williams MF. Vocal fold paralysis after anterior cervical diskectomy fusion. Laryngoscope 2000; 110:43–46.
57. Nakai S, Zielke K. Chylothorax—a rare complication after anterior and posterior spinal correction. Report on six cases. Spine 1986; 11:830–833.
58. Netterville JL, Koriwchak MJ, Winkle M, et al. Vocal fold paralysis following the anterior approach to the cervical spine. Ann Otol Rhinol Laryngol 1996; 105:85–91.
59. Newhouse KE, Lindsey RW, Clark CR, et al. Esophageal perforation following anterior cervical spine surgery. Spine 1989; 14:1051–1053.
60. Oh S, Perin NI, Cooper PR. Quantitative three-dimensional anatomy of the subaxial cervical spine: implication for anterior spinal surgery. Neurosurgery 1996; 38:1139–1144.
61. Pait TG, Killefer JA, Arnautovic KI. Surgical anatomy of the anterior cervical spine: the disc space, vertebral artery, and associated bony structures. Neurosurgery 1996; 39:769–776.
62. Pait TG, McAllister PV, Kaufman HH. Quadrant anatomy of the articular pillars (lateral cervical mass) of the cervical spine. J Neurosurg 1995; 82:1011–1014.
63. Pearl AW, Woo P, Ostrowski R, et al. A preliminary report on micronized AlloDerm injection laryngoplasty. Laryngoscope 2002; 112:990–996.
64. Pfeifer BA, Freidberg SR, Jewell ER. Repair of injured vertebral artery in anterior cervical procedures. Spine 1994; 19:1471–1474.
65. Phillips DC. Surgical treatment of myelopathy with cervical spondylosis. J Neurol Neurosurg Psychiatry 1973; 36:879–884.
66. Riley LH Jr, Robinson RA, Johnson KA, et al. The results of anterior interbody fusion of the cervical spine. J Neurosurg 1969; 30:127–133.
67. Robinson RA, Walker AE, Ferlic DC, et al. The results of anterior interbody fusion of the cervical spine. J Bone Joint Surg (Am) 1962; 44:1569–1587.
68. Schramm VL Jr, May M, Lavorato AS. Gelfoam paste injection for vocal cord paralysis: temporary rehabilitation of glottic incompetence. Laryngoscope 1978; 88:1268–1273.
69. Shen YS, Cheung CY, Nilsen PT. Chylous leakage after arthrodesis using the anterior approach to the spine. Report of two cases. J Bone Joint Surg (Am) 1989; 71: 1250–1251.
70. Smith GW, Robinson RA. The treatment of certain cervical-spine disorders by anterior removal of the intervetebral disc and interbody fusion. J Bone Joint Surg (Am) 1958; 40:607–624.
71. Smith MD, Bolesta MJ. Esophageal perforation after anterior cervical plate fixation: a report of two cases. J Spinal Disord 1992; 5:357–362.
72. Smith MD, Emery SE, Dudley A, et al. Vertebral artery injury during anterior decompression of the cervical spine. J Bone Joint Surg (Br) 1993; 75:410–415.
73. Sperry RJ, Johnson JO, Apfelbaum RI. Endotracheal tube cuff pressure increases significantly during anterior cervical fusion with the Caspar instrumentation system. Anesth Analg 1993; 76:1318–1321.

74. Stambough JL, Simeone FA. Vascular complications in spine surgery. In: Rothman RH, Simeone FA, eds. The Spine. 3rd ed. Philadelphia: W.B. Saunders Company, 1992:1877–1885.
75. Stewart M, Johnston RA, Stewart I, et al. Swallowing performance following anterior cervical spine surgery. Br J Neurosurg 1995; 9:605–609.
76. Stuart WJ. Operative injuries of the thoracic duct in the neck. Edinburgh Med J 1907; 22: 301–317.
77. Sulica L, Blitzer A. Laryngeal electromyography. In: Rubin JS, Sataloff R, Korovin G, eds. Diagnosis and Treatment of Voice Disorders. 2nd ed. New York: Thomson/Delmar Learning 2002:221–232.
78. Tew JM, Mayfield FH. Complications of surgery of the anterior cervical spine. Clin Neurosurg 1976; 23:424–434.
79. Ullman JS, Camins MB, Post KD. Complications of cervical disk surgery. Mt Sinai J Med 1994; 61:276–279.
80. Vaccaro AR, Ring D, Scuderi G, et al. Vertebral artery location in relation to the vertebral body as determined by two-dimensional computed tomography evaluation. Spine 1994; 19:2637–2641.
81. van Berge Henegouwen DP, Roukema JA, de Nie JC, et al: Esophageal perforation during surgery on the cervical spine. Neurosurgery 1991; 29:766–768.
82. Watters WC III, Levinthal R. Anterior cervical discectomy with and without fusion: results, complications, and long-term follow-up. Spine 1994; 19:2343–2347.
83. Weisberg NK, Spangler DM, Netterville JL. Stretch-induced nerve injury as a cause of paralysis secondary to the anterior cervical approach. Otolaryngol Head Neck Surg 1997; 116:317–326.
84. Welsh LW, Welsh JJ, Chinnici JC. Dysphagia due to cervical spine surgery. Ann Otol Rhinol Laryngol 1987; 96:112–115.
85. Winslow CP, Winslow TJ, Wax MK. Dysphonia and dysphagia following the anterior approach to the cervical spine. Arch Otolaryngol Head Neck Surg 2001; 127:51–55.
86. Yamamoto I, Ikeda A, Shibuya N, et al. Clinical long-term results of anterior discectomy without interbody fusion for cervical disc disease. Spine 1991; 16:272–279.
87. Zdeblick TA. Complications of anterior spinal instrumentation. Semin Spine Surg 1993; 5: 101–107.
88. Zeidman SM, Ducker TB, Raycroft J. Trends and complications in cervical spine surgery: 1989–1993. J Spinal Disord 1997; 10:523–526.
89. Zeitels SM. New procedures for paralytic dysphonia: adduction arytenopexy, Goretex medialization laryngoplasty, and cricothyroid subluxation. Otolaryngol Clin North Am 2000; 33:841–854.
90. Zeitels SM, Casiano RR, Gardner GM, et al. Management of common voice problems: committee report. Otolaryngol Head Neck Surg 2002; 126:333–348.
91. Zileli M, Naderi S, Benzel EC, et al. Preoperative and surgical planning for avoiding complications. In: Benzel EC, ed. Spine Surgery. Philadelphia: Churchill Livingstone, 1999:135–142.

16

Construct Failure in Cervical Corpectomy Surgery

Kanit Chamroontaneskul and D. Greg Anderson
University of Virginia, School of Medicine, Charlottesville, Virginia, U.S.A.

I. INTRODUCTION

Anterior cervical corpectomy has emerged as an effective method for decompression of the spinal cord for a wide variety of cervical disorders including cervical spondylotic myelopathy and radiculopathy, ossification of posterior longitudinal ligament, various fractures, neoplasms, and infectious disorders. In addition, corpectomy is useful as a salvage procedure for kyphotic deformities or vertebral collapse in patients who have undergone posterior decompressive laminectomy (10). Successful spinal reconstruction after cervical corpectomy depends on recreating the structural integrity of the anterior cervical elements using structural bone grafts or cages. In recent years, as the number of internal fixation options has increased, the use of supplemental implants to improve construct rigidity and decrease the need for postoperative immobilization has become popular (47).

One factor responsible for the proliferation of internal fixation devices for the cervical spine has been significant advances in the design and material properties of cervical implants. Despite these advances, the rate of construct failure in situations requiring multilevel corpectomy remains unacceptably high, leading in some cases to suboptimal results or the need for revision surgery. Many constructs and techniques have been used to tackle the biomechanical challenge posed by multilevel corpectomy reconstruction. This spectrum of corpectomy constructs can broadly be categorized into strut graft alone, strut graft combined with posterior fixation, strut graft combined with anterior cervical plating, or strut graft combined with both anterior and posterior instrumentations. Within these broad categories, a wide variety of technical nuances have been described, all attempting to minimize the rate of construct failure. In addition, each type of cervical corpectomy construct can be augmented with external orthoses, including cervical collars, cervical thoracic orthoses, or the halo-vest orthosis. Although the rate of success depends to some degree on the specific pathology being treated and the technical attributes of the individual surgeon, each type of reconstruction is associated with specific complications and an established rate of success within the literature.

Construct failure can be defined as strut graft dislodgement, graft or endplate fracture, graft subsidence, or failure of an internal fixation device leading to an undesirable deformity or irritation/injury of the surrounding vital or neurological structures such as the spinal cord, esophagus, trachea, and/or vascular structures. Although internal fixation devices such as cervical locking plates have improved the rate of graft dislodgement for short corpectomy constructs, long constructs (three or more levels) continue to be associated with high rates of failure despite anterior plating (10,16,27,47–49). To decrease the rate of construct failure, some surgeons have resorted to circumferential surgery (27,45,48).

Fortunately, basic science and clinical studies have improved our understanding of the biomechanical behavior of the cervical spine following corpectomy. By applying the available information, the rate of construct failure can be minimized. The goal of this chapter is to review the unique anatomy and biomechanics of the cervical region before and after corpectomy, as well as review the biomechanics of the available fixation techniques. In addition, the pertinent literature regarding the outcome of various reconstruction techniques will be reviewed with an emphasis on the success rate and specific complications for a given technique. Finally, we hope to share clinical and technical pearls that may be useful to the surgeon in dealing with these complex surgical challenges.

II. ANATOMY AND BIOMECHANICS

Vertebral body shape is similar from C3 to C7, but the vertebral body size increases as one descends in the subaxial region of the cervical spine. Over the range of C3 to C7, the average width of the vertebral body increases from 17 to 23 mm, the depth increases from 16 to 18 mm, and the height increases from 11 to 13 mm (35). The sagittal canal diameter of the normal spine remains fairly constant over this span, with an average of 15–18 mm (35). The cross-sectional area of the spinal canal is narrowest at C4 and C5 (20,32), while the spinal cord itself is largest in this area (20,32). Facet orientation changes subtly from C2 to C7, as the angulation in the sagittal plane gradually decreases from approximately 55 to about 35° (37). Spinous process length increases from C3 to C7, allowing for the increased torque needed to resist loads on the head. The neural foramen in the subaxial region measures approximately 9 mm in height, 4 mm in width, and 5 mm in length and is smallest at C5-6 and largest at C7-T1 (7,52).

During movement, the size of the spinal canal and neural foramen change. The center of rotation for cervical region is anterior to the spinal canal, and thus the canal lengthens slightly with flexion and shortens with extension (38). This necessitates sliding of the spinal cord relative to the surrounding canal. Extension of the cervical spine narrows the spinal canal relative to a flexed or neutral position (5,31). This is in part due to slight protrusion of the disks but, more importantly, to ligamentum flavum infolding, which reduces the sagittal diameter of the canal by 20–30% when compared with the flexed position. Similarly, the size of the neural foramen decreases approximately 13% when the neck is positioned in extension (51).

In spite of the changes in canal dimensions during motion, the normal spine allows a remarkable range of motion while protecting the delicate spinal cord and nerve roots from injury. Much of this motion occurs at the specialized upper cervical region (occiput C1-C2), which provides approximately 60% of the overall arc of cervical flexion-extension and rotation (34). The phenomenon of couple motions has been well documented in the spinal column, but it is most dramatic in the subaxial cervical region. This results in axial rotation in the same direction as an applied lateral bending and conversely lateral bending in the same direction as an applied axial rotation (34). Because most corpectomies are performed below the C2 level, a significant percentage of the arc or flexion-extension and rotation is generally preserved.

The cervical region is significantly different from other regions of the spine from a biomechanical prospective. Compared to other regions, the cervical vertebrae are geometrically smaller but have higher bone densities (9). In addition, the alignment of facets and disks provides for a more uniform distribution of compressive loads. Axial loads in the cervical region are evenly distributed between the anterior elements and the facet complex on each side, similar to a tripod (9). Although applied loads create a shear component across the intervertebral disk, the coexistent compression of the facets enhances cervical stability and serves to minimize the forces transmitted to the anterior column of the spine (9). Due to normal lordosis, the cervical vertebrae concentrate compressive loads towards the posterior edge of the vertebral body above C4-C5 and towards the anterior edge of the vertebral body below this level (34). The normal instantaneous axis of rotation lies in the posterior third of the disk space in the midcervical region (33,34). The normal weight-bearing axis traverses the occipitocervical joint and approximately the vertebral body of T2. Throughout the cervical region, the normal weight bearing axis falls posterior to the vertebral bodies (see Fig. 1). Any pathological process that results in a loss of physiological lordosis serves to shift the weight-bearing axis forward.

III. BIOMECHANICS OF STRUT GRAFTS AND INTERNAL FIXATION DEVICES

After anterior corpectomy, a structural strut of some sort is required to restore the integrity of the anterior column of the spine. The strut graft functions as a rigid member that resists collapse and supports the weight of the head and any applied loads. In the absence of instrumentation, the strut graft receives an increased compressive load during flexion and is partially unloaded during extension of the cervical spine. When posterior elements of the spine are deficient, such as following trauma or multilevel laminectomy, compressive loads and shear stresses transmitted to the strut graft are much greater, increasing the likelihood of failure due to graft fracture, subsidence, or dislodgement. The use of a rigid orthosis, such as halo vest, can significantly decrease mobility towards the end of the cervical spine, but allows significant motion or "snaking" of the central region of the cervical spine. Unfortunately, a halo vest orthosis does not effectively decrease axial loads in the cervical region and thus fails to totally eliminate the risk of failure (11,25,53).

Anterior cervical plate instrumentation can be used to immobilize the proximal and distal ends of the construct following cervical corpectomy. Anterior cervical plating has proven effective in short corpectomy constructs, producing a stable construct with low rates of graft dislodgement. The use of anterior plating may decrease the need for extended external immobilization or supplemental posterior procedures (8,46,48,49). Biomechanically, anterior plating decreases local motion at the corpectomy site, providing a construct that is superior to strut graft alone (8). Ideally, the strut graft and plate share the applied loads and provide an environment conducive to fusion. When a rigid anterior plate is applied, however, optimal load sharing may not be realized. Rigid anterior plates tend to shift the center of rotation of the construct to the anterior surface of the spine at the site of the plate (49). Because anterior plates are used to span the strut graft, any subsidence of the strut graft effectively removes compressive loads from the graft and transfers all compressive loads to the plate (4). In addition, an anterior plate can reverse the pattern of strut graft loading during cervical motion, producing high loads with

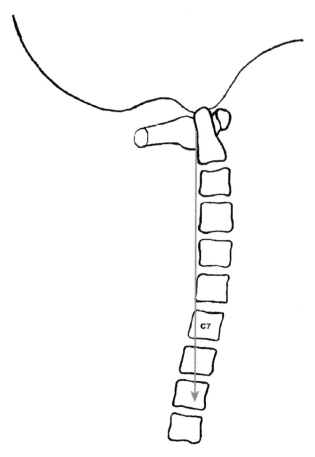

Figure 1 Normal weight-bearing axis of the cervical spine. Notice how the normal weight-bearing axis travels through the bodies of C1 and T1 and lies behind the bodies of C2-7. This relationship is important for normal cervical kinematics.

extension and partially unloading the graft during flexion (8,17,49). These high loads are seen with relatively small degrees of motion (0–10°) and may lead to endplate failure (21). Clinically, the results of anterior plating have not been universally favorable for long corpectomy constructs (≥3 levels), where the addition of an anterior cervical plate may not decrease the risk of construct failure (8,17).

The site of failure clinically occurs most commonly at the lower graft junction, often with plate and strut graft dislodgement (36). To diminish the risk of construct failure, various types of anterior cervical plates have been designed. First-generation anterior cervical plates utilized bicortical screw fixation without a mechanism to lock the screws to the plate. Because of the risks associated with bicortical screw fixation and the incidence of screw back-out, these systems have been largely supplanted by unicortical locking plates. Unicortical locking systems allowed the surgeon to gain secure fixation without the risk of spinal canal entry or screw back-out and are the standard today (10). Early unicortical locking plates produced a rigid relationship (fixed-angle device) between the screw and plate. Due to the theoretical concerns regarding stress shielding by these plates, dynamic plating systems were introduced. These systems fall into one of two categories.

The first type of dynamic plate allows the screw to rotate within the screw hole, while the second type provides a means for screws to translate in a caudad/cephalad direction. Dynamic plating systems theoretically produce better load sharing between the strut graft and anterior cervical plate (4), although well-controlled clinical studies comparing the performance of these systems to rigid, locking cervical plates have not been performed.

Posterior instrumentation using wiring or screw/plate/rod constructs is an alternative method of obtaining a mechanically stable construct following anterior corpectomy. Although interspinous wiring has been used for decades to augment stability of the cervical spine, lateral mass and pedicle screw fixation systems have gained popularity in recent years and offer enhanced construct rigidity compared to wiring (18). Some of the theoretical advantages of more rigid systems included the diminished need for supplemental halo vest immobilization and the fact that these systems can be used in situations where the laminae and/or spinous processes are fractured or absent (1,18,24,45).

When comparing posterior fixation systems to anterior plating of a multilevel corpectomy construct, Kirpatrick et al. found better construct stability using a posterior screw/plate construct (24). The authors attributed the enhanced stiffness of the posterior construct to multiple points of fixation achieved with the posterior system (10 posterior screws versus 4 anterior screws) and to the cortical bone of the lateral masses, as well as the greater moment arm of the posterior instrumentation during flexion or compression loading. Although construct stiffness is augmented by posterior internal fixation, the problem of stress concentration within the strut graft and end plates remains a concern in certain positions. As shown by Foley et al., (17) a posterior construct in conjunction with a three-level corpectomy produces high loads during flexion, approaching the force necessary to create endplate failure. In their experiment, to eliminate the tension band effect of either anterior or posterior fixation alone a circumferential construct (360° internal fixation) was required (see Fig. 2). Although biomechanically more stable, a circumferential approach is associated with increased risk, operative trauma, and time under anesthesia, which must be weighed against the risks of construct failure.

IV. INCIDENCE OF CONSTRUCT FAILURE

In clinical terms, the mechanisms of construct failure are often multifactorial and include biological, mechanical, and technical factors. Biological factors that affect the performance of a cervical construct include the underlying pathological condition, extent of disease, bone quality, and postoperative compliance. Mechanical factors include the number of levels treated, the spinal alignment, graft preload, posterior element integrity, and the material and structural properties of the strut graft and/or internal fixation devices. Technique factors include strut graft and interface carpentry, graft selection, preparation of the graft/host interface, and the application and selection of internal devices and external immobilization strategies (17). Although the relative contribution of each of these factors is difficult to ascertain in a given clinical case, general principles to achieve success are apparent in the literature. Because of wide variability between the various clinical series in the literature, direct comparison between studies is difficult.

Emery et al. (11) reviewed 108 patients with cervical spondylotic myelopathy treated over a 19-year period. Fifty-seven patients in this series underwent corpectomy and autogenous bone grafting without internal fixation devices at one to four levels. Forty-four wore rigid cervicothoracic orthoses, and 13 were placed in a halo vest orthosis

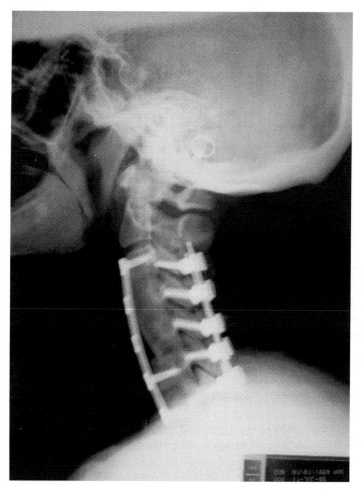

Figure 2 Multilevel cervical fixation construct with anterior and posterior instrumentation providing a balanced tension band effect.

postoperatively. Six patients (10%) in the corpectomy group sustained graft-related complications, including four who suffered displacement requiring revision surgery, one who sustained a partial graft displacement, and one who sustained an osteoporotic graft collapse. One patient in this series developed an esophageal injury as a result of graft displacement. Prior laminectomy emerged as a strong risk factor for graft-related complications and was found in four of the six patients with graft related complications ($p < 0.001$).

Saunder et al. (42) reviewed 40 cases of one- to three-level corpectomy for cervical spondylotic myelopathy. In this series collars rather than halo devices were used in most cases. Two patients sustained graft-related problems, including one graft displacement requiring revision and one fracture of the lower junctional vertebrae that was treated with bed rest and cervical traction. In another study Saunder et al. (43) reported 31 cases of four-level corpectomy performed for the same diagnosis. No internal fixation was used in these patients. Postoperative immobilization with a semi-rigid cervical collar was utilized in 25 patients, while a halo vest orthosis was used in 6 patients. Three patients (9.7%) had acute graft complications. Two gross graft displacements occurred within

48 hours of surgery, both requiring revision surgery. A third patient suffered significant graft subsidence but was managed successfully with cranial tong traction for 6 weeks.

The risk of graft-related complications is much higher following corpectomy than following discectomy, as shown by Hilibrand et al. (19), who reviewed 190 patients following multilevel anterior cervical decompression. Fifty-nine of the patients who underwent corpectomy sustained six graft displacements (10%), while 131 patients treated by discectomy sustained no graft extrusions.

Kojima et al. (25) reported 45 cases of anterior cervical corpectomy for spondylosis or ossification of the posterior longitudinal ligament. The length of the corpectomy performed in this study ranged from one to five levels. Four patients (8%) sustained bone graft extrusions, three with coexistent fracture of the lower junctional vertebrae.

A particularly difficult condition to treat is cervical myelopathy in the setting of cervical kyphosis. Zdeblick et al. (53) studied 14 patients with cervical kyphosis and myelopathy who were treated by anterior corpectomy at an average of 2.25 levels. Five patients who had kyphosis related to cervical trauma were treated with anterior decompression followed by a posterior arthrodesis using corticocancellous iliac struts with wiring. Three patients (21%) sustained strut graft dislodgment, all in the early postoperative period. None of the patients treated with supplemental posterior fixation sustained a strut graft complication.

Variable rates of strut graft dislodgement have been reported following stand-alone strut grafting without internal fixation. The rate of strut graft complications appears to depend on the length of the construct, the quality of the bone, and the presence of preoperative kyphosis. Unfortunately, the use of supplemental halo vest immobilization has not eliminated strut graft complications (11,25,53). Internal fixation devices have been used in recent years to decrease the incidence of strut graft complications (17).

Macdonald et al. (27) utilized multilevel corpectomy and fibular strut allograft in 36 patients to treat a variety of diagnosis. Anterior cervical plating was used in 15 patients. Overall, 4 patients (11%) sustained early graft displacement and 2 additional patients suffered significant graft subsidence (27). Although instrumentation was used in 15 cases, 2 of the patients (13%) who sustained graft dislodgement were treated with anterior cervical plates. In these cases, the graft displaced was associated with screw pullout.

Mohammed et al. (10) studied 185 patients following one- to three-level corpectomy using either iliac crest autograft (141 patients) or fibular allograft (44 patients). All but 6 patients received an anterior cervical plate using a nonlocking plate with bicortical fixation (Caspar) or a unicortical locking plate (CSLP). The authors found a significant difference in success rates between these two constructs with screw backout in 21% of those treated with a nonlocking plate, compared with 2% of the patients receiving the locking plate.

Vaccaro et al. (47) reviewed a series of patients treated by two- or three-level corpectomy and anterior cervical plating. Early graft dislodgement was observed in 3 of 33 (9%) two-level cases and 6 of 12 (50%) three-level cases. The difference in the rate of failure between two- and three-level corpectomy procedures was statistically significant. Surprisingly, the rate of failure for patients with three-level corpectomy did not appear to be decreased even with the use of a supplemental halo vest orthosis. The authors expressed concern regarding the high rate of failure following anterior cervical plating in three-level corpectomy procedures and suggested that supplemental posterior fixation might be warranted in these cases to decrease the rates of construct failure.

In summary, while anterior cervical plating has been effective in reducing the risk of graft dislodgement in short corpectomy constructs (27,49), the rate of strut graft complications in longer construct remains unacceptably high in spite of anterior cervical plating (17). To address this problem, alternative types of anterior cervical plates or supplemental posterior fixation have been utilized.

Epstein studied the use of a hybrid cervical plating system (Atlantis, Medtronic Sofamor Danek, Memphis, TN) that allowed screw rotation within the upper hole following one-level cervical corpectomy (14). None of the eight patients in this small study sustained graft-related complications. In another study, Epstein used the same hybrid cervical plate for one-level corpectomy in 28 patients but treated 20 patients undergoing two- to four-level corpectomies with the hybrid anterior plating plus posterior wiring (13). Two (7%) dynamic plates failed in the one-level corpectomy group, both in morbidly obese patients, but no failures were observed in the patients treated with anterior plating and posterior wiring.

Swank et al. (45) treated 15 patients with multilevel corpectomy using circumferential fixation with an anterior cervical plate and posterior lateral mass fixation (45). Although no graft dislodgements were encountered, two patients sustained hardware-related complication, one of which required a second operation to remove a displaced screw.

Epstein compared two groups of 22 patients following multilevel corpectomy treated either with or without an anterior cervical plate (15). All patients underwent posterior spinous process wiring and halo vest immobilization. Strut graft dislodgement occurred in three (14%) patients not receiving an anterior cervical plate, but none of those who were treated with anterior cervical plating.

Vanichkachorn et al. (48) reported 11 patients following multilevel corpectomy at an average of 3.36 levels treated with a junctional plate and posterior lateral mass fixation (48). The junctional plate was used to buttress the graft-vertebral bone junction of the construct and minimize the risk of graft dislodgement. In this small study, no cases of graft dislodgement were observed.

V. SPECTRUM OF COMPLICATIONS

Failure of a corpectomy construct can present in many ways such as graft extrusion, fracture, pistoning, subsidence, mortise penetration, or hardware failure. A corpectomy construct without instrumentation is most prone to graft dislodgement as the primary mode of construct failure. Although graft dislodgement can occur at either the superior or inferior end of the strut graft, dislodgement at the inferior end is much more likely due to stress concentration in this region. Most cases of graft dislodgement are encountered in the early postoperative period, often within 24 hours following surgery. In some cases, graft dislodgement may occur as the result of a technical error in graft preparation, sizing, or seating. In the three cases of early graft dislodgement reported by Saunders et al., (43) excessively long grafts and overdistraction of the corpectomy site was noted. Successful revision in these cases involved replacement with properly sized strut grafts. Others have reported graft dislodgement with fracture of the inferior vertebral junction. This type of failure may be the result of excessive removal of the endplate, the creation of stress risers from vertebral distraction pins or anterior screws or excessively long grafts. Depending on the pattern and size of the fracture fragment, revision may require removal of an extra vertebral level, which theoretically adds to the risk of further instability (see Fig. 3). Late causes of failure may include graft fracture, collapse, or subsidence. Although the direction of graft dislodgement is most commonly anterior, posterior dislodgement can occur with devastating neurological consequences (48).

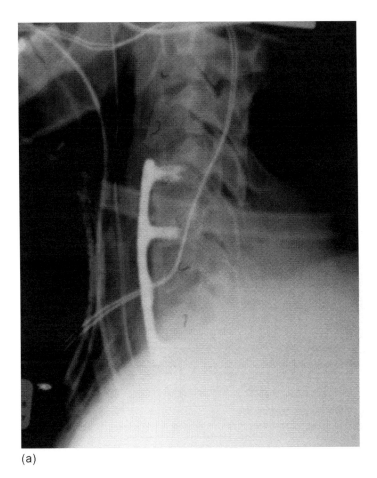

(a)

Figure 3 Construct failure requiring revision surgery. The patient initially underwent a discectomy at C4-5 and a corpectomy of C6 for the diagnosis of cervical spondylotic myelopathy (a,b). Approximately one week postoperatively, the patient noted difficulty swallowing. Radiographs revealed dislodgement of the corpectomy graft and plate at the inferior graft bone junction and a fracture of the inferior junctional vertebral body (C7) (c). The patient required revision surgery with removal of the remaining body of C7 and strut grafting from C5-T1. At the time of surgery, most of the anterior portion of C7 was noted to be fractured and thus could not be used for a graft docking site. Posterior instrumentation was placed from C4-T1 to provide stability for healing. The construct was stable and went on to successful healing (d).

Graft dislodgement may be complete or partial. Although total dislodgement generally requires another operation to correct, some cases of partial dislodgement can be closely observed, often with a change in the immobilization strategy. This may be considered if there is no evidence of compression or injury to the soft tissue structures within the neck. A high degree of vigilance is necessary to detect and treat any evidence of esophageal irritation or dysphagia that may result in esophageal penetration and a severe mediastinal infection (11).

Graft collapse has been most commonly observed with the use of osteopenic bone from the iliac crest (11,39). Osteopenic grafts are prone to fracture and collapse (43). Such a problem may require revision using a fibular strut graft. Yonenobu et al. (50)

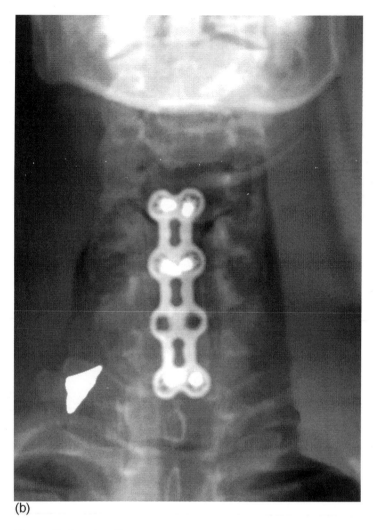

(b)

Figure 3 (*continued*)

reported such a case with fracture through the middle of an osteopenic graft 2 weeks after corpectomy causing sudden weakness of the shoulder and arm due to a C5 nerve root palsy.

Subsidence and mortise penetration may occur with loss of graft height or penetration into the end plate at the graft-vertebral junction. Slight subsidence is commonly seen and may allow a strut graft to seek a point of stability. This should not be considered a construct failure. However, subsidence that results in severe kyphosis or loss of structural integrity represents a form of construct failure. Marked kyphosis may lead to severe neck pain as a result of sagittal imbalance, creating muscle spasm as the patient attempts to support his or her head upright. In addition, kyphosis can produce neurological compromise as the spinal cord is pulled against the apex of the kyphotic deformity. Riew et al. (39) observed 3 patients in a series of 18 undergoing corpectomy who developed kyphosis of 10° or more due to subsidence of a fibular strut graft. Fortunately, none of these patients complained of neck pain at follow-up. Mortise penetration by a graft is theoretically more

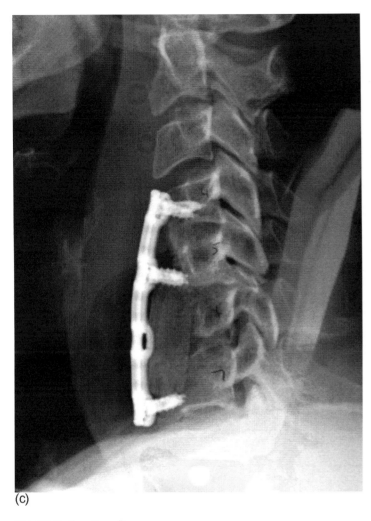

(c)

Figure 3 (*continued*)

likely when excessive endplate is removed. Another potential factor leading to graft sub-sidence is the use of a strut graft with a significantly higher modulus of elasticity than the host vertebral bone. Such a situation might arise with the use of hard cortical bone (fibula) or a titanium cage in conjunction with osteopenic vertebral bone in an elderly patient (27).

Although anterior cervical plating is commonly used to prevent strut graft extrusion, this technique is not successful in all cases (48). Screw loosening and back-out may occur under conditions of cyclic loading (52). Although minor screw back-out may be well tolerated, gross plate loosening and graft dislodgment generally require revision. When gross construct failure occurs in a corpectomy with an anterior cervical plate, a fracture of the lower vertebrae is often present (25,47). Such a fracture may traverse the endplate and communicate with screw holes, which act as stress risers, allowing displacement of the anterior, superior aspect of the lower host vertebral body. Gross displacement of the anterior cervical plate has the potential to lead to catastrophic airway complications, as noted by Riew et al. (41), who reported dislodge of a junctional plate in one patient, which

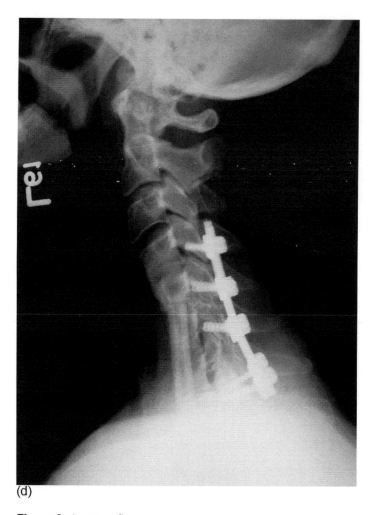

(d)

Figure 3 (*continued*)

resulted in death. Factors found to be associated with a higher rate of graft or plate dislodgement include advanced age, failure to properly lock the screws to the plate, and the use of the peg-in-hole type bone grafting technique (47).

Higher rates of graft extrusion have been observed in multilevel plated corpectomy constructs due to the high cantilever forces present at the screw/bone interface (27,47,48). Lateral mass plating has been successfully used to enhance the stability of multilevel corpectomy constructs. With posterior plating, the predominant failure mode is screw pull-out, which is less problematic compared with anterior plate loosening (23).

VI. APPROACHES

A number of factors should be taken into consideration when considering the optimal approach to use in a given case, including extent of disease, presence of deformity, any loss of stabilizing anatomy, bone quality, patient demands, and compliance. As one might expect, surgeon judgment and experience figure prominently in the decision regarding the methods to treat a given condition. The various approaches to corpectomy will be considered.

A. Anterior Stand-Alone Strut Grafting

Cervical corpectomy procedures have been successfully performed for decades to decompress the neurological structures by removal of the disks and vertebral bodies. Although the reported rate of success for this basic technique varies between authors, longer corpectomy constructs are associated with higher rates of construct failure (27). To achieve maximal construct stability, the ideal graft length, strength, and integrity of the remaining spinal anatomy is required. The halo-vest orthosis is often used with stand-alone constructs to immobilize the neck during the postoperative period. With good carpentry of the corpectomy site and graft, reasonably low rates of graft dislodgement have been reported without the use of internal fixation or a rigid orthosis (43).

B. Anterior Strut Grafting with Anterior Cervical Plating

The anterior cervical plate has been used to immobilize the fused segment and diminish the rate of graft dislodgement. Anterior cervical plating has been shown to increase the rate of successful fusion in single-level corpectomies (14). Because locked unicortical plates are biomechanically superior to unconstrained bicortical systems and are associated with fewer complications (i.e., a lower incidence of screw loosening and neurological injury), they have largely supplanted the bicortical systems (14). Although anterior plates appear to improve the results of one-level and possibly two-level corpectomies, the use of anterior plates alone with a three or more levels of corpectomy has been associated with a high rate of complications (39). Rigid locking plates do not allow load sharing with the strut graft if any significant subsidence of the graft occurs and therefore may lead to construct failure. For this reason, dynamic plates that allow axial subsidence have been designed and used clinically. The benefit of these systems is currently the subject of active debate.

C. Anterior Strut Grafting with Circumferential Internal Fixation

The most rigid, stable construct for reconstruction of a cervical corpectomy is undoubtedly achieved with a circumferential approach. The combination of anterior and posterior instrumentation and arthrodesis have demonstrated the lowest rates of construct failure for multilevel corpectomy and for situations prone to instability (e.g., postlaminectomy kyphosis) (45). Rigid segmental internal fixation with lateral mass plating provides the highest level of stability for restoration and maintenance of spinal alignment and may decrease the need for halo-vest immobilization (22,45). Patients with posterior column deficiencies and a kyphotic deformity as a result of prior injury or laminectomy are at extraordinarily high risk for construct failure and should be treated with a circumferential approach (27). Although this technique clearly involves more surgical trauma and prolonged anesthesia, performance of both the anterior decompression and the posterior procedure sequentially under the same anesthesia has been associated with a low rate of complications in skilled hands (30).

Because anterior cervical plating, when used with long corpectomy constructs, has been prone to unacceptably high rates of failure, circumferential surgery is used by some when three or more vertebral bodies are removed. There are three possible instrumentation constructs that might be used with a circumferential approach. The first is an anterior strut graft with posterior instrumentation. The second is anterior strut graft with a junctional plate and posterior instrumentation (Fig. 4). Finally, a spanning anterior cervical plating can be combined with posterior instrumentation (see Fig. 2). In a small number of reports, the use of posterior instrumentation with or without anterior instrumentation has been shown to be associated with a low rate of graft-related complications (2,15,17,22,30,39,41,45,48). Junctional plating should only be used in conjunction with posterior instrumentation due to the risk of graft and plate dislodgement, which have been reported to be associated with airway compromise (41). Theoretically, the application of anterior and posterior instrumentation counteracts the individual tension-band effect of

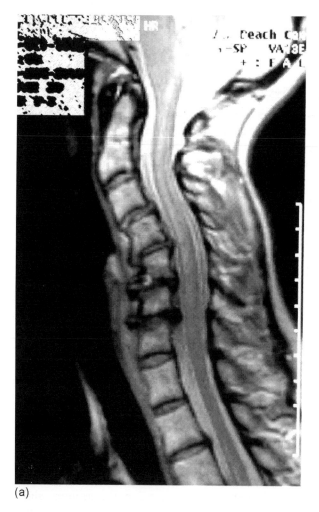

(a)

Figure 4 Cervical kyphosis. This patient presented with cervical myelopathy and a fixed kyphotic deformity (a–c). The patient was treated with anterior corpectomy of C4 and C5 and a hemicorpectomy of C6 with a discectomy performed at the C6-7 level. Anterior plating was performed to allow the plate to overlap the junction of the corpectomy graft and thus prevent anterior dislodgement of the graft during repositioning of the patient for the posterior procedure. The posterior construct consisted of lateral mass fixation from C3-6 and pedicle fixation of C7. This construct is rigid enough to allow early mobilization of the patient without the use of a halo vest orthosis.

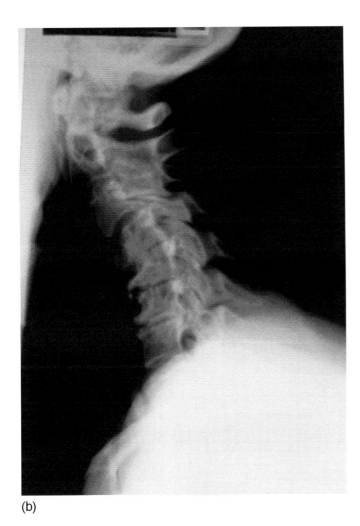

(b)

Figure 4 (*continued*)

stand-alone instrumentation, creating a rigid construct with a low chance of failure. Although biomechanically advantageous, the routine use of circumferential instrumentation cannot be justified for applications for which anterior surgery alone performs well. Therefore, the use of circumferential surgery is most commonly indicated following traumatic or neoplastic disruption of both the anterior and posterior column, with anterior spinal infections (to place the instrumentation in an unaffected compartment), with multilevel (three or more levels) corpectomy, and when treating post-laminectomy kyphosis. Some less common situations where bone quality is a major concern, such as with severe osteomalacia from renal disease, may also benefit from circumferential stabilization.

VII. STRUT GRAFT OPTIONS

Autogenous iliac crest bone remains the gold standard graft choice for one- and two-level corpectomies due to its biological and biomechanical properties and rapid

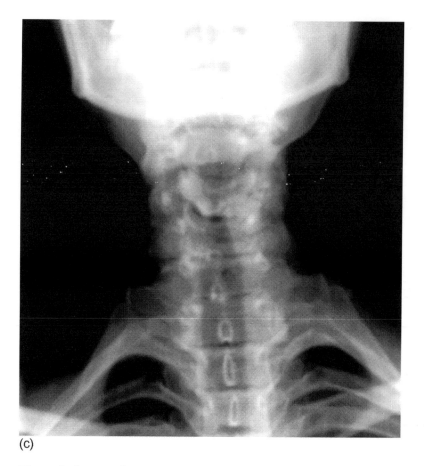

(c)

Figure 4 (*continued*)

osteointegration (10,26). However, harvest of large segments of iliac crest is associated
with a high rate of complications and persistent pain, and therefore allografts and cages
have become increasingly popular and have demonstrated generally good results. The
use of these autograft susbstitues not only eliminates the complications associated with
autograft harvest but also shortens operative times. Macdonald et al. (27) found no difference in the fusion rates between allograft and autograft cases of multilevel corpectomy,
although the allograft patients took longer to fuse and had a higher rate of complications.
Due to the curvature of the iliac crest, it becomes difficult to use this type of graft on a
more than two-level corpectomy. For longer construct, fibular shaft has proven useful
(53). Although a fibular strut shaft can be harvested from the patient, the added surgical
trauma and rate of complication for this procedure has made it less attractive when alternatives are available (12,29). Fibular allograft, due to its cortical nature, is less prone to
collapse compared with iliac crest and seems to function well in multilevel corpectomies
with or without a combined posterior instrumented fusion (2,27,45).

The use of titanium mesh cages for corpectomy reconstruction has gained popularity
in some regions. To date, relatively few studies have been published on the use of titanium
mesh in the cervical spine. The theoretical advantage of using titanium mesh is that during
corpectomy for degenerative problems, the removed corpectomy bone can be morselized

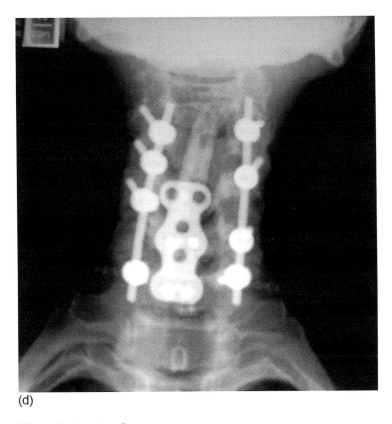

(d)

Figure 4 (*continued*)

and placed within the cage for fusion, providing the theoretical benefits of autograft without the need for a separate surgical site for graft harvest (28,40). Although some have suggested that the dramatic modulus of elasticity mismatch between a titanium cage and the vertebral endplates could lead to subsidence by allowing the cage to be a "cookie cutter," Riew et al. (40) reported using a titanium cage in 54 corpectomy constructs with good results. In this series no cage extrusions, infections, neurological deficits, or construct failure were noted. Another disadvantage with titanium cages is the relatively high cost of these devices and the difficulty of assessing fusion status. Under current investigation are cages and spacers made from other materials such as hydroxyapatite composites, PEEK, carbon fiber–reinforced polymer cages, and hydrocel (tantalum mesh), which may play a role in the future (6,44).

VIII. REVISION SURGERY

Not all graft dislodgements require revision. Partial graft dislodgement may be well toler- ated, particularly following corpectomy without instrumentation. If the construct is able to function mechanically without irritation of the surrounding soft tissue, a more rigid orthosis such as halo-vest or even bed rest with traction has been used successfully to achieve a good result (11,53). Although mild graft subsidence is not generally a problem,

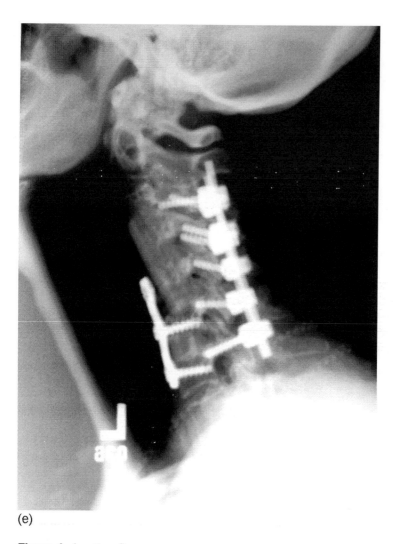

(e)

Figure 4 (*continued*)

the development of a major kyphotic deformity with collapse of an osteopenic graft can be successfully managed by revision with fibular strut graft (11,39).

Instrumentation failure is more likely to require revision surgery. While asymptomatic screw loosening has been successfully treated by observation, the risk of esophageal irritation and erosion exists (16). Gross construct failure often results in abrupt onset of neck pain, dysphagia, and in some cases neurological symptoms and mandates revision surgery. The goals of revision surgery are to ensure safety of the neural elements, obtain a mechanically competent construct, and reduce the risk of further construct problems. Because constructs incorporating a stand-alone anterior plate most often fail with a fracture of the lower vertebral endplate, revision of such a failed construct may require resection of more bone to obtain a flat, stable graft junction or mortise. It is mandatory to augment the stability of the initial construct through a different instrumentation and/or immobilization strategy to achieve success in cases where construct failure has occurred. Placement of the graft and instrumentation in this setting can be more challenging than with primary surgery due to bone loss and poor visualization. Depending on the time lapse since the initial operation, scar tissue may also be a factor with difficulty defining tissue planes and important landmarks and an increased risk of visceral, nervous, or vascular injuries (3). Patients with prior anterior surgery, posterior instability, prior laminectomy, and severe osteoporosis are at greater risk for anterior plate complications. In cases of revision surgery due to failure of an anterior construct, strong consideration should begiven to using supplemental posterior segmental fixation with or without halo immobilization.

When additional bone graft is needed, the contralateral iliac crest or allograft bone may be considered depending on the specific problem and the length of graft needed. If bone quality of the iliac crest was a contributor to the construct failure, then a stronger bone source should be sought (3). If posterior fusion is required and the prior autograft is no longer able to be used due to inadequate length, if may still be useful as morselized graft for the posterior portion of the case.

When significant time has elapsed since the original procedure, it may be desirable to approach the anterior spine from the contralateral side of the neck. Because there is a significant incidence of unrecognized recurrent laryngeal nerve injury following anterior cervical approaches, it is mandatory to determine the status of vocal cord function prior to embarking on a contralateral approach. This can be determined by an endoscopic examination of the vocal cords, generally performed by an ENT specialist or anesthesiologist. If there is evidence of vocal cord paralysis on one side, the side of the paralysis should be used for the approach to avoid the risk of bilateral vocal cord dysfunction, which can lead to respiratory embarrassment (3).

IX. AUTHORS' PREFERRED APPROACH

For one- and two-level corpectomies in patients with normal bone quality and no evidence of posterior instability or deformity, the construct of choice involves an autograft strut from the iliac crest and an anterior cervical plate. Autograft has the quickest and most reliable rate of incorporation and therefore is the author's graft of choice. Both rigid and dynamic plates seem to have similar results in this setting. Postoperative immobilization using a semi-rigid cervical collar is utilized for approximately 6–8 weeks postoperatively, followed by an active cervical rehabilitation program.

Three- or more level corpectomies have an unacceptably high rate of graft complications, therefore the author prefers using a circumferential approach with such cases. Either a spanning or a junctional cervical plate is applied anteriorly to minimize the risk of graft dislodgement when repositioning the patient for the posterior portion of the procedure. Segmental fixation using lateral mass fixation in the C3-6 levels and pedicle fixation in the C2 or C7 levels is generally employed. The graft choice for these cases usually involves a fibular allograft anteriorly. In degenerative cases, the corpectomy bone is saved and used for the posterior arthrodesis. Again using a circumferential approach with posterior facet arthrodesis with autograft provides for a quick, reliable fusion. Post-operative immobilization involves a semi-rigid cervical collar for 6–8 weeks followed by an active rehabilitation program.

In cases where the posterior ligamentous anatomy is disrupted, such as following trauma, a circumferential approach is utilized even if a shorter than three-level corpectomy is performed. An example would be a high-grade flexion tear drop injury requiring a corpectomy for decompression, which would be combined with anterior plating and posterior segmental fixation. Postlaminectomy kyphosis is always approached circumferentially. Patients with extraordinarily poor bone quality (renal osteodystrophy) or with movement disorders (athetoid cerebral palsy) are also approached with a circumferential approach.

Endplate preparation is performed by lightly burring the endplates just enough to create a posterior lip or buttress to prevent posterior graft dislodgement. An attempt is made to maintain as much of the endplate as possible to minimize subsidence and fracture. Proper graft length is felt to be extremely important. An overly long strut graft which requires excessively high distraction forces in order to seat the graft is considered to be a high risk for failure. In such a case, the graft will often subside into the endplate or create a fracture of the lower graft junction. To properly size the graft, the spine is distracted with Caspar pins or Gardner-Wells tong traction just enough to remove any slack in the soft tissues. The strut graft is then prepared to exactly fit the corpectomy space without much force required to place the graft. The width of the graft is also prepared to fit the space because gentle contact with the side walls of the trough enhances construct stability. When seating the graft, the posterior portion of the strut graft is sunk to a depth where it impacts the posterior lip of the superior endplate of the inferior host vertebra, which was created at the time of the corpectomy.

Anterior plating is performed by placing the screws as far away from the endplates as possible without entering the adjacent disk spaces. This spacing between the screw holes and the endplates is necessary to minimize the risk of a fracture propagating between the endplate and screw hole that could lead to construct failure. All distraction should be removed prior to placement of an anterior cervical plate.

During repositioning for a posterior procedure it is imperative to prevent excess extension of the cervical spine, which can lead to graft dislodgement. Segmental fixation using a lateral mass and pedicle screw construct is quick and rigid and allows the patient to be mobilized without the need for a halo in most cases.

X. CONCLUSION

Although useful for a variety of pathologies, corpectomy surgery can be associated with a number of significant complications including construct failure. Construct failure is associated with biological, mechanical, or technical factors, many of which can be avoided with a good understanding of the biomechanics of the cervical region. Modern grafting and instrumentation techniques provide a number of ways to approach the reconstructive challenge of a corpectomy. By reviewing and understanding the literature, a number of principals are evident that can help the surgeon to maximize success in these difficult cases.

REFERENCES

1. Berven S, Pedlow J. A review of recent literature on the biomechanics of spinal instrumentation. Curr Opin Orthop 1999; 10:142–147.
2. Blam OG, Albert TJ, Vaccaro AR. Surgical reconstruction of postlaminectomy cervical kyphosis. Curr Opin Orthop 2002; 13:208–213.
3. Brislin BT, Hilibrand AS. Avoidance of complications in anterior cervical revision surgery. Curr Opin Orthop 2001; 12:257–264.
4. Brodke DS, Gollogly S, Mohr A, Nguyen BK, Dailey AT, Bachus KN. Dynamic cervical plates: biomechanical evaluation of load sharing and stiffness. Spine 2001; 26(12):1324–1329.

5. Chen IH, Vasavada A, Panjabi MM. Kinematics of the cervical spine canal: changes with sagittal plane loads. J Spinal Disord 1994; 7(2):93–101.

6. Chin K, Ozuna R. Options in the surgical treatment of the cervical spondylotic myelopathy. Curr Opin Orthop 2000; 11(3):151–157.

7. Czervionke LF, Daniels DL, Ho PSP, Yu S, et al. Cervical neural foramina: correlative anatomic and MR imaging study. Neuroradiology 1988; 169:753–759.

8. DiAngelo DJ, Foley KT, Vossel KA, Rampersaud YR, Jansen TH. Anterior cervical plating reverses load transfer through multilevel strut–grafts. Spine 2000; 25(7):783–795.

9. Edward WT, Yuan HA. General considerations, evaluation, and testing. In: The Textbook of Spinal Surgery. Philadelphia: Lippincott-Raven, 1997:141–154.

10. Eleraky MA, Llanos C, Sonntag VKH. Cervical corpectomy: report of 185 cases and review of the literature. J Neurosurg 1999; 90:35–41.

11. Emery SE, Bohlman HH, Bolesta MJ, Jones PK. Anterior cervical decompression and arthrodesis for the treatment of cervical spondylotic myelopathy: two to seventeen-year follow-up. J Bone Joint Surg 1998; 80-A(7):941–51.

12. Emery SE, Heller JG, Petersilge CA, Bolesta MJ, Whitesides TE. Tibial stress fracture after a graft has been obtained from the fibula: a report of five cases. J Bone Joint Surg 1996; 78-A(8):1248–1251.

13. Epstein NE. Anterior dynamic plates in complex cervical reconstructive surgeries. J Spinal Disord 2002; 15(3):221–227.

14. Epstein NE. The management of one-level anterior cervical corpectomy with fusion using Atlantis hybrid plates: preliminary experience. J Spinal Disord 2000; 13(4):324–328.

15. Epstein NE. The value of the anterior cervical plating in preventing vertebral fracture and graft extrusion after multilevel anterior cervical corpectomy with posterior wiring and fusion: indications, results, and complications. J Spinal Disord 2000; 13(1):9–15.

16. Fessler RG, Steck JC, Giovanini MA. Anterior cervical corpectomy for cervical spondylotic myelopathy. Neurosurgery 1998; 43(2):257–265.

17. Foley KT, DiAngelo DJ, Rampersaud YR, Vossel KA, Jansen TH. The in vitro effects of instrumentation on multilevel cervical strut-graft mechanics. Spine 1999; 24(22):2366–2376.

18. Grubb MR, Currier BL, Stone J, Warden KE, An KN. Biomechanical evaluation of posterior cervical stabilization after a wide laminectomy. Spine 1997; 22(17):1948–1954.

19. Hilibrand AS, Fye MA, Emery SE, Palumbo MA, Bohlman HH. Increased rate of arthrodesis with strut grafting after multilevel anterior cervical decompression. Spine 2002; 27(2):146–151.

20. Inoue H, Ohmori K, Takatsu T, Teramoto T, Ishida Y, Suzuki K. Morphological analysis of the cervical spinal canal, dural tube and spinal cord in normal individuals using CT myelography. Neuroradiology 1996; 38(2):148–151.

21. Isomi T, Panjabi MM, Wang JL, Vaccaro AR, Garfin SR, Patel T. Stabilizing potential of anterior cervical plates in multilevel corpectomies. Spine 1999; 24(21):2219–2223.

22. Joshi AP, Pedlow FX, Hornicek FJ, Hecht AC. Surgical management of cervical spine metastatic disease. Curr Opin Orthop 2002; 13:224–231.

23. Kim DH, Pedlow FX. Advances in cervical spine instrumentation. Curr Opin Orthop 2000; 11(3):158–166.

24. Kirkpatrick JS, Levy JA, Carillo J, Moeini SR. Reconstruction after multilevel corpectomy in the cervical spine: a sagittal plane biomechanical study. Spine 1999; 24(12):1186–1191.

25. Kojima T, Waga S, Kubo y, Kanamaru K, Shimosaka S, Shimizu T. Anterior cervical vertebrectomy and interbody fusion for multi-level spondylosis and ossification of the posterior longitudinal ligament. Neurosurgery 1989; 24(6):864–872.

26. Law MD, Bernhardt M, White AA. Instructional course lectures, The American academy of orthopaedic surgeons. Evaluation and management of cervical spondylotic myelopathy. J Bone Joint Surg 1994; 76-A(9):1420–1433.

27. Macdonald RL, Fehlings MG, Tator CH, Lozano A, Fleming JR, Gentili F, Bernstein M, Wallace MC, Tasker RR. Multilevel anterior cervical corpectomy and fibular allograft fusion for cervical myelopathy. J Neurosurg 1997; 86:990–997.

28. Majd ME, Vadhva M, Holt RT. Anterior cervical reconstruction using titanium cages with anterior plating. Spine 1999; 24(15):1604–1611.

29. Malloy KM, Hilibrand AS. Autograft versus allograft in degenerative cervical disease. Clin Orthop 2002; 394:27–38.

30. McAfee PC, Bohlman HH, Ducker TB, Zeidman SM, Goldstein JA. One-stage anterior cervical decompression and posterior stabilization. A study of one hundred patients with a minimum of two years of follow-up. J Bone Joint Surg 1995; 77-A(12):1791–1800.

31. Muhle C, Weinert D, Falliner A, et al. Dynamic changes of the spinal canal in patients with cervical spondylosis at flexion and extension using magnetic resonance imaging. Invest Radiol 1998; 33(8):444–449.

32. Okada Y, Ikata T, Katoh S, Yamada H. Morphologic analysis of the cervical spinal cord, dural tube and spinal canal by magnetic resonance imaging in normal adults and patients with cervical spondylotic myelopathy. Spine 1994; 19:2331–2335.

33. Ozer AF, Oktenoglu BT, Sarioglu AC. A new surgical technique: open-window corpectomy in the treatment of ossification of the posterior longitudinal ligament and advanced cervical spondylosis: Technical note. Neurosurgery 1999; 45(6):1481–1485.

34. Panjabi MM, Crisco JJ, Vasavada A, Oda T, Cholewicki J, Nibu K, Shin E. Mechanical properties of the human cervical spine as shown by three-dimensional load-displacement curves. Spine 2001; 26(24):2692–2700.

35. Panjabi MM, Duranceau J, Goel V, Oxland T, Takata K. Cervical human vertebrae. Quantitative three-dimensional anatomy of the middle and lower regions. Spine 1991; 16(8):861–869.

36. Panjabi MM, Isomi T, Wang JL. Loosening at the screw-vertebra junction in multilevel anterior cervical plate constructs. Spine 1999; 24(22):2383–2388.

37. Panjabi MM, Oxland T, Takata K, Goel V, Duranceau J, Krag M. Articular facets of the human spine. Quantitative three-dimensional anatomy. Spine 1993; 18(10):1298–1310.

38. Reid JD. Effects of flexion-extension movements of the head and spine upon the spinal cord and nerve roots. J Neurol Neurosurg Psychiat 1960; 23:214–221.

39. Riew KD, Hilibrand AS, Palumbo MA, Bohlman HH. Anterior cervical corpectomy in patients previously managed with a laminectomy: short-term complications. J Bone Joint Surg 1999; 81-A(7):950–957.

40. Riew KD, Rhee JM. The use of titanium mesh cages in the cervical spine. Clin Orthop 2002; 394:47–54.

41. Riew KD, Sethi NS, Devney J, Goette K, Choi K. Complications of buttress plate stabilization of cervical corpectomy. Spine 1999; 24(22):2404–2410.

42. Saunders RL, Bernini PM, Shirreffs TG, Reeves AG. Central corpectomy for cervical spondylotic myelopathy: a consecutive series with long-term follow-up evaluation. J Neurosurgery 1991; 74:163–170.

43. Saunders RL, Pikus HJ, Ball P. Four-level cervical corpectomy. Spine 1998; 23(22):2455–2461.

44. Shono Y, McAfee P, Cunningham BW, Brantigan JW. A biomechanical analysis of decompression and reconstruction methods in the cervical spine. Emphasis on a carbon-fiber-composite cage. J Bone Joint Surg 1993; 75-A(11):1674–1684.

45. Swank ML, Sutterlin CE, Bossons CR, Dials BE. Rigid internal fixation with lateral mass plates in multilevel anterior and posterior reconstruction of the cervical spine. Spine 1997; 22(3):274–282.

46. Vaccaro AR, Balderston RA. Anterior plate instrumentation for disorders of the subaxial cervical spine. Clin Orthop 1997; 335:112–121.

47. Vaccaro AR, Falatyn SP, Scuderi GJ, Eismont FJ, McGuire RA, Singh K, Garfin SR. Early failure of long segment anterior cervical plate fixation. J Spinal Disord 1998; 11(5):410–415.

48. Vanichkachorn JS, Vaccaro AR, Silveri CP, Albert TJ. Anterior junctional plate in the cervical spine. Spine 1998; 23(22):2462–2467.

49. Wang JL, Panjabi MM, Isomi T. The role of bone graft force in stabilizing the multilevel anterior cervical spine plate system. Spine 2000; 25(13):1649–1654.

50. Yonenobu K, Hosono N, Iwasaki M, Asano M, Ono K. Neurologic complications of surgery for cervical compression myelopathy. Spine 1991; 16(11):1277–1282.
51. Yoo JU, Zou D, Edwards WT, Bayley J, Yuan HA. Effect of cervical spine motion on the neuroforaminal dimensions of human cervical spine. Spine 1992; 17(10):1131–1136.
52. Zaveri G, Ford M. Cervical spondylosis: The role of anterior instrumentation after decompression and fusion. J Spinal Disord 2001; 14(1):10–16.
53. Zdeblick TA, Bohlman HH. Cervical kyphosis and myelopathy: treatment by anterior corpectomy and strut–grafting. J Bone Joint Surg 1989; 71-A(2):170–182.

17

Cervical Postlaminectomy Kyphosis

Jonathan N. Grauer, John M. Beiner, Brian K. Kwon,
Alexander R. Vaccaro, and Todd J. Albert
Thomas Jefferson University and the Rothman Institute, Philadelphia, Pennsylvania, U.S.A.

I. INTRODUCTION

The cervical spine provides stability and protection to the neural elements while maintaining a high degree of flexibility. This is achieved via a precise interaction of the bony, ligamentous, and muscular elements. Perturbations to the normal anatomy can lead to imbalances which, if left uncorrected, may progress to significant deformities. Such deformities can have adverse biomechanical, clinical, and neurological sequelae.

In the cervical spine, postlaminectomy kyphosis is the most common example of imbalance leading to deformity. A typical laminectomy operation involves removal of the spinous processes, inter- and supraspinous ligaments, laminae, and the ligamentum flavum. The facet joints are usually left intact, though their capsules and possibly part of their bony anatomy can be compromised. With the loss of these posterior stabilizers and continued normal flexion forces, kyphosis can result.

II. ALTERATION OF NORMAL MECHANICS

The average cervical lordosis in the asymptomatic patient is approximately 15–35° (13,18) (Fig. 1). In this posture, Pal and Sherk (31) found 36% of the compressive load to pass through the anterior column, while 64% of the load passed through the posterior column (32% per side). The competence of both cervical spine columns is thus crucial for normal load distribution.

Complex ligamentous structures act to stabilize the cervical spine. Increased intervertebral motion has been noted after laminectomies without any violation of the facets or facet capsules by most (9,12,24), but not all authors (46). This increased motion is presumably due to disruption of the posterior ligaments. This presumption is supported by finite element analyses of Saito et al. (38), who found that kyphosis or lordosis of the cervical spine tends to develop after disruption of the posterior ligaments depending on the location of the gravitational center of the head. In the immature patient, the increased viscoelasticity of the intervertebral disks and ligamentous structures has been implicated in the pathogenesis of what has been called pseudosubluxation of the vertebral

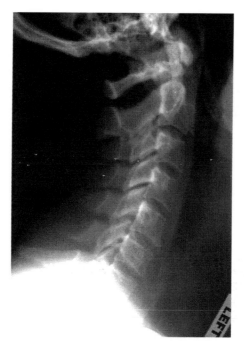

Figure 1 Lateral radiograph demonstrating normal cervical lordosis.

bodies following laminectomy procedures (43). This hypermobility of the anterior column, when no longer balanced by the posterior structures, creates kyphosis.

Biomechanical ligament sectioning studies by White and Panjabi have further linked the loss of ligamentous restraints to the loss of cervical stability (32,41). This work noted the cervical ligaments to act as a unit; the risk of instability gradually increased as more ligaments were sacrificed. From this work it was noted that there was the potential for catastrophic instability once 3.5 mm of horizontal displacement or 11° of rotational displacement was noted. As would be expected, anterior ligaments were important in resisting extension, and posterior ligaments were important in resisting flexion.

In terms of bony anatomy, Cusick et al. (8) found unilateral facetectomy to decrease the flexion-compression strength of a motion segment by 32%, while bilateral facetectomies decreased the strength by 53%. These changes were associated with anterior displacement of the instantaneous axis of rotation in the sagittal plane, leading to increased compressive loads on anterior column structures. In general, resection of 25–50% of the facet has been shown to significantly increase cervical motion in several cadaveric studies (30,46). Kumaresan et al. (23) confirmed this increased anterior loading after graded facetectomies in a finite element analysis of the cervical spine.

The facet capsules also directly contribute to cervical stability. Zdeblick et al. (47) studied cadaveric specimens that underwent graded facet capsule resections after performing a laminectomy. Increased flexion was noted after 75% of the facet capsule was resected. This was without violation of the bony facets themselves.

Muscles provide further stability to the cervical spine. In vitro experiments have shown that the osteo-ligamentous cervical spine is unable to carry the compressive load of the head without the balancing effect of muscle forces (33). The stability of the cervical spine is regained in the laboratory as muscle forces are replicated (34,35). As an example, the importance of the many muscular attachments to C2 has led many authors to recommend preserving these attachments whenever possible (29). Even if not detached, posterior cervical muscles may become denervated or fibrotic secondary to aggressive surgical retraction (10).

As kyphosis develops, the spinal cord is pulled against the apex of the kyphotic deformity, resulting in irritation or dysfunction of the cord and/or nerve roots (Fig. 2). A finite amount of spinal cord lengthening can occur without a significant rise in internal tensile stresses, such as occurs with normal cervical flexion. However, in pathological kyphosis, the posterior cord becomes stretched beyond its elastic limit. The anterior spinal cord concomitantly becomes compressed as it is pulled against the posterior vertebral osteophytes and protuberant intervertebral disks (5,36). Cord flattening, internal stresses, and compression of the anterior microvasculature may lead to cord ischemia.

Once initiated, cervical kyphosis may lead to a vicious cycle of pathological forces and the development of a progressive deformity. As the head shifts forward, the anterior column is placed under an increasing load while the posterior column is placed under increased tension (42). Posterior ligamentous structures and facet capsules subsequently become attenuated. The posterior extensor muscles are placed at a mechanical disadvantage and become less effective at holding the head upright (29) (Fig. 3).

III. CLINICAL PRESENTATION AND INCIDENCE

Instability following cervical laminectomy often follows a characteristic clinical course (1). In the early postoperative period, there is generally good resolution of radicular or myelopathic symptoms that were caused by compression of the neural elements. The patients thus experience a "honeymoon period," with excellent pain relief and return of function. As kyphosis begins to develop, the forward position of the head necessitates constant contraction of the neck extensor muscles to balance the weight of the head against gravity. This may lead to muscle fatigue and neck pain, and patients may return to using a cervical collar or may begin to manually support their chin. As a kyphotic deformity progresses, there may be a recurrence of prior neurological symptoms or onset of new neurological complaints. Gaze difficulty may also be encountered in patients with severe deformities.

It is clear that children have the highest incidence of postlaminectomy kyphosis in the cervical spine (2,4,24,44). Laminectomy in this population is most frequently performed for the treatment of Arnold-Chiari malformations, syringomyelia, and tumors. The reported incidence varies from 37% in a series of Bell et al. (4) to 95% in a series by Aronson et al. (2). Yasouka et al. (43) postulated that this is due to two main factors. First, the immature skeleton, which is particularly viscoelastic, may have an imbalance of forces after the posterior structures are compromised. Second, wedging of the anterior vertebral bodies may result from compression of the growing cartilaginous end plates. In a study of 52 pediatric patients with different kinds of spinal tumors, reoperation for deformity following laminectomy as part of resection of the tumor was the most commonly reported complication, occurring in 50% of patients (27).

Adults have a much lower incidence of kyphosis following cervical laminectomy, with a reported change in cervical curvature in 21–47% of patients (14,17,19,20,28). Zdeblick and Bohlman (45) speculated that this decreased incidence of postoperative kyphosis in adults, as compared to children, might be due to the presence of narrowed disks, osteophytes, and hypertrophied facets in the more degenerative spines.

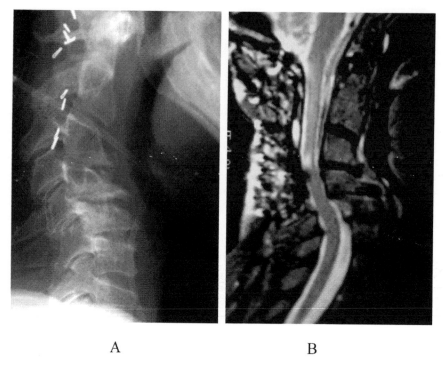

A   B

Figure 2 Lateral radiograph (A) and sagittal MRI (B) demonstrating postlaminectomy kyphotic deformity. Note the narrowing of the cervical canal with associated cord compression.

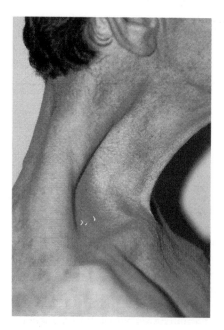

Figure 3 Extensor muscles are placed at a mechanical disadvantage as kyphotic deformities progress.

Kato et al. (20) studied patients following multilevel cervical laminectomy for ossification of the posterior longitudinal ligament. Although a postoperative change in cervical alignment (with the cervical spine becoming straight, S-shaped, or kyphotic) was seen in 47% of the patients, none of the patients had neurological worsening attributed to the presence of this deformity. Mikawa et al. (28) reviewed a series of patients following multilevel cervical laminectomy for a variety of pathologies. In their adult population, 33% demonstrated a change in cervical alignment, and a kyphotic deformity was observed in 11%. Those who developed kyphosis did not exhibit neurological worsening and thus did not require treatment.

Risk factors for the development of instability have been evaluated by many studies. Factors that consistently appear to predispose to postoperative deformity include younger age (14,21,44), lack of preoperative lordosis (17,19,21), and disruption of the posterior facet joints (21). Some have noted laminectomy of C2 to be a risk factor (14,21), whereas others have not (27,44). Some have noted that multiple-level laminectomy is correlated with increased risk of kyphosis (21), whereas others have not (4,14,26,44). Similarly, some have noted preoperative range of motion to be a risk factor (14), whereas others have not (21). Gender does not appear to be a risk factor (14,21). Katsumi et al. (21) were able to directly correlate the number of risk factors for kyphosis with the need for later stabilization procedures.

IV. PREVENTION

Prophylactic fusion should be considered at the time of the initial surgery for those who are at significant risk for developing kyphosis, as prevention is much easier than treatment of a deformity. Lateral mass fixation and fusion can be performed in conjunction with laminectomy to provide stability and prevent the development of a progressive deformity (7,21,28). Kumar et al. (22) found excellent long-term neurological improvement in 25 patients undergoing laminectomy, fusion, and lateral mass fixation for spondylotic myelopathy.

In the immature patient, the high risk of postoperative deformity is a strong indication for a concomitant instrumented posterior cervical fusion at the index procedure (Fig. 4). Some authors, however, believe that fusion can be avoided, even in children, by meticulous attention to surgical technique during the laminectomy. By strict avoidance of resection of any of the facet joints, one study reported only a 9% incidence of postlaminectomy kyphosis (26), even when done at the upper cervical levels. If a fusion is not performed, consideration for prophylactic halo immobilization or orthotic bracing should be given. In any case, careful and frequent postoperative clinical and radiological follow-up should be observed.

Laminoplasty is an alternative technique that can be considered to prevent postlaminectomy instability. Although several forms of laminoplasty have been described, the common goal of these procedures is to expand the size of the cervical canal while maintaining the integrity of the posterior vertebral arch. This is generally only considered in patients with normal cervical lordosis. Matsunaga et al. (25) reported a lower incidence of kyphosis after laminoplasty than laminectomy. Herkowitz (15) compared laminoplasty, laminectomy, and anterior decompression and found a higher rate of good and excellent outcomes in the laminoplasty group (86%) than in the laminectomy-alone group (66%).

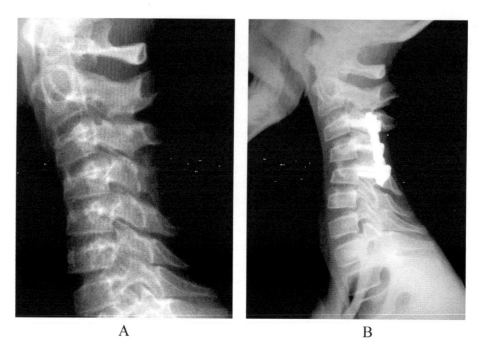

A   B

Figure 4 Preoperative (A) and postoperative (B) radiographs of a 10-year-old patient with an aneurysmal bone cyst in the lamina and spinous process of C4 who was treated with a laminectomy and instrumented posterior fusion. The tendency to kyphosis even with prophylactic fusion can be appreciated.

V. TREATMENT

In the child, once cervical kyphosis has developed, nonsurgical treatment with orthotics usually fails (43). The deformity is uniformly progressive, especially during the accelerated adolescent growth period (24). Surgical treatment is therefore indicated. The goals of correcting postlaminectomy kyphosis include decompression of the neural elements, reestablishing the normal sagittal alignment, and achieving long-term stabilization. Most authors recommend anterior cervical fusion as the treatment of choice (4,24,43). Another alternative for this deformity is posterior facet fusion (6), though loss of surface area for the fusion makes the risk of pseudarthrosis theoretically higher. Additionally, reestablishing a neutral or lordotic alignment is more difficult without anterior column correction.

In the adult, once progression of a deformity is noted, especially if accompanied by neurological deterioration or intractable neck pain, fusion is advised (4,21,39). This can be a surgical challenge. The flexibility of a curve can be assessed by flexion and extension radiographs preoperatively. If flexibility is limited, partial correction with traction can be attempted in the awake patient. Although correction of a deformity is preferred, decompression of the neural elements without causing further neurological deterioration must be the priority.

If myelomalacia and severe compression are present, the vascular supply to the spinal cord may be tenuous. For this reason, spinal cord monitoring is imperative. There is a significant risk of catastrophic deterioration if temporary hypotension occurs in this patient population. Accordingly, mean arterial pressure should be carefully observed and kept at or above the patient's waking levels.

Corpectomy was suggested for treatment of postlaminectomy kyphosis as early as 1960 by Bailey and Badgley (3). Herman and Sonntag (16) reported on 20 patients with postlaminectomy kyphosis who were treated with anterior decompression, strut grafting of an average of 3.8 levels, and anterior cervical plate stabilization. Half of the patients also received supplemental halo fixation. Kyphosis was corrected from an average of 38 degrees to an average of 16 degrees, and most patients experienced neurological improvement.

However, corpectomy in the postlaminectomy patient dissociates the left and right halves of the involved cervical segments and can lead to significant forces on the anterior strut graft. Riew et al. (37) postulated that this displacement force was responsible for the unacceptably high complication rate in their noninstrumented corpectomy/strut graft constructs. In their series of 18 patients who were treated with 1–4 level corpectomies, 9 had graft-related complications despite postoperative immobilization. These complications included graft extrusion, graft collapse, and pseudarthrosis. Based on their review, this group changed their earlier recommendation for not instrumenting postlaminectomy kyphosis correction (45) to recommending circumferential arthrodesis and instrumentation in the setting multilevel postlaminectomy kyphosis (37) (Figs. 5,6). Depending on the degree of kyphosis correction, we often add external halo immobilization in our patients.

Advocates of such circumferential fusion emphasize the biomechanical benefits of rigid posterior instrumentation in reconstructing the compromised columns of the cervical spine in the face of a deficient posterior tension band (1). In a biomechanical study,

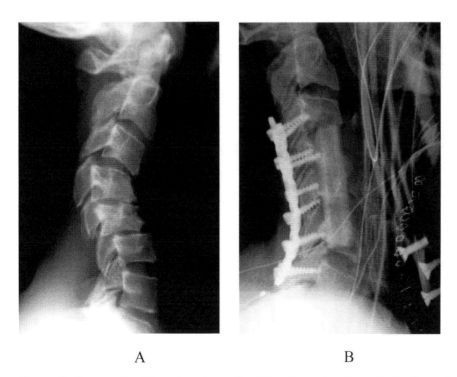

A   B

Figure 5 Preoperative (A) and postoperative (B) radiographs of a patient with postlaminectomy kyphosis which was addressed with anterior decompression and strut grafting and posterior instrumented fusion. Halo immobilization was used in the postoperative period.

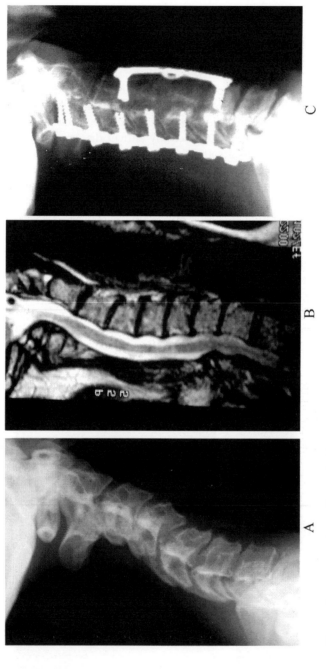

Figure 6 Preoperative radiograph (A) and sagittal MRI (B) of another patient with postlaminectomy kyphosis which was addressed with anterior decompression and strut grafting and posterior instrumented fusion (C).

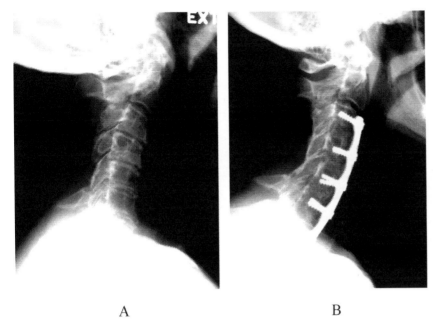

Figure 7 Preoperative (A) and postoperative (B) radiograph showing multiple interbody grafts used to restore lordosis in the setting of postlaminectomy kyphosis where there was not significant compression behind the vertebral bodies.

Foley et al. (11) showed that anterior and posterior instrumentation could significantly decrease the loading forces experienced by anterior strut grafts. Vañichkachorn et al. (40) reported no failures among 11 patients with long corpectomy constructs reconstructed for cervical myelopathy with a junctional plate and posterior instrumentation (Fig. 7).

In certain situations where decompression of the entire body is not required for decompression, segmental correction can be obtained by interbody grafting in conjunction with anterior plating (Fig. 7). Greater sagittal correction can usually be achieved with multiple interbody grafts as opposed to single longer strut grafts. However, a need for decompression behind the vertebral bodies will force the surgeon to perform longer strut grafts for reconstructive procedures. In such situations, plate fixation is generally advocated to prevent graft migration. This can be in the form either of a spanning or a kick plate, in addition to posterior cervical segmental fixation (Fig. 8).

As noted above, posterior instrumentation and facet fusion is generally recommended to decrease the rate of reconstruction failure where an attempt to correct a significant deformity is performed. C2 and C7 or T1 pedicle screws at the terminal end of the construct have additionally been recommended to enhance construct stability and decrease pullout (1). It is reasonable to consider supplemental halo fixation postoperatively for patients with circumferential instability and very large kyphosis corrections and/or poor bone quality.

VI. CONCLUSIONS

The normal function of the cervical spine requires the integrity of the posterior osteoligamentous structures to maintain the balance of forces across the region. When laminectomy

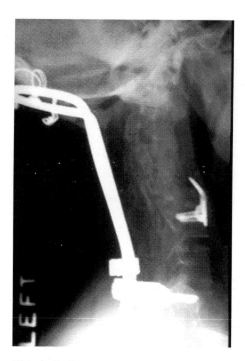

Figure 8 Postoperative radiograph showing circumferential fusion with an anterior kick plate to prevent migration of the anterior strut graft.

is performed, particularly in children, at multiple levels and higher up in the cervical spine, the potential for disruption of the balance is high and postlaminectomy kyphosis can occur. This is a devastating deformity for patients, involving pain, fatigue, and often neurological sequelae.

The best treatment is prevention. In high-risk patients undergoing laminectomy, consideration should be given to prophylactic stabilization in the form of an instrumented posterior fusion. After the deformity occurs, surgical options include anterior and circumferential reconstruction procedures. Specific surgical considerations for this complex problem have been reviewed.

REFERENCES

1. Albert TJ, Vaccaro A. Postlaminectomy kyphosis. Spine 1998; 23:2738–2745.
2. Aronson DD, Kahn RJ, Canady A. Cervical spine instability following suboccipital decompression and cervical laminectomy for Arnold-Chiari syndrome (abst). Presented at the 56th annual meeting of the American Academy of Orthopaedic Surgeons, Las Vegas, 1989.
3. Bailey RW, Bagdley CE. Stabilization of the cervical spine by anterior fusion. J Bone Joint Surg 1960; 42A:565–594.
4. Bell DF, Walker JL, O'Conner G, Tibshirani R. Spinal deformity after multiple-level cervical laminectomy in children. Spine 1994; 19:406–411.
5. Breig A, El-Nadi F. Biomechanics of the cervical spinal cord. Relief of contact pressure on and over stretching of the spinal cord. Acta Radiol Diagn 1966; 4:602–624.
6. Callahan RA, Johnson RM, Margolis RN, Keggi KH, Albright JA, Southwick WO. Cervical facet fusion for control of instability following laminectomy. J Bone Joint Surg 1977; 59A: 991–1002.

7. Cattell HS, Clark GL. Cervical kyphosis and instability following multiple laminectomies in children. J Bone Joint Surg 1967; 49A:713–720.

8. Cusick JF, Yoganandan N, Pintar F, Myklebust J, Hussain H. Biomechanics of cervical spine facetectomy and fixation techniques. Spine 1988; 13:808–812.

9. Cusick JF, Pintar FA, Yoganandan N. Biomechanical alterations induced by multilevel cervical laminectomy. Spine 1995; 20:2392–2399.

10. Epstein JA. The surgical management of cervical spinal stenosis, spondylosis and myeloradiculopathy by means of the posterior approach. Spine 1988; 13:864–869.

11. Foley KT, DiAngelo DJ, Rampersaud YR, Vossel KA, Jansen TH. The in vitro effects of instrumentation on multilevel cervical strut-graft mechanics. Spine 1999; 24:2366–2376.

12. Goel VK, Clark CR, Harris KG, Schulte KR. Kinematics of the cervical spine: effects of multiple total laminectomy and facet wiring. J Orthop Research 1988; 6:611–619.

13. Gore DR, Sepic SB, Gardner GM. Roentgenographic findings of the cervical spine in asymptomatic people. Spine 1986; 11:521–524.

14. Guigui P, Benoist M, Deburge A. Spinal deformity and instability after multilevel cervical laminectomy for spondylotic myelopathy. Spine 1998; 23:440–447.

15. Herkowitz HN. A comparison of anterior cervical fusion, cervical laminectomy, and cervical laminoplasty for the surgical management of multiple level spondylotic radiculopathy. Spine 1988; 13:774–780.

16. Herman J, Sonntag V. Cervical corpectomy and plate fixation for postlaminectomy kyphosis. J Neurosurg 1994; 80:963–970.

17. Ishda Y, Suzuki K, Ohmori K, Kikata Y, Hattori Y. Critical analysis of extensive cervical laminectomy. Neurosurgery 1989; 24:215–222.

18. Kandziora F, Pflugmacher R, Scholz M., et al. Comparison between sheep and human cervical spines: an anatomic, radiographic, bone mineral density, and biomechanical study. Spine 2001; 26:1028–1037.

19. Kaptain GJ, Simmons NE, Replogle RE, Pobereskin L. Incidence and outcome of kyphotic deformity following laminectomy for cervical spondylotic myelopathy. J Neurosurg 2000; 93:S199–S204.

20. Kato Y, Iwasaki M, Fuji T, Yonenobu K, Ochi T. Long-term follow-up results of laminectomy for cervical myelopathy caused by ossification of the posterior longitudinal ligament. J Neurosurg 1998; 89:217–223.

21. Katsumi Y, Honma T, Nakamura T. Analysis of cervical instability resulting from laminectomies for removal of spinal cord tumor. Spine 1989; 14:1171–1176.

22. Kumar VGR, Rea GL, Mervis LJ, McGregor JM. Cervical spondylotic myelopathy: functional and radiographic long-term outcome after laminectomy and posterior fusion. Neurosurgery 1999; 44:771–778.

23. Kumaresan S, Yoganandan N, Pintar FA, et al. Finite element modeling of cervical laminectomy with graded facetectomy. J Spinal Disord 1997; 10:40–46.

24. Lonstein JE. Post-laminectomy kyphosis. Clin Orthop and Rel Research 1977; 128:93–100.

25. Matsunaga S, Sakou T, Nakanisi K. Analysis of the cervical spine alignment following laminoplasty and laminectomy. Spinal Cord 1999; 37:20–24.

26. McLaughlin MR, Wahlig JB, Pollack IF. Incidence of postlaminectomy kyphosis after Chiari decompression. Spine 1997; 22:613–617.

27. Melman CT, Crawford AH, McMath JA. Pediatric vertebral and spinal cord tumors: a retrospective study of musculoskeletal aspects of presentation, treatment, and complications. Orthopedics 1999; 22:49–56.

28. Mikawa Y, Shikata J, Yamamuro T. Spinal deformity and instability after multilevel cervical laminectomy. Spine 1987; 12:6–11.

29. Nolan JP, Sherk HH. Biomechanical evaluation of the extensor musculature of the cervical spine. Spine 1988; 13:9–11.

30. Nowinski GP, Visarius H, Nolte LP, Herkowitz HN. A biomechanical comparison of cervical laminoplasty and cervical laminectomy with progressive facetectomy. Spine 1993; 14:1995–2004.

31. Pal GP, Sherk HH. The vertical stability of the cervical spine. Spine 1988; 13:447–449.
32. Panjabi MM, White AA, Keller D, Southwick WO, Friedlaender G. Stability of the cervical spine under tension. J Biomechanics 1978; 11:189–197.
33. Panjabi MM, Cholewicki J, Nubu K, et al. Critical load of the human cervical spine: an in vitro experimental study. Clin Biomech 1988; 13:11–17.
34. Panjabi MM, Miura T, Cripton PA, Wang JL, Nain AS, DuBois C. Development of a system for in vitro neck muscle force replication in whole cervical spine experiments. Spine 2001; 26:2214–2219.
35. Patwardhan AG, Havey RM, Ghanayem AJ, et al. Load-carrying capacity of the human cervical spine in compression is increased under a follower load. Spine 2000; 25:1548–1554.
36. Reid JD. Effects of flexion-extension movements of the head and spine upon the spinal cord and nerve roots. J Neurol Neurosurg Psychiatry 1960; 23:214–221.
37. Riew KD, Hilibrand AS, Palumbo MA, Bohlman HH. Anterior cervical corpectomy in patients previously managed with a laminectomy: short-term complications. J Bone Joint Surg 1999; 81A:950–957.
38. Saito T, Yamamuro T, Shikata J, Oka M, Tsutsumi S. Analysis and prevention of spinal column deformity following cervical laminectomy. I. Pathogenetic analysis of postlaminectomy deformities. Spine 1991; 16:494–502.
39. Sim FH, Svien HJ, Bickell WH. Swan-neck deformity following extensive cervical laminectomy. J Bone Joint Surg 1974; 56A:564–580.
40. Vanichkachorn JS, Vaccaro AR, Silveri CP, Albert TJ. Anterior junctional plate in the cervical spine. Spine 1998; 23:2462–2467.
41. White AA, Johnson RM, Panjabi MM, Southwick WO. Biomechanical analysis of clinical stability in the cervical spine. Clin Orthop Rel Res 1975; 109:85–96.
42. White AA, Panjabi MM, Thomas CL. The clinical biomechanics of kyphotic deformity. Clin Orthop Rel Res 1977; 128:8–17.
43. Yasuoka S, Peterson HA, Laws ES, MacCarty CS. Pathogenesis and prophylaxis of post-laminectomy deformity of the spine after multiple level laminectomy: difference between children and adults. Neurosurgery 1981; 9:145–152.
44. Yasuoka S, Peterson HA, MacCarty CS. Incidence of spinal deformity after multilevel laminectomy in children and adults. J Neurosurg 1982; 57:441–445.
45. Zdeblick TA, Bohlman HH. Cervical kyphosis and myelopathy: treatment by anterior corpectomy and strut-grafting. J Bone Joint Surg 1989; 71A:170–182.
46. Zdeblick TA, Zou D, Warden KE, et al. Cervical stability after foraminotomy: a biomechanical in vitro analysis. J Bone Joint Surg 1992; 74A:22–27.
47. Zdeblick TA, Abitol JJ, Kunz DN, McCabe RP, Garfin S. Cervical stability after sequential capsule resection. Spine 1993; 18:2005–2008.

18

Complications in the Surgical Management of Ossification of the Posterior Longitudinal Ligament Using the Anterior Approach

Kuniyoshi Abumiand
Hokkaido University, Health Administration Center, Sapporo, Japan

Manabu Ito and Yoshihisa Kotani
Hokkaido University Hospital, Sapporo, Japan

I. INTRODUCTION

The choice of surgical approach for myelopathy caused by ossification of the posterior longitudinal ligament (OPLL) has been controversial. A posterior decompressive laminectomy using a high-speed air burr has often resulted in satisfactory results (4). However, a wide laminectomy led to problems secondary to postlaminectomy kyphosis, segmental instability, and postlaminectomy membrane formation. As a response to this, many methods of laminoplasty were developed to prevent the complications resulting from laminectomy. The anterior approach for OPLL allows the direct removal of the ossified ligament (1,5) or indirect decompression by releasing the lateral margins of the ossified ligament and allowing the remainder to float forward (7,10). Satisfactory results for both the posterior and anterior approach to OPLL have been reported.

In order to select the optimal surgical procedure for OPLL, several factors must be considered, including the number of involved spinal levels, the extent of ossified ligament, the type of ossification, the sagittal alignment of the cervical spine (i.e., lordotic or kyphotic), and the surgeon's experience. In OPLL, the spinal cord is compressed anteriorly, and therefore many surgeons believe that an indirect posterior decompression procedure is less efficient in relieving neural compression. However, the cervical spine is naturally lordotic, and therefore a posterior procedure in this setting may actually provide sufficient relief of spinal cord compression as the spinal cord floats posteriorly in the majority of patients with OPLL. This may be less effective for the patients with limited ossified spinal levels in one or two motion segments. The anterior approach has several disadvantages, including risks of dural tear, bleeding from the epidural venous plexus, and direct intraoperative spinal cord injury. With an increase in the number of levels involved, the greater becomes the potential for complications using the anterior approach.

Regardless of the extent or type of OPLL, a successful direct decompression by an anterior approach often results in excellent decompression of the compressed spinal cord.

In light of the morbidity associated with the anterior approach and the adequate clinical response to the majority of posterior decompressive procedures, the anterior approach is often limited to patients with OPLL localized to the lower cervical spine involving three or fewer consecutive segments requiring one- or two-level corpectomies for decompression.

II. ANTERIOR DECOMPRESSIVE PROCEDURES FOR OPLL

A. Pathology of OPLL in the Cervical Spine

When selecting the anterior approach in the setting of OPLL, the specific anatomical pathology of OPLL must be kept in mind. The posterior longitudinal ligament (PLL) consists of a superficial and deep layer, both of which may become ossified in OPLL. In addition, the dura mater may also be involved with the process of ossification. Two lines of ossification visualized on plain lateral roentogenograms, laminograms, or computed tomograms may indicate ossification of the two layers of the PLL (Fig. 1A,C). The PLL expands laterally at the level of the intervertebral disk; therefore, the width of the ossified ligament is usually wider at the disk level than at the pedicle level. In the cervical spine there is usually room between the spinal cord and the pedicle, and it is here that the venous plexus located in the lateral portion of the cervical spinal canal becomes engorged or congested between the pedicle and the lateral border of the ossified PLL (Fig. 1C).

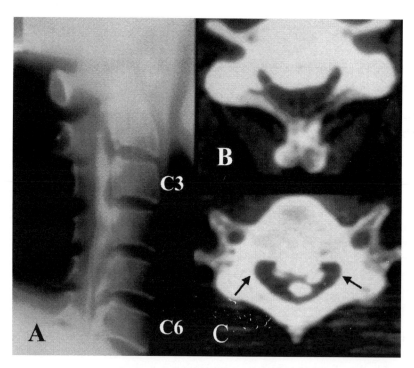

Figure 1 Two lines ossification of posterior longitudinal ligament. (A, C) Two lines of ossification visualized on plain lateral roentogenograms, laminograms, or computed tomograms indicate ossification of superficial and deep layers of the PLL. This may be specific for ossification of the dura mater. (B, C) The ossified ligament is usually wider at the disk level (B) than at the pedicle level (C). In the cervical spine there is room between the spinal cord and the pedicle. It is here that the venous plexus often becomes engorged and congested between the pedicle and the ossified PLL (arrows).

B. Anterior Decompression for OPLL

1. The Anterior Floating Method

Relieving pressure on the anterior spinal cord by allowing the ossified PLL to float anteriorly following release of the lateral margins of the OPLL has the same clinical effect as performing direct removal of the ossified ligament. Considering the risks of removal of the ossified ligament, the anterior floating procedure described by Yamaura et al. (11) is often favored. In this method the patient is placed in the supine position and the anterior aspect of the cervical spine is exposed in the standard manner. The longus colli muscles are retracted laterally, and self-retaining retractors are placed deep to the muscle margins. The intervertebral disk at all involved levels of decompression are next removed. The discectomy must be performed laterally enough to obtain good visualization of the uncovertebral joints (Luschka joint). In the initial phase of the corpectomy, a stainless steel burr is more efficient than a diamond burr to save operation time. When posterior cortex of the vertebral body and ossified ligament is encountered, the stainless steel burr may be changed to a diamond burr to minimize the risk of injury to the epidural veins and the dura mater. Following this stage of the surgery, magnification loops with a headlight or an operating microscope are recommended to obtain good visualization of the decompressive field. The posterior cortex of the vertebral body and ossified ligament are then shaved gradually using a diamond burr with continuous irrigation to prevent thermal injury to the neurological structures. The margins of this ossified mass are then released using a burr or small curette at the cranial, caudal, and bilateral lateral (gutter) margins. The released rectangular shape of ossified ligament will then begin to gradually move anteriorly (Fig. 2). During the release of the bony margins of the ossified ligament, the congested epidural venous plexus, especially at the lateral margins, may become disrupted, resulting in excessive bleeding, which may be difficult to control. Bleeding may be managed with application of hemostatic agents such as oxicellulose cotton. The use of a Kerrison rongeur is not recommended to release the ossified ligament due to the frailty of the contiguous venous plexus.

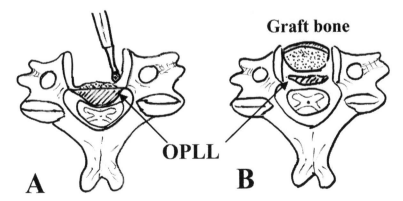

Figure 2 Anterior floating procedure. (A) The ossified ligament and the posterior vertebral cortex must be cut using a burr or small curette at the cranial, caudal, and bilateral lateral (gutter) margins of the corpectomy. (B) After cutting of four margins, the rectangular shaped ossified ligament may now begin to shift anteriorly.

One patient presenting with severe myelopathy resulting from OPLL at the C5 and C6 levels underwent decompressive surgery via the anterior floating method followed by anterior fibula strut grafting (Fig. 3). The patient's myelopathy improved satisfactorily.

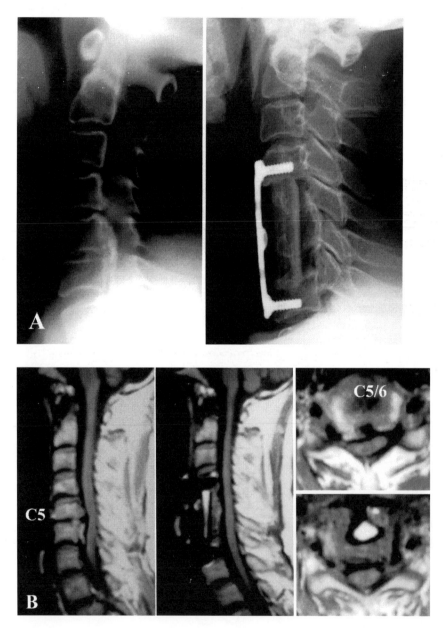

Figure 3 A patient with OPLL in the cervical spine. (A) The patient underwent decompressive surgery using the anterior floating procedure. A postoperative lateral laminogram demonstrates anterior shifting of the ossified ligament and enlargement of anteroposterior diameter of the spinal canal. (B) Pre and postoperative MR images in sagittal and transverse planes demonstrate sufficient decompression.

2. Direct Removal of the Ossified Ligament

If the surgeon intends to directly remove the ossified ligaments, the ligament must be shaved thinner than for the floating procedure. After complete release of the four margins of the ossified ligament, removal of a small portion of the ossified lesion, the caudal portion of the ossified mass, is done with a microdissector. This allows for the release of adhesions between the ossified ligament and the dura mater while retracting the ligament anteriorly. Massive bleeding may be encountered during dissection of the ossified ligament, but, the bleeding is usually adequately controlled following completion of the decompression by the packing of hemostatic agents without high pressure. After a brief pause, the packed hemostatic agents can be removed, allowing placement of the bone graft. If dissection of adhesions is excessively difficult, consideration for abandoning complete ligament removal should be undertaken in order to lessen the risk of dural tear.

3. Anterior Fusion Following Decompression

Regardless of the chosen anterior decompressive procedure, following the decompression an anterior grafting procedure is always performed. If autogenous bone graft is selected, graft bone from the iliac crest is preferable for patients who undergo a one- or two-level corpectomy. A fibula is often chosen for longer fusion spans. Usefulness of an adjunctive anterior cervical plate is surgeon specific. There have been several reports of high complication rates involving the use of long segment stand-alone plating constructs following multilevel anterior cervical corpectomies; therefore consideration of posterior stabilization is undertaken for constructs spanning three or more vertebral levels.

C. Complications of Anterior Surgery for OPLL

1. Dural Tear and Cerebral Spinal Fluid Leakage

A consistent method of decreasing the risk of dural tear is to avoid removal of the anterior ossified lesion. If the ossified ligament is adherent to the dura mater, removal of the lesion along with the dura mater may be possible while leaving the arachnoid membrane intact. However, the arachnoid membrane is extremely fragile and may easily be disrupted. Once the arachnoid membrane is disrupted with egress of cerebrospinal fluid, repair of the ruptured membrane is technically difficult due to limited visualization of the field, the small working room, and bleeding from the venous plexus. A small dural rent may be repaired by a suture combined with a small muscle or fascial patch and fibrin glue sealant. Repair of a large dural defect is usually technically impossible. Controlling cerebrospinal fluid (CSF) leakage in this situation is often accomplished by packing a thin gelfoam sheet into the gap between the lateral vertebral body borders and the grafted bone followed by placement of fibrin glue. Draining CSF in the postoperative period following unsuccessful intraoperative management often resolves spontaneously within several days. Continuous pressure suction drainage should not be used in this setting. Continuous subarachnoid drainage in the lumbar region, however, may be helpful to stop CSF leakage from the wound (3,6).

2. Injury to the Vertebral Artery

As previously described, the PLL expands laterally at the intervertebral disk level. Therefore, an anterior cervical decompression for OPLL often requires a more lateral decompression than in cases of spondylotic myelopathy. This may place the vertebral artery at risk for injury, especially if orientation of the uncinate processes as a lateral landmark is not established. Additionally, in rare cases a tortuous coursing of the vertebral artery may be present or there may be abnormal dilatation of this vessel, all of which must be identified preoperatively by imaging studies to avoid injury (Fig. 4). If vertebral arterial anomalies make an anterior approach unsafe, a posterior decompressive procedure should be strongly considered. In salvage or revision procedures, orientation of the center of the vertebral body or the location of the uncinate processes is often difficult to determine. Great care and adequate preoperative planning must be taken in these cases. A diamond burr may be used during corpectomy to minimize inadvertent violation of the vertebral artery foramen (Fig. 5). Once the artery is injured by burr, the bleeding site is covered with a hemostatic agent such as oxicellulose cotton. Usually the bleeding point cannot be found in the setting of profuse bleeding; therefore, packing of a large amount of cotton or gauze is often required. If the bleeding cannot be adequately controlled, an attempt to localize the bleeding point with direct physical compression with a spinal instrument such as a nerve root probe and a small amount of cotton is often needed. Compression often must be continued for 20–30 minutes. Packing of hemostatic agents directly into the artery lumen must be avoided due to the risk of emboli and brain infarction. The vertebral artery is generally located in the posterior half to two thirds of the anteroposterior diameter of the vertebral body when viewing the spine from the front. Therefore, injury to the vertebral artery usually occurs during the early corpectomy stage before thinning of the ossified lesion has been achieved. Once bleeding is controlled, usually with the help of direct compression by an assistant, the anterior decompression of the ossified lesion can continue. If bleeding cannot be stopped by compression of the bleeding point, the artery should

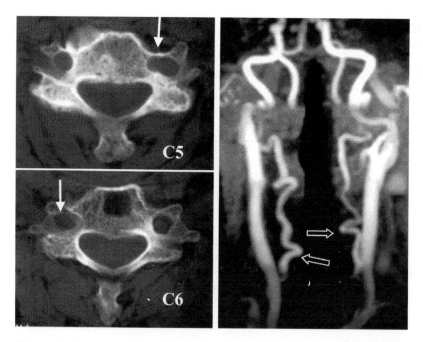

Figure 4 Tortuous course of the vertebral artery within the vertebral body. Some patients have an anomalous coursing of the vertebral artery which forms a loop or aneurysm within the vertebral body. Arrows marked on the CT scans demonstrate expansion of the foramen transversarium, and arrows on the MR angiogram demonstrate loop formation of the vertebral artery. For patients with these types of anomaly, a posterior decompressive procedure should be strongly considered.

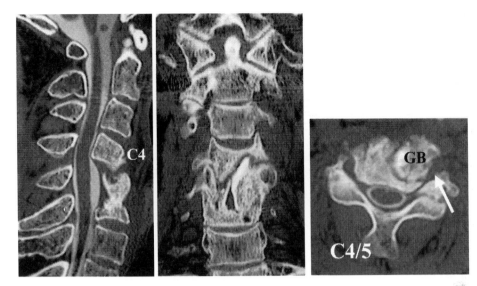

Figure 5 Difficult orientation of the vertebral artery in a salvage surgery. In salvage surgery for patients who have previously undergone anterior surgery, orientation of the center of the vertebral body or locating the uncinate process is sometimes hard. Great caution must be taken in these patients, and the early use of a diamond burr is often recommended. In the patient illustrated, the patient had undergone an anterior decompression and strut grafting for OPLL at an outside hospital and subsequently developed a pseudoarthrosis. Revision corpectomy was performed using a stainless steel burr, during which massive bleeding was encountered following injury to the vertebral artery. Bleeding was stopped with 20 minutes of direct physical compression of the bleeding vessel, and decompression was continued successfully.

be exposed at the cranial and caudal disk space or at the vertebral foramen transversarium above or below the lesion and be ligated with vascular clips. Golfinos et al. (2) has recommended direct repair of injured artery to avoid further complications related to vertebrobasilar ischemia, but, repair is very technically demanding. The incidence of neurological insufficiency caused by cerebellar ischemia fortunately is not high (8,9,10).

3. Spinal Cord Injury

Spinal cord injury may result from direct injury to the spinal cord by a burr or currette during the anterior decompression. Spinal cord injury may also result from the anterior floating method if an adequate release is not performed and the spinal cord begins to float anteriorly, impinging on a trailing ossified fragment. Additionally, the thickness of the ossified lesion must be appreciated in the anterior floating method to avoid direct impingement or compression by the graft bone during the grafting procedure. If the bone graft has a thickness equal to the antero-posterior diameter of the vertebral body, there may be the risk of spinal cord compression due to contact of the graft and floating ossified lesion at the time of bone graft insertion.

III. SUMMARY

Some surgeons believe that the complication rate in anterior cervical surgery is lower than that of posterior surgery (12). Unfortunately, several complications of anterior surgery, such as vertebral artery injury, are more common with the anterior approach. The anterior floating method in the setting of OPLL is less risky than direct extirpation of the ossified ligament and should be strongly considered in all complicated cases of OPLL. Many surgeons prefer the posterior approach in the setting of extensive OPLL due to its technical ease. The anterior approach is often reserved in patients with limited involvement of OPLL to less than two or three spinal segments.

REFERENCES

1. Epstein N. The surgical management of ossification of the posterior longitudinal ligament in 51 patients. J Spinal Disord 1993; 6:432–455.
2. Golfinos JG, Dickman CA, Zabramski JM, Sonntag VKH, Spetzler RF. Repair of vertebral artery injury during anterior cervical decompression. Spine 1994; 22:2552–2556.
3. Kitchel SH, Eismont FJ, Green BA. Closed subarachnoid drainage for management of cerebrospinal fluid leakage after an operation on the spine. J Bone Joint Surg 1989; 74A:984–987.
4. Miyazaki K, Kirita Y. Extensive simultaneous multisegmental laminectomy due to the ossification of the posterior longitudinal ligament in the cervical region. Spine 1986; 11:531–534.
5. Sakou T, Miyazaki A, Tomimura K, Maehata T, Frost HM. Ossification of the posterior longitudinal ligament of the cervical spine: subtotal vertebrectomy as a treatment. Clin Orthop Rel Res 1979; 140:58–65.
6. Shapiro SA, Scully T. Closed continuous drainage of cerebrospinal fluid fistula via lumbar subarachnoid catheter for treatment or prevention of cranial/spinal fluid fistula. Neurosurgery 1992; 30:241–245.
7. Shinomiya K, Okamoto A, Kamikozuru M, Furuya K, Yamaura I. An analysis of failure in primary cervical anterior spinal cord decompression and fusion. J Spinal Disord 1993; 6:277–288.
8. Shintani A, Zervas NT. Consequence of ligation of the vertebral artery. J Neurosurg 1972; 36:447–450.
9. Smith MD, Nmery SE, Dudley A, Murray KJ, Leventhal M. Vertebral artery injury during anterior decompression of the cervical spine. J Bone Joint Surg 1993; 75B:410–415.
10. Wright NM, Lauryssen C. Vertebral artery injury in C1-2 transarticular screw fixation: results of a survey of the AANS/CNS section on disorders of the spine and peripheral nerves. J Neurosurg 1998; 88:634–640.
11. Yamaura I, Kurosa Y, Matsuoka T, Sindo S, Shinomiya K. Anterior approach (anterior floating method) and its surgical results for cervical myelopathy caused by ossification of the ossification of the Posterior Longitudinal Ligament. In: Yonenobu K, Sakou T, Ossification of the Posterior Longitudinal Ligament. Tokyo: Springer-Verlag 1997:165–172.
12. Yonenobu K, Hosono N, Iwasaki M, Asano M, Ono K. Neurologic complications of surgery for cervical compression myelopathy. Spine 1991; 16:1277–1282.

19

Complications Encountered in the Management of Patients with Ankylosing Spondylitis

Steven C. Ludwig and Christopher M. Zarro
University of Maryland, Baltimore, Maryland, U.S.A.

I. INTRODUCTION

Ankylosing spondylitis (AS) is the third most common form of chronic arthritis in the United States. It is an inflammatory condition affecting the hips, sacroiliac joints, and the spine. AS affects about 1–3 per 1000 of the general population (1). According to the Modified New York criteria, AS is characterized by back pain in a patient younger than 40 years persisting for at least 3 months, associated with morning stiffness and improving with exercise. There is limitation of movement of the lumbar spine in the sagittal and frontal planes and decreased chest expansion compared to the normals for age and sex. On plain films of the spine there will be unilateral or bilateral sacro-iliitis. Tissue typing is not included in any set of diagnostic criteria, although there is a high degree of association between HLA-B27 positivity and definite ankylosing spondylitis (2). The site of inflammation is at the junction of fibrous tissue and bone such as tendons and ligaments. This process leads to erosion of bone and ossification of the tendons and ligaments. In the spine this occurs at the insertion of the anulus fibrosis on the vertebral body. Erosion here leads to squaring of the vertebrae, while ossification leads to syndesmophytes and the classic "bamboo spine" caused by calcification of the longitudinal ligaments (3). This fusion of the spinal column causes a decrease in movement and elasticity resulting in altered biomechanics of the spine, rendering it susceptible to a variety of disorders including fracture, dislocation, progressive spinal deformity, atlanto-occipital or atlanto-axial subluxation, and spinal stenosis. The rigidity and immobility of the AS spine has a propensity to develop osteoporosis, further increasing the risk of fracture (4).

II. SPINAL FRACTURES

Diffuse paraspinal ossification and inflammatory osteitis creates a fused, brittle spine that is susceptible to fracture even by minor trauma. The fused or "bamboo spine" becomes osteopenic following long-term immobility making the spine vulnerable. Three recognized patterns of vertebral fractures exist: simple vertebral compression fractures, transversely oriented shear fractures, and stress fractures associated with pseudo-arthrosis. Simple vertebral compression fractures are injuries that occur early in the course of disease and are related to osteoporosis. They typically result in stable kyphosis. Transversely oriented shear fractures are acute fractures that disrupt the ossified supporting ligaments and usually traverse the disk space. Stress fractures associated with pseudoarthrosis are subacute injuries that tend to occur in the thoracolumbar region. The inflammatory process may play a role, but many are caused by the nonunion of stress fractures.

Fractures in AS patients can occur at all levels of the spine. The magnitude of the forces necessary to fracture the spine of an AS patient are much less than those of a patient with a normal spine. Normally, preload is absorbed by spinal ligaments, disks, and facet joints. In patients with AS, these ossified structures, along with exaggerated spinal kyphosis and decreased lumbar lordosis, create a rigid, brittle spine that is prone to fracture. Additionally, other factors that make the ankylosed spine more prone to fracture include osteoporosis as well as impaired mobility. This causes the patient to have an increased vulnerability to falls due to an unstable kyphotic posture.

In the AS patient, calcification of the anulus fibrosis reduces the movement and elasticity of the intervertebral disk, making it the point of least resistance when the spine is involved in trauma (5). It is important to note the difficulty in making the initial diagnosis of spinal fractures in this patient population. This is due to several factors, such as increased density of ossified ligaments, distortion of the normal anatomy by the kyphotic angles and ossification, poorly outlined disk spaces, and increased osteopenia.

Many patients with AS do not realize their injuries due to their baseline pain. Therefore, when an injury of the spine is suspected in these patients, imaging should include the entire spine and not just the symptomatic region. Since there is such difficulty making the diagnosis, there must be a high index of suspicion and realization of the drastic consequences that may occur (5).

Due to the difficulty in diagnosis using plain radiographs, the physician should employ the use of advanced imaging techniques. Magnetic resonance imaging (MRI) allows the visualization of intramedullary edema, disk space injury, spinal cord injury, and epidural hematoma. Bone scans can be used, but it is difficult to differentiate degenerative changes from acute trauma (1). Thin cut computed tomography (CT) scans with coronal and saggital reconstruction can allow visualization of the fracture (Fig. 1). Once diagnosed, vertebral fractures should be managed with three basic principles in mind: reduction of fracture and realignment, early stabilization, and minimization of patient transfers.

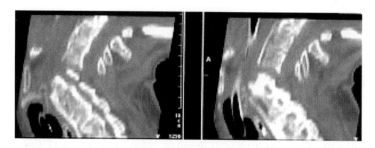

Figure 1   Computed tomography scan of the extension–distraction injury.

III. CERVICAL FRACTURES

Cervical fractures are a serious and possibly life-threatening complication of ankylosing spondylitis. It has been reported that 57–71% of cases result in neurological deficits compared to 44% of patients with normal spines. There is a 35% mortality rate, which is nearly double that of normal fractured spines (6). It is important to evaluate any change in neck pain and head position in these patients because there may be minimal or a remote history of trauma. It is unfortunate that the often minor nature of the trauma and frequency of pain symptoms in these patients result in costly delays in the recognition and management of cervical fractures.

The cervical spine is the most common site of spinal fracture in AS patients. These injuries account for up to 75% of all spine fractures in AS patients. Fractures at all cervical levels have been reported, but the lower cervical segments (fifth through seventh cervical spine segments) are the most susceptible to injury. The most frequent mechanism of spinal cord injury in AS patients is hyperextension of the neck (Fig. 2). This occurs due to the position of the head and neck in relation to the thoracic spine. The forwardly flexed neck due to kyphosis is at risk with both falling forward and backward. It is important to note the frequency and ease of hyperextension injuries in these patients when performing endotrachial intubation. In this situation the anesthesiologist will often place the normal patient in the neutral to hyperextended neck position. This poses a problem to the AS patient with a rigid cervical spine. Another area of concern is with EMS personnel and the application of cervical collars in the acute setting. These collars keep the normal neck in a neutral position, which for the AS patient is a position of dangerous hyperextension. This hyperextension can result in an iatrogenically induced fracture through the ossified intervertebral disks (Fig. 3) (7,8). Due to the instability of these fractures, collars, orthoses, and neutral axial halo vest traction are not adequate for immobilization. These conventional mechanisms of immobilization have led to failed union, fracture displacement, and progression of neurological deficit. Thus, when faced with a patient with AS

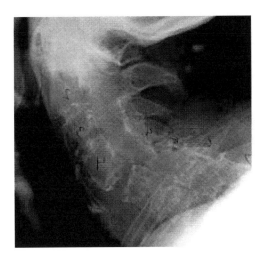

Figure 2 A 68-year-old male who presented after a motor vehicle accident. The lateral cervical spine films shows the extension distraction injury of the C4-5 disk space. At the time of this radiograph the patient had motion in all extremities.

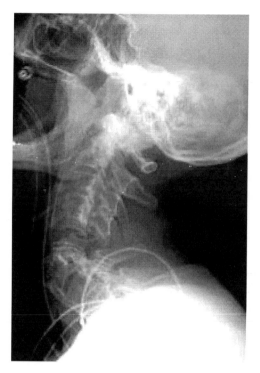

Figure 3 Lateral cervical spine of the same patient after being intubated for respiratory distress showing complete 3-column extension-distraction shearing fracture of C4-5 disk space resulting in quadriplegia.

and with a suspected cervical spine injury, the spine should be immobilized in the position it typically presents in. Modification of standard technique, such as elevation of the head with sandbags on each side, as well as halo cast immobilization with kyphotic bars will assist in safely immobilizing the patient. Fracture reduction, when necessary, can be applied through halo traction in line with the original deformity. The original deformity is most often in the position of flexion (8). The vector of traction should be superior and anterior, and most cases can be reduced with less than 10 pounds of weight (5).

IV. THORACOLUMBAR FRACTURES

Thoracic and lumbar fractures occur less frequently than cervical fractures, at 14% and 5%, respectively. Fractures of the thoracic and lumbar spines in ankylosing spondylitis patients can be of three types: shearing/distraction-extension injuries (Fig. 4), wedge compression (Fig. 5), and pseudoarthrosis associated. Each has a unique clinical stability, neurological sequelae, and mode of treatment. In general, upper thoracic fractures in the presence of a rigid sternum and ribcage are relatively stable but should be followed since they can lead to a progressive kyphotic deformity. About 25% present initially with neurological deficits, but most present with increasing pain (10). There has been much confusion between fractures of the thoracolumbar spine and inflammatory changes in these patients. Radiological features of the fracture commonly occur through

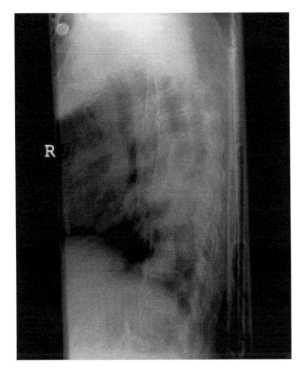

Figure 4 Lateral plain radiograph of an ankylosing spondylitis patient with a hyperextension injury showing mid thoracic spine disk space widening at T7-T8 consistent with an extension-distraction thoracic fracture.

the intervertebral disk or vertebral body. The mechanism of injury is through a distraction-extension force. Bony deformation and stress fracture occur most likely in the thoracolumbar and lumbosacral junctions (11). This occurs due to increased stress in the region resulting from a progressive loss of lumbar lordosis and subsequent vertebral flattening with an axial load to the lumbar spine. This flattening causes the posterior elements to experience tensile stresses as opposed to the normal compressive forces. As this happens, the apex of the normal kyphosis migrates distally to the thoracolumbar junction, placing it at the center of a two-lever arm—the thoracic spine and rib cage above and the lumbar spine and sacrum below (3). A rare complication of thoracolumbar vertebral fractures is the occurrence of visceral complications such as a laceration of the aorta. This is a potentially devastating complication with a mortality rate of 90%. In patients with ankylosing spondylitis, the aorta is at risk because there may be early elastic tissue weakening or a predisposition to aortitis (12).

V. PREOPERATIVE SURGICAL CONSIDERATIONS

Due to the fragility of the spinal column, all prestabilization patient transfers should be carefully supervised by a knowledgeable medical care provider. Preoperative anesthesia consultation should be sought due to the difficulty with intubation as a result of the kyphotic deformity and inability to extend the neck. Fiberoptic intubation should be

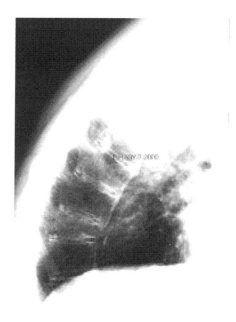

i. Sitzer

Figure 5 Lateral plain radiograph showing calcification of the anterior longitudinal ligament. This is often referred to as the "bamboo spine." Also evident in this radiograph is the presence of a compression fracture and kyphotic deformity.

employed by the anesthesiologist to avoid any forward movement of the cervical spine. Due to the deformity of the spine, surgical positioning on a standard operating room table may not be possible. Modifications using bolsters, rolls, and pillows may be required. Moreover, the kyphotic posture may make anterior exposure, especially to the cervical spine, challenging. In patients with a cervical fracture and chin-on-chest deformity that has been previously reduced and stabilized back to their prefracture posture, surgical stabilization is often performed posteriorly with multiple points of fixation proximal and distal to the fracture site (Figs. 6,7). This allows the surgeon to close down the fracture site and avoid an anterior approach.

VI. PULMONARY COMPLICATIONS

Due to fibrotic upper lung fields, ankylosed ribs, and an exaggerated thoracic kyphosis, patients with ankylosing spondylitis often have a fixed rib cage, restricting pulmonary and diaphragmatic expansion. This places the pulmonary system at great risk for severe complications such as difficulties with postoperative extubation, pulmonary toileting, atelectasis, and pneumonia (4). Due to these risks, patients should have preoperative pulmonary evaluations, which include a careful history and physical exam, a chest x-ray, pulmonary function tests, and evaluation by an anesthesiologist.

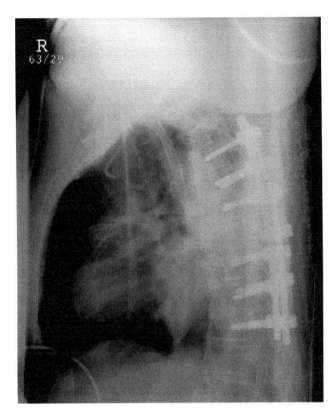

Figure 6 Lateral plain radiograph of thoracic spine showing pedicle screw and rod fixation from T3-T11.

VII. FRACTURE TREATMENT

Fractures in ankylosing spondylitis lead to instability in flexion, extension, and rotation. Therefore, surgical procedures must control all directions of instability. When surgically stabilizing fractures in the setting of AS, at least three segments above and below the lesion should be fixated. Careful preoperative evaluation of the patient's spine in both the coronal and sagittal plane should be performed so as not to end a point of fixaton at a level where a significant deformity exists.

Due to the patient's osteoporosis, obtaining solid fixation using conventional surgical techniques may be problematic. Wiring into osteoporotic bone is not advisable, as the wires may cut through the osteopenic posterior elements. Hooks, when utilized, may pull out. A contemporary popular means of fixation is pedicular screw fixation (Figs. 6,7).

Osteoporotic bone reduces screw mechanical fixation stength and can lead to clinical failure. In order to enhance mechanical fixation in osteoporotic bone, various techniques can be implemented. These techniques include augmentation using polymethylmethacrylate (PMMA). When used in small amounts (3 cc/screw) prior to screw insertion, PMMA has been shown to reinforce the screw/bone interface strength (9). Hasegawa et al. (12a) has shown that the combination of a pedicle screw with sublaminar hook leads to an

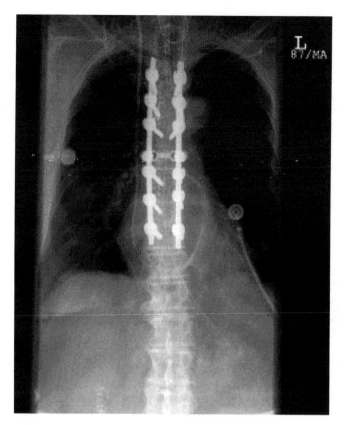

Figure 7 Thoracic spine radiograph of postoperative patient who underwent posterior stabilization of extension-distraction injury.

increase in stiffness compared to pedicle screws alone in osteoporotic bone. This technique may be implemented at the terminal end of the construct. Finally, an expandable pedicle screw has been shown to increase biomechanical stability without the risk of bicortical fixation (18).

Anterior instrumentation is fraught with technical challenges resulting from underlying osteoporosis, which can lead to its loosening. Subsequent loosening of the anterior instrumentation may lead to potential catastrophic vascular injuries of the aorta as well as damage to the esophagus from pressure necrosis (13). Additionally, the anterior approach is extremely difficult in these patients due to the kyphotic angle and forward flexion of the spine. Modification of standard operative positioning may be required. In patients who require anterior surgery, in order to avoid the potential catastrophic complications of hardware loosening, posterior stabilizaton and fusion should be implemented (Fig. 8).

VIII. SPINAL EPIDURAL HEMATOMA

Spinal epidural hematoma occurs rarely compared to intracranial epidural hematoma, but in AS its incidence is much higher. Its etiology may be traumatic or nontraumatic, resulting from coagulopathy, vascular lesion, and iatrogenic or idiopathic causes. Spinal

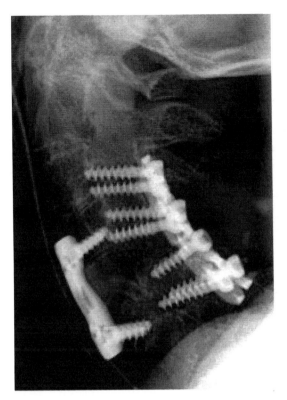

Figure 8 Postoperative lateral cervical spine radiograph showing anterior and posterior fixation and stabilization.

epidural hematoma complicating AS may result from trivial neck trauma and usually presents as incomplete spinal cord injury with rapidly progressive deterioration. The speculated mechanism is often due to bleeding from disrupted epidural veins, diseased hypervascular epidural soft tissue, or fractured bone, which leads to an expanding hematoma confined within a rigid spinal canal. Clinically, the hematoma follows a rapid course, manifesting as an incomplete cord injury with rapidly deteriorating neurological status. Most patients experience ascending weakness and numbness within several hours after injury as a result of external compression from the enlarging hematoma. The prognosis is poor due to several factors. These include multiple medical comorbidities, instability of the fracture site, multiple fractures of the osteoporotic spine, the extent of the hematoma, and delay in seeking medical attention. CT with or without myelography, as well as MRI can be used to demonstrate the presence of a spinal epidural hematoma. MRI can detect ligamentous injuries, herniated disks and hemorrhage, or edema within the cord, but its use may be limited by the inability to use monitoring devices or traction equipment that is typically required in these patients (14,15). The treatment of a patient with a clinically significant epidural hematoma is emergent evacuation followed by stabilization of the injured segments. Clinically insignificant hematomas associated with fractures should be monitored carefully in an ICU setting for any evolving neurological deficit. Strict avoidance of anticoagulation medications should be adhered to due to the propensity for these patients to develop epidural hematomas in the acute traumatic setting.

IX. EXCESSIVE BLOOD LOSS DURING SURGERY

During posterior spinal surgery the patient is placed in the prone position, which allows the abdomen to hang freely, putting minimal pressure on the ventral thorax in order to decrease the impact of the prone position on ventilation and thoracolumbar bleeding. Tetzlaff et al. (16) described difficulty with obtaining the prone position leading to increased intra-abdominal pressure, decreasing inferior vena cava flow and increasing azygous flow. This led to an increase in flow through the valveless epidural plexus and subsequently an increased risk of blood loss with damage to these vessels. Additionally, the pathophysiology of AS leads to infiltration of granulation tissue into the bony insertion of ligaments and joint capsule. This causes areas of intense fibroblastic proliferation, reactive bone formation, and neovascularization. The long-term consequences are osteoporosis and heterotopic bone formation, which increases bleeding with manipulation of the spine. The combination of these factors can lead to the devastating consequence of massive hemorrhage in a patient with AS (16). Intraoperatively controlled hypotension, use of cell saver, and judicious use of hemostatic agents may assist with the control of bleeding. The skin and soft tissues may be injected with 1:500,000 epinephrine:saline to minimize bleeding along with thrombin-soaked raytecs to control bleeding during exposure.

X. CONCLUSION

Patients with ankylosing spondylitis are at increased risk for spinal fractures and subsequent neurological deterioration. These patients must be informed of the risks and propensity towards osteopenia. Once recognized, judicious use of appropriate medications as well as an axial loading exercise regimen early in life may minimize the degree of osteoporosis (17). When evaluating patients for possible fracture, physicians must realize that many injuries will be missed with plain radiographs and advanced imaging techniques should be considered. Once a fracture is identified, the physician must ensure proper immobilization and care with all patient transfers. When operative stabilization is indicated, the patient must be evaluated by the anesthesiologist in order to address difficulties with intubation, coexistent lung disease, and any cardiac abnormalities. During preoperative planning the surgeon must be aware of coexistent osteoporosis to avoid the pitfall associated with standard fixation techniques. Ultimately, the patient with AS must be instructed to have his or her spine evaluated after even minor trauma, since many injuries are overlooked due to chronic pain.

REFERENCES

1. Finkelstein JA, Chapman JR, Mirza S. Occult vertebal fractures in ankylosing spondylitis. Spinal Cord 1999; 37:444–447.
2. Goei The, Steven, Van Der Linden, Cats: evaluation of diagnostic criteria for ankylosing spondylitis: a comparison of the Rome, New York and Modified New York criteria in patients with a positive clinical history screening test for ankylosing spondylitis. Br J Rheumatol 1985; 24:242–249.
3. Bridwell K, DeWald R. The Textbook of Spinal Surgery. Philadelphia: Lippincott-Raven, 1997.

4. Fox M, Onofrio B, Kilgore J. Neurological complications of ankylosing spondylitis. J Neurosurg 1993; 78:871–878.

5. Detwiler K, Loftus C, Godersky J, et al. Management of cervical spine injuries in patients with ankylosing spondylitis. J Neurosurg 1990; 72:210–215.

6. Fast A, Parikh S, Marin E. Spine fractures in ankylosing spondylitis. Arch Phys Med Rehab 1986; 67:595–597.

7. Murray G, Persellin R. Cervical fracture complicating ankylosing spondylitis: a report of eight cases and review of the literature. Am J Med 1981; 70:1033–1041.

8. Broom M, Raycroft J. Complications of fractures of the cervical spine in ankylosing spondylitis. Spine 1988; 13(7):763–766.

9. Cook SD, Salkeld SL, Whitecloud TS. Biomechanical evaluation and preliminary clinical experience with an expansive pedical screw design. J Spinal Disord 2000; 13(3):230–236.

10. Trent G, Armstrong GWD, O'Neil J. Thoracolumbar fractures in ankylosing spondylitis: high risk injuries. Clin Orthop Rel Res 1988; 227:61–66.

11. Gelman M, Umber J. Fractures of the thoracolumbar spine in ankylosing spondylitis. Am J Roentgenol 1978; 130:485–491.

12. Savolaine E, Ebraheim N, Stitgen S, et al. Aortic rupture complicating a fracture of an ankylosed thoracic spine. Clin Orthop Rel Res 1991; 272:136–140.

12a. Hasegawa K, Takahashi HE, Uchiyama S, et al. An experimental study of a combination method using a pedicle screw and laminar hook for the osteoporotic spine. Spine 1997; 22(9):958–962.

13. Exner G, Botel U, Kluger P, Richter M, Eggers C Ruidisch. Treatment of fracture and complication of cervical spine with ankylosis spondylitis. Spinal Cord 1998; 36:377–379.

14. Wu C, Lee S. Spinal epidural hematoma and ankylosing spondylitis: case report and review of the literature. J Trauma 1998; 44(3):558–561.

15. Foo D, Rossier A. Post traumatic spinal epidural hematoma. Neurosurgery 1982; 11:25–32.

16. Tetzlaff J, Yoon H, Bell G. Massive bleeding during spine surgery in a patient with ankylosing spondylitis. Can J Anaesth 1998; 45(9):903–906.

17. Wade W, Salstein R, Maiman D. Spinal fractures complicating ankylosing spondylitis. Arch Phys Med Rehabil 1989; 70:398–401.

18. Wittenberg RH, Lee K, Shea M, et al. Effect of screw diameter, insertion technique, and bone cement augmentation of pedicular screw fixation strength. Clin Orthop Rel Res 1993; 296:278–287.

20

Complications of Closed Skeletal Reduction for Cervical Spinal Instability

Farhan N. Siddiqi, Victor M. Hayes, and Jeff S. Silber
Long Island Jewish Medical Center, New Hyde Park, New York, U.S.A.

I. BACKGROUND

Cervical traction devices such as Cone's, Blackburn's, Crutchfield's, and Gardner-Wells tongs were utilized as external spine manipulation devices for many years prior to halo use. The first use of skull tongs for cervical spine manipulation is credited primarily to Howard H. Hepburn, who developed skull tongs specifically for cervical spine traction at the University of Alberta. Hepburn, the first neurosurgeon at the university, developed the hypothesis that traction would promote healing in cervical spine injuries based on his experience treating wounded soldiers during World War I. Hepburn designed his skull tongs based on common ice tongs and used automobile tire tubing as an elastic to keep the tongs applied to his patient's head. These tongs were first utilized in the mid-1920s and began to receive acknowledgement by the 1930s. In 1933 W. G. Crutchfield popularized his own cervical traction tongs. Crutchfield described his application of extension tongs to the calvaria of a 23-year-old woman with a traumatic C2-C3 fracture, and from that point on their use became widespread throughout the United States.

Today, cervical fracture/dislocation reduction and immobilization with traction is falling out of favor secondary to systemic complications from prolonged bed rest. However, the use of traction devices in emergent reduction of cervical fracture dislocations as well as for maintenance of cervical alignment prior to definitive treatment has current applications in modern spinal trauma management.

II. INTRODUCTION

Closed reduction of cervical injuries can decrease the complexity of subsequent surgical procedures, improve acute stability preventing further neurological deterioration, and dramatically improve neurological status (1–3). Prompt reduction of cervical dislocation within 2 hours of injury has been reported to dramatically improve neurological function and even reverse tetraplegia (4).

Attainment of physiological skeletal alignment may increase potential long-term neurological recovery and help to acutely decrease the enticing factors of the secondary

291

cascade in spinal cord injury. Acute decompression by reduction of fracture/dislocations may lessen spinal cord edema, hematoma, and membrane depolarization, which have been shown to lead to delayed and continued neurological compromise.

Emergent closed reduction of cervical fracture/dislocations has been recommended in the absence of a distracting injury in the awake and cooperative patient (5,6). Weight application in excess of 140 lb has been reported, and up to 70% of body weight has been advocated as safe (7–9). In cooperative patients magnetic resonance imaging (MRI) should not delay reduction, but in an unresponsive or uncooperative patient MRI is advocated to assess any neural compromise from a protruding disk into the spinal canal prior to any attempt at reduction (10,11).

Traction has also been advocated for the maintenance of spinal alignment in unstable fracture patterns with or without neurological injury to promote early callus formation prior to mobilization in an upright halo fixator (12). Cervical traction with reduction for up to 3 weeks followed by halo immobilization with return to traction for loss of reduction has been advocated for unstable injuries such as C1 burst (Jefferson) fractures, odontoid fractures, and C2 traumatic spondylolisthesis (hangman's fractures).

Despite the obvious efficacy of cervical traction for acute fracture/dislocation as well as use in unstable fracture patterns, the use of Gardner-Wells and other cervical skeletal traction devices have been associated with significant local and systemic complications.

III. SYSTEMIC COMPLICATIONS

Systemic complications from cervical traction usage stem mainly from prolonged bed rest. This often results from dysfunctional motor, sensory, and vital function control secondary to spinal cord injury. Extended bed rest increases morbidity and mortality risk in spinal cord–injured patients, mainly in the form of respiratory compromise including pneumonia, global neurological compromise, thromboembolism, sepsis, and decubiti (13–15).

A. Pulmonary

Acute respiratory compromise has been reported in the literature during cervical traction and reduction of Type II posterior displaced odontoid fractures. Harrop et al. (16) reported 155 patients with C2 fractures, of which 32 were specifically Type II odontoid fractures with posterior displacement of the proximal (dens) fragment. Forty percent of these patients experienced acute respiratory compromise during cervical traction and reduction that required the cervical spine to be placed in a flexed position. Three patients could not be subsequently intubated and expired. The results of this study concluded that acute retropharyngeal swelling may lead to the inability to be intubated with the cervical spine placed in the flexed position. Based on these findings, the authors recommended prereduction nasotracheal intubation with posteriorly displaced Type II odontoid fractures that require reduction in a flexed position (16).

B. Neurological

Neurological deterioration after admission to a spinal cord injury center is a well-documented and devastating entity. Worsening of neurological status after all types of spinal cord injury was studied by Farmer et al. (17), who retrospectively reported on 1031 patients over a 16-year period. Results demonstrated that worsening of neurological status occurred a mean of 4 days after initial injury. This finding was seen with increased frequency when surgery was performed within 5 days after injury, in patients with ankylosing spondylitis, in the setting of sepsis, and/or in patients requiring intubation. In this review the authors found that halo application, cervical traction, and Stryker frame use were all risk factors for neurological deterioration in this population (17). In another study, Harrop et al. (18) examined ascending neurological compromise in patients with complete spinal cord injury in the acute setting. The authors found a significant correlation between ascending neurological injury and mortality during the hospital course. One hundred and eighty-two patients with complete spinal cord injury [acute spinal injury association (ASIA) Class A] were identified from 1904 spinal cord injuries over a 7-year period. Twelve patients had ascending compromise within 30 days of injury. Three temporal subsets were identified as increasing the risk for ascending neurological compromise:

1. Early deterioration (< 24 h) was associated with cervical traction and was related to unrecognized disk protrusion prior to reduction.
2. Delayed deterioration (24 h to 7 days) was related to sustained hypotension in the ICU setting.
3. Late deterioration (> 7 days) was observed in patients with vertebral artery injuries.

Based on these findings, the authors recommended attempts to recognize and manage these risk factors in order to help prevent or lessen their temporal effects on ascending injury (18).

C. Thromboembolic

Thromboembolic phenomena are a cause of significant morbidity and mortality in the spinal cord–injured patient. The use of anticoagulation for thromboembolic prophylaxis has been associated with epidural hematoma formation, and therefore mechanical prophylaxis has been the mainstay of treatment anecdotally (19). No long-term studies have been reported evaluating the efficacy of inferior venacaval filters, both permanent and removable, and their effects on thromboembolism in the spine injury patient.

Systemic complications of cervical traction in the spinal cord–injured patient are common and are significant contributors to the increased morbidity and mortality in these patients. Strict adherence to intensive care protocols and further studies to evaluate management and prevention of these complications are needed. Strict management and prevention protocols can be safely and effectively used, but the physician and nursing care teams must be intimately aware of systemic complications that can occur outside of the cervical spine region.

IV. LOCAL COMPLICATIONS

Local complications of cervical tongs include calvarial dural pin penetration, pin tract infection, brain abscess, meningitis, propagation of skull fracture, occipital decubitus formation, loss of pin fixation, hanging weight complications, arterial injury, missed distraction injury, overdistraction, traction-related disk protrusion, and misapplication of pins leading to possible canal compromise or fracture malalignment (14,15,19).

A. Pin Penetration

Cervical traction devices are designed to exert a constant compressive load to the outer skull table without penetration of the inner skull table. The Gardner-Wells tongs achieve this by way of spring-loaded pins designed to exert a constant force once the spring indicator engages. A model by Lerman et al. found the average force applied with a 1 mm pin indicator protrusion to be 30 lb, whereas the average force to penetrate cadaveric skulls was 162 lb (20). Ideally, the force of the pins should remain constant throughout the duration of treatment. Krag et al. (21) studied cadaveric skulls in order to identify ideal pin-placement sites in order to avoid possible skull penetration. The authors' findings indicated that ideal pin sites with the thickest skull bone were located just above the external auditory meatus bilaterally (21). If flexion or extension moments are to be applied to the traction device, pin sites may be moved 1 cm anterior or posterior to apply those forces (21). If moved substantially anteriorly, direct cutdown to bone should be utilized to avoid temporal artery laceration.

However, even with identified ideal application sites, pin tract infection, loosening, or pathologically softer skull bones may allow penetration of pins and subsequent complications. Littleton et al. (22) studied various cervical tong pin pressures in cadavers to examine consequences of overtightening. Forces generated at recommended settings were 141 N from PMT tongs, 132 N from Gardner-Wells tongs, and negligible forces from Depuy Ace tongs. Overtightening of Gardner-Wells tongs by as little as 0.3 mm beyond recommendations led to forces in excess of 448 newtons. Failure of temporal bone specimens ranged from 636 ± 351 N for Depuy Ace tongs to 956 ± 227 N for Gardner-Wells tongs. Thus, even small increments of overtightening of Gardner-Wells tongs may lead to skull penetration (22).

Overtightening has led to a specific constellation of symptoms, as reported by Choo et al. (23) This is based on a report of a 42-year-old patient who had application of Gardner-Wells tongs for a C6 burst fracture with an accompanied C6-C7 anterior fracture/dislocation. Thirty-seven days after cervical traction application, a pin site became inflamed and the patient was started on parenteral antibiotics. On day 42 the patient felt a sudden movement of the tongs and developed a severe headache, fever, and vomiting. A radiograph demonstrated a 5 mm penetration of the infected pin beyond the inner table of the skull. Removal of the tongs led to resolution of the symptoms, but the next day the patient sustained two transient ischemic attacks localized to the area of pin penetration. Although these symptoms resolved without sequelae, they demonstrate a symptom constellation related to skull penetration by a halo pin site (23).

B. Pin Site/Intracranial Infection

Pin site infections commonly occur and are treated with local cleansing, debridement, and antibiotics; rarely, however, they may lead to the possible complication of a brain abscess and/or meningitis. A brain abscess carries a mortality rate of 24%, making its early diagnosis and treatment critical, especially in patients in the intensive care unit who may be sedated (24). The symptoms and signs of an intracranial abscess includes pin tract infection (which may be occult), unexplained headache, vomiting, and neurological changes that do not coincide with the site of spinal injury. These symptoms and the subsequent diagnosis of a brain abscess have been reported in all age groups (25). Loosening of pins in the face of infection is common, but these pins should not be retightened secondary to the high risk of inner skull cave penetration. Radiological investigation in select cases and repositioning of pins is the appropriate management in these cases. Avoidance of pin site infection is the goal of nursing care and should be undertaken daily with sterile dressing changes and cleansing. Occasional local debridement may be necessary (26).

C. Pin Loosening

Loss of fixation of cervical tong pins can lead to disastrous consequences. Spontaneous release of pins can lead to sudden loss of cervical fracture reduction and spinal alignment leading to potential neurological compromise from spinal cord, nerve root, or vascular injury. Failure usually occurs at the pin-bone interface. Institutions commonly reuse tongs, whereas halo devices are commonly discarded after one use. In a biomechanical comparison, Lerman et al. (27) compared pin site pullout strengths with new, rarely used, and heavily used Gardner-Wells tongs. Findings revealed that the pullout strength of new and rarely used tongs exceeded the maximum weight clinically used in traction and reduction. However, heavily utilized tongs secondary to wear in spring mechanisms did not have pullout strengths able to withstand the high weights often used clinically. Thus, tong recalibration and replacement is needed for repeatedly used tongs in order to avoid pullout during reduction and management (27).

The use of MRI-compatible graphite tongs has become commonplace in the initial emergency room setting to allow further imaging after fracture/dislocation reduction. Blumberg et al. (28) examined the pullout strength of titanium alloy MRI-compatible Gardner-Wells tongs in comparison to stainless steel non–MRI-compatible Gardner-Wells tongs in a cadaver model. The titanium alloy pins failed secondary to plastic deformation at the tips in excess of 50 lb of traction. Their results demonstrated the need to change to stainless steel tongs if weights in excess of 50 lb are needed for reduction to avoid potential loss of fixation (28). Carbon fiber MRI-compatible tongs have also been studied and have been found to fail above 80 lb of traction and should be used with caution or exchanged for stainless steel if higher weights are needed (19).

D. Pulley Systems

Cervical traction systems often use hanging weights to hold reductions maintaining spinal alignment. These pulley and weight systems can cause complications based on the amounts and types of pulleys used. Furthermore, these cumbersome set-ups can inhibit patient care as well as hinder patient transportation. Commonly, multiple pulleys are utilized in order to establish an increased biomechanical advantage, decreasing the weight needed to maintain and hold reductions. However, Nystrom et al. (29) demonstrated that frictional forces are transmitted to the ropes causing errors in estimation of the weight applied. Their findings indicated a 10–21.5% change in total weight transmitted to the cervical spine based on the type of pulley used in a one-pulley system. However, in a three-pulley system, total weight transmitted to the cervical spine was dampened as much as 65% of expected. Their important findings indicate that weight application may be in error secondary to types and numbers of pulleys used. Thus, types and amounts of pulleys used should be taken into account when changing weights during cervical traction therapy. Additionally, Nystrom et al. also demonstrated that during transportation of patients with hanging weight traction, swinging of the weights can lead to energy transfer to the cervical spine with loss of fracture alignment and/or redislocation. The authors advised that transportation be done with strict avoidance of weight swinging. The authors also concluded that spring traction devices may offer better force characteristics than hanging weight systems during transportation (29).

E. Arterial Injuries

Arterial injuries from cervical traction devices have been described both intracranially and extracranially. Injuries to the temporal artery from direct laceration, intracranial artery injury from pin site invasion, and vertebral artery injury from traction have all been described. Temporal artery laceration can occur with initial percutaneous insertion of tong pins. Avoidance of the area directly anterior and superior to the ear tragus for percutaneous pin placement is recommended unless direct cutdown to bone is made. Nimityongskul et al. (30) reported a case of recurrent pulsitile bleeding from a pin site that developed after initial insertion of pins. This bleeding became intermittently severe and chronic, necessitating surgical ligation of the temporal artery for hemostasis. Hirsh (31) described an intracranial aneurysm secondary to pin site penetration from cervical skull calipers. In his description, a fusiform intracranial aneurysm followed the placement of skull calipers and resulted in rupture and bleeding with cerebral mass effect that required surgical drainage. Finally, vertebral artery injury has been well described in cervical trauma. Vertebral artery injury can occur in cervical trauma patients sustaining a facet joint dislocation or transverse foramen fracture and can result in fatal neurological sequellae (32). If injury to the vertebral artery has occurred from the initial trauma event, cervical traction may in some cases worsen the injury, but stabilization of fracture/ dislocations may help avoid propagation and embolization of vertebral artery clots (32). Furthermore, cervical traction has been associated with vertebral artery injury in some nontraumatic cases as well. Horsley et al. (33) reported a cervical traction–induced rupture of a vertebral artery aneurysm in a patient with neurofibromatosis. He recommended arteriography of patients with medical histories consistent with possible aneurysmal lesions. Dickinson et al. (34b) reported bilateral vertebral artery dissections leading to stroke after the use of 8 lb of cervical traction used to reduce a myelopathic patient with severe basilar impression. Cervical traction in the face of possible vertebral artery injury or with a history consistent with possible arterial disease should be carefully considered and studied prior to application of traction.

V. OVERDISTRACTION

Overdistraction of cervical spine injuries with cervical skeletal traction can be a devastating complication. Reports have shown erroneous placement of cervical traction on distracting-type injuries leading to spinal cord overdistraction and subsequent death (19). Jeanneret et al. (35) reported five cases of overdistraction and offered recommendations to avoid this disastrous complication. Injuries including occipitocervical dislocations, fractures of the odontoid process, C2 traumatic spondylolisthesis (hangman's fractures), hyper-extension/distraction injuries, and bilateral fracture/dislocations all may represent rupture of both anterior and posterior ligamentous complexes. These injuries are especially vulnerable to overdistraction, and the authors recommended the use of much less weight than that commonly utilized for reduction of these injuries with frequent radiological confirmation. Furthermore, the authors recommended beginning reduction with 2 kg and adding additional weight under continuous neurological and radiological observation, with a return to 2 kg once reduction is achieved. Any change in neurological symptoms or breathing pattern (Cheyne-Stokes reported in one case) should prompt immediate reduction in weight to previously tolerated amounts. Reduction in weight after neurological deterioration generally leads to a return in neurological function to predistraction levels (35).

VI. POSTREDUCTION NEUROLOGICAL DETERIORATION

Acute reduction of cervical fracture/dislocations in the emergency setting has been advocated to theoretically improve neurological outcome. However, in cases of uncooperative, sedated, or unresponsive patients, acute reduction has rarely been associated with sudden neurological deterioration. This is commonly due to an unrecognized traumatic cervical disk protrusion from the dislocation resulting in sudden canal compromise (10,11,17). Harrop et al. demonstrated early (< 24 h) ascending neurological deterioration in complete spinal cord injuries in a small percentage of patients due to unrecognized disk protrusion. Mahale et al. reported 18 patients with neurological deterioration after acute reduction of cervical dislocations. Four patients were reduced with traction, four with manipulation, and seven with open reduction. Neurological deterioration was not related to age, sex, mechanism, level, or type of dislocation. Thirteen patients made a full recovery, one made a partial recovery, and one remained completely paralyzed and died 3 months later. The authors recommended early MRI or computed tomography (CT) myelogram to diagnose a disk protrusion in the unresponsive or uncooperative patient (36). If imaging can be done immediately, there may be efficacy in imaging prior to reduction in many cases.

VII. TRACTION VECTORS

Traction in a flexed position has been advocated for the reduction of cervical facet dislocations. Flexion and extension moments are utilized in reduction of fractures with angulation such as odontoid fractures. Inadvertent positioning of cervical tong pins anterior or posterior of the central axis of the head may lead to unwanted flexion or extension of the cervical spine and can lead to spinal misalignment with resultant spinal canal compromise. Ching et al. (37) demonstrated in a cadaveric model that traction of cervical burst fractures in an extended or compressed (flexed) position leads to compromise of the spinal canal. Increased compression of the spinal cord in a compromised canal may lead to a more extensive neurological deficit, and thus the authors advocate placement of the head in a neutral position with pin placement directly superior or above the external auditory meatus. Confirmation of neutrality should be done with immediate radiological imaging to avoid the extended or compressed positioning (37).

VIII. CONCLUSION

The use of closed skeletal cervical traction in the United States as a definitive management approach has declined since the advent of the halo device as well as improved surgical techniques of internal fixation. However, traction is often a necessary initial treatment intervention in many types of unstable cervical fractures and dislocations for both reduction and temporary spinal stabilization. Unfortunately, the use of cervical traction necessitates prolonged bed rest, extended use of external skull pins, and a large amount of traction weight. Complications from the use of these devices are many and include both systemic and local problems. Even so, these traction devices can be safely utilized to provide adequate initial and at times definitive management. However, a strict care plan must be maintained by both physicians and nurses and must address both the local and systemic complications associated with these devices.

REFERENCES

1. Subin B, Liu JF, Marshall GJ, et al. Transoral anterior decompression and fusion of chronic irreducible atlantoaxial dislocation with spinal cord compression. Spine 1995; 20:1233–1240.
2. Mahale YJ, Silver JR. Progressive paralysis after bilateral facet dislocation of the cervical spine. J Bone Joint Surg 1992; 74B:219–223.
3. Shrosbree RD. Neurological sequelae of reduction of fracture dislocations of the cervical spine. Paraplegia 1979; 17:212–221.
4. Gillingham J. Letter. J Neurosurg 1976:766–767.
5. Shanmuganathan K, Mirvis SE, Levine AM. Rotational injury of cervical facets: CT analysis of fracture patterns with implications for management and neurologic outcome. AJR 1994; 163:1165–1169.
6. Star AM, Jones AA, Cotler JM, et al. Immediate closed reduction of cervical spine dislocations using traction. Spine 1990; 15:1068–1072.
7. Kleyn PJ. Dislocations of the cervical spine: closed reduction under anaesthesia. Paraplegia 1984; 22:271–281.
8. Sabiston CP, Wing PC, Schweigel JF, et al. Closed reduction of dislocations of the lower cervical spine. J Trauma 1988; 28:832–835.
9. Delamarter RB, Sherman J, Carr JB. Pathophysiology of spinal cord injury. Recovery after immediate and delayed decompression. J Bone Joint Surg 1995; 77A:1042–1049.
10. Lee AS, MacLean JC, Newton DA. Rapid traction for reduction of cervical spine dislocations. J Bone Joint Surg 1994; 76B:352–356.
11. Metz CM, Kuhn JE, Greenfield ML. Cervical spine alignment in immobilized hockey players: radiographic analysis with and without helmets and shoulder pads. Clin J Sports Med 1998; 8:92–95.
12. Schweigel JF. Management of the fractured odontoid with halothoracic bracing. Spine 1987; 12:838–839.
13. Bednar DA, Parikh J, Hummel J. Management of type II odontoid process fractures in geriatric patients; a prospective study of sequential cohorts with attention to survivorship. J Spinal Disord 1995; 8:166–169.
14. Garfin SR, Botte MJ, Waters RL, et al. Complications in the use of the halo fixation device. J Bone Joint Surg 1986; 68A:320–325.
15. Glaser JA, Whitehill R, Stamp WG, et al. Complications associated with the halo-vest. A review of 245 cases. J Neurosurg 1986; 65:762–769.
16. Harrop JS, Vaccaro A, Przybylski GJ. Acute respiratory compromise associated with flexed cervical traction after C2 fractures. Spine 2001; 26:E50–E54.
17. Farmer J, Vaccaro A, Albert TJ, Malone S, Balderston RA, Cotler JM. Neurologic deterioration after cervical spinal cord injury. J Spinal Disord 1998; 11:192–196.
18. Harrop JS, Sharan AD, Vaccaro AR, Przybylski GJ. The cause of neurologic deterioration after acute cervical spinal cord injury. Spine 2001; 26:340–346.
19. Rockwood C, Green D, Bucholz R, Beaty J. Rockwood & Green's Fractures in Adults. 5th ed. Philadelphia: Lippincott Williams & Wilkins, 2000.
20. Lerman JA, Dickman CA, Haynes RJ. Penetration of cranial inner table with Gardner-Wells tongs. J Spinal Disord 2001; 14:211–213.

21. Krag MH, Monsey RD, Fenwick JW. Cranial morphometry related to placement of tongs in the temporoparietal area for cervical traction. J Spinal Disord 1988; 1:301–305.
22. Littleton K, Curcin A, Novak VP, Belkoff SM. Insertion force measurement of cervical traction tongs: a biomechanical study. J Orthop Trauma 2000; 14:505–508.
23. Choo JH, Liu WY, Kumar VP. Complications from the Gardner-Wells tongs. Injury 1996; 27:512–513.
24. Williams FH, Nelms DK, McGaharan KM. Brain abscess: a rare complication of halo usage. Arch Phys Med Rehabil 1992; 73:490–492.
25. Martinez-Lage JF, Perez-Espejo MA, Masegosa J, Poza M. Bilateral brain abscesses complicating the use of Crutchfield tongs. Childs Nervous System 1986; 2:208–210.
26. Soyer J, Iborra JP, Fargues P, Pries P, Clarac JP. Brain abscess following the use of skull traction. Chirurgie 1999; 124:432–434.
27. Lerman JA, Haynes RJ, Koeneman EJ, Koeneman JB, Wong WB. A biomechanical comparison of Gardner-Wells tongs and halo device used for cervical spine traction. Spine 1994; 19:2403–2406.
28. Blumberg KD, Catalano JB, Cotler JM, Balderston RA. The pullout strength of titanium alloy MRI-compatible and stainless steel MRI-incompatible Gardner-Wells tongs. Spine 1993; 18:1895–1896.
29. Nystrom B, Allard H, Karlsson H. Analysis of the traction forces in different skull traction systems. Neurosurgery 1988; 22:527–530.
30. Nimityongskul P, Bose WJ, Hurley DP Jr. Anderson LD. Superficial temporal artery laceration. A complication of skull tong traction. Orthop Rev 1992; 21:761,764–765.
31. Hirsh LF. Intracranial aneurysm and hemorrhage following skull caliper traction. Review of skull traction complications. Spine 1979; 4:206–208.
32. Veras LM, Pedraza-Gutierrez S, Castellanos J, Capellades J, Casamitjana J, Rovira-Canellas A. Vertebral artery occlusion after acute cervical spine trauma. Spine 2000; 25:1171–1177.
33. Horsley M, Taylor TK, Sorby WA. Traction-induced rupture of an extracranial vertebral artery aneurysm associated with neurofibromatosis. Spine 1997; 22(2):225–227.
34. Dickinson LD, Tuite GF, Colon GP, Papadopoulos SM. Vertebral artery dissection related to basilar impression: case report. Neurosurgery 1995; 36(4):835–838.
35. Jeanneret B, Magerl F, Ward JC. Over distraction: a hazard of skull traction in the management of acute injuries of the cervical spine. Arch Orthop Trauma Surg 1991; 110:242–245.
36. Mahale YJ, Silver JR, Henderson NJ. Neurological complications of the reduction of cervical spine dislocations. J Bone Joint Surg 1993; 75(Br):403–409.
37. Ching RP, Watson NA, Carter JW, Tencer AF. The effect of post-injury spinal position on canal occlusion in a cervical spine burst fracture model. Spine 1997; 22:1710–1715.

21

Complications of Posterior Occipitocervical Instrumentation

Rick C. Sasso
Indiana Spine Group, Indianapolis, Indiana, U.S.A.

In the past 10 years enormous progress has been made in our ability to stabilize the cervical spine. Specifically, posterior cervical instrumentation has profoundly advanced with screw-fixation techniques, allowing us to anchor very well into every segment of the occipito-cervical-thoracic spine, and the introduction of rod-based systems that connect these various screws to a stable platform. Associated with these new techniques are very specific challenges and potential complications. This chapter will detail these possible problems as well as outline preoperative strategies to avert complications and suggest techniques to minimize the severity of injury if a complication occurs.

I. OCCIPITAL FIXATION

The evolution of occipitocervical fixation with advancing technology and progressive construct stability has allowed treatment of more complex craniocervical instabilities with a higher success rate and less cumbersome postoperative immobilization. Initial on-lay fusion and simple wire techniques required periods of traction followed by a halo. Rod and wire constructs were more stable, but continued to have difficulty preventing axial loads due to the rods pistoning through the sublaminar wires. Plate and screw constructs (1) were the first truly stable types of occipitocervical fixation, but depended upon fixed hole-hole distances in the plate, which made proper insertion of the screws sometimes difficult. Modern screw-rod devices allow independent insertion of the screw anchors as well as stable connection to the longitudinal rod (2).

Biomechanical evaluation of occipitocervical instrumentation demonstrates occipital wire-rod devices to be least stable, especially under axial loads (3,4). Occipital screws are the strongest method of occipital fixation. The most significant complications of using other types of occipital fixation such as wire and hooks are the risk of loss of fixation and the risks of halo immobilization. Especially in elderly patients, the risk of pulmonary complications and death is very real with the use of halos (5,6).

The most common causes of occipitocervical instability are rheumatoid arthritis with vertical migration of the odontoid and trauma to the ligamentous structures of the craniocervical junction. Tumors and infections may also cause destruction of the stabilizing elements. The patient is positioned prone with a Mayfield pin headrest. Attention to intraoperative positioning is critical in order to not allow occipitocervical kyphosis. The vertebral artery emerges from the transverse foramen of the atlas and courses medially on the anterior portion of the superior surface of the posterior ring. Dissection on the cephalad aspect of the posterior aspect of C1 should not extend more than 12 mm lateral to the midline.

Occipital screws at the cephalad end of a fusion may limit problems associated with occipital fixation. Further cranial settling of the upper cervical spine following odontoid-ectomy has been reported with nonrigid posterior occipitocervical instrumentation (7). Occipital screws are the strongest method of occipital fixation. Bicortical screws are 50% stronger than occipital wire (8,9). Occipital wire and rod constructs are less stable, especially under axial loads. In conditions with significant occipitocervical instability where axial forces must be neutralized, such as vertical migration of the odontoid, occipital screw plate or rod instrumentation is optimal. Extensive destruction of the occiput may make this technique very difficult. It is optimal, depending on the spinal system, to place three occipital screws on each side of the midline (total of six). Six occipital screws demonstrate the highest construct stiffness in human cadaveric biomechanical studies (10). They should be positioned just below the superior nuchal line, as close to the external occipital protuberance as possible (Fig. 1). If cerebrospinal fluid (CSF) is encountered, simply apply the screw and it will stop.

Occipital screw length ranges from 6 to 14 mm, with the average screw measuring 10 mm. Immediately lateral to the external occipital protuberance (EOP) will accommodate up to a 14 mm screw. The best zone for screw insertion is up to 20 mm lateral to the EOP along the superior nuchal line decreasing to 5 mm lateral to the EOP at 20 mm inferior to the superior nuchal line. This forms a V-type configuration.

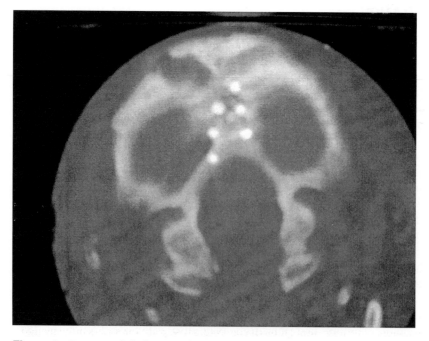

Figure 1   Proper occipital screw placement close to the midline.

The occipital screws should be placed last, after the C2 and subaxial screws are inserted, which are applied with much less variability than the occipital screws. The rod or plate should first be bent to the appropriate occipitocervical sagittal lordotic angle with enough room along the occipital longitudinal member to place three screws (Fig. 2). If the rod or plate is to run over the superior nuchal line, a reverse bend should be made to allow it to lie flat on the occiput. The C2 screw (pedicle or transarticular C1-2) is placed first, and then the subaxial lateral mass screws are applied. If a rod is used, it will want to pivot on its apex at the occipitocervical junction, with the cephalad aspect of the rod angling either lateral or medial. Allow it to angle medial before tightening the connectors in the cervical spine (Fig. 3). If a plate is used, a coronal plane bend can be applied to angle the occipital portion medially. Screws aligned in the midline on one longitudinal member are a weak construct under torsional loads.

Bicortical occipital fixation is desired. First, it provides for stronger purchase than unicortical screws or wire. Second, if the far cortex is not drilled or tapped and a screw is applied that reaches the far cortex, it will strip its threads due to its tip abutting the hard cortical bone. This will result in very poor purchase. The drill stop should be set to 10 mm and the far cortex felt with the drill at high revolution and drilled through. The hole must be tapped. The occipital cortex is very hard (thus allowing for excellent fixation), but if threads are not tapped into this cortical bone, the screw may not even get started.

Inadequate occipital thickness may be a pitfall. This usually occurs if screws are attempted too close to the foramen magnum. Also, in this position it is difficult to place the screw perpendicular to the plate or rod because of the steep angle necessary to drill, tap, and screw close to the foramen magnum. Thus, make sure the occipital screws are positioned closer to the superior nuchal line.

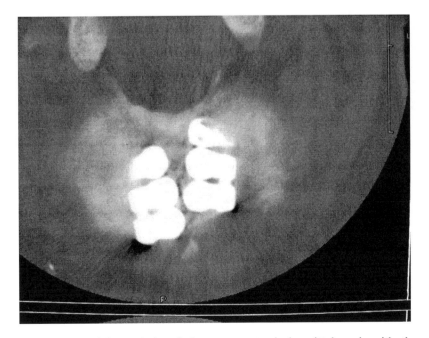

Figure 2 Occipitocervical rods bent to anatomical sagittal angle with three occipital screws attached to each longitudinal member through offset connectors that place the screws medially into the thickest bone.

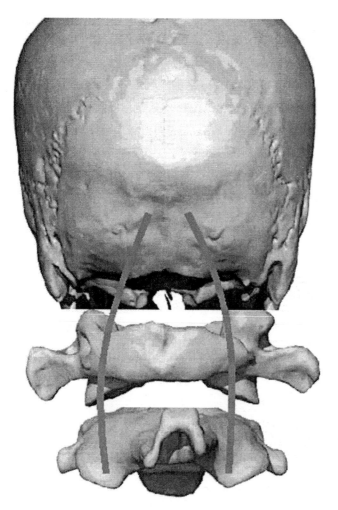

Figure 3 O-C rods pivot on apex at C1 with cephalad angulation toward the midline to allow the
screws medial position.

If a significant amount of the occiput is resected for decompression or it is destroyed
for other reasons, placing three screws below the superior nuchal line may not be possible.
Screws may be applied cephalad to the superior nuchal line, but the transverse sinus must
be considered. This venous sinus is usually just deep to the superior nuchal line. If this
venous sinus is encountered, simply place the screw. Attempting to formally repair this
sinus is fraught with complications.

II. TRANSARTICULAR C1-C2 SCREWS

In 1985 Magerl and Seeman (11) described the posterior C1-C2 transarticular screw
fixation technique that Magerl had been performing since the 1970s. This alternative in
the surgical management of patients with atlantoaxial instability profoundly increases

the stability of fixation compared to traditional wire constructs and eliminates the need for halo immobilization postoperatively. Traditional methods of atlantoaxial arthrodesis (AAA) include posterior C1-C2 wiring constructs such as the Gallie (12), Brooks-Jenkins (13), or interspinous method (14). Because of the significant mobility of the C1-C2 segment, most reported studies have been performed utilizing supplemental halo-vest immobilization with these techniques in order to improve fusion rates, however, failure rates for AAA with these methods have subsequently ranged from 3 to 80% (15–18). While biomechanical studies have demonstrated the Brooks-type fixation, with its wedge-compression grafting and sublaminar wire position at C2, to be more stable than the modified Gallie methods (19,20), all posterior C1-C2 wiring constructs loosen after cyclical loading and allow significant increases in C1-C2 rotational and translational motion (21). Flexible cables have increased the ease of sublaminar wire passage, and their use may thus decrease the rate of iatrogenic neurological deficit during wire passage, reported to be 5–7% (15,17). Concomitant atlas fractures or a deficient C1 posterior arch completely prevents utilization of these AAA methods. Transarticular screw fixation of C1-C2 avoids these complications of wire fixation.

This method requires an anatomical reduction intraoperatively to avoid-complications of vertebral artery (VA) injury, neurological deficit, or inadequate bony purchase. A precise drill trajectory is needed, entering at the posterior cortex of the C2 inferior articular process approximately 2 mm above the C2-C3 facet joint and 2–3 mm lateral to the medial border of the C2-C3 facet. This is then directed superiorly, down the axis of the C2 pars interarticularis, aiming toward the anterior arch of C1 (as viewed in a lateral image), with a 0–10 degree medial angulation. This is performed under biplane fluoroscopic imaging or with the use of a frameless stereotactic image-guidance system. This method of internal fixation does not require an intact posterior arch of C1 but, when used in conjunction with a posterior C1-C2 wiring, creates a very rigid three-point fixation system, providing immediate multidirectional stability. Biomechanical studies have demonstrated this method of internal fixation to be more rigid than posterior wiring techniques, particularly in rotation, where transarticular screws were noted to be 10-fold stiffer (22). Clinical results have reported fusion rates up to 100% with this method of AAA, along with the additional advantage that it avoids the need for any supplemental halo-vest immobilization (23,24).

C1-C2 transarticular screws are potentially the most dangerous screw inserted by spine surgeons because of the possibility of vertebral artery injury. They may be contraindicated unilaterally in up to 18% due to anomalous VA anatomy (25). Song and coworkers noted a 95% fusion rate among patients who underwent unilateral transarticular screw fixation due to anatomical constraints (26). Grob et al. (24), in one of the largest series of transarticular screw AAAs, reported no instance of VA or spinal cord injury, 6% other screw-related complications, and a pseudarthrosis rate of less than 1%. Despite its clinical and biomechanical advantages, this technique is technically demanding. In one recent survey, the risk of VA injury with this method was 4%, although the risk of subsequent neurological deficit after vascular injury was reported to be only 0.2% (27).

The C2 vertebral artery groove is anatomically highly variable. Because the C2 body is relatively narrow, the VA is more medial in the axis than in the subaxial spine. The artery travels in an almost transverse lateral direction into the transverse foramen of the atlas, crossing immediately anterior to the C2-C3 facet joint. The vertebral artery is located anterior to the pars interarticularis of C2, along the inferior portion of the superior facet. With an anomalous VA position forming a high-riding transverse foramen that significantly narrows the pars of C2, this would effectively preclude safe placement of a posterior C1-C2 transarticular screw. This is of great concern if transarticular C1-C2 screw fixation is considered. Before this technique of atlantoaxial fixation is performed, spiral computed tomography (CT) scanning with sagittal reconstructions is useful to look for this vascular anomaly (Fig. 4).

Vertebral artery injury may occur without an anomaly. A shallow trajectory or a lateral trajectory may injure a normally placed artery. Since the VA runs from medial to lateral just anterior to the entry point, a shallow (flat) trajectory could jeopardize the artery. If C1 is not anatomically reduced and slipped anterior to C2, a shallow trajectory is required to obtain entry into the lateral mass of C1, which risks injury to the artery. The VA is subject to injury in C2 at the beginning of the screw path. Lateral placement of the transarticular screw also places the VA at risk (Fig. 5). The optimal path is a very steep cephalad angulation with a slight [10°] medial path. Unilateral VA injury is usually tolerated without difficulty; however, bilateral VA injury can be fatal.

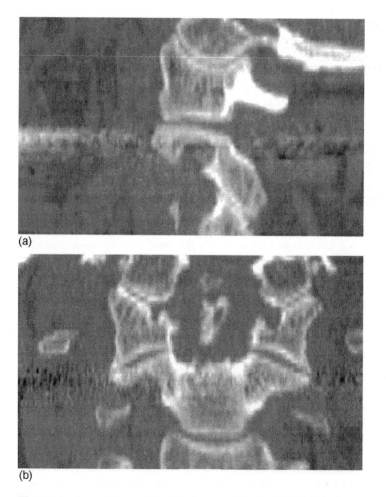

(a)

(b)

Figure 4 Anomalous vertebral artery position in C2. (a) Spiral computed tomography (CT) scan with sagittal reconstruction demonstrating a high-riding VA groove. (b) Coronal reconstruction with the high-riding VA groove and contralateral normal pars interarticularis of C2.

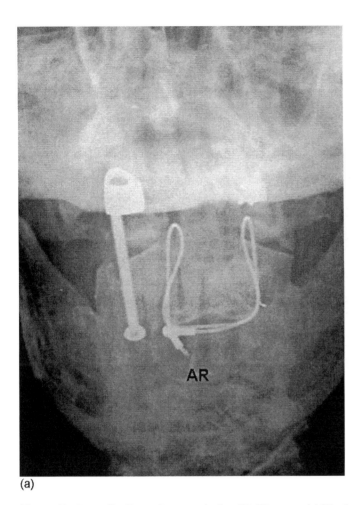

(a)

Figure 5   Laterally directed transarticular C1-C2 screw. (a) The laterally directed screw placed the VA at risk in C1. The contralateral side had a high-riding VA groove and was not appropriate for transarticular C1-C2 Screw insertion. (b) Postoperative CT scan demonstrating the screw in the lateral aspect of the lateral mass of C1.

A common problem after drilling across the C1-C2 joint occurs if a tap is then threaded across the joint. If significant instability is present, the tap will not enter the lateral mass of C1, but will simply push C1 cephalad and anterior. To avoid this problem, after drilling across the joint, the drill is kept in place to stabilize the segment while the contralateral side is drilled and tapped. If the first drill injures the vertebral artery, however, this may not be apparent with the drill bit blocking the hole. Thus, the first drill bit should be removed to look for injury and then replaced across the joint to stabilize it before drilling and tapping the contralateral side. If a VA injury occurs, place the screw across the joint (this will usually stop the bleeding) and obtain an angiogram postoperatively. It is extremely important to not drill across the contralateral joint if the VA is hit.

The hypoglossal nerve is at risk if the screw length is too long. The internal carotid artery also passes anterior to the C1 lateral mass on its way to the carotid foramen in the

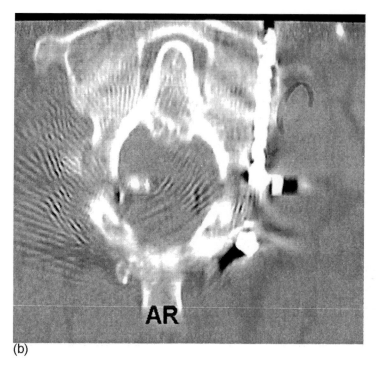

(b)

Figure 5 (*continued*)

base of the skull. Currier (27a) has recently shown in an anatomical study that the distance between the internal carotid artery and the anterior cortex of the center of the C1 lateral mass is 2–4 mm with the head and neck in neutral rotation.

III. OCCIPITOCERVICAL INSTRUMENTATION

A key principle to remember is that internal fixation only functions as an internal splint while the bone graft incorporates. The goal is to provide an environment that facilitates a solid occipitocervical arthrodesis. Autograft bone is the gold standard. Cement should not be used unless life expectancy is very short (< 6 weeks). An occipitocervical structural bone graft should be applied to optimize an early and exuberant fusion.

Intraoperative positioning is critical. Do not allow occipitocervical kyphosis. The patient is placed prone with a Mayfield pin headrest. Bicortical iliac crest autograft is harvested through a longitudinal incision over the posterior superior iliac spine. The occipitocervical spine is decorticated with a high-speed burr. The posterior cortex of the midline occiput is removed to expose bleeding cancellous bone. This thick area of the occiput has the optimal bone to serve as a foundation for the fusion. The posterior elements of C1 and C2 are also decorticated before the bicortical graft is laid down.

If a large area of the midline occiput is resected or if a laminectomy of C1 and C2 is performed, cancellous autograft slush can be placed laterally over the atlantoaxial joint extending cephalad onto the lateral aspect of the occiput. This bone graft is applied underneath and lateral to the plate or rod. A major advantage of screw-rod constructs is the extensive area available for the graft.

The bicortical iliac crest autograft plate is placed against the bleeding cancellous surface of the midline occiput between the two plates or rods. The caudal end of the graft is notched to allow it to straddle the posterior spinous process of C2. A bicortical occipital screw is drilled in the midline cephalad to the graft (just caudal to the superior nuchal line and underlying transverse sinus). A cable or wire is wrapped around the midline screw (two revolutions from being fully seated) and around the C2 posterior spinous process. The cable or wire is tightened over the bone graft plate to keep it in position. The midline occipital screw is then fully seated producing the final tightening of the construct. Alternatively, the midline occipital screw may be placed directly through the bone graft.

If a suboccipital decompression is performed, it is important to assure that the bone graft does not drop into the laminectomy defect because this may cause neurological comprise. The graft must be well seated on stable cancellous occipital bone and caudally onto solid lamina and posterior spinous process of C2. As the cable or wire is tightened down on top of the bicortical bone graft, the graft/host interface must have a large surface area and be very stable cephalad and caudad. If the graft is unstable or not long enough to span the defect, do not leave this potentially dangerous piece of bone over the dura. Morselize the bone graft plate and pack the cancellous graft over decorticated host bone safely, lateral to the spinal canal. As long as the occipitocervical instrumentation provides a stable environment, the morselized graft will heal.

IV. C1 LATERAL MASS SCREWS

Segmental fixation in the C1 lateral mass has recently gained wide interest due to the introduction of cervical polyaxial screw/rod instrumentation (28). In the 1980s Professor F. Magerl placed AO 3.5 mm cortical screws into the C1 lateral mass, but had no stable way to connect this anchor to C2 other than wrapping a wire around the screw head and the posterior arch of C2 (F. Magerl, personal communication). Due to the anatomy of the C2 nerve root, a plate/screw device cannot be tightened down onto the posterior elements without compressing the nerve under the plate. With the advent of screw/rod devices that rigidly attach the screw to the rod, a stable construct can be applied across the C1-C2 joint without damaging the C2 nerve. These constructs do not rely on the longitudinal member to be compressed onto the posterior elements by bicortical screws for stability, but are positioned posteriorly off of the bone with room for bone graft and the C2 nerve underneath the construct.

The exposure of the entry point for the C1 lateral mass screw requires precise knowledge of the anatomy of the occipitocervical junction. Although most spine surgeons are very comfortable exposing the C1-C2 joint from a caudal to cephalad orientation because this is the transarticular C1-C2 screw approach, exposing the joint from cephalad to caudal is not a traditional experience. The three-dimensional relationship between the lateral mass of C1 and its posterior arch is extremely important to understand, as is the neurovascular anatomy of C1-C2. The vertebral artery emerges from the transverse foramen of the atlas and courses medially on the anterior portion of the superior surface of the posterior ring. Dissection on the cephalad aspect of the posterior aspect of C1 should not extend more than 12 mm lateral to the midline. The dissection laterally on the posterior arch of C1 should be on the middle to caudal aspect to avoid the vertebral artery. Dissection caudally to the joint requires a significant anterior course from the lateral aspect of the posterior arch to the lateral mass of C1 (Fig. 6). During this exposure, the extensive venous plexus surrounding the C2 nerve root may be the source of

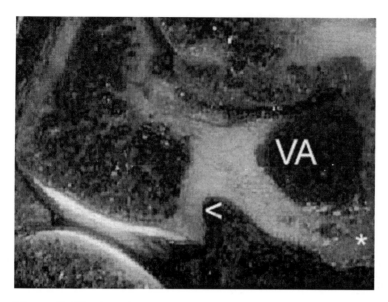

Figure 6 The lateral mass of C1 ($<$) is extremely far anterior to the posterior arch (*).
VA = vertebral artery.

significant bleeding. Subperiosteal dissection to the joint, which is far anterior from the lateral aspect of the posterior arch of C1, is mandatory to mobilize the C2 nerve with its venous plexus. Once exposure of the posterior aspect of the C1 lateral mass is achieved, the C2 nerve with its venous leash can be pulled caudally to expose the joint. The proper entry point for the screw is at the cephalad aspect of the lateral mass, at the base of the posterior arch (Fig. 7). In order to allow a more horizontal trajectory for the screw and to position the screw head cephalad to the C2 nerve, the inferior aspect of the posterior arch of C1 is burred away. This creates a home to nestle the polyaxial screw head. Do not remove too much of the C1 posterior arch because the vertebral artery is positioned in the cephalad groove (Fig. 8). After a recess is created in the caudal aspect of the dorsal arch of C1 and the C2 nerve root is retracted inferiorly, aim for the midpoint of the C1 tubercle. Bicortical purchase is optimal. Connect this screw to a C2 pars or pedicle screw through a longitudinal connector (Fig. 9).

V. C2 PARS VERSUS PEDICLE SCREWS

Before detailing the potential complications of inserting various types of instrumentation into C2, it is mandatory to differentiate between a screw placed into the C2 pars interarticularis and one placed into the C2 pedicle. This has not been clear in previous literature and has been used interchangeably to describe the same screw position. These screw sites, however, are not identical and possess distinct challenges of insertion and different potential complications.

The confusion between the positions of these screw types lies in the unique anatomy of the C2 vertebra. As long as the standard definitions of pars interarticularis and pedicle are kept in mind, however, the differentiation of these two structures is very clear. The pars

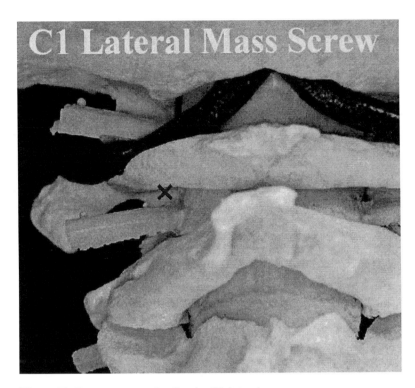

Figure 7 Proper entry point for the C1 lateral mass screw.

interarticularis is the region of bone between the superior and inferior articular processes. The pedicle is the region of bone that connects the posterior elements to the vertebral body. Because the superior articular process of C2 is extremely far anterior, the pars interarticularis is very large. This anterior position of the superior articular process also creates a very narrow and short window for connection to the C2 body—the pedicle (Fig. 10).

The C2 pars interarticularis screw is in the exact same position as a transarticular C1-C2 screw, detailed above, except that it stops short of the joint. The entry point is the same (2–3 mm superior and 2–3 mm lateral to the medial aspect of the C2-3 facet joint). Since the greatest danger for injury to the vertebral artery is in C2 when a transarticular C1-2 screw is placed, the exact same incidence of injury is present for C2 pars screws. It is a shorter version of the transarticular screw.

The C2 pedicle screw follows the path of the pedicle into the vertebral body. For a screw to be inserted into the C2 vertebral body from the posterior elements, it by definition has to pass through the pedicle. The entry point is significantly cephalad to the entrance for the pars screw and slightly lateral. The medial angulation is significantly more than that of the pars screw, approximately 30 degrees, while the pars screw is placed almost straight ahead. This cephalad starting point and medial angulation makes the pedicle screw less likely to injure the vertebral artery. The artery runs from medial to lateral in front of the C2-3 facet joint. Since the pedicle screw starts cephalad, the artery is more likely to have traveled lateral to the starting point compared to the pars screw (where the artery may be medial or just anterior to the starting point), and the screw is running away (medial) from the artery as it enters the pedicle. The pars screw does not have a steep medial trajectory and is thus closer to the artery as it moves toward the superior articular process (Fig. 11).

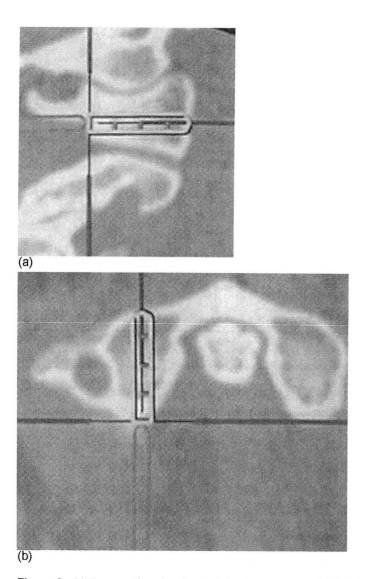

(a)

(b)

Figure 8   (a) Preoperative plan for C1 lateral mass screw. (b) Axial view of preoperative plan.

Another advantage of the C2 pedicle screw is that because the cephalad trajectory is not as steep (approximately 30° compared to >45° with the pars screw), the pedicle screw can usually be placed through the incision. The pars and transarticular screws need to have a very steep cephalad trajectory to keep them away from the vertebral artery. This usually requires them to be placed through percutaneous stab incisions at the cervicothoracic junction.

VI. SUBAXIAL LATERAL MASS SCREWS

Several techniques for placement of lateral mass screws have been published (29–31). The Roy-Camille technique starts the screw in the center of the lateral mass and directs

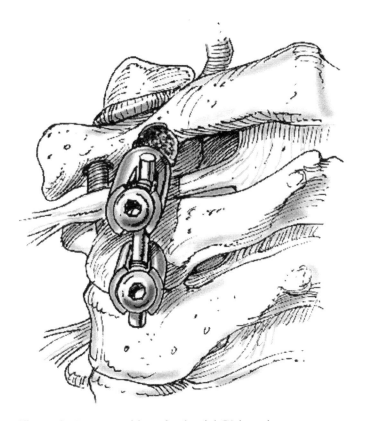

Figure 9 Proper position of polyaxial C1 lateral mass screw connected to a C2 anchor.

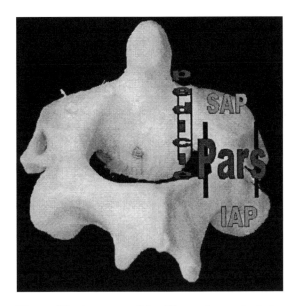

Figure 10 Anatomy of the C2 pars interarticularis and pedicle (SAP = superior articular process; IAP = inferior articular process).

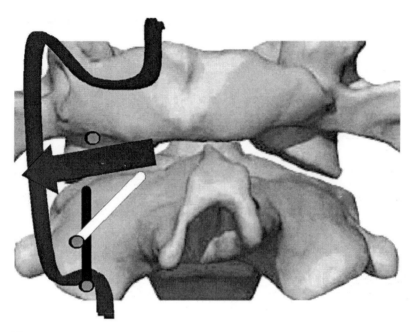

Figure 11 The starting points and trajectory for C2 pars (dark) and pedicle (white) screws. The curved line is the vertebral artery. The arrow is the C2 nerve root. The gray dot above the arrow is the starting point for the C1 lateral mass screw.

it 10 degrees laterally and perpendicular to the posterior cortex of the articular mass. With Magerl's technique, the screw is inserted 2–3 mm medial and superior to the center of the lateral mass. This screw is directed 25 degrees laterally and oriented superiorly 40–60 degrees (parallel to the articular surface of the facet joint). Bicortical fixation is advised (32). An et al. (31) set out to find the screw trajectory that would be safest for the nerve roots. They found that the nerve root exits at the anterolateral portion of the superior facet. They postulated that the ideal exit point of the drill should be the juncture between the foramen transversarium and the facet. They recommended that the screw be inserted 30 degrees lateral and 15 degrees cephalad, starting 1 mm medial to the center of the lateral mass for C3-C6 to avoid the nerve root and the facet joint. Heller et al. (33) compared the Roy-Camille and Magerl techniques during simulated operating room conditions. They found that both techniques were quite safe in terms of injury to the spinal cord or to the vertebral artery. The Roy-Camille technique had less risk of injury to the nerve root, and the Magerl technique had less risk of violation of the facet joint.

Posterior cervical plating systems have enjoyed success spanning short segments with a strong biomechanical profile (34–38). They are relatively easy and safe to apply in the lateral mass, with minimal complications reported in the subaxial cervical spine (39–41). When spanning long or transitional segments such as the occipitocervical or cervico-thoracic junctions, however, profound technical difficulties can occur. The necessity of placing multiple screws in very specific locations at steep and various angles away from the plane of the plate make these traditional posterior cervical devices ineffective.

Posterior cervical screw/rod systems were developed to address the inadequacies of plate constructs. The fundamental problems of posterior cervical plates are:

1. Fixed hole-to-hole distance with difficulty placing anchors (screws) along the length of the plate when it spans multiple segments.
2. Limited ability to direct screws divergent from the screw holes, especially when screws are placed into different structures (lateral mass and pedicle) along the same plate.
3. Non-rigid connection between the screw and longitudinal member (plate).
4. Lack of adequate space for bone graft over the facet joints after the plate is screwed down onto the dorsal surface of the lateral mass.
5. Inability to capture an anchor that is medial or lateral to the longitudinal member (the screw has to go through the plate hole).
6. Requirement of removing and replacing the screw if a plate change occurs.
7. The inability to compress or distract the screws relative to each other once they have been placed.

The ideal posterior stabilization device allows the screw to be driven into the perfect position at the proper trajectory and then not removed as the longitudinal member is attached. This can only be accomplished with a rod-based system.

Placement of screws in appropriate cervical anatomical structures such as the lateral mass and pedicle is more precise with less tolerance for error than in the lumbar pedicles. Techniques and instrumentation that allow perfect application of screws in the posterior cervical spine will decrease the incidence of screw-related complications. A major disadvantage of plate-based systems is the necessity of screws traversing through the plate holes with fixed hole-to-hole distance and trajectory. This characteristic of plate systems may lead to higher screw misplacement. Graham et al. (42) reported a 6.1% lateral mass screw malposition rate using a plate-based system with a 1.8% per screw rate of radiculopathy. Rod-based systems theoretically should improve on this malposition rate due to the ability to place the screws anywhere along the rod without the constraint of driving the screws through fixed holes. Rod-based systems that allow screws to be fixed at any of a range of orientations relative to the rod should also improve the malposition rate by permitting proper trajectory of the screw. Interfacet variability is a significant anatomical factor. Even with a large choice of plates, it may not be possible to place a screw in each lateral mass, and screw position, on occasion, may not be optimal. Plates with oblong rather than circular holes were created to accommodate the variability in interfacet distance, but this is still restrictive. A screw-rod connection permits the screws to be inserted in the ideal position with regard to interfacet distance and not constrained by plate-hole distances.

The biomechanical characteristics of a posterior cervical screw/rod device have been carefully evaluated by Grubb et al. (43). An in vitro biomechanical investigation with nondestructive and destructive testing in a human cadaveric model determined the relative stability of a posterior cervical spinal rod system and posterior cervical screw/plate construct. Significantly greater stability was noted in the cervical rod construct during nondestructive and destructive flexural testing despite unicortical screw fixation in the cervical rod group and bicortical fixation in the reconstruction plate group. Gill et al. (36) have shown that bicortical lateral mass screw fixation is stiffer than unicortical fixation. Despite the biomechanical disadvantage of unicortical purchase in the rod group, no detectable differences in stability between the reconstruction plate and the cervical rod could be found during torsional and lateral bending nondestructive testing. With nondestructive and destructive flexural bending, however, the cervical rod construct showed improved stability. As a result of the design of the lateral mass connector, the cervical rod sits approximately 3-4 mm dorsal to the lateral mass. This feature gives the construct a greater bending moment of inertia in the sagittal plane and allows space for bone graft.

Modern posterior cervical systems (2) allow insertion of the lateral mass screws completely independent of the longitudinal member. This assures that the screw is placed in the most ideal position according to the local anatomy. Once the screw is seated, it does not have to be modified. The rod is simply dropped onto the screws. It is important to be able to capture the rod directly onto the screw or in any manner medial or lateral. Changes of height and alignment between the screws need to be accommodated by the system (polyaxial screws and offset connectors) rather than by changing position of the screws. Complications of the instrumentation such as rod fracture or screw breakage are extremely rare with current systems.

VII. SUBAXIAL PEDICLE SCREWS

Lateral mass screws are extremely strong and are the safest screws that spine surgeons implant. In rare instances, however, subaxial pedicle screws may be appropriate, such as in cases of destruction of the lateral mass. Therefore, spine surgeons should be very knowledgeable about the proper application of cervical subaxial pedicle screws and also understand the potential significant complications associated with their insertion. Transpedicular fixation of the cervical spine poses a particular challenge to surgeons due to the close proximity of the cervical pedicle to the spinal cord, nerve roots, and vertebral arteries. Due to the small margin of error allowed for ideal cervical pedicle screw placement, even small miscalculations can result in a vascular or neural injury. Therefore, intimate knowledge of the cervical pedicles is important. Ludwig et al. compared the accuracy of three different techniques for placing pedicle screws in cadaveric specimens (44). With screws placed based on morphometric data alone, 12.5% of the screws were placed entirely within the pedicle; 21.9% had a noncritical breach; and 65% had a critical breach. In this study, "critical" is defined as encroachment of the vertebral artery, nerve root, or spinal cord by the screw, while "noncritical" is violation of the pedicle cortex without injury to surrounding vital structures. In the second technique (lamino-foraminotomy), 45% of the screws were within the pedicle; 15.4% had a noncritical breach; and 39.6% had a critical breach. In the third technique (computer-assisted surgical guidance system), 76% of the screws were placed entirely within the pedicle; 13.4% had a noncritical breach; and 10.6% had a critical breach.

Abumi et al. in 1994 was the first to report placement of pedicle screws in the subaxial spine (45). Thirteen patients with fractures/dislocation of the middle and lower cervical spine underwent transpedicular screw fixation. The angle of Abumi's cervical pedicle screws ranged from 25 degrees to 45 degrees medial to the midline in the transverse plane. All patients had solid fusion without loss of correction at an average of 22 months follow-up. Despite three cortical breaches of the 52 screws that were placed, no neurological or vascular complications were observed. This study demonstrated that safe and successful placement of cervical pedicle screws was possible. Nevertheless, current data seem to indicate that unless one is intimately familiar with cervical pedicle anatomy and is well versed in cervical pedicle screw placement, this fixation option should be performed sparingly.

A significant problem with cervical pedicle screw insertion is medial angulation. Whereas lateral mass screws are angulated laterally so that your hand is toward the midline, profound lateral dissection of the soft tissues is required to allow the proper medial trajectory for the pedicle screw. The soft tissues tend to force your hand medial, thus decreasing the medial angulation. This may place the lateral vertebral artery at risk.

Pedicle screw insertion at C7 is much more reasonable because the pedicle is larger and the foramen transversarium usually does not contain the vertebral artery. Also, the lateral mass is slightly smaller. Note, however, that 10% of the population has a VA in the C7 foramen transversarium.

ANNOTATED BIBLIOGRAPHY

Occipitocervical Fusion Technique

Sasso RC, Jeanneret B, Fischer K, Magerl F. Occipitocervical fusion with posterior plate and screw instrumentation: a long-term follow-up Study. Spine 1994; 19:2364–2368.

> 32 patients with average 50-month follow-up
> OC fusion with plates and screws—Magerl transarticular C1–C2 technique
> No halos
> All fused with no neurological complications

Apostolides PJ, Dickman CA, Golfinos JG, Papadopoulos SM, Sonntag VK. Threaded Steinman pin fusion of the craniovertebral junction. Spine 1996; 21:1630–1637.

> 39 patients with average 38-month follow-up
> OC fusion with Steinman pin wired to occiput and cervical laminae
> Postoperative halo—34 patients; only 5 patients treated without postoperative halo
> 35 fused; 2 "fibrous union"; 1 nonunion; 1 death

Song GS, Theodore N, Dickman CA, Sonntag VK. Unilateral posterior atlantoaxial transarticular screw fixation. J Neurosurg 1997; 87:851–855.

> 19 patients with atlantoaxial instability
> Unilateral transarticular screw with interspinous bone graft wiring and Philadelphia collars
> 18 patients—solid fusion
> No operative, postoperative neurovascular complications

Robertson SC, Menezes AH. Occipital calvarial bone graft in posterior occipitocervical fusion. Spine 1998; 23:249–255.

> 25 patients with split-thickness, autologous calvarial bone grafts with contoured loop and
>   cable
> 7 halo, 12 Minerva vest, 6 Philadelphia collar
> 22 of 25 "stable"
> No complications from harvest site

Casey AT, Hayward RD, Harkness WF, Crockard HA. The use of autologous skull bone grafts for posterior fusion of the upper cervical spine in children. Spine 1995; 20:2217–2220.

> 7 pediatric patients
> Autologous calvarial bone secured with sublaminar wires
> Halo for 3 months
> 100% fusion
> No morbidity due to graft harvest

Lowry DW, Pollack IF, Clyde B, Albright AL, Adelson PD. Upper cervical spine fusion in the pediatric population. J Neurosurg 1997; 87:671–676.

> 25 pediatric patients
> Os odontoideum (11), rotatory subluxation (5), Down syndrome (4), odontoid fracture (2), atlanto-occipital dislocation (2), other (1)
> 21 of 25 solid fusion
> Failures due to wire cut-through of C1 arch in 2; halo complication in 2

Dormans JP, Drummond DS, Sutton LN, Ecker ML, Kopacz KJ. Occipitocervical arthrodesis in children. JBJS 1995; 77A:1234–1240.

> 16 pediatric patients
> OC fusion with autogenous iliac crest and postoperative halo
> 15 of 16 patients fused
> Complications in 7 patients

Subaxial Pedicle Screws

Kotani Y, Cunningham BW, Abumi K, McAfee PC. Biomechanical analysis of cervical stabilization systems. An assessment of transpedicular screw fixation in the cervical spine. Spine 1994; 19:2529–2539.

> Anterior plating methods provided less stability than that of posterior constructs under axial, torsional, and flexural loading conditions.
> Exclusive posterior procedures provided increased stability compared with the intact spine in one level fixation.

Abumi K, Itoh H, Taneichi H, Kaneda K. Transpedicular screw fixation for traumatic lesions of the middle and lower cervical spine: description of the technique and preliminary report. J Spinal Disord 1994; 7:19–28.

> Thirteen patients with traumatic injuries of the middle or lower cervical spine were treated with transpedicular screw fixation using the Steffee variable screw system. Nerve function and correction of deformity was satisfactory in all the patients. Solid fusion and correction of deformity occurred in all 13.

Ebraheim NA, Xu R, Knight T, Yeasting. Morphometric evaluation of lower cervical pedicle and its projection. Spine 1997; 22:1-6.

> This study evaluated the lower cervical pedicle from C3 to C6 to provide information for accurate transpedicular screw fixation in this area. The authors found statistically significant differences in the dimensions of the C6 pedicle height and the pedicle sagittal angle of C4 when comparing males and females, suggesting that standard screw application techniques cannot be advocated and preoperative detailed imaging is necessary to avoid screw misplacement.

Jeanneret B, Gebhard JS, Magerl F. Transpedicular screw fixation of articular mass fracture-separation: results of an anatomical study and operative technique. J Spinal Disord 1994; 7:222–229.

> After placing 33 screws in cadaver cervical spine pedicles, Jeanneret and colleagues concluded that transpedicular screw fixation of the lower cervical spine is safe and effective using an entry point 3 mm below the facet joint on a vertical line in the middle of the articular mass with the drill angled medially approximately 45°.

Miller RM, Ebraheim NA, Xu R, Yeasting RA. Anatomic consideration of transpedicular screw placement in the cervical spine. Spine 1996; 21:2317–2322.

> Using 40 cervical vertebrae from eight cadaveric specimens, the authors compared the effectiveness of blind transpedicular screw placement and transpedicular screw placement using partial laminectomy and tapping technique. Although still relatively high, they found a decrease in the incidence of screw violations using the laminectomy and tapping technique. They concluded that this technique should not be used routinely.

REFERENCES

1. Sasso RC, Jeanneret B, Fischer K, Magerl F. Occipitocervical fusion with posterior plate and screw instrumentation: a long-term follow-up study. Spine 1994; 19:2364–2368.
2. Mummaneni PV, Haid RW, Traynelis VC, Sasso RC, Subach BR, Fiore AJ, Rodts GE. Posterior cervical fixation using a new polyaxial screw and rod system: technique and surgical results. Neurosurg Focus 2002; 12:Article 8 (1-5).
3. Hulbert RJ, Crawford NR, Choi WG, Dickman CA. A biomechanical evaluation of occipitocervical instrumentation: screw compared with wire fixation. J Neurosurg 1999; 90:84–90.
4. Sutterlin CE 3rd, Bianchi JR, Kunz DN, Zdeblick TA,Johnson WM, Rapoff AJ. Biomechanical evaluation of occipitocervical fixation devices. J Spinal Disord 2001; 14(3): 185–192.
5. Bednar D, Parikh J, Hummel J. Management of type II odontoid process fractures in geriatric patients: a prospective study of sequential cohorts with attention to survivorship. J Spinal Disord 1995; 8:166–169.
6. Seybold EA, Bayley JC. Functional outcome of surgically and conservatively managed dens fractures. Spine 1998; 23:1837–1846.
7. Naderi S, Pamir MN. Further cranial settling of the upper cervical spine following odontoidectomy. Report of two cases. J Neurosurg. 2001; 95(2 suppl):246–249.
8. Roberts DA, Doherty BJ, Heggeness MH. Quantitative anatomy of the occiput and the biomechanics of occipital screw fixation. Spine 1998; 23:1100–1108.
9. Haher TR, Yeung AW, Caruso SA, Merola AA, Shin T, Zipnick RI, Gorup JM, Bono C. Occipital screw pullout strength: a biomechanical investigation of occipital morphology. Spine 1999; 24:5–9.
10. Oda I, Abumi K, Sell LC, Haggerty CJ, Cunningham BW, McAfee PC. Biomechanical evaluation of five different occipito-atlanto-axial fixation techniques. Spine 1999; 24:2377–2382.
11. Magerl F, Seeman PS. Stable posterior fusion at the atlas and axis by transarticular fixation. In: Kehr P, Weidner A, eds. Cervical Spine I. New York: Springer-Verlag, 1985:322–327.
12. Gallie WE. Fracture and dislocations of the cervical spine. Am J Surg 1939; 46:495–499.
13. Brooks AL, Jenkins EB. Atlantoaxial arthrodesis by the wedge compression method. J Bone Joint Surg 1978; 60A:279–284.
14. Dickman CA, Papadopoulos SM, Sonntag VK, et al. The interspinous method of posterior atlanto-axial arthrodesis. J Neurosurg 1991; 74:190–198.
15. Fielding JW, Hawkins RJ, Ratzan SA. Spine fusion for atlanto-axial instability. J Bone Joint Surg 1976; 58A:400–407.
16. Fried LC. Atlanto-axial fractures. Failure of posterior C1 to C2 fusion.. J Bone Joint Surg 1973; 55B:490–496.
17. Griswold DM, Albright JA, Schiffman E. Atlantoaxial fusion for instability. J Bone Joint Surg 1978; 60A:258–292.
18. Dickman CA, Crawford NR, Paramore CG. Biomechanical characteristics of C1-C2 cable fixations. J Neurosurg 1996; 85:316–321.

19. Grob D, Crisco JJ, Panjabi MM, Wang P, Dvorak J. Biomechanical evaluation of four different posterior atlanto-axial fixation techniques. Spine 1992; 17:480–490.
20. Hajeck PD, Lipka J, Hartline P, Saha S, Albright JA. Biomechanical study of C1-C2 posterior arthrodesis techniques. Spine 1993; 18:173–177.
21. Crawford NR, Hurlbert RJ, Choi WG, Dickman CA. Differential biomechanical effects of injury and wiring at C1-C2. Spine 1999; 24:1894–1902.
22. Hanson PB, Montesano PX, Sharkey NA, et al. Anatomic and biomechanical assessment of transarticular screw fixation for atlanto-axial instability. Spine 16 1991; 1141–1145.
23. Marcotte P, Dickman CA, Sonntag VK, et al. Posterior atlantoaxial screw fixation. J Neurosurg 1993; 79:234–237.
24. Grob D, Jeanneret B, Aebi M, et al. Atlantoaxial fusion with transarticular screw fixation. J Bone Joint Surg 1991; 73B:972–976.
25. Paramore CG, Dickman CA, Sonntag VKH. The anatomic suitability of the C1/C2 complex for transarticular screw fixation. J Neurosurg 1996; 95:221–224.
26. Song GS, Theodore N, Dickman CA, Sonntag VK. Unilateral posterior atlantoaxial transarticular screw fixation. J Neurosurg 1997; 87:851–855.
27. Wright NM, Lauryssen C. Vertebral artery injury in C1/C2 transarticular screw fixation: results of a survey of the AANS/CNS section on disorders of the spine and peripheral nerves. J Neurosurg 1998; 88:634–640.
27a. Currier BL, Todd LT, Maus TP, Fisher DR, Yaszemski MJ. Anatomic relationship of the internal carotid artery to the C1 vertebra: a case report of cervical reconstruction for chordoma and pilot study to assess the risk of screw fixation of the atlas. Spine 2003; 28(22):E461–E467.
28. Harms J, Melcher P. Posterior C1-C2 fusion with polyaxial screw and rod fixation. Spine 2001; 26:2467–2471.
29. Magerl F, Grob D, Seemann P. Stable dorsal fusion of the cervical spine (C2-T1) using hook plates. In: Kehr P, Weidner A, eds. Cervical Spine I. Urenna: Springer-Verlag, 1987:217–221.
30. Roy-Camille R, Saillant G, Mazel C. Internal fixation of the unstable cervical spine by a posterior osteosynthesis with plates and screws. In: Shork MM, ed. The Cervical Spine. 2nd ed. Philadelphia: J.B. Lippincott Company, 1989:390–403.
31. An HS, Gordin R, Renner K. Anatomic considerations for plate-screw fixation of the cervical spine. Spine 1991; 16:S548–S551.
32. Heller JG, Estes BT, Zaouali M, Fliers RD, Diop A. Biomechanical study of screws in the lateral masses: variables affecting pullout resistance. J Bone Joint Surg (Am) 1996; 78:1315–1321.
33. Heller JG, Carlson GD, Abitbol JJ, Garfin SR. Anatomic comparison of the Roy-Camille and Magerl techniques for screw placement in the lower cervical spine. Spine 1991; 16:S552–S557.
34. Ulrich C, Woersdoerfer O, Kalff R, Claes L, Wilke H. Biomechanics of fixation systems to the cervical spine. Spine 1991; 16:S4–S9.
35. Sutterlin CE III, McAfee PC, Warden KE, Rey RM, Farey D. A biomechanical evaluation of cervical spinal stabilization methods in a bovine model: static and cyclical loading. Spine 1988; 13:795–802.
36. Gill K, Paschal S, Corin J, Ashman R, Bucholz W. Posterior plating of the cervical spine: a biomechanical comparison of different posterior fusion techniques. Spine 1988; 13:813–816.
37. Montesano PX, Juach MS, Anderson PA, Benson DR, Hanson PB. Biomechanics of cervical spine internal fixation. Spine 1991; 16:S10–S16.
38. Coe JD, Warden KE, Sutterlin III CE, McAfee PC. Biomechanical evaluation of cervical stabilization methods in a human cadaveric model. Spine 1989; 14:1122–1131.
39. Swank ML, Sutterlin CE, Bossons CR, Dials BE. Rigid internal fixation with lateral mass plates in multilevel anterior and posterior reconstruction of the cervical spine. Spine 1995; 22:274–282.
40. Heller JG, Silcox DH, Sutterlin CE. Complications of posterior cervical plating. Spine 1995; 20:2442–2448.
41. Wellman BJ, Follett KA, Traynelis VC. Complications of posterior articular mass plate fixation of the subaxial cervical spine in 43 consecutive patients. Spine 1998; 23:193–200.

42. Graham AW, Swank ML, Kinard RE, Lowery GL, Dials BE. Posterior cervical arthrodesis and stabilization with a lateral mass plate: clinical and computed tomographic evaluation of lateral mass screw placement and associated complications. Spine 1996; 21:323–328.

43. Grubb MR, Currier BL, Stone J, Warden KE, An KN. Biomechanical evaluation of posterior cervical stabilization after a wide laminectomy. Spine 1997; 22:1948–1954.

44. Ludwig SC, Kowalski JM, Edwards CC, In: Heller JG ed. Cervical pedicle screws: comparative accuracy of two insertion techniques. 2nd ed. Spine 2000; 25:2675–2681.

45. Abumi K, Itoh H, Taneichi H, Kaneda K. Transpedicular screw fixation for traumatic lesions of the middle and lower cervical spine: description of the techniques and preliminary report. J Spinal Disord 1994; 7:19–28.

22
Complications Relating to the Treatment of Odontoid Fractures

Gannon B. Randolph and Darrel S. Brodke
University of Utah, Salt Lake City, Utah, U.S.A.

I. INTRODUCTION

Fracture of the odontoid process of the second cervical vertebra is a common injury encountered by the spine surgeon. A recent multicenter study of 33,922 blunt trauma admissions demonstrated cervical spine injuries in 2.4% (1). Of those patients, up to 10% may have an injury of the odontoid process or atlantoaxial complex (2). It is likely that all surgeons managing cervical trauma will be faced with this type of injury and will need to counsel patients on the risks of complications in their selected treatment. In this chapter we hope to shed light on the risks and complications involved in odontoid fractures and in their management by nonoperative, posterior operative, and anterior operative based treatment strategies.

The study of the pathophysiology and treatment of odontoid fractures is not new. Orfila is reported to have described the fracture pattern in cadaveric hanging studies he conducted in 1848. Organized evaluation, treatment, and classification of odontoid fractures would not be undertaken until over 100 years later with the seminal work of Anderson and D'Alanzo in 1974 (3). They described three types of injuries to the odontoid process that form the basis of the most commonly used classification system of odontoid fractures. We will use their classification for descriptive purposes throughout the remainder of this chapter (Fig. 1).

Treatment of odontoid fractures has undergone radical change in the 30 years since Anderson and D'Alanzo's work. Whereas most fractures were historically treated with immobilization methods, surgical intervention is now becoming the preferred treatment option. This stems from the greater success of surgical treatment, especially anterior screw fixation, in achieving bony union while preserving some motion in the atlantoaxial joint (4–7). However, posterior cervical fusion remains the gold standard against which the success and complication rate of anterior procedures must be measured. Nonoperative treatment also remains a viable option in selected types of odontoid fractures. It avoids the inherent risks assumed with incision, dissection, and hardware placement.

Type I

Type II

Type III

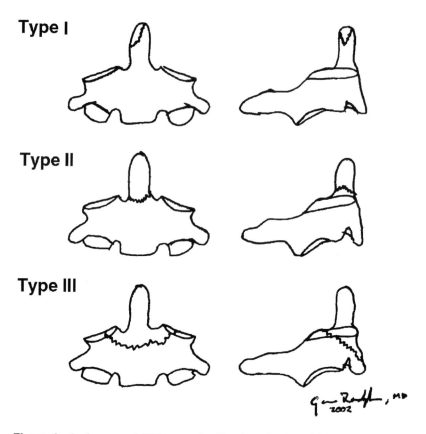

Figure 1 Anderson and D'Alanzo classification of odontoid fractures.

II. ANATOMY AND BIOMECHANICS OF AN ODONTOID FRACTURE

The C2 vertebra (axis) is the strongest cervical vertebra (8). The tooth-shaped odontoid process, or dens (Greek for tooth), is a superior process that intimately articulates with the anterior arch of the C1 vertebra (atlas). This articulation provides roughly 50% of the rotation in the cervical spine. Normal rotation from midline averages 43° to either side, with >65° of rotation required for dislocation of the atlantoaxial joint. Several strong ligaments, including the transverse, alar, and apical ligaments, hold the odontoid in close approximation with the atlas. These ligaments and their vectors of restraint are responsible for the differing fracture patterns of the odontoid.

The Anderson and D'Alanzo classification system describes three main fracture patterns (3). A great deal of work, most recently using supercomputer-aided finite element analysis, has been done in an attempt to elucidate the mechanism of injury in these three fracture types. Type I fractures are felt to be due to traumatic force applied in lateral shear or compression with the head in an extended position and caused by alar ligament avulsion at their insertion onto the odontoid (9). Type II fractures have been reproduced by axially rotating the head and applying a traumatic force in the lateral or oblique directions (~45°) (4,9,10). The exact mechanism of type III fractures remains poorly understood but has been reproduced with traumatic extension of the neck (4,9,10).

It is known that traumatic flexion can cause odontoid fracture as well, but there is no consistent type of injury that occurs with this mechanism.

III. DEFINITION OF COMPLICATIONS

A complication is defined as "a morbid process or event occurring during a disease that is not an essential part of the disease, although it may result from it or from independent causes" (11). In surgery the added connotation involves those morbid processes or events that are due to unexpected technical errors occurring before, during, or after a therapeutic or diagnostic procedure. This includes failure of the procedure to achieve the desired result. The potential number of complications in difficult injuries, such as the odontoid fracture, is nearly limitless. However, there is a spectrum of complications that are well defined and frequently associated with the injury and its treatment. In the surgical literature, the prevention of some of these complications, namely nonunion and neurological injury, are paramount in measuring the success of treatment.

Most scientific observations of complications associated with the natural history and treatment of odontoid fractures are divided into two broad categories: major and minor complications. There is no general consensus as to which complications fit into each of these categories. Some authors call a wound infection that required a return to the operating suite but did not require revision or removal of hardware a minor complication. We, however, believe any complication that requires a return to surgery and the concomitant risks of anesthesia to be a major complication. In general, major complications relate to injuries that are permanent or life-threatening (e.g., death or unresolving neurological injury), require another operation, or injure other organ systems (e.g., brain, GI, or vascular) (Table 1). Minor complications are usually self-limited, although they may require pharmacological treatment (e.g., pain or minor infection), or associated with

Table 1   Major Complications of Odontoid Fracture and Treatment

Nonunion
Malunion
Dural tear requiring reoperation
Death
Respiratory compromise
Failure of hardware or brace
Permanent neurological injury
Stroke
Spinal cord injury
Vascular injury
Gastrointestinal injury
Infection requiring reoperation
Major bleeding
Shock
Outcome with loss of independence or significant change in ADL's
Missed injury
Major anesthesia complications

Table 2 Minor Complications of
Odontoid Fracture and Treatment

Pain
Infection not requiring reoperation
Resolving or temporary neurological injury
Minor bleeding
Dural tear not requiring reoperation
Minor anesthesia complications
Decreased range of motion
Delayed union
Adjacent segment arthritis
Excessive length of procedure
Hygiene problems
Dysphagia
Pseudo arthrosis of C1 on C2
Pin loosening
Maceration or ulceration of skin

small technical errors at the time of surgery (e.g., minor bleeding or dural tear not requiring reoperation) (Table 2).

IV. NATURAL HISTORY OF AN ODONTOID FRACTURE

A minority of odontoid fractures that present to the spinal surgeon have resultant neurological injury. These few neurological injuries are likely often catastrophic in terms of respiratory function and result in death at the scene of the accident. Most authors feel that the majority of patients who suffer injuries to the odontoid process survive long enough to be medically evaluated. There may be a higher risk of neurological injury in a patient with an odontoid fracture that goes on to pseudoarthrosis, especially in the setting of reinjury. Evidence comes from studies of patients who present remote from their causitive injury with complications. In 1993 Crockard et al. evaluated 16 patients who presented with late complications 4–540 months after their original injury (12). Fifteen of 16 patients had moderate to intractable neck pain upon presentation. Eleven patients had evidence of myelopathy on neurological exam. Other neurological findings included bulbar palsy and profound tetraplegia. It is important to note that after treatment only 4 of 11 patients (36%) had complete resolution of their neurological deficits.

In 1996 Fairholm et al. evaluated a series of 51 patients from Tapei, China, who presented late with neurological deterioration from undiagnosed traumatic odontoid fractures (13). The majority of these patients also presented with neck pain. None of the patients had a neurological deficit at the time of their original injury, which averaged 4.1 years prior to evaluation (range 2 months to 40 years). There was a broad spectrum of neurological injury. To quote the original article, "Although a few presented with unilateral or focal long tract involvement, a progressive continuum of change led to tetraparesis or tetraplegia with respiratory failure." Twenty-four of the patients had tetraparesis (47%), and 8 (18%) had tetraplegia with respiratory complications. Four patients died, and a significant number had residual neurological dysfunction after treatment. These studies illustrate the risk of major complications associated with failure to diagnose and treat odontoid fractures. They also highlight the limited neurological recovery that can be expected if the injury is not treated acutely.

V. NONOPERATIVE MANAGEMENT

Prior to modern surgical approaches to the upper cervical spine and current instrumentation, nonoperative management was the only tool available for the treatment of odontoid fracture. This type of management and its complications are the most thoroughly covered in the academic literature. Today, nonoperative management remains a reasonable treatment choice, particularly in young patients with type III odontoid fractures, some patients with nondisplaced type II fractures, patients who are poor surgical candidates, and all patients who have type I odontoid fractures in the absence of occipital-cervical instability (2,3,14–25). Nonoperative management may involve use of multiple different bracing strategies, including but not limited to soft collars, rigid neck collars, Minerva bracing, and halo vest bracing. Traction only for treatment of odontoid fractures is mostly of historical interest as the significant complications associated with prolonged immobilization are well documented. Although a nonoperative strategy avoids the complications commonly associated with incision, dissection, and internal hardware placement, it is not without significant risk of complication.

In their series of 60 patients, Anderson and D'Alonzo reported on two type I fractures. Both healed in cervical collars (3). Nonoperative management of type II and III fractures in this series was performed with traction followed by bracing with halo devices or Minerva bracing. Of the 32 type II fractures, 14 nondisplaced fractures were treated in traction with a 36% nonunion rate. Three of eight (38%) displaced type II fractures went on to nonunion; the remainder all had union with an average time to heal being 5.6 months. Of the 25 patients with type III fractures, 24 were treated nonoperatively. One hundred percent of patients with nondisplaced fractures went on to union with an average time to union of 5.5 months. Eight of nine displaced type III fractures went on to union at an average time of 4 months. The ninth had three reported complications: nonunion, dysphagia, and pain. The authors also identified one patient who died within one week of traction being placed. No other complications are noted in this series. The series highlights the extended treatment time that may be required for fusion with this method of nonoperative management. It also demonstrates the difficulty of treating type II fractures, especially displaced fractures, with nonoperative methods.

In 2000 Govender et al. reported their series of 183 patients (109 type II and 74 type III) treated nonoperatively in South Africa with Minerva and SOMI (sterno-occipito mandibular immoblizer) bracing (14). Of the 109 type II fractures, 46% went on to nonunion, with 17% having a fibrous union. Malunion occurred in 17% of patients who had union. All type III fractures united, but malunion was noted in 28%, and delayed union (defined as greater than 16 weeks) occurred in 22%. Pain was reported in 64% of patients, but was not statistically associated with one type of fracture over another. The authors also reported loss of range of motion in those 152 patients who went on to union. Of the patients evaluated, 31% had some but less than 25% decrease in range of motion and 15% had a greater than 25% loss in range of motion. Two patients were tetraparetic at presentation; both had complete resolution of paresis. This study also evaluated the vascular anatomy of the odontoid. It was once believed that poor union rates of odontoid fractures were related to a relative watershed area at the location of type II fractures (odontoid waist). It is now believed that failure of union at this site is likely due to the paucity of cancellous bone contact at the mostly cortical waist of the odontoid. This is an important consideration in the management of this type of fracture and may explain the higher rates of pseudoarthrosis with type II fractures.

Lennarson et al. evaluated 60 patients with type II odontoid fractures in a case control study reported in 2000 (15). This study defined cases as nonunions. The complication of nonunion was evaluated for statistical association with neurological deficit, gender, associated illness (e.g., diabetes mellitus), degree of fracture displacement, direction of fracture displacement, age, length of hospital treatment, and length of follow-up. The only significant finding was that individuals over 50 years of age had increased risk of nonunion. This association has been demonstrated in many studies (19,20,22–27).

Dunn and Seljeskog evaluated 128 patients with odontoid fractures in 1986 (24). Sixteen patients had a delayed or misdiagnosis of their injury. Sixteen patients died during the acute phase, 8 had severe cord injuries (often with associated cervical spine fractures), and one had pneumonia with sepsis. Eighty patients were treated nonoperatively with halo fixation followed by collar immobilization or SOMI bracing. Nonunion occurred in 19 of 80 patients (24%); all of these patients had type II odontoid fractures. Other reported complications included loss of pin fixation in 9 patients (11%), fracture redislocation in 5 patients (6%), pin site cellulitis in 4 patients (5%), occipital scalp decubitus ulceration in one patient (1%), and early removal of bracing by patients in 2 cases (2.5%). This study demonstrates that nonoperative management can result in significant motion at the site of fracture. In fractures prone to nonunion, this may result in higher rates of complication. Also, nonoperative management requires careful scrutiny to maintain optimum function of halo devices and avoid pin complications.

Clark and White compiled the results of a large Cervical Spine Research Society multicenter study in 1985 (25). They noted a general trend towards missed injury in patients with odontoid fractures due to concomitant substance use or head injury. The study had 96 type II odontoid fractures. Complications in this group included three patients with exacerbation of pretreatment neurological deficit. Multiple treatment modalities were used. In the nonoperative group managed by halo device, 18% went on to nonunion, 5% displaced significantly in the halo device and had nonunion, and 8% had delayed or malunion. Of the 48 type III fractures evaluated, 42 were treated nonoperatively with a combination of nonoperative modalities including bed rest, skeletal traction, orthosis, and halo device. The halo group demonstrated an 81% union rate with a single nonunion and one case of nonunion with fracture displacement. There was also one death from cardiopulmonary arrest while in a halo device. A patient treated in an orthosis had a malunion associated with myelopathy as a complication. This patient had to undergo a posterior spinal decompression and fusion as a result of the treatment complication.

The studies evaluated reveal much about the complications associated with nonoperative-based treatment strategies of odontoid fractures. Type I fractures do very well with nonoperative treatment and have few complications. Type II fractures treated nonoperatively do poorly, especially if displaced, with a high complication rate. The most common complication is nonunion, a major complication. A fracture nonunion can go on to displacement and subsequent neurological injury, which may not resolve. Type III fractures can be managed with nonoperative means, most effectively in halo devices. Nonunion can still be a problem, but is much less frequent than in nonoperative management of type II fractures, even if the type III fracture is displaced. Commonly encountered complications include pin tract infections, loosening of pins, and hygiene problems. Sudden death has occurred in patients treated nonoperatively. In many instances it is hard to discern the cause of death, but it is likely that in some cases catastrophic neurological injury from displacement of the odontoid fracture caused respiratory failure. It is important to keep this in mind when counseling patients.

VI. POSTERIOR SPINAL FUSION

Posterior spinal fusion was the first operative treatment strategy for odontoid fractures to show consistent fusion rates with an acceptable risk-to-benefit ratio. This technique is widely considered the gold standard against which other operative procedures must be compared. It is also commonly used as the salvage procedure if another treatment strategy fails to obtain fusion or results in a complication that precludes continuation of that method. There are many different techniques for obtaining a posterior spinal fusion at the atlantoaxial articulation, including wire constructs, screw constructs, and plate constructs, all with autograft or allograft bone.

It should be understood that a posterior spinal fusion does not specifically fixate the odontoid fracture; rather it fuses the C-1 vertebrae to the C-2 vertebrae (Fig. 2). This halts all motion at the atlantoaxial articulation resulting in an environment where motion at the fracture site is minimized and union can occur. Reduction of C-1 on C-2 can be performed intraoperatively, and this usually allows for reduction of a displaced odontoid. Fusion of C1-C2 results in a significant decrease in rotational range of motion in the cervical spine; herein lies one of the major critiques of posterior spinal fusion as a treatment for odontoid fracture. It should be noted that loss of range of motion can occur with all treatment options, including nonoperative care.

Any operative treatment carries the risk of complications, and posterior cervical fusion is no exception. Several large studies have demonstrated both major and minor complications associated with this operative strategy. Coyne et al. performed a retrospective review of their results with posterior spinal fusion for disease at the C1-C2 level in 1995 (28). They had 18 odontoid fractures in their series, 15 type II fractures, and 2 type III fractures. Multiple different fusion procedures were performed, including Gallie, Brooks-Jenkins, Halifax clamping, and transarticular screw fixation. Complications for the entire series included a 6% rate of neurological complications, including new-onset myelopathy and exacerbation of preexistent myelopathy. They also had a 19% failure of fusion rate with the primary fusion techniques (Gallie and Brooks-Jenkins). Both patients who had neurological complications had sublaminar wire passage, a commonly described complication in this type of procedure (29). No description of minor complications was given in this article. This may be construed as indicating there were no minor complications. However, minor complications certainly outnumber major complications, and the more rational interpretation is that minor complications were simply not reported. It is important to counsel patients that the risk of neurological injury is possible with treatment of odontoid fractures by a primary posterior spinal fusion.

Bednar et al. evaluated 11 patients with type II odontoid fractures who were recruited and treated prospectively in 1995 (30). The impetus for this study was an internal institutional review that demonstrated an unacceptably high rate of mortality in non-operatively treated geriatric patients with type II odontoid fractures. All patients were neurologically intact, and the mean age was 74 years. The Brooks and Jenkins technique of posterior spinal fusion was performed. No cases of death either in hospital or postdischarge were attributed to the surgery. All but one of the fractures initially demonstrated displacement, but after surgery only 9% had failure of fusion. The salvage procedure for

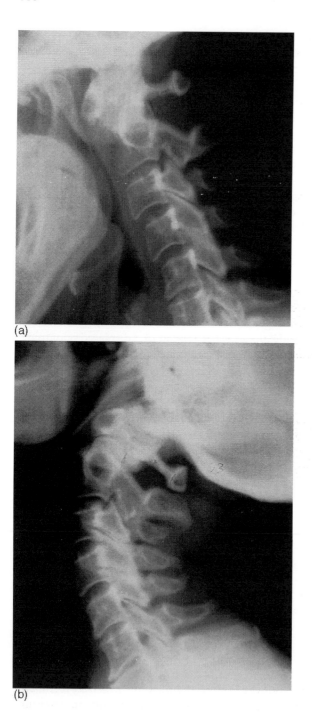

(a)

(b)

Figure 2 Type II odontoid fracture treated with transarticular screw fixation, bone grafting, and sublaminar wires. (a) Preoperative lateral flexion radiograph; (b) preoperative lateral extension radiograph; (c) preoperative coronal CT scan; (d) postoperative AP radiograph; (e) Postoperative lateral radiograph.

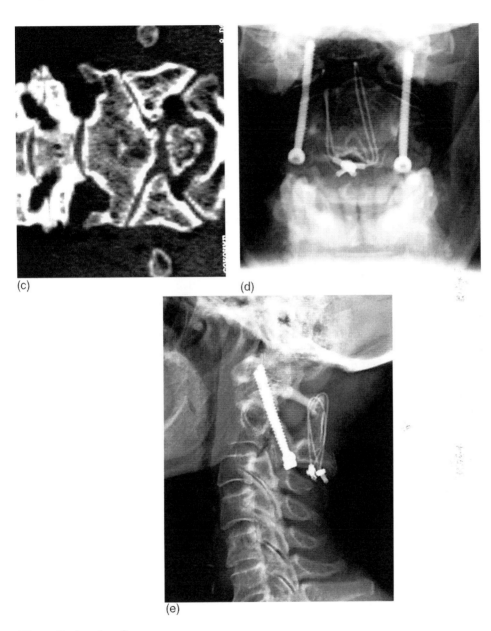

(c)

(d)

(e)

Figure 2 *(continued)*

failure of fusion in this study was anterior odontoid screw fixation, which in this case did result in ultimate fusion for all patients. Minor complications were not reported in this series.

Maiman and Larson reported their retrospective series of odontoid fractures in 1982 (31). They had 51 total patients, and over half of the patients were under 40 years of age. Two types of fractures were evaluated: 49 patients had type II fractures and 2 had type III fractures. Three patients presented with significant neurological deficit before treatment, and 4 patients had odontoid fractures that were initially missed on plain radiographs. Fifteen patients with type II fractures were treated nonoperatively; all of these patients failed to fuse the fracture, and they were salvaged with a posterior spinal fusion. All patients treated surgically were reported to have evidence of bone healing at 4–10 weeks postoperatively. However, at 6 months 34% of patients who had failed nonoperative management and were salvaged with a posterior spinal fusion demonstrated delayed union. The study highlights the fact that a posterior spinal fusion works effectively as a salvage procedure for odontoid nonhealing. One patient was reported to have hardware failure, but a stable fusion. One patient had a minor wound infection at an iliac crest bone graft donor site (2%). Pain was reported as moderate to severe in 11 (22%) patients at follow-up postoperatively. Evaluation of rotational motion was recorded in this study, and 7 patients (14%) had a clinically significant loss of motion. Of note, there was a correlation in this series with loss of range and post-operative pain syndromes.

Clark and White's series of odontoid fractures included patients treated both operatively and nonoperatively (25). In the operative portion of their series, they had 26 patients with type II odontoid fractures who were initially treated with a posterior spinal fusion. Only one (4%) failed to unite. Posterior spinal fusion was successfully used as a salvage treatment in 20 patients who failed to fuse with nonoperative treatment.

While posterior spinal fusion remains an excellent choice in the treatment of odontoid fractures, it is not without risk of complications. Evaluation of the available data reveals little about the minor complications associated with this type of surgical management. We believe this is due to a paucity of recorded complications rather than their absence. The most prevalent major complications associated with posterior spinal fusion are nonunion and neurological injury to the patient. Loss of motion is felt by many to be a considerable drawback to posterior spinal fusion, although the major studies detailing results of posterior spinal fusion in odontoid fracture do little to shed light on this subject.

VI. ANTERIOR ODONTOID SCREW FIXATION

The anterior screw fixation approach was separately described by Nakanishi in 1980 and Bohler in 1982 (32,33). These reports shifted the focus from transoral approaches to direct anterior approaches, with a resultant decrease in surgical morbidity. The majority of spinal surgeons are comfortable with the Smith-Robinson approach to the cervical spine. Advantages of anterior screw fixation include direct fixation of the fracture and maintenance of atlantoaxial motion. However, the procedure is not without complications and is technically challenging. Interest in this form of fixation and its advantages has produced a significant volume of literature in recent years. Evaluation of this literature demonstrates the myriad of complications inherent in this form of treatment.

Henry et al. reviewed their series of 81 patients treated with anterior screw fixation in 1999 (5). Twenty-nine patients had type II fractures, and 52 patients had type III fractures. The mean age of the patients was 57 years. Follow-up for a mean of 16.6 months was performed on a total of 61 patients. Only 8% of patients failed to unite their fracture. The mean time to union was 14.1 weeks. Three of the patients diagnosed with nonunion refused further surgery and had clinically excellent results. Attention was paid in this study to range of motion after surgery. Full range of motion was maintained in 70% of patients, limitation of less than 25% in 20%, and limitation of greater than 25% in 10%. Pain at rest occurred in 2% and occasional pain in 7%. This study showed that anterior screw fixation could result in fusion rates comparable with posterior spinal fusion. It also shows that range of motion can be significantly compromised in some patients treated this way.

A major complication directly attributed to the anterior approach occurred in an 83-year-old woman who was tetraparetic after the surgery and died from respiratory failure 6 days later. Postoperative dysphagia was noted in two patients and pharyngeal edema in one. Failure of fixation occurred in three patients (5%). Nine patients died in this study as a result of generalized physiological insults including respiratory failure, thromboembolism, cardiac failure, and sepsis. The authors attributed this to preexistant risk factors in the patients whose mean age was 79. Other minor complications noted were deep vein thrombosis and pressure sores.

In another large and well-documented series, Apfelbaum et al. reported on 147 patients in 2000 (6). They were able to follow 133 patients, 7 being lost to follow-up and 7 having died in the immediate postoperative period. Patients were divided into two groups for purpose of outcome evaluation: those with recent fractures and those with a remote history of trauma. There were 129 patients with recent fractures. Immediate postoperative imaging demonstrated suboptimal placement of screws in 3%, highlighting the technical difficulties of the surgery even in experienced hands. Failure of fusion occurred in 12% of patients treated, and asymptomatic malunion was present in 3% (Fig. 3). There were other complications in this group. Hardware-related failures occurred in 9% of patients, the most common problem being screw pullout (cutout) of the C2 vertebral body, which occurred in 5 patients. Two of these patients had to undergo revision surgery, and the remainder were managed nonoperatively. Screw backout along its insertion tract was the second most common hardware complication in the acute treatment group (Fig. 4). This again occurred at the insertion site in the C2 body in 4 patients. Two patients were salvaged successfully with reoperation, and one was managed nonoperatively. The last patient died of respiratory failure following displacement of the unfixed odontoid. Other noted complications included superficial wound infections treated with oral antibiotics in 2% of patients. There was a subset of patients in this study, 6%, who died of non–surgery-related complications in the immediate postoperative period. This group is similar to the group reported on by Henry et al. (5).

In the 18 patients treated remotely, successful positioning of surgical hardware was more difficult with 11% of patients having suboptimal placement of hardware. Both patients with this complication required reoperation, and in one the screw was too long and perforated the superior cortex of the dens, although no neurological injury occurred. Nonunion was noted in 31% of patients and fibrous union in 44%. Hardware complications occurred in this group as well, but the major mechanism is different than in the recent fracture group. Three patients had screw fracture at the site of bone fracture (Fig. 5). One patient had screw backout. The other interesting complication noted in this group was esophageal perforation. This was treated by making the patient NPO for 3 days. The lesion spontaneously resolved. Obviously this complication is unique to the anterior approach, and must be considered in the patient with dysphagia and pain.

El Saghir and Böhm prospectively evaluated a cohort of 30 patients in 2000 (7). All patients evaluated had type II fractures, and the mean age was 45 years. One patient who had preoperative high-level tetraplegia died in the immediate postoperative period from his injuries. The 29 remaining patients went onto union, demonstrated radiographically at 6 months. No hardware failure occurred in this series, but screws were extracted in 8 patients due to concerns about C2-3 degeneration after 4 patients, 13.3%, were found to have osteophytes at the antero-inferior border of C2. In one of these patients, spontaneous fusion developed. Chronic pain remained problematic in one patient. Three patients had dysphagia in the immediate postoperative period, but all had resolution by 3 months.

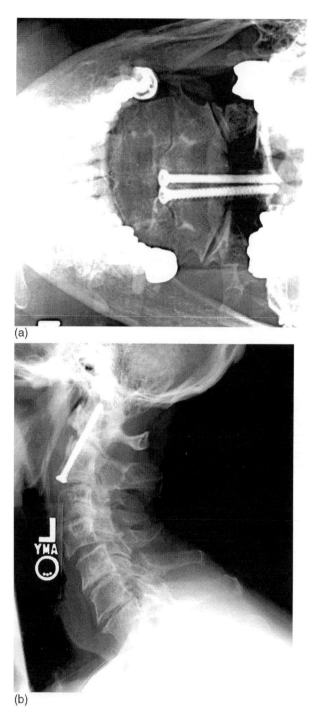

(a)

(b)

Figure 3 Stable psedoarthrosis after failure of union with anterior odontoid screw fixation. The patient refused further treatment. (a) AP radiograph; (b) lateral radiograph; (c) flexion lateral radiograph; (d) extension lateral radiograph.

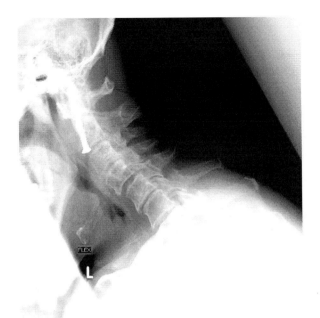

(c)

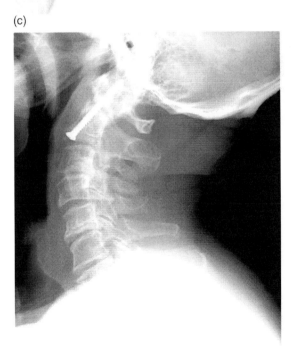

(d)

Figure 3 *(continued)*

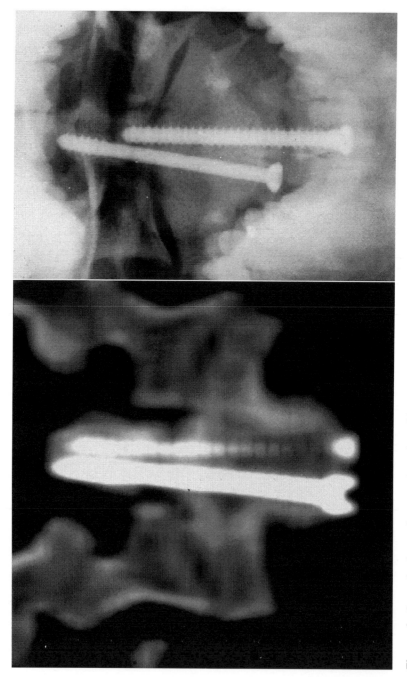

Figure 4 Screw backout after anterior odontoid screw fixation with two screws.

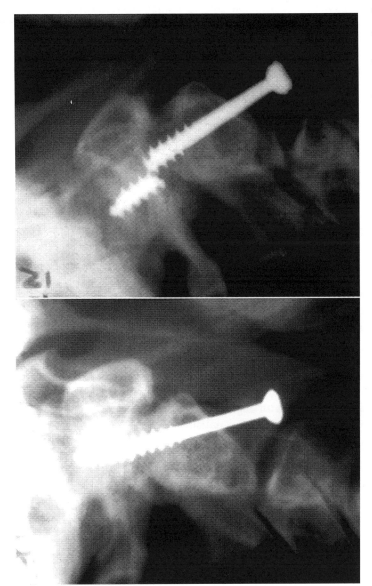

Figure 5 Lateral and extension lateral radiographs of a patient with screw failure and pseudo-arthrosis after fixation of a remote type II odontoid fracture.

These studies are by far the largest series on odontoid fracture treatment by anterior screw fixation in the literature. Smaller studies demonstrate other complications and their causes. Suboptimal placement of screw fixation is regularly felt to be a complication of the difficulty in obtaining good intraoperative images of the fracture (34). Wound hematomas, poorly selected fracture types (extremely oblique fractures) for anterior screw fixation, pneumothorax, and isolated paresthesias are also reported complications (34–36).

Evaluation of this literature demonstrates several pitfalls that occur during treatment of odontoid fractures with anterior screw fixation. As with the other forms of treatment reviewed, fractures that occur remote from the time of treatment have a much higher rate of nonunion. Patients should be warned of this complication. In addition, both Apfelbaum and Henry had a patient die as a result of failure of fixation in the early postoperative period. This reveals the danger involved in failure to fixate the odontoid and the importance of attention to detail in this approach. It may be wise to use some form of external immobilization until good postoperative radiographic evaluation of fixation can take place. Also highlighted in the complications occurring from anterior fixation are the risks to the anterior structures of the neck and the close proximity to the respiratory organs. By and large, complications are relatively rare with this treatment form, and success rates of fusion are comparable to those of posterior spinal fusion.

VIII. CONCLUSIONS

In this chapter we have evaluated the existing literature in an attempt to understand the types of complications associated with odontoid fractures. Several conclusions can be drawn from the findings. Most importantly, regardless of treatment choice, both major and minor complications occur and should be discussed with patients. Some fracture types, particularly type II fractures, seem to have a higher complication rate of nonunion when treated with nonoperative treatment strategies. Fractures that occurred remote to the time of treatment also seem to have higher complication rates. There seems to be a trade-off in anterior versus posterior treatment options. The anterior approach puts the structures at the anterior of the neck at risk for injury but may have superior results compared to posterior fixation with regards to maintenance of range of motion and, assumedly, function. The fact that many patients with odontoid fractures are elderly must be acknowledged, as the compromised physiology of these individuals puts them at greater risk for postoperative complications related to organ system failure. Due to the success of both anterior and posterior based treatment strategies in salvage, good options exist for the surgeon who has had failure of his or her initial treatment choice. Finally, it is encouraging that there seems to be a good chance for patients who are neurologically impaired prior to treatment to have a partial or even full recovery.

REFERENCES

1. Goldberg W, Mueller C, Panacek E, Tigges S, Hoffman JR, Mower WR. Distribution and patterns of bunt traumatic cervical spine injury. Ann Emerg Med 2001; 38(1):17–21.
2. Vaccaro AR, Madigan L, Ehrler DM. Contemporary management of adult cervical odontoid fractures. Orthopedics 2000; 23(10):1109–1113.
3. Anderson LD, D'Alanzo RT. Fractures of the odontoid process of the axis. J Bone Joint Surg (Am) 1974; 56:1663–1674.

4. Doherty BJ, Heggeness MH, Esses SI. A biomechanical study of odontoid fractures and fracture fixation. Spine 1993; 18(2):178–184.

5. Henry AD, Bohly J, Grosse A. Fixation of odontoid fractures by anterior screw. J Bone Joint Surg (Br) 1999; 81(3):472–477.

6. Apfelbaum RI, Lonser RR, Veres R, Casey A. Direct anterior screw fixation for recent and remote odontoid fractures. J Neurosurg 2000; 93(2 suppl):227–236.

7. El Saghir, Böhm H. Anderson type II fracture of the odontoid process: results of anterior screw. J Spinal Disord 2000; 13(6):527–530.

8. Moore KL. Clinically Oriented Anatomy. 3rd ed. Baltimore: Williams and Wilkins, 1992.

9. Puttlitz CM, Goel VK, Clark CR, Tranyelis VC. Pathomechanisms of failures of the odontoid. Spine 2000; 25(22):2868–2876.

10. Graham RS, Oberlander EK, Stewart JE, Griffiths DJ. Validation and use of a finite element model of C-2 for determination of strength patterns of anterior odontoid loads. J Neurosurg 2000; 93(1 suppl):117–125.

11. Spraycar M. Stedman's Medical Dictionary. 26th ed. Baltimore: Williams and Wilkins, 1995.

12. Crockard HA, Heilman AE, Stevens JM. Progressive myelopathy secondary to odontoid fractures: clinical, radiological, and surgical features. J Neurosurg 1993; 78(4):579–586.

13. Fairholm D, Lee ST, Lui TN. Fractured odontoid: the management of delayed neurological symptoms. Neurosurgery 1996; 38(1):38–43.

14. Govender S, Maharaj JF, Haffajee MR. Fractures of the odontoid process. J Bone Joint Surg (Br) 2000; 82(8):1143–1147.

15. Lennarson PJ, Mostafavi H, Traynelis VC, Walters BC. Management of type II dens fractures. Spine 2000; 10:1234–1237.

16. Vieweg U, Meyer B, Schramm J. Differential treatment in acute upper cervical spine injuries: a critical review of a single-institution series. Surg Neurol 2000; 54(3):203–210.

17. Hart R, Saterbak A, Rapp T, Clark C. Nonoperative management of dens fracture nonunion in elderly patients without myelopathy. Spine 2000; 25(11):1339–1343.

18. Chutkan NB, King AG, Harris MB. Odontoid fractures: evaluation and management. J Am Acad Orthop Surg 1997; 5(4):199–204.

19. Seybold EA, Bayley JC. Functional outcome of surgically and conservatively managed dens fractures. Spine 1998; 23(17):1837–1845.

20. Stoney J, O'Brien J, Wilde P. Treatment of type-two odontoid fractures in halothoracic vests. J Bone Joint Surg (Br) 1998; 80(3):452–455.

21. Anderson PA, Budorick TE, Easton KB, Henley MB, Salciccioli GG. Failure of halo vest to prevent in vivo motion in patients with injured cervical spines. Spine 1991; 16(10 suppl): 501–505.

22. Polin RS, Szabo T, Bogaev CA, Replogle RE, Jane JA. Nonoperative management of types II and III odontoid fractures: the Philadelphia collar versus the halo vest. Neurosurgery 1996; 38(3):450–456.

23. Bucholz RD, Cheung KC. Halo vest versus spinal fusion for cervical injury: evidence from an outcome study. J Neurosurg 1989; 70(6):884–892.

24. Dunn ME, Seljeskog EL. Experience in the management of odontoid process injuries: an analysis of 128 cases. Neurosurgery 1986; 18(3):306–310.

25. Clark CR, White AA. Fractures of the dens. J Bone Joint Surg (Am) 1985; 67(9): 1340–1348.

26. Schweigel JF. Halo-thoracic brace management of odontoid fractures. Spine 1979; 4(3): 192–194.

27. Cooper PR, Maravilla KR, Sklar FH, Moody SF, Clark WK. Halo immobilization of cervical spine fractures. J Neurosurg 1979; 50(5):603–610.

28. Coyne TJ, Fehlings MG, Wallace MC, Bernstein M, Tator CH. C-1-C2 posterior cervical fusion: long-term evaluation of results and efficacy. Neurosurgery 1995; 37(4):688–692.

29. Lundy DW, Murray HH. Neurological deterioration after posterior wiring of the cervical spine. J Bone Joint Surg (Br) 1997; 79(6):948–951.

30. Bednar DA, Parikh J, Hummel J. Management of type II odontoid process fractures in geriatric patients; a prospective study of sequential cohorts with attention to survivorship. J Spinal Disord 1995; 8(2):166–169.
31. Maiman DL, Larson SJ. Management of odontoid fractures. Neurosurgery 1982; 11(4): 471–476.
32. Nakanishi T. Internal fixation of odontoid fracture (in Japanese). Orthop Traumatic Surg 1980; 23:399–406.
33. Bohler J. Anterior stabilization for acute fractures and nonunions of the dens. J Bone Joint Surg (Am) 1982; 64(1):18–27.
34. Esses SI, Bednar DA. Screw fixation of odontoid fractures and nonunions. Spine 1991; 16(10S):S483–S485.
35. Pasquale XM, Anderson PA, Schlehr F, Thalgott JS, Lowrey G. Odontoid fractures treated by anterior odontoid screw fixation. Spine 1991; 16(3S):S33–S37.
36. Etter C, Coscia M, Jaberg H, Aebi M. direct anterior fixation of dens fractures with a cannulated screw system. Spine 1991; 16(3S):S25–S32.

23

Complications Related to the Surgical Treatment of Cervical Myelopathy

John M. Rhee
The Emory Spine Center, Emory University School of Medicine, Atlanta, Georgia, U.S.A.

K. Daniel Riew
*Washington University School of Medicine and Barnes-Jewish Hospital,
St. Louis, Missouri, U.S.A.*

I. INTRODUCTION

Cervical myelopathy can develop secondary to disk herniations, spondylotic changes, and ossification of the posterior longitudinal ligament (OPLL). Often these causes become pathological in the setting of a congenitally stenotic spinal canal. Because the natural history is typically one of stepwise progression (1), most authors recommend surgery for progressive or severe symptoms. In virtually all cases, decompression of the spinal cord is required to halt progression or induce recovery. Decompression can be performed anteriorly through a corpectomy and fusion approach, or posteriorly via laminoplasty or laminectomy approaches, with or without fusion.

Despite the fact that surgery for cervical myelopathy can be highly successful, neurological complications are not uncommon. One series involving 384 patients demonstrated a 3.4% incidence of early postoperative C5 nerve root deterioration and a 2% incidence of early postoperative spinal cord dysfunction (2). Other authors have noted a 1–2% incidence of neurological injury with anterior decompression and fusion (3). In order to minimize the incidence of neurological injury in these patients with already tenuous spinal cord function, extreme caution and attention to detail must be exercised not only intraoperatively, but also during preoperative planning, positioning, and postoperative care.

II. POSITIONING COMPLICATIONS

Proper patient positioning is critical to successful surgery for cervical myelopathy (Fig. 1). Failure to do so can lead to catastrophic neurological complications, make surgery technically more difficult to perform, and increase bleeding. Extra time and care taken during positioning will more than pay off in facilitating surgery and reducing complications (Fig. 2). In general, the neck is somewhat extended for anterior operations, being careful

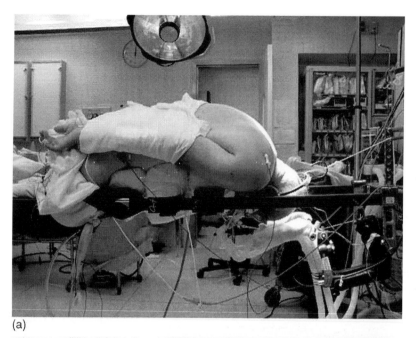

(a)

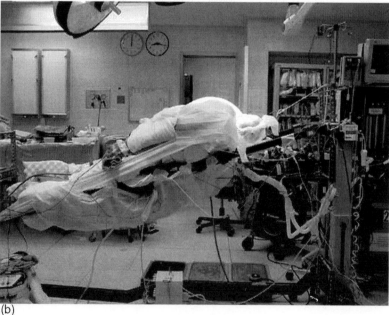

(b)

Figure 1 (a) A man with ankylosing spondylitis and severe cervical kyphosis has been placed on a Jackson frame with his head suspended using Gardner-Wells tongs. This keeps the face and eyes completely free but allows for the repositioning of the neck intraoperatively without someone having to adjust the Mayfield headrest. The head is suspended with 15–20 lb of Gardner-Wells tong traction. (b) The patient is then placed in a reverse Trendelenburg position. A body-warming blanket is taped to the undersurface of the table such that the hot air rises and keeps the patient warm. The shoulders are gently taped down and the arms are tucked. Using three bolsters on either side decompresses the abdomen, which reduces intraoperative bleeding.

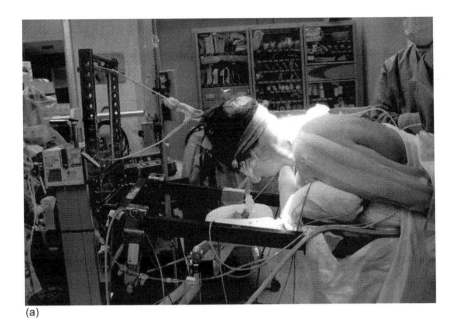

(a)

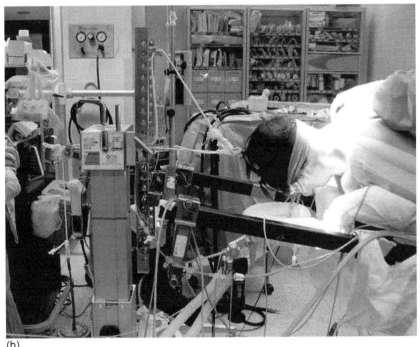

(b)

Figure 2   (a) When the patient requires a posterior cervical foraminotomy as well as a fusion, we use two ropes to suspend the head and neck. In this figure the head is being suspended from the lower of the two ropes. This places the neck into a more flexed position, opening up the facet joints so that it is easier to perform a foraminotomy. (b) Following the foraminotomy, the weight is switched to the top rope. This restores the neck to a normal lordotic position, in which the fusion should be performed.

to avoid excessive extension (see below), whereas the neck is neutral to slightly extended or flexed for most posterior operations.

Because the anterior-posterior dimension of the spinal canal decreases with extension of the neck, excessive extension should be avoided in all patients with cervical myelopathy, regardless of whether an anterior or posterior procedure is being performed. The surgeon should preoperatively check the amount of extension tolerated by the patient and avoid extending the neck any further than that during positioning. In addition, awake, fiberoptic intubation should be considered in myelopathic patients to avoid iatrogenic spinal cord injury during intubation. After intubation, the patient's motor function is assessed prior to putting the patient to sleep to confirm that a spinal cord injury has not occurred. A baseline set of spinal cord monitoring data should also be obtained after induction of anesthesia but prior to positioning. These baseline data are then compared to postpositioning data to ensure that the patient has been properly positioned without compromising an already tenuous spinal cord. If the patient is so myelopathic that adequate baseline monitoring data cannot be obtained, the patient may be positioned awake. Prior discussion with the patient regarding the possibility of awake positioning is important to facilitate cooperation and minimize patient anxiety.

When positioning patients for either an anterior or posterior approach, it is common to tape the shoulders down in order to assist in intraoperative radiographic visualization, particularly of the caudal segments of the cervical spine. However, excessive downward force on the shoulders can lead to a brachial plexopathy. If a patient has a short neck and a stocky body habitus, it may not be possible to safely visualize C7 or T1. In such situations, rather than taping the shoulders with excessive force throughout the entire case, it is advisable to tape the shoulders more loosely and then scrub out or have unscrubbed assistants briefly pull longitudinally on the arms while radiographs are being taken. Somatosensory evoked potential (SSEP) monitoring data should be obtained prior to draping, so that if problems related to shoulder taping are detected they can be more easily corrected. Typically, SSEP degradation related to positioning manifests early on rather than later during the case, unless the position of the patient has changed during the course of the operation. However, because SSEP data cannot absolutely be relied upon to detect positioning-related problems, judgment must be used in determining how much force to apply in taping the shoulders. We recommend erring on the side of caution and using less force. Care must also be taken during positioning to avoid peripheral nerve compression from improper padding of the arms and legs (e.g., ulnar or peroneal nerves).

During posterior cervical operations, improper positioning can also lead to excessive bleeding. The abdomen should be free of compression with the patient placed into reverse Trendelenburg to reduce venous pressure in the neck. Although bleeding from posterior cervical operations is rarely of the magnitude to cause hemodynamic embarrassment, undue bleeding may hinder visualization and, in particular, the performance of foraminotomies, during which foraminal bleeding is often encountered even in the best of circumstances. Usually, if the patient is properly positioned, foraminal bleeding can be readily controlled with the brief application of gelfoam and cottonoids, allowing decompression to proceed. In contrast, if the patient is not positioned properly and venous pressure is unduly high, foraminal bleeding may obscure safe visualization during foraminotomy despite attempts at hemostasis. When positioning a patient into reverse Trendelenburg, care must be taken to avoid the inadvertent application of traction on the neck and spinal cord. This can occur with the use of tongs (especially Mayfield) because the head is relatively fixed while the body may slide caudally due to gravity. This problem can be avoided by putting the knees at the break point of the operating table such that the tibias prevent caudal migration as the table is placed into reverse Trendelenburg. A sling placed behind the buttocks with an upward-directed vector may also be beneficial.

Miscellaneous tong-related complications—such as pin site infection, cerebrospinal fluid (CSF) leak, and slippage of tongs—can occur but are rare if proper attention to detail is used during application. Pressure on the eyes and face should be avoided in the prone position because this can lead to visual complications and pressure necrosis. Extreme care should be exercised if a horseshoe headrest is used. It is preferable instead to suspend the face with tongs. Air embolism has been reported with the seated position for posterior cervical surgery, but in most cases surgery for cervical myelopathy can be performed in a prone position without invoking the risks associated with the seated position.

III. HEMODYNAMIC COMPLICATIONS

Especially when operating on myelopathic patients, it is critical to maintain adequate spinal cord perfusion during the procedure. Patients with cervical spondylotic myelopathy may have impairment of anterior spinal cord circulation due to compression from ventral osteophytes or OPLL. In the setting of already compromised cord perfusion, intraoperative drops in blood pressure can have catastrophic neurological consequences. The anesthesiologist should be alerted to the importance of maintaining adequate blood pressure, and arterial lines may be recommended to allow for continuous monitoring of hemodynamic parameters, especially in patients who exhibit cardiovascular lability. Pressors, such as neosynephrine, may also be needed intraoperatively. Hypotensive anesthesia should be avoided, as it is potentially detrimental to cord perfusion and is not generally necessary to limit bleeding in cervical spine procedures if a patient has been properly positioned. Hypotension can occur during surgery for a number of reasons, but it is most commonly encountered during posterior cervical operations as the patient is positioned prone and put into reverse Trendelenburg. Therefore, it is critical for the anesthesiologist to be alerted to the possibility and vigilant even prior to incision.

It is unclear exactly at what level the blood pressure should be maintained during surgery for cervical myelopathy. The goal is to maintain an adequate spinal cord perfusion pressure, analogous to the cerebral perfusion pressure targeted in patients with head injury. However, whereas cerebral perfusion pressure in head trauma patients can be readily monitored by comparing mean arterial pressure (MAP) to intracranial pressure obtained from an intracranial pressure bolt, the same is not true in the cervical spine, where measurement of intraspinal pressure is not clinically feasible. Empirically, keeping the MAP in the mid to high 70s appears to be adequate in most cases. In addition, the hematocrit should be > 30 to maximize spinal cord oxygenation and the oxygen saturation kept at 100%.

IV. TRACTION COMPLICATIONS

Intraoperative traction is commonly used in the surgical treatment of cervical spine pathology. However, in patients with cervical myelopathy who have ventral cord compression from spondylotic bars, OPLL, or disk herniations, the application of traction to the spine can result in stretching or tethering of the spinal cord and subsequent neurological compromise. It is recommended to avoid any significant amount of traction on the spine until the spinal cord has been decompressed. If anterior corpectomy is being performed, tongs can be placed with a minimal amount of traction (e.g., 5 lb) to gently stabilize the head and neck until decompression is completed. After decompression, weight can be placed as necessary to facilitate graft placement. Similarly, longitudinal distraction on vertebral body distraction pins over areas of spinal cord compression should be avoided until those segments have been decompressed.

V. DIRECT SPINAL CORD TRAUMA

Direct trauma to the spinal cord is a rare but potential complication of cervical spine surgery (4). In one report, intraoperative trauma was identified as being causative of postoperative spinal cord injury in 0.05% (38 of 82,114) of anterior cervical discectomy and fusions (5). This report did not specify the proportion of the patients operated on for myelopathy versus radiculopathy. Theoretically, the incidence of direct spinal cord trauma during surgery for cervical myelopathy should be higher than that for nonmyelopathy, because spinal cord decompression is necessary in these patients, which presumably carries a higher risk for inadvertent injury.

Inadvertent slippage of instruments is one mechanism by which direct spinal cord trauma can occur. Stabilization of all instruments passed near the spinal cord is mandatory to minimize the incidence of such complications. The hand holding the instrument should be stabilized on the patient's own body in order to prevent plunging into the spinal canal and also to protect against bucking movements of the patient (Fig. 3). Suction devices should be held with a "palm-up" technique, with the hand resting on the patient's body. Particularly when using a high-speed burr, surgical assistants and scrub personnel should be careful to avoid jostling the tubing, which could transmit unwanted forces to the burr itself (Fig. 4).

Spinal cord trauma can also occur during the placement of bone grafts. One should never apply excessive force in order to get a graft to fit. It is advisable instead to downsize the graft, use traction, or perform endplate carpentry to achieve the desired fit. In general, no more than gentle tapping forces should be used to impact the graft, even if the endplates have been cut with a posterior ridge to avoid posterior graft extrusion during anterior cervical fusion. Graft sizers used to size ACDFs should be inserted with the same degree of caution (Fig. 5). The same principle applies when inserting rib struts to keep laminoplasty hinges open posteriorly.

Graft-related spinal cord trauma can also occur if a graft is excessively deep, leading to cord impingement. The depth of the graft should be less than that of the vertebral body, particularly if countersinking is desired. The appropriate depth can be estimated by measurements taken from preoperative lateral radiographs (accounting for magnification), magnetic resonance imaging (MRI), or computed tomography (CT). One can also estimate the depth of the disk space based on preoperative imaging, then place a spinal needle bent to just less than that depth before performing a localizing lateral radiograph (Fig. 6). By comparing the known length of the bent needle with that of the disk space on the localizing film, the depth of the disk space and thus that of the graft can be estimated. Alternatively, the depth of the corpectomy or discectomy site can be directly measured with a wooden or metal probe after decompression and prior to graft placement.

Direct spinal cord injury can also occur with the placement of screws. Although pull-off strength is greater with bicortical screws than with unicortical screws and locking plates (6), in most cases the advantage of improved fixation with bicortical purchase is

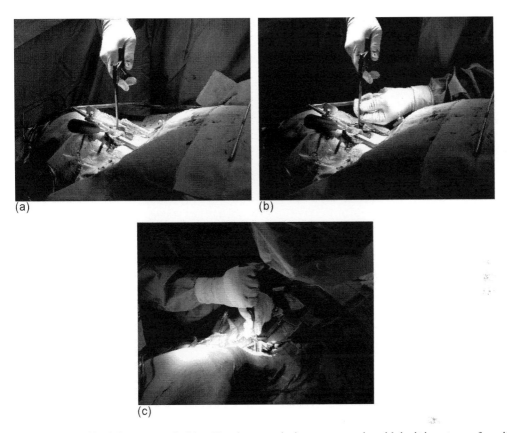

Figure 3 (a, b) If the surgeon holds a Kerrison or pituitary rongeur in midair, it is not as safe as if it is stabilized by the opposite hand, which rests on the patient. In addition, one can hold a sponge in the stabilizing hand and clean the instruments. This is the most efficient and safe technique to remove debris. Handing the instrument off to the nurse to be cleaned each time requires much more arm motion as well as time. (c) Instruments such as curettes should be stabilized with the opposite hand to prevent inadvertent plunging into the spinal cord.

outweighed by the risks. Modern locking plate designs are sufficiently strong for most applications. Even with unicortical fixation, however, care must be taken to prevent spinal cord injury. Screw and drill length can be estimated in the manner described above for graft depth. Most anterior cervical plate systems are equipped with drill stops that limit the depth of drilling to a predetermined amount. However, it is imperative that the surgeon always double check the length of any drills being used in order to avoid inadvertent spinal cord trauma. If in doubt, lateral fluoroscopy can be used during drilling and screw insertion.

When performing spinal cord decompression, either anteriorly or posteriorly, downward pressure should not be exerted onto the spinal cord with instruments used to perform the decompression. Large Kerrison rongeurs should be avoided, as their footplates may be unduly thick and cause spinal cord compression with insertion. The preferred technique is to use a high-speed burr to create a thin shell of bone that can gently be lifted off of the spinal cord using a microcurette. We prefer the use of the operative microscope, which greatly assists in performing a safe and effective decompression. Unwanted downward pressure on the spinal cord may also occur while attempting to

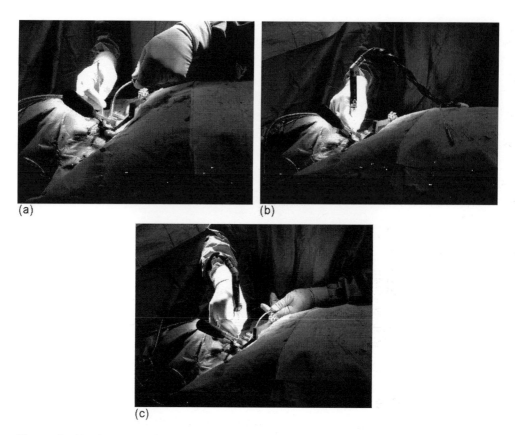

Figure 4   (a) The surgeon is holding the suction device in midair. If the surgeon is bumped from behind or the patient bucks, the suction can inadvertently traumatize the structures in the neck, including the spinal cord. (A safer way is demonstrated in Fig. 4c.) (b) If the hose of the air drill is inadvertently pulled by someone while the surgeon has it running, it can result in catastrophic injury to the patient. (A safer way is to wrap the cord underneath the hand of the surgeon as in Fig. 4c.) This way, if the hose is accidentally pulled by one of the assistants, it is tethered by the surgeon's hand. (c) The left hand of the surgeon is holding the suction device with the hand resting on the patient. This minimizes the risk of inadvertent injury to the spinal cord.

tamponade bleeding. Foraminal bleeding encountered during anterior or posterior foraminotomy is readily controlled with a small piece of gelfoam and cotton pledget without resorting to excessive force. In contrast, if a vertebral artery laceration occurs, massive bleeding can ensue that can be extremely difficult to control. If pressure is necessary to tamponade the bleeding, it should be directed laterally towards the lacerated artery rather than posteriorly towards the spinal cord.

VI. VERTEBRAL ARTERY INJURY

Although the true incidence of vertebral artery injury during anterior cervical decompression is unknown, one series estimated it to be as high as 0.5% (7). Unilateral injury may not have clinically apparent neurological sequelae in patients with normal vertebrobasilar and posterior cerebral artery circulations. However, 10% of patients have an atretic unilateral vertebral artery which does not contribute significantly to brainstem bloodflow.

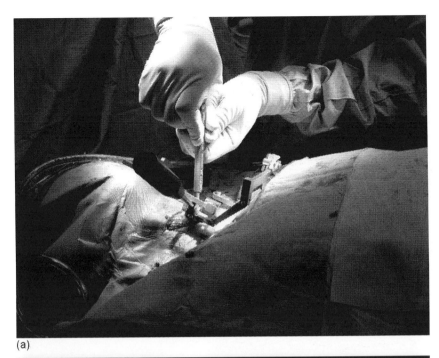

(a)

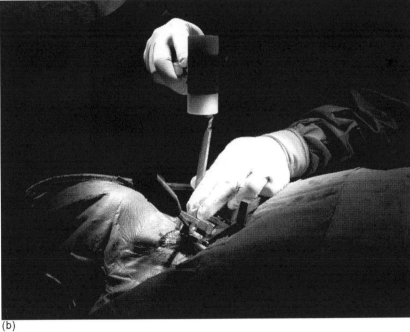

(b)

Figure 5 (a, b) A graft sizing device should never be pushed into the disk space. If it suddenly gives, it can result in injury to the spinal cord. Instead, it should be gently placed in between the disk space, and the disk space should be distracted using either tongs or distraction pins. The sizing device can be gently tapped with a mallet.

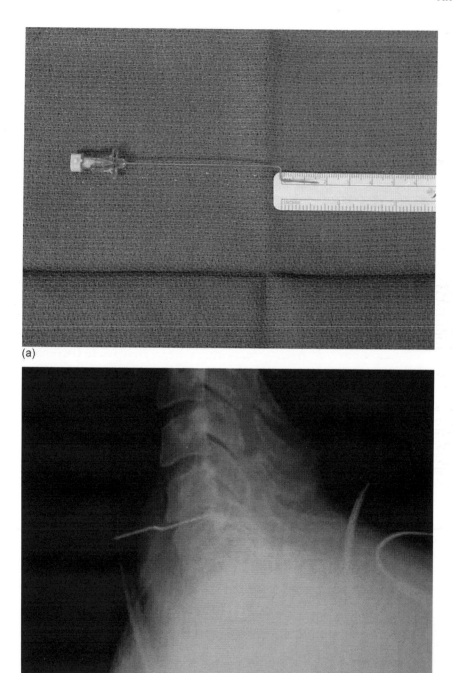

(a)

(b)

Figure 6 (a) Needles that are placed into the wound to localize a disk level should be bent at the tip to prevent inadvertent migration into the cord. (b) Needle marking the disk space. With the needle bent to a known length, one can estimate what the screw length should be.

In such patients, the consequence of injury to the dominant artery can be devastating. Cerebellar ischemia or, in worse cases, infarction can occur, which may be manifested as Wallenberg's syndrome (lateral medullary syndrome). The clinical picture of cerebellar ischemia or infarction can be protean depending on the specific structures involved, but may include sensory changes, ataxia, vertigo, nausea, vomiting, nystagmus, diplopia, Horner's syndrome, dysphagia, hoarseness, and paralysis (8).

In order to minimize the incidence of vertebral artery complications, it is prudent to scrutinize the preoperative MRI or CT scan to rule out the presence of an anomalous vertebral artery coursing medial to its usual position within the intertransverse foramen and lateral to the lateral border of the uncinate (Fig. 7). If anomalies are suspected, angiography should be considered preoperatively. One should confine the decompression within the lateral borders of the uncinate processes in the middle third of the disk space or vertebral body, because this is the depth at which the vertebral artery typically lies. The width of spinal cord decompression can be estimated on preoperative imaging but will rarely if ever need to extend lateral to the uncinates. Further lateral decompression of foraminal stenosis, if necessary, can be done by undercutting within the posterior third of the disk space, which is usually dorsal to the location of the artery. In this manner, sufficient foraminal decompression can be safely achieved out laterally at the level of the disk space while reducing potential risks of vertebral artery laceration.

Vertebral artery lacerations during anterior cervical surgery can occur if the usual landmarks are not appreciated or if an anomalous artery exists that is medial to the usual safe zones. Because in most cases a preoperative angiogram will not have been obtained to assess vertebral artery dominance or sufficiency of posterior cerebral collateral circulation, a lacerated artery should be repaired rather than ligated if at all possible. If repair

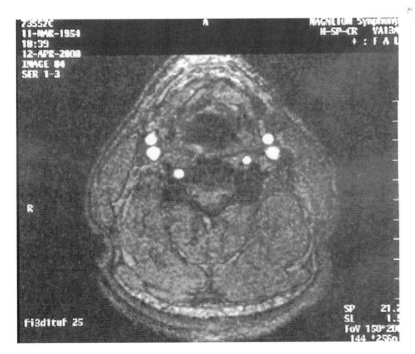

Figure 7 Note the anomalous vertebral artery on the left side in this case. It is anterior to the foramen transversarium, where it belongs, and is prone to injury during the dissection of the longus colli.

cannot be performed, options include ligation or temporary tamponade followed by endovascular stenting. Nerve root injuries have been reported with the "blind" placement of sutures during attempts to ligate the vertebral artery (7) and thus should be avoided except in desperate circumstances.

Vertebral artery injury during posterior cervical spine surgery may occur at the level of C1, where the two arteries traverse toward the midline en route to ascending into the foramen magnum. Excessive lateral dissection of the posterior ring of C1 should be avoided. If lateral exposure is necessary, for example, in order to expose the C1-2 facet joint or the C1 lateral mass, it is safer to dissect subperiosteally on the undersurface of the C1 ring towards the joint and the C1 lateral mass because the artery lies away on the cephalad surface of C1.

VII. HEMATOMA FORMATION

The formation of an expanding epidural hematoma can lead to neurological compromise, as well as other deleterious consequences, including infection, wound dehiscence, and airway obstruction. Prevention of hematoma formation begins by achieving meticulous hemostasis prior to closure. Most foraminal bleeding can be controlled by the judicious application of gelfoam, pledget, and gentle suction, as described above. Large epidural bleeding may require bipolar coagulation. When placing anterior cervical grafts within a disk space, small spaces should be left bilaterally to allow for any residual epidural bleeding to seep around the graft rather than collect and create pressure within the epidural space. Drains should be placed into the deep wound during posterior cervical surgery whenever possible. During anterior decompression and fusion, a deep drain should be placed into the retropharyngeal space just anterior to the spine. The drain should also be placed as caudally as possible within this space in order to prevent hematoma collection in the dependent portion of the wound.

VIII. ROOT LEVEL PALSIES

Segmental root level palsy has been reported after decompression for cervical myelopathy, most commonly after cervical laminoplasty. Though rarer, cases have also occurred after anterior decompression: the incidence of postoperative radiculopathy from anterior cervical discectomy and fusion has been estimated to be 0.17% (5). The incidence of segmental root palsy after laminoplasty ranges from 5 to 12% (9) and most commonly affects the C5 root, resulting in deltoid and biceps weakness. The palsies tend to be motor-dominant, although sensory dysfunction and radicular pain are also possible. The problem may arise at any point postoperatively, from immediately to 20 days later (9), complicating what otherwise appeared to be a successful decompression of the spinal cord. Recovery to useful function usually occurs over weeks to months in the majority of patients, but has been reported to take as long as 6 years (10).

The cause of segmental root palsy after laminoplasty is unknown but may be related to nerve root traction as the decompressed cord floats posteriorly. Anatomically, the C5 root has a direct, short course, with little redundancy as it exits the spinal cord. Thus, as the spinal cord drifts posteriorly after laminoplasty, the C5 root may be stretched beyond its limits of tolerance. Another reason for the preferential involvement of C5 may arise from the fact that C5 is typically near the apex of lordosis—thus the extent of postoperative spinal cord shift and root traction will generally be greatest at that level. Finally, because the deltoid is innervated by a single root, lesions involving that root will have a profound effect on function. Strategies to combat the development of postoperative C5 root palsy include prophylactically performing foraminotomies, which has been recommended, but not proven, to prevent this complication (11). Also, less aggressive opening of the laminoplasty, with an angle of the lamina between 45 and 60°, may be sufficient for spinal cord decompression yet prevent excessive posterior spinal cord drift and therefore segmental root palsy (9).

However, C5 is not the only level that has been reported to suffer injury after spinal cord decompression. In order of frequency, C6, C7, and, very rarely, C8 palsies can also occur. An alternative mechanism of injury may be direct root trauma intraoperatively, which was reported to be problematic early in the technical evolution of laminoplasty (12). However, this mechanism seems implausible in the majority of cases given that many of the palsies occur in a delayed fashion postoperatively, and the incidence of root palsy has not diminished despite refinements in surgical technique. A recently proposed mechanism relates to the development of segmental edema within the gray matter of the spinal cord after decompression, leading to dysfunction of root levels served by that (those) segment(s) of the cord (13). According to this hypothesis, segmental palsy may be mediated by a reperfusion-like injury to a chronically ischemic spinal cord.

IX. SPINAL CORD MONITORING

Intraoperative spinal cord monitoring with SSEP is the standard of care when performing spinal deformity surgery (14). The primary benefit of monitoring deformity patients is to identify neurological compromise associated with curve correction. In addition, monitoring has been reported to be of value in surveillance of the upper extremities during deformity operations, where the brachial plexus and arms may be left in one position for a prolonged period of time (15,16). During spinal instrumentation, EMG monitoring can help identify malpositioned pedicle screws (17). Despite its utility in deformity surgery, spinal cord monitoring is not a universally accepted standard of care during cervical spine surgery. However, monitoring may be helpful in myelopathic patients to identify impending neurological compromise due to improper positioning of the neck, excessive traction, or intraoperative hypotension. In both myelopathic and nonmyelopathic patients, monitoring may also be of value in detecting brachial plexus injury due to shoulder taping or arm positioning during anterior cervical surgery (18).

As noted above, a baseline set of SSEPs is recommended after intubation and prior to positioning. Another set of data is then obtained to confirm proper positioning. The commonly accepted warning criteria are a 50% decrease in amplitude and a 10% increase in latency of SSEPs. Other authors have found that raising the warning criteria to a 60% decrease in amplitude can result in a lower false-positive rate (0.96% vs. 3.5% with 50% criteria) without raising the false-negative rate (0.16% for both 50% and 60% criteria). Using these criteria, Roh et al. (19) noted a 2% incidence ($n = 17$) of patients meeting the warning criteria for potential neurological dysfunction in a series of 809 consecutive cervical spine operations, which included both myelopathic and non-myelopathic patients. None of the patients in this series sustained a permanent neurological deficit, and these authors found SSEP data to be useful in prompting intervention and affecting outcome. Normalization of SSEP data with intraoperative intervention (e.g., release of shoulder tape or cervical traction, repositioning, decompression, or termination of surgery) was associated with the absence of a postoperative neurological deficit in 13 of the 17 meeting warning criteria. Only one patient who had recovery of SSEP data after intervention awoke with a postoperative deficit, which was transient. In contrast, persistent SSEP degradation despite intraoperative intervention was associated with a postoperative neurological deficit (again, transient) in the remaining 3 patients. Other authors also corroborate the utility of SSEP monitoring during surgery for cervical myelopathy. Epstein et al. found a 3.7% incidence of quadriplegia in a series of 218 unmonitored operations, compared to a 0% incidence in a series of 100 monitored cases.

Although baseline abnormalities in spinal cord monitoring data have been demonstrated in myelopathic patients (20–22), and the severity of myelopathy has been correlated with the severity of spinal cord monitoring abnormality (23–25), intraoperative improvements in data during decompression do not appear to reliably predict long-term prognosis. Bouchard et al. (26) found that, at one week, patients who had intraoperative improvement in SSEP data did exhibit greater clinical recovery, but at long-term follow up there was no difference in clinical outcome between those with and without intraoperative improvement.

In addition, other authors have found that obtaining longitudinal follow-up electrophysiological data postoperatively is poorly correlated with individual clinical outcome (27). It appears that monitoring data should not be relied upon to determine the adequacy of decompression or to provide prognostic information, but rather as an intraoperative indicator of impending harm to the spinal cord.

Controversy also exists as to the necessity of obtaining motor-evoked potentials (MEPs) during cervical spine surgery (28,29). During deformity surgery, neurogenic motor-evoked potentials (NMEPs) have been reported to detect impending cord injury before SSEPs, allowing intervention at an earlier, potentially more reversible stage (30). Furthermore, SSEPs only monitor the function of the dorsal columns and extrapolates their function onto the function of the cord as a whole. In patients with cervical spondylotic myelopathy or OPLL, where ventral cord compression typically predominates, it is theoretically preferable to directly monitor anterior motor column function. Monitoring of the ventral motor tracts is even more desirable when performing anterior cervical decompressions, where the anterior portion of the spinal cord is subjected to greater risk than the posterior columns.

However, MEPs may be more difficult to consistently and reliably obtain than SSEPs. A variety of methods are available for obtaining motor data, including electrical versus magnetic and spinal versus cortical stimulation. Methods of obtaining MEPs include percutaneous-translaminar, spinous process (where two electrodes are placed on consecutive spinous processes cephalad to the area of interest), disk, and transcranial. For most anterior cervical operations, percutaneous-translaminar electrodes are preferred, followed by disk stimulation if the percutaneous route is unsuccessful. Posterior spinous process electrodes require an open approach and are reserved for posterior surgery. Transcranial elicitation has recently been reported to be of benefit in cervical spine surgery (31). Currently available data indicate that if MEPs are available, they may provide useful adjunctive information to that obtained through SSEPs.

If intraoperative monitoring meets warning criteria, several actions should be considered. The mean arterial pressure should be elevated in order to maintain proper spinal cord perfusion. The hematocrit should be raised to 30 or more to provide proper oxygen-carrying capacity, and the oxygen saturation should be maintained at or near 100%. Consideration can be given to instituting the spinal cord injury steroid protocol (bolus 30 mg/kg intravenous methylprednisolone, followed by 5.4 mg/kg/h for 23 hours), although this protocol was established in the treatment of traumatic blunt spinal cord injury and has never been proven to be of benefit in the setting of intraoperative spinal cord injury. Cervicaltraction, if present, should be released. The surgeon should also consider early termination of the operation if hemodynamic instability or a potential stroke is causative.

REFERENCES

1. Lees F, Turner JW. Natural history and prognosis of cervical spondylosis. Br Med J 1963; 2:1607–1610.
2. Yonenobu K, et al. Neurologic complications of surgery for cervical compression myelopathy. Spine, 1991; 16(11):1277–1282.
3. Emery SE, et al. Anterior cervical decompression and arthrodesis for the treatment of cervical spondylotic myelopathy: two to seventeen year follow-up. J Bone Joint Surg 1998; 80A: 941–951.
4. Graham JJ. Complications of cervical spine surgery. A five-year report on a survey of the membership of the Cervical Spine Research Society by the Morbidity and Mortality Committee. Spine 1989; 14(10):1046–1050.
5. Flynn TB. Neurologic complications of anterior cervical interbody fusion. Spine 1982; 7(6):536–539.
6. Spivak JM, Chen D, Kummer FJ. The effect of locking fixation screws on the stability of anterior cervical plating. Spine 1999; 24(4):334–338.
7. Smith MD, et al. Vertebral artery injury during anterior decompression of the cervical spine. A retrospective review of ten patients. J Bone Joint Surg Br, 1993; 75(3):410–415.
8. Kistler JP, Ropper AH, Martin JB. Cerebrovascular diseases. In: Isselbacher KJ, ed. Harrison's Principles of Internal Medicine. New York: McGraw-Hill, 1994:2233–2256.
9. Uematsu Y, Tokuhashi Y, Matsuzaki N. Radiculopathy after laminoplasty of the cervical spine. Spine 1998; 23(19):2057–2062.
10. Satomi K, et al. Long-term follow-up studies of open-door expansive laminoplasty for cervical stenotic myelopathy. Spine, 1994; 19:507–510.
11. Yonenobu K, Yamamoto T, Ono K. Laminoplasty for myelopathy: indications, results, outcome and complications. In: Clark C, ed. The Cervical Spine, 3rd ed. Philadelphia: Lippincott-Raven, 1998:849–864.
12. Hirabayashi K, Satomi K, Toyama Y. Surgical management of OPLL: anterior versus posterior approach—part II. In: Clark C, ed. The Cervical Spine, 3rd ed. Philadelphia: Lippincott-Raven, 1998:876–887.
13. Chiba K, et al. Segmental motor paralysis after expansive open-door laminoplasty. Spine, 2002; 27(19):2108–15.
14. Padberg AM, Bridwell KH. Spinal cord monitoring: current state of the art. Orthop Clin North Am, 1999; 30(3):407–433, viii.
15. O'Brien MF, et al. Evoked potential monitoring of the upper extremities during thoracic and lumbar spinal deformity surgery: a prospective study. J Spinal Disord 1994; 7:277–284.
16. Schwartz DM, et al. Prevention of positional brachial plexopathy during surgical correction of scoliosis. J Spinal Disord 2000; 13:178–182.
17. Darden BV, 2nd, et al. Evaluation of pedicle screw insertion monitored by intraoperative evoked electromyography. J Spinal Disord, 1996; 9(1):8–16.
18. Schwartz D, et al. Neurophysiologic identification of impending neurologic injury from positioning for anterior cervical spine surgery. Presented at 29th annual meeting of the Cervical Spine Research Society, November 29, 2001, Monterey, California.
19. Roh M, et al. The utility of somatosensory evoked potential monitoring during cervical spine surgery: How often does it prompt intervention and affect outcome? Presented at Scoliosis Research Society 2002 annual meeting, Seattle, WA.

20. Kotani H, et al. Evaluation of cervical cord function in cervical spondylotic myelopathy and/or radiculopathy using both segmental conductive spinal-evoked potentials (SEP). Spine 1986; 11(3):185–190.

21. Perlik SJ, Fisher MA. Somatosensory evoked response evaluation of cervical spondylytic myelopathy. Muscle Nerve 1987; 10(6):481–489.

22. Yu YL, Jones SJ. Somatosensory evoked potentials in cervical spondylosis. Correlation of median, ulnar and posterior tibial nerve responses with clinical and radiological findings. Brain 1985; 108(pt 2):273–300.

23. Chang MH, et al. "Numb, clumsy hands" and tactile agnosia secondary to high cervical spondylotic myelopathy: a clinical and electrophysiological correlation. Acta Neurol Scand, 1992; 86(6):622–625.

24. Chistyakov AV, et al. Motor and somatosensory conduction in cervical myelopathy and radiculopathy. Spine 1995; 20(19):2135–2140.

25. Kotani H, et al. Evaluation of cervical cord function using spinal evoked potentials from surface electrode. Spine 1992; 17(3):339–344.

26. Bouchard JA, Bohlman HH, Biro C. Intraoperative improvement of somatosensory evoked potentials—correlation to clinical outcome in surgery for cervical spondylitic myelopathy. Spine 1996; 21:589–594.

27. Bednarik J, et al. The value of somatosensory- and motor-evoked potentials in predicting and monitoring the effect of therapy in spondylotic cervical myelopathy. Prospective randomized study. Spine 1999; 24(15):1593–1598.

28. Darden BV, Hatley MK, Owen JH. Neurogenic motor evoked potential monitoring in anterior cervical surgery. J Spinal Disord 1996; 9:485–493.

29. Gokaslan ZL, et al. Intraoperative monitoring of spinal cord function using motor evoked potentials via transcutaneous epidural electrode during anterior cervical spinal surgery. J Spinal Disord 1997; 10:299–303.

30. Padberg AM, et al. Somatosensory- and motor-evoked potential monitoring without a wake-up test during idiopathic scoliosis surgery. An accepted standard of care. Spine 1998; 23(12):1392–1400.

31. Sethuraman V, et al. The utility of transcranial motor-evoked potential monitoring as an indicator of impending cervical spinal cord injury. Presented at 29th annual meeting, Cervical Spine Research Society, November 29, 2001, Monterey, California.

24

Complications Related to the Surgical Management of Intradural Spinal Cord Tumors

Aaron S. Dumont, John A. Jane, Jr., and John A. Jane, Sr.
University of Virginia School of Medicine, Charlottesville, Virginia, U.S.A.

I. INTRODUCTION

The surgical management of intradural spinal cord tumors has evolved considerably over time, particularly over the past three decades with the widespread implementation of the operating microscope with its unparalleled magnification and illumination. Refinements in technique, equipment, monitoring, neuroprotection, and other adjuncts continue into the present. Prior to the 1970s many clinicians managing patients harboring intrinsic spinal cord tumors advocated conservative observation given the significant morbidity and mortality associated with operative intervention. Even the basic philosophy of surgical management has radically changed from the antiquated goal of open biopsy for diagnosis only, to one of radical and complete excision whenever possible complemented by stabilization when indicated. All clinical, pathological, and radiological data should be considered in each case among a neuro-oncological team, with the goal of appropriate but aggressive surgical removal of the tumor in the hope of achieving a cure.

The ensuing discussion will address the pathological entities comprising spinal cord tumors (as different considerations pertain to different lesion categories) in addition to important clinical and radiological features that help to guide individualized management of patients and operative strategies with emphasis on complication avoidance.

II. PATHOLOGICAL SPECTRUM

Intradural spinal tumors are comprised of a diverse spectrum of pathological lesions. Intradural spinal cord tumors may be broadly categorized into two large groups: extramedullary and intramedullary tumors (each with its own distinct subset of tumors and unique considerations for management) (Table 1).

The majority of extramedullary lesions are meningiomas, nerve sheath tumors, and filum ependymomas. Meningiomas arise from arachnoid cap cells in the dura near the

Table 1 Spinal Cord Tumors

Extramedullary (2/3)		Intramedullary (1/3)	
Meningioma	(40%)	Ependymoma	(45%)
Nerve sheath tumor	(40%)	Astrocytoma	(40%)
Ependymoma of filum	(15%)	Hemangioblastoma	(5%)
Miscellaneous	(5%)	Miscellaneous	(10%)

sleeve of the nerve root (accounting for their frequent lateral location, although those arising in the upper cervical spine and foramen magnum are often situated in a ventral or ventrolateral position). Meningiomas occur predominantly in females (75–85%), and most are thoracic in location (80%) (1–3). Most are entirely intradural, although approximately 10% are either intradural and extradural or entirely extradural (2). Bony involvement is usually not seen. Nerve sheath tumors include both schwannomas and neurofibromas. Schwannomas are grossly found as eccentric masses arising from the nerve with a discrete attachment that typically do not enlarge the nerve, while neurofibromas produce fusiform (plexiform) enlargement of the involved nerve root making delineation between tumor and normal nerve impossible. These tumors affect men and women equally, most commonly in the fourth to sixth decades, throughout the spine. Most nerve sheath tumors are intradural, but some may extend in a "dumbbell" fashion through the dural root sleeve and include both intradural and extradural components. Like nerve sheath tumors elsewhere, the vast majority arise from the sensory root. Additionally, some (10%) may be epidural or paraspinal in location or, rarely (< 1%), may be intramedullary (4). Malignancy may be found in some 2.5% of lesions (5), with 50% occurring in those with neurofibromatosis portending a poor prognosis. Filum terminale ependymomas, most of which are of the myxopapillary type, are most common in the third to fifth decades, with a slight predilection for males. Almost all are histologically benign. The remainder of extramedullary lesions are indeed rare but may include lipomas, dermoids, epidermoids, teratomas, paragangliomas, and various cysts.

The majority of intramedullary spinal cord tumors are primary glial neoplasms, including astrocytomas and ependymomas, in addition to less common tumors of glial nature, including oligodendrogliomas, gangliogliomas, and subependymomas (6–11). Astrocytomas of the spinal cord are most prevalent in the first three decades of life. Indeed, astrocytomas are the most common pediatric intramedullary spinal cord tumor. There is a predilection for involvement of the cerivical and cervicothoracic segments (60% of cases) (4). In pediatric patients, nearly 90% are benign lesions largely of the grade 1 and 2 fibrillary and pilocytic varieties, while the remaining 10% are malignant (8). In adults, fibrillary astrocytomas are most common, while pilocytic astrocytomas are confined to early adulthood. Malignant astrocytomas are seen in 25% of cases in adults (4). Ependymomas represent the most common intramedullary tumor in adults. There is no sex predominance, and they are found most frequently in middle-aged adults. Most ependymomas are benign and well circumscribed and do not infiltrate adjacent spinal cord parenchyma (10,12–14). Hemangioblastomas account for 3–8% of intramedullary tumors. Approximately 15–25% of hemangioblastomas of the spinal cord occur in association with von Hippel-Lindau syndrome (4). They occur at any age (rare in pediatric patients), are benign and vascular in origin, and are almost always found to have a pial attachment. Most arise from a dorsal or dorsolateral position. Other rare intramedullary tumors include metastases, nerve sheath tumors, inclusion tumors and cysts, melanocytomas, and neurocytomas. In addition, a myriad of lesions of nonneoplastic origin, including infections, sarcoidosis, multiple sclerosis, and other conditions leading to transverse myelitis, must be considered.

III. CLINICAL AND RADIOLOGICAL FEATURES

The clinical and radiological features of spinal cord tumors are important in deciding upon a specific treatment and when it should be implemented. Extramedullary tumors are usually slow-growing masses, and symptoms referable to these lesions are reflective of this. Symptoms, of course, depend upon specific location. Those arising around the foramen magnum and upper cervical regions are usually ventral in location and typically present with suboccipital and posterior cervical pain in addition to affecting the muscles of the distal arm (especially hand intrinsics), producing atrophy and discoordination. The symptoms usually progress in a characteristic fashion affecting the ipsilateral arm, followed by the ipsilateral leg, contralateral leg, and then the contralateral arm. Symptoms of hydrocephalus and raised intracranial pressure [presumably due to increased protein in the cerebrospinal fluid (CSF), impairing circulation] may also occur, particularly with those tumors producing complete myelographic block or with schwannomas that increase CSF protein. Long tract signs are typical of mid- and caudal cervical tumors with asymmetry of early signs and symptoms (ascribed to the lateral location of most of these tumors). A Brown-Sequard–type picture is reasonably common. Thoracic tumors are also dominated in presentation by long tract signs with early distal weakness. Posterior column involvement producing ataxia may also be seen with midline tumors. Filum lesions typically present with back pain with possible asymmetrical lower extremity radiation. Increased pain with recumbency may be seen with many extramedullary tumors, especially with large cauda equina tumors.

The mainstay of diagnosis in extramedullary tumors remains magnetic resonance (MR) imaging with and without gadolinium enhancement. Occasionally, myelography with postmyelographic computed tomography (CT) may also be useful. On noncontrasted images, extramedullary tumors typically demonstrate spinal cord or cauda equina displacement, CSF capping, and signal abnormalities. Most of these tumors are mildly hypointense to cord parenchyma on T1-weighted images, while nerve sheath tumors are more likely to be hyperintense to cord parenchyma on T2-weighted sequences compared to meningiomas. The majority of these tumors exhibit some degree of contrast enhancement, with meningiomas typically demonstrating uniform uptake and sometimes enhancement of adjacent dura (a so-called dural tail). More heterogeneous contrast uptake is usually seen with nerve sheath tumors and filum lesions.

The clinical features of intramedullary spinal cord tumors are quite variable. Initial symptoms are usually nonspecific and may progress insidiously with time, with a time to diagnosis of one to several years. More malignant lesions, however, may manifest symptoms over a span of weeks to months, and intratumoral hemorrhage may present acutely (more commonly with ependymomas). Pain, rarely radicular in nature, is the most common presenting symptom in adults. Motor and sensory symptoms are the initial manifestation in about one third of patients. With cervical cord lesions, upper extremity symptoms are typical, often with asymmetrical involvement. Sensory complaints usually consist of dysesthesias rather than numbness. A central cord syndrome may also be encountered.

Thoracic tumors most commonly produce sensory changes and spasticity, which often begins distally with proximal progression. Lumbar and conus medullaris tumors usually present with back pain and leg pain with early bowel and bladder involvement. On examination, patients with intramedullary tumors often demonstrate objective evidence of neurological dysfunction. A mild neurological deficit accompanied by evidence of cord enlargement on spinal imaging is indicative of most benign intramedullary tumors. Malignant tumors typically present with a more accelerated onset of symptoms with only mild cord enlargement on imaging evaluation.

The mainstay in the diagnosis of intramedullary tumors is also MR imaging. The majority of intramedullary tumors are isointense or slightly hypointense to normal cord on T1-weighted images, often accompanied by indiscrete cord enlargement. T2-weighted sequences are more sensitive in the detection of these lesions as most are hyperintense to normal cord. The true extent of the tumor (versus edema or polar cysts), however, is more specifically defined with contrasted images, with almost all tumors demonstrating some contrast uptake (Fig. 1). Ependymomas may demonstrate uniform contrast enhancement with symmetrical location within the cord. Most are accompanied by polar cysts. Heterogeneous enhancement may be seen with intratumoral cysts or necrosis. The appearance of astrocytomas is more heterogeneous, often exhibiting ill-defined margins with variable (and often irregular) contrast uptake. In some instances, particularly with presumed vascular intramedullary tumors such as hemangioblastomas, preoperative angiographic evaluation is warranted to facilitate pre-operative planning and guide intraoperative treatment by defining feeding and draining vessels.

Clinical and radiological follow-up of all patients remains an essential component of management in all patients harboring spinal cord tumors. Changes ascertained in clinical and/or radiological data may represent an indication for initial intervention, more frequent assessment, or adjuvant therapy/repeat intervention.

IV. MANAGEMENT PARADIGMS: AN INDIVIDUALIZED APPROACH

The tenets of contemporary management are founded upon an emphasis of complete surgical excision whenever possible with most spinal cord tumors (15,16). Although surgical management has advanced tremendously and is generally safe in experienced hands, it is associated with serious potential risks to neurological function in addition to the general risks of any surgical procedure. Proper patient selection remains a critical initial means of complication avoidance. It is imperative to consider all available clinical, radiological, and pathoanatomical data in each case in formulating a management decision. It is common to arrive at an initial misdiagnosis when assessing patients with symptoms suggestive of an intramedullary lesion. In some instances cervical degenerative disease has produced cord signal changes that may mimic the appearance of an intramedullary lesion. These lesions may resolve with treatment of the cervical spondylosis. In other cases, further work-up may reveal a Chiari malformation and syrinx rather than a tumor. In still other instances, work-up for multiple sclerosis, such as CSF studies, brain imaging, etc., have provided the diagnosis and obviated the need for operative intervention. Of course, the same principles apply to patients followed long term posttreatment. Abnormalities on follow-up imaging may represent simple post-operative changes, which can be followed with repeat imaging or other modalities to prove that this is truly the case rather than

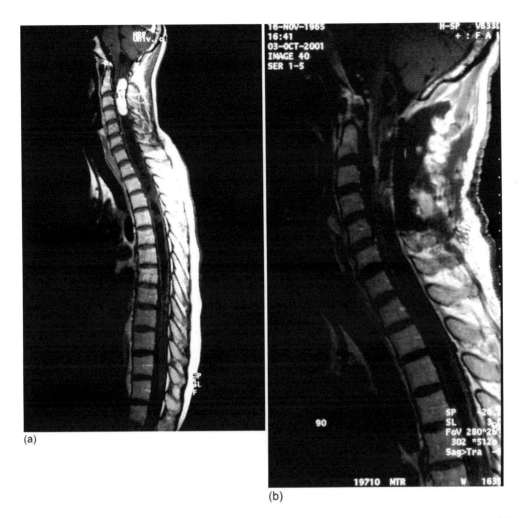

Figure 1 Cervical hemangioblastoma: 35-year-old female who presented with progressive right hand and subsequent arm numbness. (a) Preoperative MRI demonstrating a C2-4 hemangioblastoma. The tumor was resected completely while the patient was kept unparalyzed and allowed to breathe while being carefully monitored. (b) Postoperative MRI demonstrating complete resection of tumor and the patient had an excellent postoperative outcome.

residual tumor or recurrence. Unnecessary adjuvant and/or operative intervention can hence be minimized.

V. OPERATIVE INTERVENTION AND COMPLICATION AVOIDANCE

Most patients with clinical and radiological evidence of spinal cord tumors are offered surgical therapy. As discussed above, patient selection is critical as an initial step in complication avoidance. Some patients such as those with uncontrolled primary disease (disseminated glioblastoma or metastatic cancer), moribund medical conditions, or extremely elderly patients with minimal symptoms and lesions unlikely to grow substantially in their expected life expectancy (e.g., small meningiomas) in addition to patients afflicted with cord changes secondary to other processes (as discussed above) are not candidates for surgical intervention.

Preoperatively, patients are evaluated in the same fashion as all patients undergoing major neurosurgical procedures. Routine laboratory studies (complete blood counts, chemistries and coagulation tests) are performed with appropriate ancillary testing (chest x-rays, electrocardiograms) and medical clearance (in elective cases) as indicated. Frank discussions of the risks, benefits, alternatives, nature of the surgery with goals and expected outcomes are undertaken before surgery, and written informed consent is obtained.

All diagnostic studies, including MR imaging, myelography, angiography, electromyography (EMG), and cystomyography (CMG), are interpreted with all clinical data in a multidisciplinary neurosurgical conference, after which a definitive plan is formulated. Intraoperative monitoring decisions are also made here. In addition, following surgery almost all cases are discussed at neuroscience grand rounds where clinical, radiological, and pathological data are discussed among house staff and attendings from neurology, neuroradiology, neuropathology, medical neuro-oncology, radiation oncology, and neurosurgery to discuss the management of each case and follow-up/potential potential future therapy.

Preoperatively the authors administer high-dose corticosteroids (i.e., 6–10 mg of intravenous dexamethasone or 160 mg of intramuscular methylprednisolone acetate and 250 mg of intravenous methylprednisolone) with continuation of a dexamethasone taper regimen into the postoperative period. Some surgeons use on rare occasions the methylprednisolone 24-hour acute spinal cord injury protocol perioperatively. This may help to decrease perioperative edema and inflammation, although there is a lack of objective data to support its routine use. Prophylactic antibiotics are given in all cases and are continued into the perioperative period in the rare instance where a postoperative drain is used. Daily surveillance CSF analysis is performed in every patient with a lumbar drain.

Intraoperative monitoring is used on a selective basis using several different modalities. For patients with foramen magnum or high cervical cord lesions, paralytics are typically avoided, and the patient is allowed to breathe spontaneously. The operating team then watches carefully for changes in respiration during the surgery. Somatosensory-evoked potentials are used sparingly in selected cases. Intraoperative motor stimulation has proven to be useful for tumors of the conus and cauda equina, especially in patients with tethered cords and lipomas/lipomyelomeningoceles.

In every case intraoperative x-ray confirmation of the level in question is obtained prior to bony removal. Intraoperative ultrasonography is also employed to ensure complete exposure of the tumor (both cranial-caudal and lateral exposure) prior to dural opening (Fig. 2). These simple measures have ensured that the exposure of the tumor has been optimal and hemostasis can be meticulously achieved prior to opening of the dura, thereby minimizing introduction of blood into the subarachnoid space. The operative microscope is used in every case and the tumor is dissected, largely sharply, under high magnification. Prior to dural opening, the end-tidal PCO_2 is kept at an acceptable level (25–30) to slacken the spinal cord.

Different surgical considerations exist for each type of intradural tumor. Extramedullary lesions are first considered. In the vast majority of cases, benign nerve sheath tumors can be resected completely using a standard posterior laminectomy (although one may employ laminoplasty in children). Most nerve sheath tumors are dorsal or

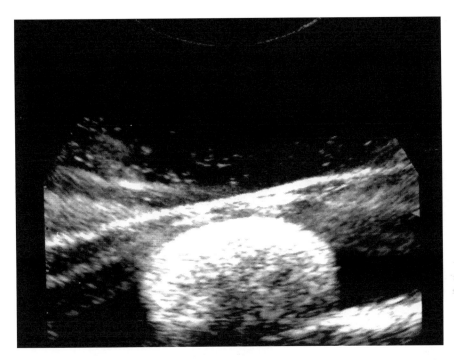

Figure 2 Intraoperative ultrasound — 85-year-old patient who presented with progressive paraparesis and diminished sensation. Intraoperative ultrasound performed before dural opening, illustrating the intradural extramedullary lesion, which proved to be a T1-2 meningioma.

dorsolateral in location and immediately apparent upon dural opening. Ventrally situated lesions may require transection of the dentate ligament for adequate exposure. In those lesions originating in the region of the cauda equina, the nerve roots must carefully be dissected off the tumor to allow access. One may attempt to displace the nerves to one side whenever possible, rather than attempting to work between displaced nerve roots on either side. Dissection proceeds directly on the tumor surface where one often encounters an arachnoid membrane, which is opened sharply and then reflected. The tumor capsule is then coagulated to diminish vascularity and shrink overall size. Attachment of the tumor to the nerve root of origin is identified, a step that may first require internal debulking of the tumor in cases of large tumors. Except in the case of small tumors (where preservation of some fasicles is possible), the nerve root of origin is taken to allow complete tumor removal. The ventral nerve root may be preserved, however. Sacrifice of the nerve root rarely produces detectable neurological deficit likely due to preexistent compensation by adjacent nerve roots. With lateral extension of the tumor beyond the foramen in the cervical spine, a complete unilateral facetectomy may be performed to facilitate exposure and safe removal. An important consideration during lateral dissection is the position of the vertebral artery, which is typically displaced anteriorly and medially and is separated from the tumor capsule by periosteum and a venous plexus. When total unilateral face-tectomy is performed, the authors have performed contralateral lateral mass plate fusion of the intact facet. With lateral extension in thoracic and lumbar tumors, an extended posterolateral approach (lateral extracavitary) is often used; only rarely is a combined anterior and posterior approach used. For malignant peripheral nerve sheath tumors, the treatment involves total excision followed by postoperative radiation.

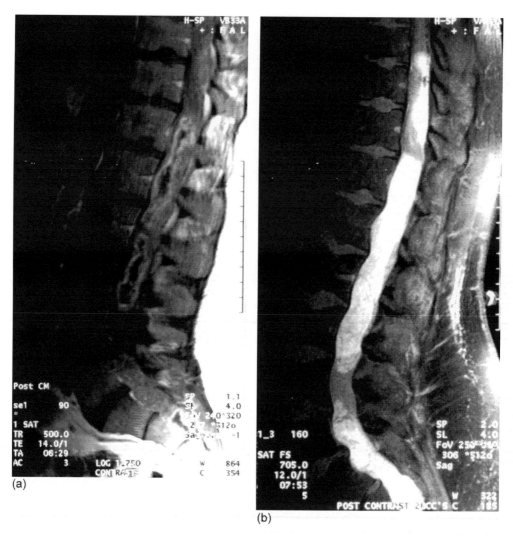

Figure 3 Extensive ependymoma with subarachnoid seeding—30-year-old male who presented with a long history of leg pain and diminished reflexes in his left lower extremity. Upon initial evaluation the patient was found to have an extensive intradural tumor from T9-S2. An extensive debulking was performed but was subtotal as the tumor had broken out from its capsule and infiltrated adjacent nerves (preoperative MRI; a, b). The patient subsequently presented 3 years later with blurred vision and visual loss. MR imaging demonstrated a parasellar tumor, which was resected via a frameless stereotactically guided craniotomy with pathology matching the spinal specimen (myxopapillary ependymoma) (c, d).

Total surgical resection of spinal meningiomas is the preferred and usually attainable goal for treatment of these intradural extramedullary lesions. Total resection, however, is not synonomous with cure as there is still a 10–15% recurrence rate at 10 years after gross total or near-total removal of spinal meningiomas (17). Standard posterior approaches (laminectomy, laminoplasty) are sufficient in most cases. Even in large, ventrally positioned tumors a posterior approach (with possible dentate ligament sectioning) is adequate as the tumor, during its growth, has provided the necessary exposure itself.

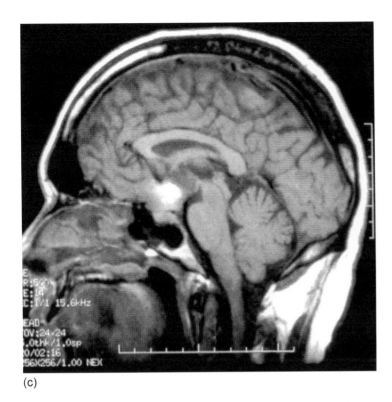

(c)

Figure 3 (*continued*)

The tumor is dissected along its surface after opening the investing arachnoid membrane. This plane is especially important in some ventral tumors where the tumor/spinal cord interface is less than optimally visualized. Preservation of this arachnoid plane increases the safety and ease of removal. The tumor surface is typically coagulated, and the tumor is excised en bloc (for smaller tumors) or debulked centrally and then pulled down on its sides for complete removal. There is some controversy about the management of the dural base, with options including coagulation of the attachment or total excision with dural graft. Some authors have reported no difference between methods (3). Many surgeons coagulate the attachment for ventral tumors and in tumors removed in the elderly (where the chance of symptomatic recurrence is less than the predicted morbidity of total dural excision), while for most dorsal and dorsolateral tumors (especially in younger patients) the dural attachment is excised.

For tumors of the filum terminale (e.g., ependymomas) several considerations for removal exist. Total en bloc resection is possible for small to moderate-sized tumors which are separate from the nerve roots of the cauda equina. There is often an afferent and efferent limb of normal filum that may be sectioned for total tumor removal. Some surgeons attempt to avoid internal decompression when possible to minimize the risk of CSF dissemination of tumor. Large filum terminale ependymomas carry the risk of CSF dissemination, and complete MR imaging of the brain and spine is probably warranted preoperatively (Fig. 3). These tumors may also be tenaciously adherent to neighboring nerve roots, at which point tumor debulking and subtotal removal becomes the realistic goal. Tumors in which piecemeal total or near-total removal

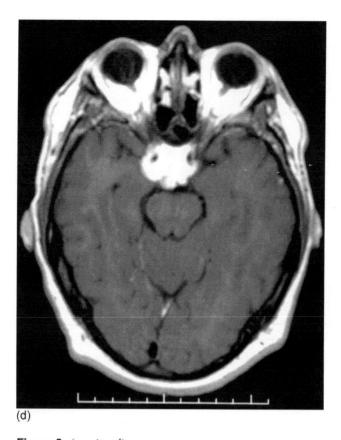

(d)

Figure 3 (*continued*)

has been achieved may be followed postoperatively with serial MR imaging. For those with subtotal removal, postoperative radiation therapy may be warranted, especially with known CSF dissemination, although this makes potential future surgery more difficult.

Surgery is a critical diagnostic and therapeutic step in the management of intramedullary spinal cord tumors. The goal of surgical therapy remains long-term tumor control with minimal morbidity. The aggressiveness of resection is particularly guided by the intraoperatively observed interface between tumor and spinal cord. Benign and well-circumscribed lesions can be totally excised with minimal morbidity, while in cases of poor demarcation of tumor boundaries, more conservative debulking is accomplished to minimize potential morbidity. Long-term tumor control or cure can be achieved for hemangioblastomas, most ependymomas, and some benign astrocytomas. Intraoperative neuropathological analysis can play an important role in guiding resection and minimizing potential morbidity to the patient. In cases of malignant intramedullary neoplasm of glial origin, aggressive surgical resection is not warranted and carries a significant risk of morbidity. An exception to this generally tenet involves mid-thoracic and lower malignant astrocytomas at the time of first recurrence associated with profound deficit (Fig. 4). Some surgeons have considered and performed excision of the spinal cord en bloc. Radiation becomes the mainstay of therapy in most patients with

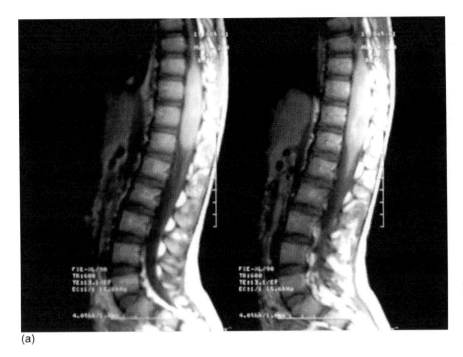

(a)

Figure 4 Reccurent malignant astrocytoma—9-year-old male who initially presented with progressive difficulty with gait (a). Preoperative MRI demonstrates a T9-12 enhancing intramedullary tumor that was aggressively resected. The patient improved postoperatively, but declined and presented with recurrence and profound deficit (b). Detailed discussions were held with the patient and family and radical resection with spinal cord removal from T7 to L1 was performed. Postoperative MRI revealed no residual tumor or recurrence at most recent follow-up (c).

malignant astrocytomas, however, and may also play a role in other subsets of patients (e.g., adult low-grade tumors, which tend to be more diffusely infiltrative than their pediatric counterparts, although efficacy is not entirely clear). Two general strategies are employed for tumor removal depending upon the nature of the lesion. For ependymomas and some astrocytic tumors, the general strategy for removal is one of central debulking followed by pulling down of the sides of the tumor with careful microdissection. However, for vascular tumors such as hemangioblastomas, the strategy is distinctly different, as inadvertent employment of the former strategy may be fraught with torrential hemorrhage that is often difficult to control. For hemangioblastomas, the surgeon must work around the lesion along the tumor surface while meticulously avoiding entrance into the tumor. En bloc resection is the goal, and indeed, piecemeal removal or incomplete resection would be extremely difficult to perform. It is always important to differentiate feeding vessels from vessels in transit along the tumor surface. Preoperative or intraoperative angiography can often be useful. Inadvertent sacrifice of vessels in transit can be devastating because of the nature of the blood supply to the spinal cord.

Attention to closure in all cases of intradural spinal cord tumor surgery is paramount. Significant morbidity can arise from complications of wound closure. The dura is closed in watertight fashion primarily, on occasion with a dural graft substitute.

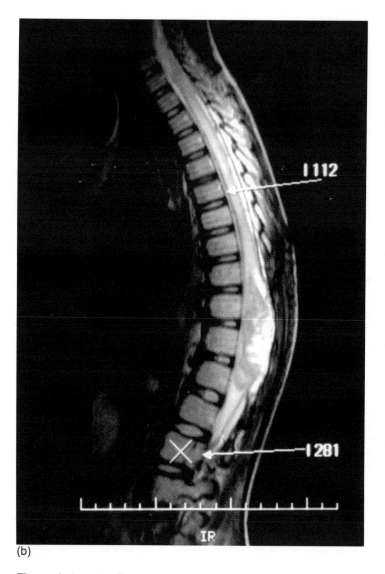

(b)

Figure 4 (*continued*)

The fascia is also closed in a meticulous watertight fashion, and the skin is closed with running nylon suture (or running absorbable suture in pediatric patients). More recently, some surgeons have selected a subcuticular running closure technique in certain pediatric patients.

Complications related to surgery of intradural spinal tumors include worsening of neurological deficits or production of new neurological symptoms, CSF leak, postoperative hematomas, postoperative infection (superficial, paraspinal, epidural/subdural, subdural, meningitis), and spinal instability and/or delayed deformity. Strategies discussed in the preceding sections have been refined and implemented by many surgeons to minimize morbidity to the patient and maximize preservation or improvement in postoperative neurological function.

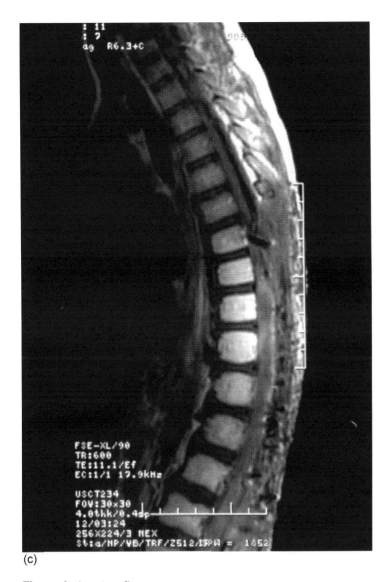

(c)

Figure 4 (*continued*)

VI. CONCLUSIONS

Tremendous progress has been made in the surgical management of spinal cord tumors with time. The dawning of the microsurgical era nearly three decades ago provided impetus for the evolution of surgical techniques. Continued refinements in technique, monitoring, and pharmacological and other adjuncts have helped direct surgical resection of intradural spinal cord tumors to its present state. The philosophy of management has evolved from conservative observation to biopsy only and to its contemporary form of aggressive resection with the goal of total removal whenever possible. Complications associated with surgery for intradural spinal cord tumor removal are numerous, but fortunately may be minimized through careful patient selection, preoperative planning, intraoperative decision making, meticulous technique, and careful postoperative management. The overall goal of surgical management remains long-term tumor control/cure with minimal morbidity, and in many cases this long sought-after goal may now come to fruition.

REFERENCES

1. Levy WJ, Bay J, Dohn DF. Spinal cord meningioma. J Neurosurg 1982; 57:804–812.
2. Nittner K. Spinal meningiomas, neurinomas, and neuofibromas, and hour glass tumours. Vinken PH, Bruyn GW, eds. Handbook of Clinical Neurology. Amsterdam: Elsevier North-Holland, 1976:177–322.
3. Solero CL, Fornari M, Giombini S, Lasio G, Oliveri G, Cimino C, Pluchino F. Spinal meningiomas: review of 174 operated cases. Neurosurgery 1989; 125:153–160.
4. McCormick PC, Stein BM. Spinal cord tumors in adults. In: Youmans JR, ed. Neurological Surgery. 4th ed. Philapelphia: W.B. Saunders Company, 1996:3102–3122.
5. Seppala MT, Haltia MJJ. Spinal malignant nerve sheath tumor or cellular schwannoma? A striking difference in prognosis. J Neurosurg 1993; 79:528–532.
6. Cooper PR. Outcome after operative treatment of intramedullary spinal cord tumors in adults: intermediate and long-term results in 51 patients. Neurosurgery 1989; 25:855–859.
7. DeSousa AL, Kalsbeck JE, Mealey J Jr, Campbell RL, Hockey A. Intraspinal tumors in children. A review of 81 cases. J Neurosurg 1979;51:437–45.
8. Epstein FJ, Farmer JP. Pediatric spinal cord tumor surgery. Neurosurg Clin North Am 1990; 1:569–590.
9. Fisher G, Mansuy L. Total removal of intramedullary ependyomas: follow-up study of 16 cases. Surg Neurol 1980; 14:243–290.
10. McCormick PC, Stein BM. Intramedullary tumors in adults. Neurosurg Clin North Am 1990; 1:609–630.
11. Stein BM, McCormick PC. Intramedullary neoplasms and vascular malformations. Clin Neuorsurg 1992; 39:361–387.
12. McCormick PC, Torres R, Post KD, Stein BM. Intramedullary ependymoma of the spinal cord. J Neurosurg 1990; 72:523–533.
13. Mork SJ, Loken AC. Ependymoma: a follow-up study of 101 cases. Cancer 1977; 40:907–915.
14. Russell DS, Rubenstein LJ. Pathology of Tumors of the Nervous System. 5th ed. Baltimore: Williams and Wilkins, 1989.
15. El-Mahdy W, Kane PJ, Powell MP, Crockard HA. Spinal intradural tumors: Part I — extramedullary. Br J Neurosurg 1999; 13:550–557.
16. Kane PJ, El-Mahdy W, Singh A, Powell MP, Crockard HA. Spinal intradural tumors: Part II — intramedullary. Br J Neurosurg 1999; 13:558–553.
17. Mirimanoff RO, Dusoretz DE, Linggood RM, Ojemann RJ, Martuza RL. Meningioma: analysis of recurrence and progression following neurosurgical resection. J Neurosurg 1985; 62:18–24.

25

Vascular Injury, Epidural Fibrosis, and Arachnoiditis

John C. France and Frank Fumich
West Virginia University Health Science Center, Morgantown, West Virginia, U.S.A.

Jeffery Hogg
West Virginia University, Morgantown, West Virginia, U.S.A.

I. VASCULAR INJURY

A. Introduction

Fortunately, the devastating occurrence of a significant vascular injury is a rare event in lumbar spine surgery. Although Mixter and Barr described lumbar discectomy as an operative technique to treat prolapse of the intervertebral disk herniation in 1934 (1), it was not until 1945 that published reports began to emerge regarding vascular injury as a complication of lumbar discectomy (2). In 1948 Holscher reported five cases of injury to the great vessels, pointing out the potential grave consequences of this type of injury (3). In his report a case of a pseudoaneurysm is described in detail and other cases are alluded to, some of which resulted in death. Since then numerous reports have been published describing arterial and venous injury as well as the formation of ateriovenous fistulas (4,5).

Direct vascular injury during an anterior approach to the spine can result from exposure, retraction, or in the course of applying instrumentation. An incidence of vascular injury as high as 15.6% has been reported by Baker et al. (6), although the rate of vascular injuries vary between other papers on anterior lumbar surgery (7–12). The venous system is much more prone to injury due to the thinner walls of these vessels and local anatomical factors such as the ascending lumbar vein on the left. The usual treatment strategy for a major vessel is direct repair or vein grafting. In spite of a successful repair, the risk of vascular thrombosis is high. In the trauma literature, for instance, the incidence of postrepair thrombosis has been noted to be as high as 58% (13–16). Less invasive surgical techniques, such as laparoscopic approaches for anterior spinal surgery, have done little to reduce the incidence of vascular injuries (17,18). Vascular injuries can also result as a complication of spinal instrumentation and have been noted acutely during the insertion of screws (19) and as a late complication due to aortic erosion (20). For this reason, care should be taken to prevent contact between a pulsating vessel and sharp edges on a spinal implant.

From the posterior approach a vascular injury can occur during insertion of pedicle screws (21,22), removal of a broken implant (23), or discectomy. Discectomy appears to be the procedure most prone to a vascular injury when an instrument such as a curette or pituitary rongeur exits the disk space anteriorly, causing direct injury to one of the great vessels (24,25). Vascular injuries cased by a pituitary rongeur are particularly difficult to manage because a portion of the vessel wall is often removed (24). In these cases, bleeding can be catastrophic, requiring a quick laparotomy and vascular control to save the life of the patient. In contrast, vascular injuries due to a misplaced implant may not be immediately recognized until the patient begins to have signs of hypovolemia. Because treatment of vascular injuries during posterior spinal surgery is difficult, prevention of these injuries is of the upmost importance. This requires careful placement of implants and the use of radiographic control to ensure that an implant is in an acceptable location. In addition, "plunges" with sharp instruments can usually be avoided if the surgeon steadies his or her hands against the patient's back. Finally, great care must be taken when cleaning out the disk space to avoid violation of the anterior disk.

B. Anatomy

Familiarity with vascular anatomy is key to avoiding vascular injuries. The inferior vena cava lies to the right of the aorta and along the right anterior aspect of the vertebral body and disk. In contrast, the aorta lies more along the midline of the anterior surface of the spine (Fig. 1). The aorta and inferior vena cava bifurcate into the common iliac arteries and veins, respectively, at approximately the level of the L4-5 level, although variations in the level of bifurcation are common. The left common iliac vein courses posterior to

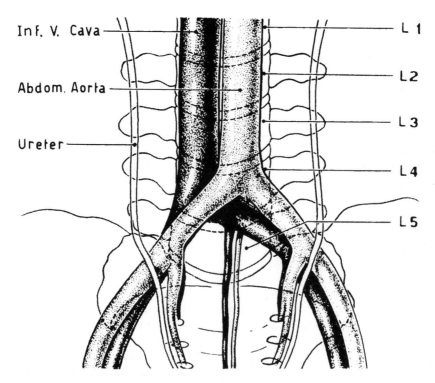

Figure 1 Relationship of the vascular anatomy to the corresponding lumbar disk level. (From Ref. 24.)

the aortic bifurcation and often extends just caudal to the axilla of the aortic bifurcation. The right iliac vein is shorter than the left and runs more vertically. The central sacral vein and artery exit the inferior vena cava and aorta, respectively, at their bifurcations then travel in the midline over the L5 vertebral body, L5-S1 disk, and sacral prominence. Because the vascular structures lie immediately anterior to the vertebral body and disk and because they are adherent to the spine, they are vulnerable to injury if the anterior anulus or anterior cortex of the vertebral body is penetrated. The risks of vascular injury appears to be greatest at the L4-5 level (Fig. 2a), where about 65% of the vascular injuries occur, perhaps due to the large surface area covered by vascular anatomy at this level and to the critical position of the left common iliac vein, which is entrapped between the anterior surface of the anulus and the firmer common iliac artery. The next most frequent level of vascular injury is the L5-S1 (Fig. 2b) level, which accounts for about 21% of the total.

By far the most commonly injured vessels are the common iliac artery and vein, although injuries to the inferior vena cava and distal aorta have also been reported (Fig. 3). Less frequent sites of injury include the internal iliac vessels (26–28), inferior mesenteric artery (29), and the middle sacral vessels (30). Vascular injury does not always occur on the side of the surgical approach (31) and may be the result of an indirect mechanism such as a traction injury as a result of adhesions between the anulus and the vein (32).

Other soft tissue injuries can occur in conjunction with a vascular injury, including injuries to the ureter (34,38), urethra (35,36), or intestines (29,39). It is important to take this into consideration during exploration and repair of a vascular injury as the result of a lumbar spinal procedure.

C. Incidence

Although vascular injuries during anterior surgery are not particularly uncommon, vascular injuries with posterior surgery have been rare. The precise incidence of a major vascular complication during lumbar disk surgery is unknown, but a survey of 3500 members of the American Academy of Orthopedic Surgeons (with a 33% response rate) found 59 arterial injuries (25). Similarly, Harbison polled 100 surgeons who performed lumbar discectomies as a significant portion of their practice and found 25 cases of vascular injury (40). DeSaussure polled 739 neurosurgeons and 2288 orthopedic surgeons and accumulated 106 cases of vascular injury with a mortality rate of 47% (41). Gurdjian et al. reported 1176 lumbar discectomies with only a single inferior vena cava tear, giving a vascular injury incidence of 0.085% (42). The larger series of Wildforster estimated the incidence of vascular injury to be 0.045% in a series of 68,329 lumbar cases (43). Using an average vascular injury rate of 0.05%, the approximately 200,000 lumbar discectomies performed annually in the United States would be complicated by 100 vascular injuries (44).

D. Presentation and Diagnosis

The early literature reports a mortality rate from vascular injury between 23 and 59% (29,40,41), although these figures predate many of the more modern vascular surgery techniques and were collected during the time period when surgeons were only beginning to recognize vascular injury as a potential complication of lumbar spinal surgery (45–50). A review of the literature between 1970 and 2002 revealed a mortality rate of 10% (4 deaths out of 40 cases) as a result of a vascular injury during spinal surgery. This

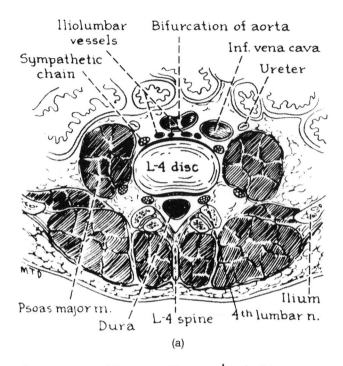

Iliolumbar vessels
Bifurcation of aorta
Sympathetic chain
Inf. vena cava
Ureter
L-4 disc
Psoas major m.
Dura
L-4 spine
4th lumbar n.
Ilium
MTD
(a)

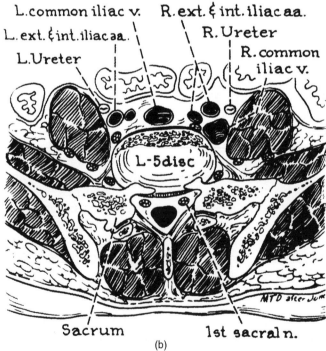

L.common iliac v.
R. ext. & int. iliac aa.
L. ext. & int. iliac aa.
R. Ureter
L. Ureter
R. common iliac v.
L-5disc
Sacrum
1st sacral n.
MTD after Jom
(b)

Figure 2 (a) Cross-sectional anatomy at the L4-5 disk level. (b) Cross-sectional anatomy at the L5-S1 disk level. (From Ref. 29.)

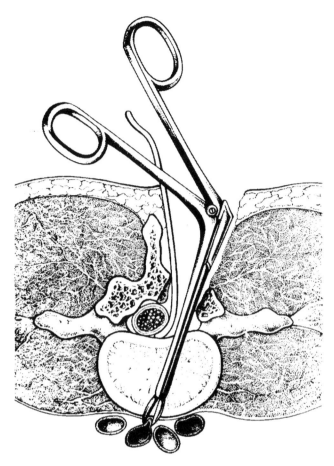

Figure 3 Schematic representation of mechanism of vascular injury during lumbar discectomy. (From Ref. 24.)

lower mortality rate may be more related to advances in vascular surgery rather than early detection since more than half the cases of reported vascular injuries had delays in diagnosis of 1–8 years. Of the 40 cases of vascular injuries reviewed, 6 were immediately recognized during the operation when the patient suffered a sudden drop in blood pressure. Surprisingly, only 3 patients were noted to have a gush of blood from the disk space (27,32,51–53). In some cases the diagnosis was made by observing a protuberant abdomen or bruit when the patient was rolled supine following surgery, while other cases were confirmed with CT scanning and arteriogram (53). All of the patients recognized early were treated successfully by surgical exploration. In contrast, a patient with intraoperative cardiovascular collapse without abnormal bleeding was thought to have suffered a coronary event but was found at the time of autopsy to have suffered a vascular injury (54).

Delayed recognition of a vascular injury following posterior lumbar spine surgery is not atypical. In the above-mentioned literature, 10 of 40 patients were recognized to have a probable vascular injury in the early postoperative period (recovery room). Only 2 of these patients had any indication of a problem intraoperatively, but they were stabilized with fluid administration. In some cases, profound hypotension was the presenting sign leading to immediate surgical intervention (55–57), although other patients were stabilized and treated first by arteriography (Fig. 4) (58). For these delayed cases, presenting symptoms included an unexplained drop in their hematocrit (33,59), abdominal pain, an expansile or tender masses, and/or a bruit or palpable thrills. Two patients exhibited signs of lower extremity edema or ischemia (60,61). Another patient demonstrated an expanding wound hematoma (30).

In rare cases, a vascular injury has not been recognized for many years and may present as an arteriovenous fistula. The presenting symptoms in these cases can include shortness of breath, congestive heart failure, claudication, or hepatosplenomegally (28,62–64) (Fig. 5). Abdominal pain with a palpable mass may be present, but perhaps the most consistent finding is an audible bruit upon auscultation of the abdomen. Applying direct pressure to the abdomen to occlude an arteriovenous fistula and then recording a decrease in pulse rate and a rise in diastolic blood pressure has been described as Branham's sign for this condition. Table 1 outlines various signs and symptoms of a vascular injury occurring as a result of spinal surgery.

Awareness of the possibility of a vascular complication and vigilance in its prevention and diagnosis is critical to a satisfactory outcome. Holscher summarized this condition well in 1948 when he wrote: "The ease with which this complication can occur can only be appreciated by the surgeon in whose hands such an unfortunate incident has happened" (3).

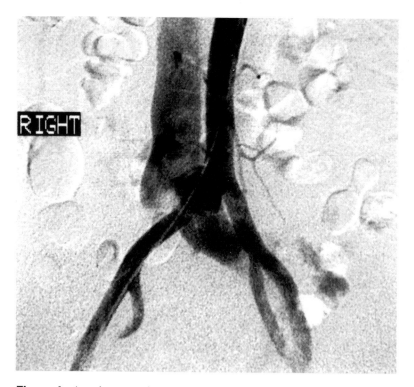

Figure 4 Arteriogram taken several days following a far lateral L4-5 discectomy demonstrating early filling of the inferior vena cava from the right common iliac artery due to an iatrogenic arteriovenous fistula.

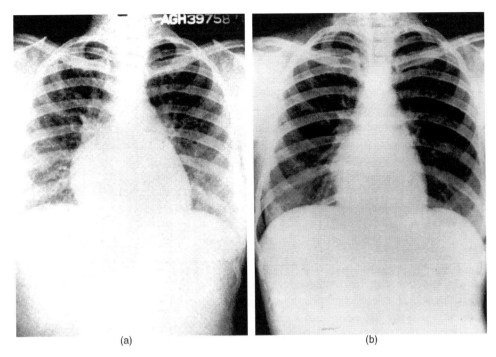

(a) (b)

Figure 5 (a) Enlargement of the cardiac shadow on a chest x-ray obtained 5 months post-operatively from an L4-5 discectomy. The patient's initial course was unremarkable until she developed lower extremity swelling and shortness of breath shortly before this film. An arteriovenous fistula was identified as the cause of her congestive heart failure. (b) Chest x-ray revealing resolution of the cardiac enlargement following surgical correction of the arteriovenous fistula. (From Ref. 40.)

Table 1 Diagnostic Indicators of Vascular Injury

Immediate (intraoperative)
Sudden hypotension, tachycardia
Bleeding from within the disk space
May be uneventful

Early (24–48 h postop)
Hypotension, tachycardia
Abdominal pain
Palpable abdominal mass, palpable thrill
Abdominal bruit
Ischemic extremity

Late (>48 h)
Abdominal mass, palpable thrill
Abdominal bruit
Hepatosplenomegaly
Congestive heart failure (chest pain, shortness of breath, murmur, abnormal x-ray)
Fatigue
Extremity edema
Assymetrical ankle brachial index
Extremity ischemia

E. Treatment, Prevention, and Medicolegal Implications

The spectrum of treatments applied to vascular injuries during spine surgery has ranged from vessel ligation with or without sympathectomy to vascular patches or grafts to direct repair (63). Fortunately, the mortality rate from this complication has decreased over the last several decades (34). Today, one risk for mortality seems to be a delay in diagnosis or failure to suspect a vascular injury (54). Therefore, early diagnosis of these injuries is imperative to avoid or minimize the risk of mortality. Once a vascular injury has been diagnosed, surgical intervention is the mainstay of treatment for those injuries involving the great vessels (51,56).

In the setting of less invasive techniques that do not allow for direct visualization of the operative field, prevention of these injuries may be even more difficult. Kanter and Friedman studied preoperative CT scans (65) to look at surgical trajectories in minimally invasive spine surgery that would minimize the risk to the surrounding vascular structures. Gower et al. studied the depth of safe disk penetration accounting for magnification on plain lateral radiographs (66). During discectomy, a variety of technical tips have been postulated to prevent vascular injury (3). These include (a) patient positioning, emphasizing that the abdomen should be allowed to hang free to decrease venous congestion and avoid compressing the vascular structures against the anterior aspect of the anulus (67), (b) awareness of the depth of instrument penetration into the disk space, even marking the pituitary to better visualize that depth, (c) measuring the dimensions of the disk on preoperative imaging studies, (d) maintaining hemostasis in the epidural space to improve exposure and make it more apparent that new bleeding is from within the disk space itself, perhaps indicating a vascular injury, and (e) pulling tissue out of the disk slowly (24).

The issue of partial versus complete discectomy has been considered, hypothesizing that attempting to remove the entire disk is more dangerous in terms of potential vascular injury. Intuitively this seems to be true, since the more passes made into the disk space, the greater the chance that one may result in overpenetration of the annulus fibrosis. The literature, however, is abundant with cases of partial discectomies that have resulted in vascular injury. Birkeland and Taylor suggested that once the pituitary enters the disk, it should be advanced forward only with the jaws open to minimize the risk of violating the anterior anulus (Fig. 6) (29). Simmons suggested that the pituitary should be tilted against the endplates to allow the surgeon tactile feedback, confirming that the instrument was contained within the disk space. (E. H. Simmons, personal communication).

Because of the devastating nature of many vascular injuries and the litigious nature of our society, it is not surprising that malpractice litigation often follows. Goodkin and Laska reviewed 17 such legal cases that reached jury verdicts (68). Although their discussion emphasizes the importance of early recognition, they acknowledge that in some injuries this is not possible. They also emphasize the importance of the informed consent process and conclude that this complication, detected and treated appropriately, does not constitute malpractice.

II. EPIDURAL FIBROSIS

A. Introduction

Failed back surgery syndrome may be defined as the presence of persistent or worsened lower back, buttock, thigh, or leg pain in a patient who has undergone at least one prior

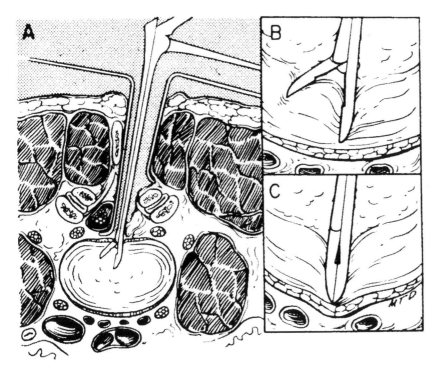

Figure 6 A schematic illustration of one technique to avoid anterior anulus penetration with the pituitary rongeur. Upon entering the disk space, the jaws of the rongeur are opened (A), then the pituitary is advanced while the jaws remain open (B), making anterior anular penetration less likely than would be the case if the jaws remain shut forming a point (C). (From Ref. 29.)

back surgery. The issue of failed back surgery is complex and includes issued related to residual spinal pathology, chronic pain behavior, and in some cases secondary gain.

There are multiple etiologies of the failed back surgery syndrome (FBSS). These may include failure to establish the correct diagnosis or a failure in the technical performance of the operation (69). In other cases, the patient has pathology that simply is not amenable to a surgical solution. Some of the organic causes for FBSS include epidural scarring, arachnoiditis, spinal stenosis, spinal instability, retention or recurrence of disk herniation, infection, and pseudoarthrosis (70). These anatomical causes of the FBSS are often compounded by psychosocial factors, such as workers' compensation claims and pending legal claims where secondary financial and or emotional gain are significant factors.

Although epidural fibrosis and arachnoiditis have been studied for over 60 years, they remain a controversial cause of spinal pain and have eluded a successful treatment method (71). Depending on how epidural fibrosis is defined, the incidence of this condition at repeat lumbar surgery ranges from 37 to 100% (72,73).

B. Etiology

Epidural fibrosis is part of the natural healing and scar formation that accompanies any surgical procedure. Although the effect of this scarring has been the subject of much research and controversy, the exact role that it plays in spinal pain is uncertain. The first animal study dedicated to the problem of epidural fibrosis was performed by Key and

Ford in 1948 (74). In this study, they demonstrated that following an insult to the anulus fibrosis in dogs, epidural scar tissue formed. To minimize the formation of scar, minimizing iatrogenic injury to the anulus has been encouraged (75). Another source of epidural scar formation was shown to be the overlying injured paraspinal muscles proposed by LaRocca and MacNab in 1974 (Fig. 7) (76). Using a rabbit model, they demonstrated that fibroblasts migrated from injured erector spinae musculature around the neural structures in a laminectomy defect and coined the term "laminectomy membrane" to describe this adherent scar tissue. In an effort to prevent this process, a number of barrier devices have been suggested or tested.

Several factors in the surgical technique have been implicated in leading to excessive postoperative epidural scarring. These include prolonged nerve root retraction, poor wound hemostasis, and retention of foreign bodies or surgical debris within the wound (71). Hoyland et al. found microscopic debree from surgical swabs within epidural scar and emphasized the need to remove all foreign material (77) (Fig. 8).

The consequences of epidural scar formation in pain and clinical improvement following surgery have been debated. Mixter and Barr believed that epidural fibrosis develops as nature's spontaneous but inefficient attempt to stabilize the spine following surgery (1). Others have argued that scar formation may lead to recurrent pain. Some studies have found a correlation between extensive epidural scarring, as measured by MRI, and suboptimal clinical outcomes including recurrent radicular symptoms (78–80). In one study patients having extensive peridural fibrosis were 3.2 times more likely to experience recurrent radicular pain than those patients with less extensive peridural scarring (92).

One factor hypothesized to result from scarring is tethering of nerve root to surrounding structures. Hypothetically, this could lead to nerve tension and ichemic effects with spinal motion when tension is placed on the root (71). Additionally, abundant scar could produce a mass effect leading to compression of neural structures. Finally, the mechanoreceptors entrapped within scar tissue may be activated, leading to pain (71).

The presence of epidural scar alone as a cause of postoperative pain is not universally accepted. Vogelsang et al. found no correlation between the degree of radicular

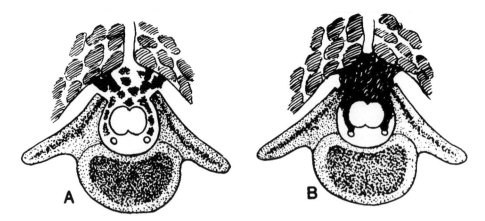

Figure 7 The laminectomy membrane. (A) Fibroblast migration from the undersurface of the overlying erector spinae musculature extending into the postoperative hematoma. (B) Dense fibrous scar binding the undersurface of the muscle to the posterior and lateral surfaces of the dura and nerve roots extends through the surgical defect. (From Ref. 76.)

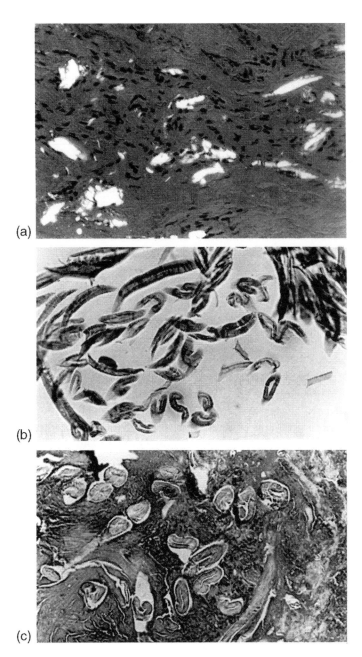

Figure 8 Surgical swab debris. (a) Peridural tissue viewed with polarizing microscopy show fragments of fibrillar, birefringment foreign material within fibrous tissue and in close association with chronic inflammatory cells (haematoxylin and eosin ×380). (b) Section of surgical swab material showing characteristic flattened-tube appearance. (c) Perineural biopsy of fibrous tissue containing foreign material which has the same flattened tube appearance as the swab (Grocotts Gomori ×90). (From Ref. 77.)

pain and the extent of epidural scarring present on MRI following lumbar micro-discectomy (81). Nygaard et al. had similar finding in their study of postoperative epidural scar formation with MRI following microdiscectomy (82). Others have also failed to demonstrate any correlation between a poor surgical outcome and increased scar formation (83,84).

C. Assessment

The initial assessment of a FBSS patient begins with a thorough, unbiased history and physical examination. In addition to the usual historical data obtained from a patient, a detailed sequence of the events of previous surgical procedures should be sought. A history of initial clinical improvement with later recurrence of symptoms can suggest an organic cause such as postoperative infection or recurrent disk herniation (85). Imaging of the spine plays an important role in these difficult cases, looking for signs of a correctable condition. Although epidural fibrosus or arachnoiditis is not generally amenable to a surgical solution, recurrent disk formation may be treated successfully with a surgical approach.

Historically, myelography and, subsequently, CT following myelography were the mainstay of spinal imaging for spinal patients. Although noncontrast CT is less specific than either contrast-enhanced CT or MR, contrast-enhanced CT can effectively distinguish peridural fibrosis from recurrent disk herniation in 80% of cases. Peridural fibrosis/scar demonstrates homogeneous contrast enhancement, whereas recurrent disk herniation is recognized as tissue with lower attenuation and a peripheral rim of contrast enhancement (86,87). A disk herniation may be suggested by the following factors: mass effect, contiguity with the disk space, a density above 90 Hounsfield units, calcification or gas within the tissue, and a polypoid or nodular configuration in the epidural space. Peridural fibrosis often demonstrates a more linear configuration (Fig. 9) and may be situated above or below the disk level. In general, scar lacks a significant mass effect.

Magnetic resonance imaging has become the preferred imaging modality of the spine in most regions of the country. In the absence of ferromagnetic instrumentation, it achieves multiplanar images with superior soft tissue contrast. With or without gadolidium contrast, MRI is able to distinguish between recurrent disk herniation and peridural fibrosis in many cases (88,89). MRI also allows the diagnosis of other conditions relevant to FBSS such as lateral recess stenosis, arachnoiditis, fat graft compression on the thecal sac, postoperative hematoma, or infection (90).

Peridural fibrosis is best evaluated by MR imaging performed before and immediately following intravenous gadolinium contrast material. To obtain maximal enhancement, fast spin-echo T2-weighted sagittal and axial images and pre- and post-contrast T1-weighted images are often obtained. The postcontrast T1-weighted images need to be obtained within approximately 2 minutes of the contrast injection in order to maximize the value of the injected contrast agent as the contrast between scar and disk diminishes with time, becoming negligible by 30 minutes postinjection (94).

Pre- and postcontrast MRI has a 96% accuracy in differentiating peridural fibrosis from disk herniation. For patients 6 or more weeks past surgery, sagittal and axial T1-weighted MR imaging before and after administration of gadopentetate dimeglumine is an effective method of evaluating the postoperative lumbar spine (91). The degree of enhancement of scar tissue relates to the length of time elapsed since surgery. Patients less than 9 months after surgery exhibit the greatest degree of enhancement, while patients many years from an operation may show minimal enhancement (93).

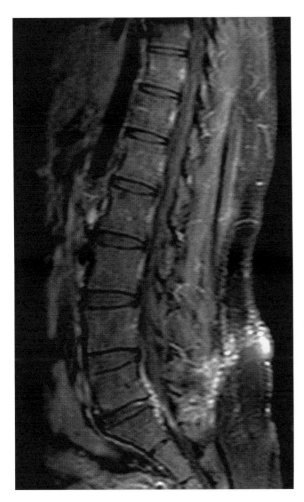

Figure 9 A sagittal postcontrast T1-weighted image showing linear enhancement in the peridural tissue at, above, and below the disk level in a 41-year-old woman 8 months postoperative after a L4-5 microdiscectomy.

Precontrast T1-weighted imaging of a recurrent disk herniation typically results in the appearance of a low-signal extradural mass of tissue isointense with disk material in the intervertebral space. Postcontrast T1-weighted images often show a rim of enhancing tissue surrounding the disk fragment. Using MR imaging, both recurrent disk herniation (Fig. 10) and peridural fibrosis (Fig. 11) have similar signal intensity on unenhanced T1-weighted images. It is important to recognize that both processes may coexist to variable degrees (Fig. 12).

Other findings on MRI included nerve-root enhancement (whether focal or intradural) and thickening of the nerve root postoperatively. In combination with a disk herniation or nerve-root displacement, these two signs may strengthen the indication for repeat surgery if a patient does not respond to nonoperative measures. However, root enhancement for the first 6 months following surgery may be a normal post-operative finding (93).

D. Treatment

The best treatment for arachnoiditis and peridural fibrosis is prevention. Damage to the dura and nerve roots from overretraction may be minimized by gentle handling of neural tissue during retraction and exposure (97,98). Frequent relief of retracted neural tissue lessens the potential injury to these structures and minimizes postoperative occurrence of arachnoiditis and epidural fibrosis. Surgical instruments should be in good condition, without small defects in their surface composition that may abrade the dura, leading to scarring. Blood and foreign material that may promote inflammation and scarring should be eliminated prior to closure.

In accordance with LaRocca's theory that fibroblast migration from roughened erector spinae musculature is a potential inciting event for the development of epidural

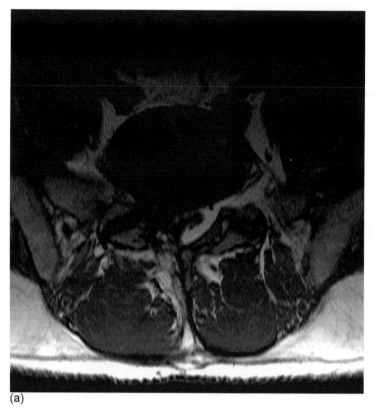

(a)

Figure 10 Recurrent disk herniation. (a) Precontrast T1-weighted image shows large right central zone extradural soft tissue mass ipsilateral to the right L5 laminectomy defect. Note the absent ligamentum flavum. (b) Fat suppression postcontrast T1-weighted image shows the right S1 nerve root sleeve posteriorly displaced against the right inferior articular facet of L5 and absence of enhancement within the bulk of extradural tissue. The nonenhancing extradural tissue is the migrated portion of an extruded disk. Some ring enhancement around this herniated disk material represents granulation tissue, and the remaining enhancement is likely a small degree of peridural fibrosis. (c) Sagittal postcontrast T1-weighted image shows a recurrent disk herniation at L5-S1 level. The inferior migration of the herniated disk material at the S1 suprapedicular level indicates this herniation is an extrusion. No visible enhancement is seen within the disk itself.

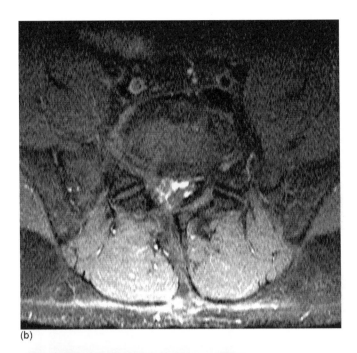

(b)

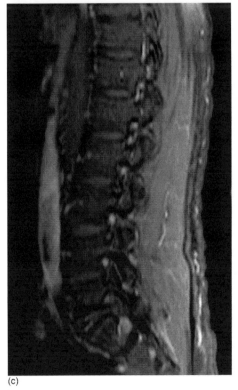

(c)

Figure 10 (*continued*)

scar formation, several laminectomy barriers have been tested. Biological substances such as autologous fat grafts, ligamentum nuchae, and nonbiological materials including gelfoam, silastic, polylactic acid, steroid preparations, and gelatin are some of the materials tested for this purpose (99,100).

LaRocca and MacNab tested the ability of gelfoam and silastic tubing to prevent epidural fibrosis in dogs by placing these materials into the laminectomy defect adjacent to the dura (76). The gelfoam effectively served as an interposing membrane preventing the formation of postoperative epidural scar even after its resorption by the 6-week time point, although the long-term benefit of this substance has been questioned (105). The silastic tubing also performed well in preventing scar formation and, like gelfoam, did not alter nerve conduction.

Other investigators have suggested that free fat graft makes an ideal interpositional membrane (101,102,105,106). The fat graft is harvested from the subcutaneous tissues and positioned over the dura, extending beyond the edges of laminectomy (Fig. 13). Although the free fat graft has been shown to block epidural scar formation, potential complications

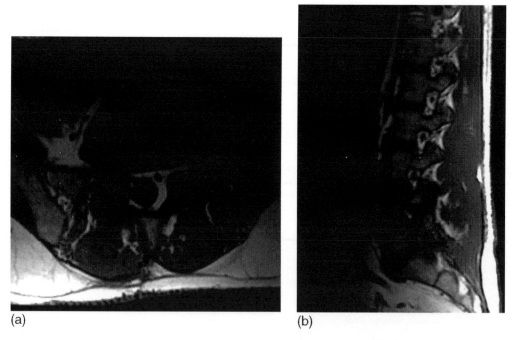

(a)   (b)

Figure 11 Peridural fibrosis. (a) Precontrast axial T1-weighted image shows an abnormal extradural soft tissue isointense with the intervertebral disk in the right subarticular and foraminal zone of the L5-S1 disk. The extradural fat in the foramen remains on the left and is absent on the symptomatic right side. Note surgical change of prior right side laminotomy. (b) Precontrast right sagittal T1-weighted image shows absence of epidural fat in the right L5-S1 neural foramen, extending both above and below the disk level. (c) Postcontrast axial T1-weighted image shows diffuse homogeneous enhancement in the abnormal tissue, which is isointense to the disk in the precontrast axial image at this level (a), indicating the enhancing tissue represents peridural fibrosis. (d) Right sagittal postcontrast T1-weighted image shows a subtle abnormality, which only becomes strikingly apparent when compared to the right sagittal precontrast T1-weighted image (b). With contrast the tissue that replaces the normal foraminal fat now has a characteristic homogeneous enhancement of peridural fibrosis.

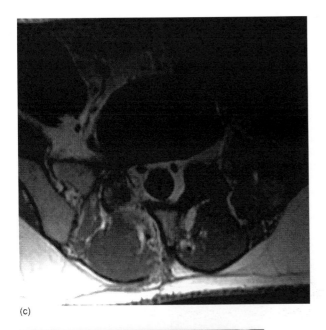

(c)

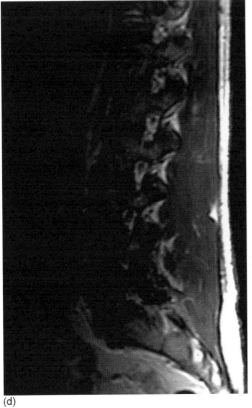

(d)

Figure 11 *(continued)*

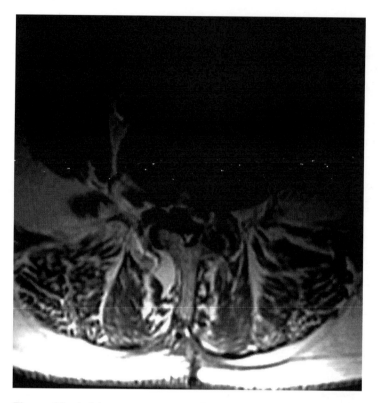

Figure 12 Axial postcontrast T1-weighted image shows the rim of enhancing granulation tissue surrounding the disk material, which does not demonstrate enhancement. The full extent of this combined process is best appreciated with scrutiny of multiple planes of pre- and postcontrast images.

such as nerve root or cauda equina compression can occur when packed tightly adjacent to these neural structures (103). Fat grafts have been shown to decrease in size over time, but in most studies maintain tissue planes at the laminectomy site. The infrequent incidence of hypertrophic scarring adjacent to a free fat graft has been observed, although this is rare (104). Ligmentum nuchae has been also used to inhibit epidural fibrosis following laminectomy (105).

The role of steroids in inhibiting scarring has also been investigated, but this has led to an increased incidence of wound breakdown and delayed healing in some cases (106). Other bioabsorbable materials such as polylactic acid have also been used to inhibit scar formation.

The barrier substance ADCON-L, designed for the prevention of epidural scar formation, was received with much enthusiasm in the mid-1990s after extensive testing in Europe and the United States (95,107–115). Significantly decreased epidural scarring was observed following lumbar disk surgery with the use of ADCON-L (116–118). Studies to quantitate the amount of postoperative epidural scar formation with MRI showed that those with decreased scar formation also had less postoperative back pain. This product eventually was removed from the market due to its association with persistent dural leaks following inadvertent durotomies. This was probably the result of the product's anti-inflammatory effects, which prevented healing of these small leaks (119).

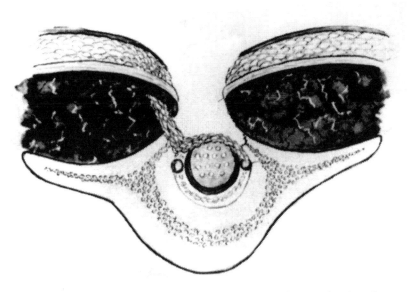

Figure 13 Placement of pedicle fat graft. Transverse diagram showing placement of the graft as it is brought over the dural sac and tucked under the nerve root, but not around it. It is held with a very fine suture of silk. (From Ref. 101.)

Neurolysis of epidural scar excision has been discouraged due to the often unsatis-factory clinical outcome following this procedure (71,73,120–122). Scar tissue excision associated with a revision spinal reconstructive procedure has resulted in the complete relief of symptoms in only a few cases (69). The risk of nerve root injury and durotomy are increased in revision surgery due to tethering and adherence of delicate and sometimes friable neural structures within scar tissue (Figs. 14,15). Removal of scar tissue alone as a reason for surgical intervention should only be considered in the presence of sphincter dysfunction or progressive motor weakness. Previous attempts to excise epidural scar have resulted in clinical failure in the majority of cases due to the reformation or abundant recurrence of scar tissue and keloid (98). A negative outcome from repeat lumbar disk surgery has been associated with surgery primarily performed for neurolysis, a diagnosis of predominantly fibrosis at the time of repeat surgery, and the absence of a pain-free interval following the initial surgery. Even stronger associations with negative outcomes following repeat surgery include a history of prior psychiatric treatment, current involvement in a compensation or a legal claim, or a history of having undergone two or more operations on the lumbar spine. Salvage therapy for the multiply operated back has trended toward the use of pain clinics, physical therapy, and psychosocial support. Return to work is hampered by psychological stressors, family and financial issues, and a lack of motivation in some individuals.

E. Conclusion

Epidural fibrosis is an unavoidable and natural process of the healing process following lumbar disk surgery. The association between the development and quantity of postoperative epidural scar formation and pain has been both supported and refuted by studies. Our ability to eliminate this factor following lumbar disk surgery has not yet been

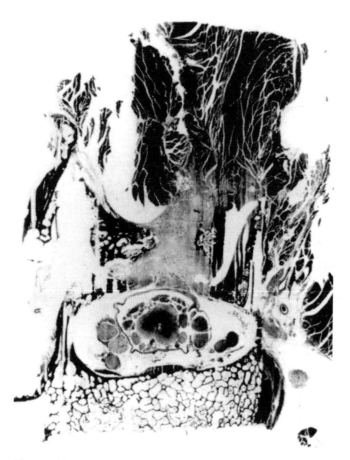

Figure 14 Low-power view of peridural fibrosis. Low-power cross-sectional view demonstrates peridural fibrosis within the laminectomy site that extends from the dural surface toward the fascial layer (Masson's trichrome; original magnification × 1). (From Ref. 122a.)

achieved and is compounded by several other organic, societal, and psychosocial issues that will continue to plague the spine surgeon treating lumbar disk disease. Our best treatment is prevention through gentle and meticulous surgical technique. The role of barrier substances is not entirely clear at the time of this writing.

III. ADHESIVE ARACHNOIDITIS

A. Introduction

Spinal arachnoiditis is a pathologic entity whose earliest description is credited to Quincke in 1893 (123) and by Spiller in 1903 (124). In the last 100 years the descriptive terminology, possible etiological agents, and methods of therapy have varied greatly, demonstrating the challenge of understanding and treating this spinal condition. The descriptive terminology has varied from meningitis serosa circumscripta spinalis, meningitis serosa spinalis, chronic spinal meningitis, and spinal meningitides with radiculo-myelopathy (125).

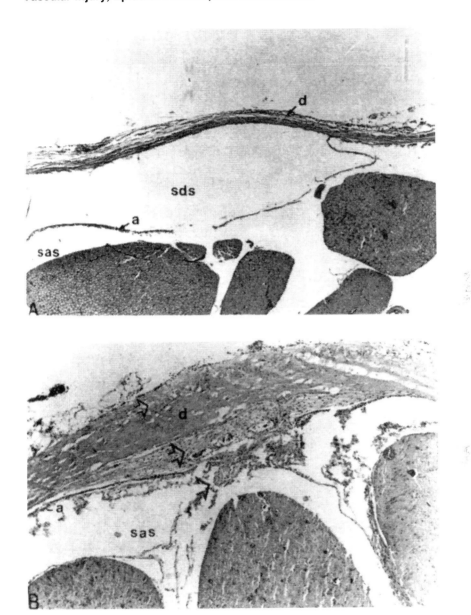

Figure 15 Normal and fibrotic changes in monkey meninges. Photomicrograhs illustrating (A) the normal meninges in a control animal and (B) the fibrotic changes in a treated animal. The subarachnoid space (sas), arachnoid (a), dura mater (d), and subdural space (sds) are labeled. (From Ref. 122b.)

B. Definition

Spinal arachnoiditis is an inflammation of the pia-arachnoid membrane surrounding the spinal cord or cauda equina (126). Arachnoiditis results from the intrathecal introduction of chemical irritants, radiographic contrast agents, and hemorrhage, all of which settle in dependent parts of the thecal sac, possibly accounting for the geographic location of intrathecal fibrosis (127). Degrees of severity vary from mild thickening of the membranes to solid adhesions obliterating the subarachnoid space, blocking cerebrospinal fluid flow and injected contrast agents (128). Arachnoiditis has been observed following myelography in patients without undergoing surgery as well as following spinal surgery (129).

C. Etiologies

Many causes of arachnoiditis have been posited. The suspected etiological agents include infections such as syphilis, gonorrhea, and tuberculosis, trauma, herniated nucleus pulposis, spinal surgery, exposure to myelographic dyes, spinal anesthesia, and predisposing conditions such as spinal stenosis (130). The majority of reported cases in the literature have involved the introduction of oil-based contrast material into the subarachnoid space or spinal surgery (131–133). Oil-based preparations, including Pantopaque, have had the highest correlation with the development of arachnoiditis.

Animal studies performed by Howland and Hoffman on dogs demonstrated arachnoiditis following the injection of Pantopaque contrast in combination with autologous blood into the subarachnoid space (134–136). Surgically, discectomy and laminectomy with extensive canal exploration have demonstrated the highest incidence of arachnoiditis (71,137). In 1924 Lear and Harvey demonstrated that injury to the pia-arachnoid, without obvious injury to the dura, may occur in surgery and is followed by dense adhesions of the pia-arachnoid and dural tissue (138). This is due to the bi-potential nature of the dural lining cells participating in the inflammatory response producing dural-leptomeningeal adhesions. The presence of blood or contrast material and traumatic insults such as surgery may all contribute to the genesis of arachnoiditis. The timing of surgery is also of importance following contrast myelography. Spinal surgery performed soon after the introduction of contrast into the leptomeninges has been correlated with a higher incidence of postoperative arachnoiditis as shown in Jorgensen et al.'s 1975 report (139).

D. Pathophysiology

Initially the subarachnoid space fills with a fibrinous exudate containing negligible cellular components. Within this medium, which is devoid of vascularization, few enzyme-producing leukocytes exist. Fibrinous bands may then proliferate in the absence of enzymes and leukocytes, which if present may have been beneficial in controlling this progression. As a result the fibrin-covered roots and redundant arachnoid membranes stick together during the resolution of inflammation. These fibrinous bands act as bridges for the fibrocytes to lay down collagen, thus converting the fibrin into collagenized adhesions. The end result is adhesive arachnoiditis, the end stage of arachnoid inflammation (Fig. 16).

The stenosis created by scarring of the nerve roots probably decreases local blood flow by increasing tension on the nerve roots. This factor may influence local nerve root metabolism and nerve root degeneration (140–142). The actual correlation between pain and the presence of arachnoiditis is not fully understood. It has been postulated that chronic arachnoiditis decreases nociceptor thresholds through an interruption of cerebrospinal fluid circulation (143). Fibrotic scarring of the nerve roots may increase mechanical sensitivity and decrease the nociceptor threshold.

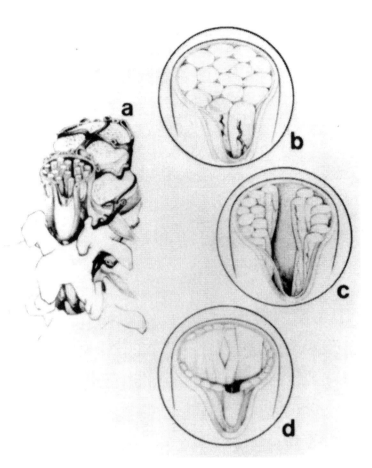

Figure 16 Anatomical relationships and progression of arachnoiditis. (a) Normal anatomical relationships in the lumbar area. (b) Radiculitis phase of lumbosacral arachnoiditis. (c) Arachnoiditis phase of lumbosacral arachnoidits. (d) Adhesive arachnoiditis phase of lumbosacral arachnoiditis. (From Ref. 140.)

E. Clinical Presentation and Diagnosis

Intadural adhesions seen on imaging studies do not always correlate with patients symptoms. However, in patients thought to be symptomatic from arachnoiditis, back pain and sciatica seem to be the predominant symptoms. In the postsurgical cases, the radicular leg pain may be recurrent or persistant or symptoms of neurogenic claudication may be present. The magnitude of back pain is often significantly greater in comparison to the expected level of postoperative pain. As Auld showed in a group of seven patients who went on to develop arachnoiditis, the level of pain experienced was significantly more severe than the expected level of postoperative pain following routine lumbar laminectomy (144). Along with the increased intensity and duration of back pain, episodes of violent bilateral leg muscle spasm and cramping have also been observed. In many cases the symptoms related to arachnoiditis often have a gradual onset. These symptoms usually appear 1–6 months following an operative lumbar spine procedure.

At the time of symptom onset, an elevated body temperature may occur along with rare chills. Peripheral white blood counts are usually within normal limits. Erythrocyte sedimentation rates are usually also within normal range but may occasionally exceed 30 mm/h. Examination of cerebrospinal fluid is usually clear, with blood present only following traumatic taps. Cerebrospinal fluid obtained early in the course of arachnoiditis usually reveals a paucity of leukocytes and an elevation of spinal fluid protein. Spinal fluid protein averages 50 mg/100 mL, but ranges of 11–126 mg/mL have been recorded.

Physical examination characteristically shows grossly limited spine motion and painful straight leg raising over 70° of hip flexion. The presence of objective bilateral

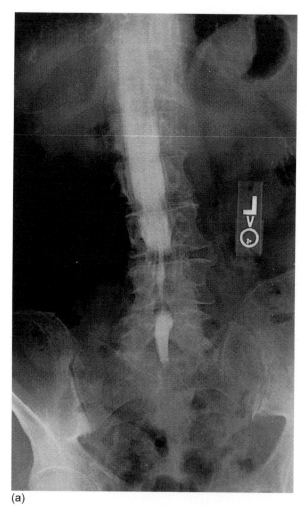

(a)

Figure 17 Spinal arachnoiditis in an 85-year-old woman who had undergone Pantopaque myelography 31 years prior to this study. (a) Note absent visibility of nerve roots and essentially featureless, distorted thecal sac at the level of the caudal L4 endplate. (b) The axial postmyelogram CT shows markedly diminutive contrast column due to adhesive arachnoiditis with clumping on lumbosacral nerve roots and adhesion of roots to the inner surface of the thecal sac. (c) A sagittal reconstruction from a postmyelogram CT reveals clumping and adhesions of lumbosacral nerve roots within the thecal sac, diffusely, and especially from the mid to the lower L4 through L5 levels.

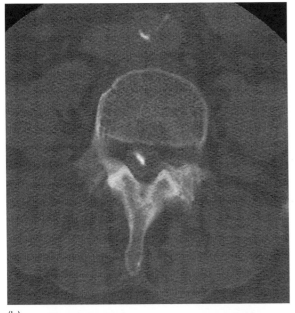

(b)

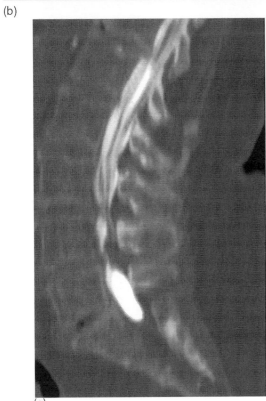

(c)

Figure 17 (*continued*)

sensory, motor, and reflex abnormalities often represent significant involvement of multiple root levels. Less than 25% of patients with symptomatic arachnoiditis have been reported to have sphincter involvement. Complete incontinence has been rarely observed.

Myelograms in the setting of arachnoiditis often demonstrates filling defects and/or an irregular, tapering, streaking of the oil column in the presence of an oil-based dye. Elkington described the classic picture of "candle gutterings" on oil-based myeolography in 1951 (145). Other descriptions have been used, but all describe decreased flow of contrast material through the leptomeninges that results from the adhesive reaction between the dural and pia-arachnoid layers. Myelography and CT/myelography clearly depict the changes associated with spinal arachnoiditis (Fig. 17). However, some cases of localized involvement may mimic a disk herniation if non-filling of only a single nerve root sleeve is present.

Three patterns of arachnoiditis have been described with MR imaging: (a) matted or clumped nerve roots (Fig. 18), (b) an "empty" thecal sac, in which nerve roots are diffusely scarred and adherent to the inner surface of the thecal sac (Fig. 19), and (c) a myelographic block due to filling of the thecal sac by a mass phenomenon, the end stage of the inflammatory response (Fig. 20) (146,147). The physical limit or boundary of arachnoiditis

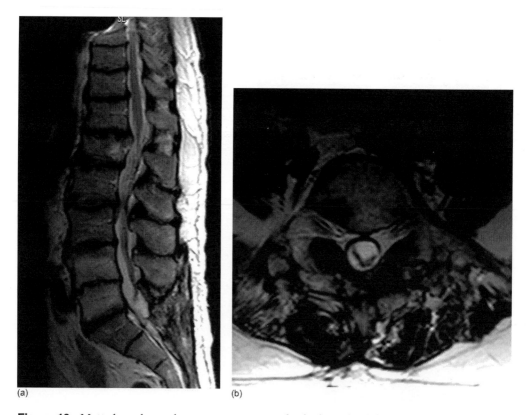

(a)   (b)

Figure 18 Matted or clumped nerve root pattern of spinal arachnoiditis occuring after a L5-S1 laminectomy. (a) Sagittal fast spin echo T2-weighted image suggests adhesions and clumping of lumbosacral nerve roots from inferior L2 endplate, extending caudally. However, accurate evaluation for this condition requires use of both sagittal and axial images. (b) Axial fast spin echo T2-weighted image confirms the clumping and adhesion of nerve roots characteristic of spinal arachnoiditis.

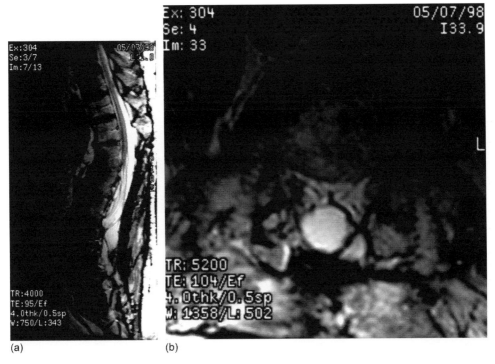

(a)   (b)

Figure 19 "Empty" thecal sac appearance of spinal arachnoiditis in an elderly man who had undergone multiple lumbar procedures, including instrumentation with transpedicular screws, which required subsequent removal due to postoperative infection. (a) Sagittal fast spin echo T2-weighted image demonstrated a paucity of visible nerve roots in the lumbar spinal canal caudal to the T12 level. The visible roots are adherent in a bizarre, distorted configuration, some attaching at multiple locations. (b) Axial fast spin echo T2-weighted image shows completely absent visibility of nerve roots at the L5 vertebral level. Note the laminectomy and screw tracks, which remain visible after their removal.

is demonstrated by the absence of adhesions, the presence of dural pulsations, and/or the free flow of cerebrospinal fluid.

Computed tomograpy may illustrate the presence of arachnoid calcification/ ossification and is recommended prior to myelography to avoid artifacts that may obscure any calcium-based structure or bone fragments impinging on the spinal cord or nerve roots.

Gross pathological findings of adhesive arachnoiditis include meningeal thickening and absent dural pulsations or CSF flow. Fibrous tissue coursing through the sub-arachnoid space obliterates the intradural space and some of the epidural space (Fig. 21). Histological specimens display fibrosis and/or hyalinization of the arachnoid. Chronic inflammatory cells, calcium depositions, osseous metaplasia, and intradural bone are much less common findings.

F. Classification

Adhesive arachnoiditis may present either gradually following the first 6 months of surgery or with a more delayed onset. Segmental arachnoiditis is defined as adhesions

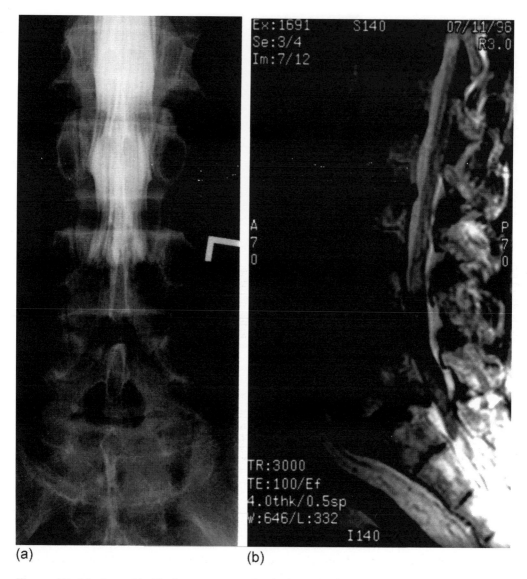

(a)   (b)

Figure 20 Myelographic block appearance of spinal arachnoiditis. (a) Anteroposterior lumbar myelogram shows complete obstruction to the passage of water soluble nonionic subarachnoid contrast at the mid-L4 level. (b) Sagittal fast spin echo T2-weighted image shows a low signal intensity mass of fibrotic tissue displacing cerebrospinal fluid intensity from the spinal canal in the same patient. (c) Axial postmyelogram CT image at the level of a transition between normal subarachnoid space and the fibrotic mass at L4.

at a single level. Diffuse arachnoiditis extends beyond one segment and usually is present caudally to the end of the dural sac.

Jorgensen et al. classified arachnoiditis into two types (139). Type I involves root sleeve adhesions or adhesions within the caudal thecal sac. Type II describes the presence of adhesive proliferation.

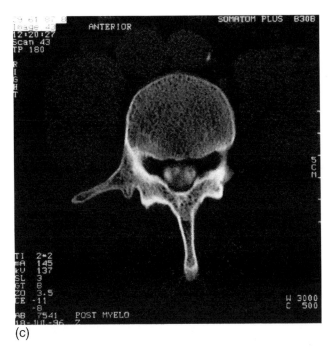

(c)

Figure 20 (*continued*)

A second radiological classification of adhesive arachnoidal disease has been described by Benner and Ehni (148). Type 0 describes extradural compression (spondylosis/stenosis) or a form of pseudoarachnoiditis, Type I is the presence of local postoperative changes, Type II consists of a single level of arachnoiditis, Type III of multiple levels, Type IV is a complete CSF block secondary to arachnoiditis, and Type V is arachnoiditis ascending greater than two levels above the operative site.

G. Treatment

There is no surgical treatment for the postoperative syndrome of adhesive arachnoiditis. In fact, surgery runs the risk of making the patient's symptoms worse. Only a few reports of success following durotomy and nerve root lysis of adhesions have been reported. The best treatment is the prevention of intradural scarring by careful handling of the neural structures. Any trauma to the dura allowing blood to penetrate the subarachnoid space may be an inciting event leading to the development of postoperative adhesive arachnoiditis. Dural tears created either by trauma or at the time of surgery necessitate repair to prevent this postoperative syndrome (97). If an acceptable closure technique is utilized at the time of the incidental durotomy, there does not appear to be any additional long-term increased risk of arachnoiditis following dural laceration (149–153).

Postoperative back braces to minimize nerve root motion for patients with symptoms of arachnoiditis have been tried with minimal success. Intrathecal steroids have occasionally been used with success to decrease symptoms of pain. Aggressive pain management and physical therapy are often the mainstay of treatment. The use of narcotic medications on a chronic basis for these patients remains controversial. All attempts

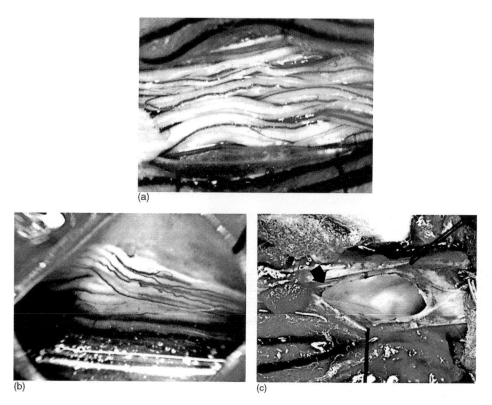

Figure 21 (a) Photograph at surgery of swollen and hyperemic nerve fibers that have herniated out of the dural incision to fill the operative field, indicating the previous increased tension within the dura. (b) The opened dura and the presence of nerve fibers of the cauda equina held by collagenous scar tissue to each other and to the dura. Small globules of Pantopague are floating in the cerebrospinal fluid at the bottom. (c) An opened dura exposing an apparently empty cavity. The atrophied nerve roots are enmeshed in solid collagenous scar tissue and are plastered to the dura and to each other. Thinned nerve roots are seen running along the edges of the dural opening (arrow). A piece of Gelfoam is on the right. (From Ref. 140.)

should be made to maximize patient activity and strengthening and progress towards normal activities of daily living. However, many patients fail to reach this goal. Dorsal spinal column stimulators, though not commonly used in the treatment of adhesive arachnoiditis, have had success rates as high as 35–60%. De La Porte recommends the use of spinal cord stimulators only following the exhaustion of all other treatments (154).

H. Conclusion

Adhesive arachnoiditis is a postoperative clinical syndrome with a poor prognosis and few treatment options. The prevention of postoperative scarring will depend on limiting the number of back operations to those most likely to be beneficial based on the patient's symptoms and specific mechanical findings. Further research into intrathecal scar prevention and the continued use of gentle surgical technique may decrease the incidence of this difficult syndrome.

ACKNOWLEDGMENTS

We express our gratitude to April McClay RN, Suzanne Smith, and Nina Clovis for their assistance in the collection and organization of reference material used in this chapter.

REFERENCES

1. Mixter WJ, Barr JS. Rupture of the intervertebral disk with involvement of the spinal cord. N Engl J Med 1934; 211:210–215.
2. Linton RR, White PD. Arteriovenous fistula between the right common iliac artery and the inferior vena cava. Arch Surg 1945; 50:6.
3. Holscher EC. Vascular complications of disk surgery. J Bone Joint Surg 1948; 39A:968–970.
4. Stambough JL, Simeone FA. Vascular complications in spine surgery. In: Herkowitz HN, Garfin SR, Balderston RA, Eismont FJ, Bell GW, Wiesel SW, eds. The Spine. Philadelphia: WB Saunders Company, 1999:1711–1724.
5. Ford LT. Symposium: Complications of lumbar-disc surgery, prevention and treatment. J Bone Joint Surg 1968; 50-A:382–393.
6. Baker JK, Reardon PR, Reardon MJ, Heggeness MH. Vascular injury in anterior lumbar surgery. Spine 1993; 18:2227–2230.
7. Harmon PH. Anterior Extraperitoneal lumbar disk excision and vertebral body fusion. Clin Orthop 1960; 18:169–182.
8. Flynn JC, Hoque MA. Anterior fusion of the lumbar spine. J Bone Joint Surg 1979; 61A:1143–1150.
9. Raugtstad TS, Harbo K, Hogberg A, Skeie S. Anterior interbody fusion of the lumbar spine. Acta Orthop Scand 1982; 53:561–565.
10. Westfall SH, Merenda JT, Naunheim KS, Conners RH, Kaminski DL, Weber TR. Exposure of the anterior spine:technique, complications, and results in 85 patients. Am J Surg 1987; 154:700–704.
11. Haas N, Blauth M, Tscherne H. Anterior plating in thoracolumbar spine injuries: indications, techniques, and results. Spine 1991; 16:S100–S111.
12. Kostuik JP. Anterior fixation for burst fractures of the thoracic and lumbar spine with or without neurologic involvement. Spine 1988; 13:286–293.
13. Hobson Rw, Yeager RA, Lynch TG, Lee BC, Jain K, Jamil Z, Padberg FT Jr. Femoral venous trauma: techniques for surgical management and early results. Am J Surg 1983; 146:220–224.
14. Pasch AR, Bishara RA, Schuler JJ, Lim LT, Myer JP, Merlotti G, Barrett JA, Flanigan DP. Results of venous reconstruction after civilian vascular trauma. Arch Surg 1986; 121:607–611.
15. Meyer J, Walsh J, Schuler J, Barrett J, Durham J, Eldrup-Jorgensen J, Schwarcz T, Flanigan DP. The early fate of venous repair after civilian vascular trauma. Ann Surg 1987; 206:458–464.
16. Aitken RJ, Matley PJ, Immelman EJ. Lower limb vein trauma: a long term clinical and physiological assessment. Br J Surg 1989; 76:585–588.
17. Nordestgaard AG, Bodily KC, Osborne Jr RW, Buttorff JD. Major vascular injuries during laparoscopic procedures. Am J Surg 1995; 169:543–545.
18. McAfee PC, Regan JR, Zdeblick T, Zuckerman J, Picetti GD, Heim S, Geis WP, Fedder IL. The incidence of complications in endoscopic anterior thoracolumbar spinal reconstruction surgery. Spine 1995; 20:1624–1632.
19. Matsuzaki H, Tokuhashi Y, Wakabayashi K, Kitamura S. Penetration of a screw into the thoracic aorta in anterior spinal instrumentation. Spine 1990; 15:1159–1165.
20. Jendrisak MD. Spontaneous abdominal aortic rupture from erosion by a lumbar fixation device: a case report. Surgery 1986; 99:631–633.

21. Blumenthal s, Gill K. Complications of the Wiltse pedicle screw fixation system. Spine 1993; 18:1867–1871.

22. Whitecloud TS, Butler JC, Cohen JL, Candelora PD. Complications with variable spinal plating system. Spine 1989; 14:472–476.

23. Vanichkachorn JS, Vaccaro AR, Cohen MJ, Cotler JM. Potential large vessel injury during thoracolumbar pedicle screw removal: a case report. Spine 1997; 22:110–113.

24. Montorsi W, Ghiringhelli C. Genesis, diagnosis, and treatment of vascular complications after intervertebral disk surgery. Int Surg 1973; 78:233–235.

25. Hohf RP. Arterial injuries occurring during orthopedic operations. Clin Orthop 1963; 28:21–37.

26. Shumaker HB, King H, Campbell R. Vascular complications from disk operations. J Trauma 1961; 1:177–185.

27. Bass J, Lach J, Fegelman RH. Vascular injuries during lumbar laminectomy. Am Surg 1980; 46:649–650.

28. Quigley TM, Stoney RJ. Arteriovenous fistulas following lumbar laminectomy: the anatomy defined. J Vasc Surg 1985; 2:828–833.

29. Birkeland IW, Taylor TKF. Major vascular injuries in lumbar disk surgery. J Bone Joint Surg 1969; 51B:4–19.

30. Kiev J, Dupont JR, Kerstein MD. Injury of a medial sacral vessel during lumbar laminectomy. Ann Vasc Surg 1996; 10:63–65.

31. Chiache K, Tsuji HK, Schobinger R, Kneisel J, Cooper P. Arteriovenous fistula between the common iliac vessels. Arch Surg 1960; 80:258–261.

32. Bolesta MJ. Vascular injury during lumbar discectomy associated with peridiscal fibrosis: case report and literaure review. J Spinal Disord 1995; 8:224–227.

33. Smith DW, Lawrence BD. Vascular complication of lumbar decompression laminectomy and foraminotomy: a unique case and review of the literature. Spine 1991; 16:387–390.

34. Fruhwirth J, Koch G, Amann W, Hauser H, Flaschka G. Vascular complications of lumbar disk surgery. Acta Neurochir 1996; 138:912–916.

35. Moore CA, Cohen A. Combined Arterial, venous, and ureteral injury complicating lumbar disk surgery. Am J Surg 1968; 115:574–577.

36. Sandoz I, Hodges CV. Ureteral injury incident to lumbar disk operation. J Urol 1965; 93:687.

37. Borski AA, Smith RA. Ureteral injury in lumbar disk operation. J Neurosurg 1960; 17:525.

38. McKay HW, Baird HH, Justis HR. Management of ureteral injuries. JAMA 1954; 154:202.

39. Smith EB, DeBord JR, Hanigan WC. Intestinal injury after lumbar discectomy. Surg Gyn Ob 1991; 173:22–24.

40. Harbison S. Major vascular complications of intervertebral disk surgery. Ann Surg 1954; 140:342–348.

41. DeSaussure R. Vascular injury coincident to disk surgery. J Neurosurg 1959; 16:222–229.

42. Gurdjian FS, Ostrowski AZ, Hardy WG, Lindner DW, Thomas LM. Results of operative treatment of protruded and ruptured lumbar discs. J Neurosurg 1961; 18:783–791.

43. Wildforster U. Intraoperative complications in lumbar intervertebral disk operations. Cooperative study of the spinal group of the German Society of Neurosurgery. Neurochirurgia 1991; 34:53–56.

44. Taylor MV, Deyo RA, Cherkin DC, Kreuter W. Low back pain hospitalization: recent United States trends and regional variations. Spine 1994; 19:1207–1213.

45. Seeley SF, Hughesw CW, Jahnke EJ. Major vessel damage in lumbar disk operation. Surgery 1954; 35:421–429.

46. Spittell JA, Palumbo PJ, Love JG, Ellis FH. Arteriovenous fistula complicating lumbar disk surgery. N Engl J Med 1963; 268:1162–1165.

47. Taylor H, Williams E. Arteriovenous fistula following disk surgery. Br J Surg 1962; 50:47–50.

48. Glass BA, Ilgenfritz HC. Arteriovenous fistula secondary to operation for ruptured intervertebral disc. Ann Surg 1954; 140:122–127.

49. Debakey ME, Cooley DA, Morris GC, Collins H. Arteriovenous fistula involving the abdominal aorta: report of four cases with successful repair. Ann Surg 1958; 147:646–658.

50. Fortune C. Arterio-venous fistula of the left common iliac artery and vein. Med J Austria 1956; 1:660–661.

51. Brewster DC, May ARL, Darling RC, Abbott WM, Moncure AC. Variable manifestations of vascular injury during lumbar disk surgery. Arch Surg 1979; 114:1026–1030.

52. Franzini M, Altana P, Annessi V, Lodini V. Iatrogenic vascular injuries following lumbar disc surgery: a case report and review of the literature. J Cardiovasc Surg 1987; 28:727–730.

53. Kelly JJ, Reuter KL, Waite RJ. Vascular injury complicating lumbar discectomy: CT diagnosis. AJR 1989; 153:1233–1234.

54. Ewah B, Calder I. Intraoperative death during lumbar discectomy. Br J Anesth 1991; 66:721–723.

55. Alvarez H, Cazarez JC, Hernandez A. An alternative repair of major vascular injury inflicted during lumbar disk surgery. Surgery 1987; 101:505–507.

56. Sagdic K, Ozer ZG, Senkaya I, Ture M. Vascular injury during lumbar disk surgery: report of two cases; a review of the literature. VASA 1996; 25:378–381.

57. Ezra E, Richenberg JL, Smellie WAB. Major vascular injury during lumbar laminectomy. J R Soc Med 1996; 89:108–109.

58. Salander JM, Youkey JR, Rich NM, Olson DW, Clagett GP. Vascular injury related to lumbar disk surgery. J Trauma 1984; 24:628–631.

59. Jarstfer BS, Rich NM. The challenge of arteriovenous fistula formation following disc surgery: a collective review. J Trauma 1976; 16:726–733.

60. Serrano Hernando FJ, Martin Paredero VM, Solis JV, Del Rio A, Lopez Parra JJ, Orgaz A, Aroca M, Tovar A, Paredero Del Bosque V. Iliac arteriovenous fistula as a complication of lumbar disk surgery: a report of two cases and review of literature. J Cardiovasc Surg 1986; 27:180–184.

61. Raptis S, Quigley F, Barker S. Vascular complications of elective lower lumbar disk surgery. Aust NZ J Surg 194 ; 64:216–219.

62. Hildreth DH, Turcke DA. Postlaminectomy arteriovenous fistula. Surgery 1977; 81:512–520.

63. Marks C, Weiner SN, Reyman M. Arteriovenous fistula secondary to intervertebral disk surgery. Surgery 1992; 32:417–424.

64. Duque Ac, Merlo I, Janeiro MJC, Madeira EN, Pinto-Ribeiro R. Postlaminectomy arteriovenous fistula: the Brazilian experience. J Cardiovasc 1991; 32:783–786.

65. Kanter SL, Friedman WA. Percutaneous discectomy: an anatomical study. Neurosurgery 1985; 16:141–146.

66. Gower DJ, Culp P, Ball M. Lateral lumbar spine roentgenograms: potential role in complications of lumbar disk surgery. Surg Neurol 1987; 27:316–318.

67. Eie N, Solgaard T, Kleppe H. The knee-elbow position in lumbar disk surgery: a review of complications. Spine 1983; 8:897–900.

68. Goodkin R, Laska LL. Vascular and visceral injuries associated with lumbar disk surgery: medicolegal implications. Surg Neurol 1998; 49:358–372.

69. Barr JS. Low-back and sciatic pain. J Bone Joint Surg 1951; 33A:633–649.

70. Greenwood J, McGuire TH, Kimbell F. A study of the causes of failure in the herniated intervertebral disk operation. An analysis of sixty-seven reoperated cases.. J Neurosurg 1952; 9:15–20.

71. Benoist M, Ficat C, Baraf P, Cauchoix J. Postoperative lumbar epiduro-arachnoiditis: diagnostic and therapeutic aspects. Spine 1980; 5:432–436.

72. Finnegan WJ, Fenlin JM, Marvel JP, Nardini RJ, Rothman RH. Results of surgical intervention in the symptomatic multiply-operated back patient. Analysis of sixty-seven cases followed for three to seven years. J Bone Joint Surg Am 1979; 61A:1077–1082.

73. Cauchoix J, Ficat C, Girard B. Repeat surgery after disk excision. Spine 1978; 3:256–259.

74. Key JA, Ford LT. Experimental intervertebral disk lesions. J Bone Joint Surg Am 1948; 30A:621–630.
75. Ether DB, Cain JE, Yaszemski MJ, Glover JM, Klucznik RP, Pyka RE, Lauerman WC. The influence of anulotomy section on disk competence. A radiographic, biomechanical, and histologic analysis. Spine 12994 ; 19:20712–2076.
76. LaRocca H, MacNab I. The laminectomy membrane. Studies in its evolution, characteristics, effects and prophylaxis in dogs. J Bone Joint Surg Br 1974; 56B:545–550.
77. Hoyland JA, Freemont AJ, Thomas AM, McMillan JJ, Jayson MI. Retained surgical swab debris in post-laminectomy arachnoiditis and peridural fibrosis. J Bone Joint Surg Br 1988; 70B:659–662.
78. Dullerud R, Graver V, Haakonen M, Haaland AK, Loeb M, Magnaes B. Influence of fibrinolytic factors on scar formation after lumbar discectomy. A magnetic resonance imaging follow-up study with clinical correlation performed 7 years after surgery. Spine 1998; 23: 1464–1469.
79. Maroon JC, Abla A, Bost J. Association between peridural scar and persistent low back pain after lumbar discectomy. Neurol Res 1999; 21:S43–S46.
80. Ross JS, Robertson JT, Frederickson RC, Petrie JL, Obuchowski N, Modic MT, deTribolet N. Association between peridural scar and recurrent radicular pain after lumbar discectomy. Magnetic resonance evaluation. Neurosurgery 1996; 38:855–863.
81. Vogelsang JP, Finkenstaedt M, Vogelsang M, Markakis E. Recurrent pain after lumbar discectomy: the diagnostic value of peridural scar on MRI. Eur Spine J 1999; 8:475–479.
82. Nygaard OP, Kloster R, Dullerud R, Jacobsen EA, Mellgren SI. No association between peridural scar and outcome after lumbar microdiscectomy. Acta Neurochir 1997; 139: 1095–1100.
83. Tullberg T, Grane P, Isacson J. Gadolinium-enhanced magnetic resonance imaging of 36 patients one year after lumbar disk resection. Spine 1994; 19:176–182.
84. Annertz M, Jonsson B, Stromqvist B, Holtas S. No relationship between epidural fibrosis and sciatica in the lumbar postdiscectomy syndrome: a study with contrast-enhanced magnetic resonance imaging in symptomatic and asymptomatic patients. Spine 1995; 20:449–453.
85. Fischgrund JS. Use of ADCON-L for epidural scar prevention. J Am Acad Orthop Surg 2000; 8:339–343.
86. Osborn AG. Diagnostic Neuroradiology. St. Louis: Mosby, 1994.
87. Gundry CR, Fritts HM. Magnetic resonance imaging of the musculoskeletal system. Part 8. The Spine, section 1. Clin Orthop 1997; 338:275–287.
88. Ido K, Urushidani H. Fibrous adhesive entrapment of lumbosacral nerve roots as a cause of sciatica. Spinal Cord 2001; 39(5):269–273.
89. Djukic S, Lang P, Morris J, Hoaglund F, Genant H. The postoperative spine. Magnetic resonance imaging. Orthop Clin North Am 1990; 21(3):603–624.
90. Ross JS, Masaryk TJ, Schrader M, Gentili A, Bohlman H, Modic MT. MR imaging of the postoperative lumbar spine: assessment with gadopentetate dimeglumine. Am J Roentgenol 1990; 155:867–872.
91. Ross JS, Obuchowski N, Modic MT. MR evaluation of epidural fibrosis: proposed grading system with intra- and inter-observer variability. Neurol Res 1999; 21(suppl 1):S23–S26.
92. Glickstein MF, Sussman SK. Time-dependent scar enhancement in magnetic resonance imaging of the postoperative lumbar spine. Skeletal Radiol 1991; 20(5):333–337.
93. Jinkins JR. Posttherapeutic Neurodiagnostic Imaging. Philadelphia: Lippincott-Raven, 1997.
94. Haughton V, Schreibman K, DeSmet A. Contrast between scar and recurrent herniated disk on contrast-enhanced MR images. AJNR Am J Neuroradiol 2002; 23:1652–1656.
95. BenDebba M, Augustus van Alphen H, Long DM. Association between peridural scar and activity-related pain after lumbar discectomy. Neurol Res 1999; 21(suppl 1):S37–S42.
96. Grane P, Lindqvist M. Evaluation of the post-operative lumbar spine with MR imaging. The role of contrast enhancement and thickening in nerve roots. Acta Radiol 1997; 38(6): 1035–1042.

97. Pheasant HC. Sources of failure in laminectomies. Orthop Clin North Am 1975; 6:319–329.

98. Fager CA, Freidberg SR. Analysis of failures and poor results of lumbar spine surgery. Spine 1980; 5:87–94.

99. Kiviuoto O. Use of free fat transplants to prevent epidural scar formation. An experimental study. Acta Orthop Scand 1976; 3:S21–S75.

100. Lee CK, Alexander H. Prevention of postlaminectomy scar formation. Spine 1984; 9:305–312.

101. Gill GG, Scheck M, Kelley ET, Rodrigo JJ. Pedicle fat grafts for the prevention of scar in low-back surgery. A preliminary report on the first 92 cases. Spine 1985; 10:662–667.

102. Langenskiold A, Kiviluoto O. Prevention of epidural scar formation after operations on the lumbar spine by means of free fat transplants. Clin Orthop Rel Res 1976; 115:92–95.

103. Stromqvist B, Jonsson B, Annertz M, Holtas S. Cauda equina syndrome caused by migrating fat graft after lumbar spinal decompression: a case report demonstrated with magnetic resonance imaging. Spine 1991; 16:100–101.

104. Martin-Ferrer S. Failure of autologous fat grafts to prevent postoperative epidural fibrosis in surgery of the lumbar spine. Neurosurgery 1989; 24:718–721.

105. Yon-Hing K, Reilly J, de Korampay V, Kirkaldy-Willis WH. Prevention of nerve root adhesions after laminectomy. Spine 1980; 5:59–64.

106. Jacobs RR, McClain O, Neff J. Control of postlaminectomy scar formation: an experimental and clinical study. Spine 1980; 5:223–229.

107. de Tribolet N, Porcet F, Lutz T, Gratzel O, Brotchi J, van Alphen A, van Acker RE, Benini A, Strommer KN, Bernays RL, Goffin J, Beuls EA, Ross JS. Clinical assessment of a novel anti-adhesion barrier gel: prospective, randomized, multicenter, clinical trial of ADCON- L to inhibit postoperative peridural fibrosis and related symptoms after lumbar discectomy. Am J Orthop 1998; 17:111–120.

108. Lo H, Frederickson RCA. Use of ADCON in neurosurgery: preclinical review. Neurol Res 1999; 21:S27–S32.

109. Robertson JT, Maier K, Anderson RW, Mule JL, Palatinsky EA. Prevention of epidural fibrosis with ADCON-L in presence of a durotomy during lumbar disk surgery: experiences with a pre-clinical model. Neurol Res 1999; 21:S61–S66.

110. Robertson JT, Petrie JL, Frederickson RCA, de Tribolet N, Hardy R. ADCON L symposium round table discussion. Eur Spine J 1996; 5:S26–S28.

111. Brotchi J, Pirotte B, De Witte O, Levivier M. Prevention of epidural fibrosis in a prospective series of 100 primary lumbo-sacral discectomy patients: follow-up and assessment at re-operation. Neurol Res 1999; 21:S47–S50.

112. Geisler FH. Prevention of peridural fibrosis: current methodologies. Neurol Res 1999; 21(suppl 1):S9–S22.

113. Schwicker D. Cost effectiveness of lumbar disk surgery and of a preventive treatment for peridural fibrosis. Eur Spine J 1996; 5:S21–S25.

114. de Tribolet N, Robertson JT. Lack of postdiscectomy adhesions following application of ADCON L: a case report. Eur Spine J 1996; 5:S18–S20.

115. Petrie JL, Ross JS. Use of ADCON L to inhibit postoperative peridural fibrosis and related symptoms following lumbar disk surgery: a preliminary report. Eur Spine J 1996; 5:S10–S17.

116. Einhaus SL, Robertson JT, Dohan FC, Wujek JR, Ahmad S. Reduction of peridural fibrosis after lumbar laminectomy and discectomy in dogs by a resorbable gel (ADCON L). Spine 1997; 22:1440–1447.

117. Ross JS, Robertson JT, Frederickson RC, Petrie JL, Obuchowski N, Modic MT, deTribolet N. Association between peridural scar and recurrent radicular pain after lumbar discectomy. Magnetic resonance evaluation. Neurosurgery 1996; 38:855–863.

118. Porchet F, Lombardi D, de Preux J, Pople IK. Inhibition of epidural fibrosis with ADCON-L: effect on clinical outcome one year following re-operation for recurrent lumbar radiculopathy. Neurol Res 1999; 21:S51–S60.

119. Le AX, Rogers DE, Dawson EG, Kropf MA, DeGrange DA, Delamarter RB. Unrecognized durotomy after lumbar discectomy: a report of four cases associated with the use of ADCON-L. Spine 2001; 26:115–118.

120. Waddell G, Kummel EG, Lotto WN, Graham JD, Hall H, McCulloch JA. Failed lumbar disk surgery and repeat surgery following industrial injuries. J Bone Joint Surg 1979; 61A:201–207.

121. Finnegan WJ, Fenlin JM, Marvel JP, Nardini RJ, Rothman RH. Results of surgical intervention in the symptomatic multiply operated back patient: analysis of 67 cases followed for three to seven years. J Bone Joint Surg 1979; 61A:1077–1082.

122. Law JD, Lehman RAW, Kirsch WM. Reoperation after lumbar discectomy. J Neurosurg 1978; 48:259–263.

122a. Gerszten PC, Moossy JJ, Flickinger JC, Gerszten K, Kalend A, Martinez AJ. Inhibition of peridual fibrosis of after laminectomy using low-dose external beam radiation in a dog model. Neurosurgery 2000; 46(6):1478–1485.

122b. Haughton VM, Nguyen CM, Ho. K-C. The etiology of focal spinal arachnoiditis: an experimental study. Spine 1993; 18:1193–1198.

123. Horrax G. Generalized cisternal arachnoiditis simulating cerebellar tumor: surgical treatment and end results. Arch Surg 1924; 9:95.

124. Spiller WG, Musser JH, Martin E. Arachnoidal cysts. Univ Penn Med Bull 1903; 16:27–30.

125. Benner B, Ehni G. Spinal arachnoiditis. The postoperative variety in particular. Spine 1978; 3:40–44.

126. Wiesel SW. The multiply operated lumbar spine. Instruct Course Lect 1985; 34:68–77.

127. DeVilliers PD, Booysen EL. Fibrous spinal stenosis. A report on 850 myelograms with a water-soluble contrast medium. Clin Orthop Rel Res 1976; 115:140–144.

128. Gabriel EM, Friedman AH. The failed back surgery syndrome. In: Wilkins RH, Rengachary SS. Neurosurgery 2nd ed. New York: McGraw-Hill 1996: 3863–3870.

129. Simeone FA. Lumbar disk disease. In: Wilkins RH, Rengachary SS, eds. Neurosurgery. 2nd ed. New York: McGraw-Hill, 1996:3805–3816.

130. Cooper RG, Mitchell WS, Illingworth KJ, St. Clair Forbes W, Gillespie JE, Jayson MI. The role of epidural fibrosis and defective fibrinolysis in the persistence of postlaminectomy back pain. Spine 1991; 16:1044–1048.

131. Delamarter RB, McCulloch JA. Microdiscectomy and microsurgical laminotomies. In: Frymoyer JW, ed. The Adult Spine: Principles and Practice. 2nd ed. Philadelphia: Lippincott, 1997:1961–1988.

132. Ghormley RK. The problem of multiple operations on the back. Instr Course Lect AAOS 1957; 14:56–63.

133. Long DM. Failed back surgery syndrome. Neurosurg Clin North Am 1991; 2:899–919.

134. Hoffman GS. Spinal arachnoiditis. What is the clinical spectrum? I. Spine 1983; 8:538–540.

135. Hoffman GS, Ellsworth CA, Wells EE, Franck WA, Mackie RW. Spinal arachnoiditis: What is the clinical spectrum? II. Arachnoiditis induced by pantopaque/autologous blood in dogs, a possible model for human disease. Spine 1983; 8:541–551.

136. Howland WJ, Curry LJ. Experimental studies of pantopaque arachnoiditis. Radiology 1966; 87:253.

137. Quiles M, Marchisello, Tsairis P. Lumbar adhesive arachnoiditis. Etiologic and pathologic aspects. Spine 1978; 3:45–50.

138. Lear M, Harvey S. The regeneration of the meninges. Ann Surg 1924; 80:536–544.

139. Jorgensen J, Hansen PH, Steenskow V, Ovesen N. A clinical and radiological study of chronic lower spinal arachnoiditis. Neuroradiology 1975; 9:139–144.

140. Burton CV. Lumbosacral arachnoiditis. Spine 1978; 3:24–30.

141. Burton CV, Kirkaldy-Willis WH, Yong-Hing K, Heithhoff KB. Causes of failure on the lumbar spine. Clin Orthop Rel Res 1981; 157:191–197.

142. Yamagami T, Matsui H, Tsuji H, Ichimura K, Sano A. Effects of laminectomy and retained extradural foreign body on cauda equina adhesion. Spine 1993; 18:1774–1781.

143. Cooper RG, Mitchell WS, Illingworth KJ, Forbes WS, Gillespie JE, Jayson MIV. Epidural fibrosis and defective fibrinolysis. Spine 1991; 15:1044–1048.
144. Auld AW. Chronic spinal arachnoiditis: a postoperative syndrome that may signal its onset. Spine 1978; 3(1):88–91.
145. Elkington JStC. Arachnoiditis. Mod Trends Neurol 1951; 1:149–161.
146. Castillo M, Harris JH. Imaging of the Spine: A Teaching File. Baltimore: Williams & Wilkins, 1998.
147. Bowen BC. Case Review: Spine Imaging. St. Louis: Mosby, 2001.
148. Benner B, Ehni G. Spinal arachnoiditis. Spine 1978; 31:40–44.
149. Bosacco SJ, Gardner MJ, Guille JT. Evaluation and treatment of dural tears in lumbar spine surgery: a review. Clin Orthop 2001; 389:238–247.
150. Cammisa FP Jr, Girardi FP, Sangani PK, Parvataneni HK, Cadag S, Sandhu HS. Incidental durotomy in spine surgery. Spine 2000; 25:2663–2667.
151. Wang JC, Bohlman HH, Riew KD. Dural tears secondary to operations on the lumbar spine: management and results after a two-year-minimum follow-up of eighty-eight patients. J Bone Joint Surg Am 1998; 80A:1728–1732.
152. Jones AAM, Stambough JL, Balderston RA, Rothman RH, Booth RE JR. Long-term results of lumbar spine surgery complicated by unintended incidental durotomy. Spine 1989; 14:443–446.
153. Eismont FJ, Wiesel SW, Rothman RH. Treatment of dural tears associated with spinal surgery. J Bone Joint Surg Am 1981; 63A:1132–1136.
154. De La Porte C, Siegfried J. Lumbosacral spinal fibrosis (spinal arachnoiditis); its diagnosis and treatment by spinal cord stimulation. Spine 1983; 8:593–603.

26
Complications of Thoracic and Lumbar Pedicle Screw Fixation

Se-Il Suk and Sang-Min Lee
Seoul Spine Institute, Inje University, Sanggye Paik Hospital, Seoul, Korea

I. INTRODUCTION

Pedicle screw fixation has become one the most widely used fixation methods in modern spinal surgery. This is due in part to the superior mechanical properties of the pedicle screw, which provides the strongest fixation site in most situations. When correctly placed, pedicle screws avoid encroachment into the spinal canal and thus prevent neural irritation. Pedicle screws are an integral component of rigid internal fixation that allows early mobilization without external bracing. Pedicle screws can be used in regions of the spine following laminectomy where wire and sublaminar hook constructs may not be used. Finally, pedicle fixation has successfully been employed over the entire spine and in a wide variety of pathological conditions, making the pedicle screw a very flexible form of internal fixation. When compared with hooks, pedicle screws offer enhanced three-dimensional correction of deformities and can be used to preserve motion segments.

Despite the advantages of pedicle screw fixation over other types of spinal implants, usage of pedicle screws has been limited by concerns over the risk of screw misplacement, which can lead to serious neurological injuries. Misplaced screws not only are useless in terms of fixation, but also pose a serious neurovascular risk. In certain regions of the spine, pedicle screws are thought to pose a particularly high risk. For example, screws placed on the concave side at the apex of a coronal spinal deformity are in close proximity to the spinal cord that is tethered by the spinal deformity. In this setting, even a minor screw breech can lead to a cord injury. Likewise, cervical pedicle screws in the C3-6 regions have been associated with encroachment into the transverse foramen, in some cases leading to vascular injury. This chapter will address the anatomy and technical aspects of pedicular fixation in the thoracolumbar spine and review the literature associated with pedicle screw placement. Our overall goal will be to stress complication avoidance.

II. PEDICLE AND PEDICLE SCREW FIXATION

A. Anatomy

For safe and reliable pedicle screw usage, a thorough understanding of spinal anatomy is mandatory. This anatomical knowledge must be specific to various regions of the spine where screw fixation is employed.

The pedicles in the thoracic and lumbar regions of the spine are short and relatively thick and project dorsally from the upper (cranial) portion of the vertebral body. The angle formed by the pedicle and the vertebral body in the coronal and sagittal planes varies depending on the spinal location. The overall shape of the pedicle forms an oval cylinder in cross section with a wall of cortical bone that is thicker medially than laterally. Immediately medial to the pedicle are the neural elements in most regions of the spine. The superior and inferior aspects of the pedicles are adjacent to the intervertebral foramen and close to the exiting nerve roots and segmental blood vessels. In particular, the nerve roots traverse the foramen just inferior to the pedicles, making them vulnerable to an inferior breech of the pedicle. The anterolateral surface of the spine is adjacent to great vessels and internal organs, which could be injured by instrument "plunges" or overly long pedicle screw implants.

The shapes, dimensions, and orientations of the pedicles vary significantly from region to region within the spine (1). Vertical (sagittal) diameter of the pedicle in adults is the most narrow at the T1 vertebra measuring 9.9 mm on average (range 7.0–14.5 mm) and is the widest at T11, measuring 17.4 mm on average (range 12.5–24.1 mm). The transverse diameter of the pedicle is the narrowest dimension of the pedicle and determines the diameter of pedicle screw that can be used. The transverse diameter is widest at L5 (avg. 18 mm; range 9.1–29.0 mm) and narrowest at T4 or T5 (avg. 4.5 mm; range 3.0–7.0 mm). The diameter decreases gradually from the T1 to T4 or T5 and then gradually increases as one moves caudad to the L5 level. The transverse angle of the pedicles, which is the angle formed by the axis of the pedicle and a vertical (parallel to the spinous process), is important to consider when preparing a pilot hole for screw placement. The transverse angle of the pedicles gradually decreases from a mean of 30 degrees at T1 vertebra to negative 5 degrees (range $-17°$–14.5°) at T12 and then increases to 30 degrees at the L5 level (range 19°–44°). The sagittal angle, which is the angle formed by the axis of the pedicle and a horizontal line paralleling the lower vertebral endplate, is the largest (cephalad direction) at T2 (17.5 degrees on average) and is the least at L5, where it averages -1.8 degrees. The depth from the dorsal surface of the pedicle to anterior cortex is the shortest at T1, measuring 36.9 mm on average (range 26–52 mm), and longest at the L2 or L3 vertebra, measuring 51.9 mm on average (range 42–62 mm). These anatomical parameters should be considered during screw preparation and implant selection and are especially critical in spinal deformity surgery where radiographic guidance is obscured by rotational or angular deformities of the spinal column.

B. Clinical Applications of Pedicle Screws

Despite the biomechanical and theoretical advantages of pedicle screw instrumentation, many surgeons hesitate to use pedicle screws, especially in certain regions of the spine (e.g., the cervical or thoracic spine), for fear of causing a neurological deficit due to improperly placed implants. Placement of pedicle screws is especially demanding when operating on very young patients or those with severe spinal deformities. However, in recent years the use of pedicle screws in the thoracic region of the spine has increased in popularity.

With regards to planning for a thoracic pedicle screw case, Cinotti et al. (2) suggested measuring the width of the pedicles in the T4–T8 region on CT scans prior to surgery, as the widths may not be suitable for pedicle instrumentation. Fortunately, in nondeformity cases there appears to be a 2 mm lateral epidural space along the medial boarder of the pedicle as shown by Reynolds et al. in a study employing radiographic contrast (3). Gertzbein and Robbins hypothesized that a maximal "safe zone" for medial encroachment of a pedicular implant would be about 4 mm, including 2 mm of epidural space and the 2 mm subarachnoid space in thoracic region lateral to the actual spinal cord tissue (4).

The anatomical factors, i.e., transverse pedicle widths and angle, may vary in the deformed spine depending on the etiology, magnitude, and rotation of the deformity. A meaningful analysis of transverse screw angle requires a fundamental knowledge of segmental pedicle morphometry and a consistent association between the screw entry point and the pedicle axis (1). Liljenqvist et al. (5,6) reported that the endosteal transverse pedicle width was significantly smaller on the concavity of a coronal deformity in the thoracic spine. These authors suggested using caution when considering the use of pedicle screws in the apical region on the concave side of a coronal deformity due to the increased theoretical risk in cord injury. Despite the challenges of placing pedicular implants in deformity patients, O'Brien et al. (7) found no pedicles that would not accept a pedicular implant among 512 thoracic morphologies in 29 adults with thoracic idiopathic scoliosis. Using Computed tomography (CT) scans, the pedicle transverse widths in this study were found to range between 4.6 and 8.25 mm.

In children the pedicles are smaller than in adults, but the relative pedicle dimensions and orientations remain similar those in the adult. Despite the general concerns regarding pedicle breeches, pedicle screw fixation is feasible in the immature spine. The spinal canal reaches 80–90% of the adult size at the time of birth and reaches the adult size by age 2. After the age of 3, the growth of the pedicle occurs mostly from the lateral aspect of the pedicle rather than the medial pedicle along the spinal canal. The pedicle may accept a screw in pediatric patients that is larger than the outer diameter of the pedicle without violation of the cortex due to plastic deformation (8–10). Zindrick et al. reported the safe use of pedicle screw implants in immature patients with carefully preoperative assessment (11).

III. COMPLICATIONS OF PEDICLE SCREW

Complications of spinal implants can be divided into three categories according to the point at which the complication is encountered. The first category consists of complications that occur during spinal exposure and includes soft tissue injury, adjacent facet damage, and fractures of the transverse process. The second category consists of complications encountered during preparation of the implant site and includes pedicle penetration, drill or tap overpenetration, pedicle fractures, and misplacement of screws. The third category includes complications encountered after placement of the implant such as screw cutout. The second category of complication is most characteristic of pedicle screws as opposed to other type of implants.

A. Screw Misplacement

Screw misplacement is the most common complication encountered with pedicle screw fixation. Several reports detail wide variability in the incidence of this occurrence, with a range from 0 to over 40% (Fig. 1a). Vaccaro et al. reported an overall rate of cortical penetration of 41% (23% medially, 18% laterally) for 90 pedicle screws placed in the T4–T12 region without radiographs (12,13). Roy-Camille et al. found a 10% rate of screw misplacement using intraoperative radiographs (14). Lonstein et al. reported a 5.1% incidence of screw misplacement in 4790 pedicles (15). Gertzbein and Robbins noted that 81% of the screws in his study were placed within 2 mm of the medial border of the pedicle but observed 6% that had 4–8 mm of medial canal encroachment (4). Belmont et al. (16) reported a rate of 43% wall perforation for thoracic pedicle screws but that noted 99% of the screws had less than 2 mm of medial cortical penetration. Amiot et al. (17) noted that

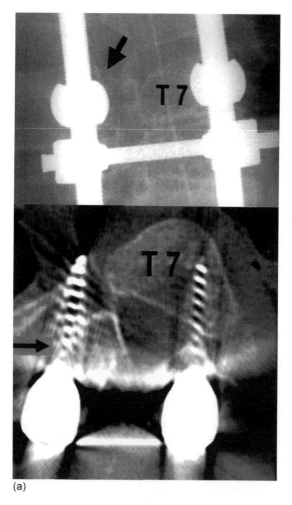

(a)

Figure 1   Complications of pedicle screw. (a) The postero-anterior radigraph and CT scan of a patient with idiopathic scoliosis demonstrated lateral cortical penetration of a screw put into the left pedicle of T7. (b) A surgeon unexperienced with pedicle screw fixation used thoracic pedicle screws to stabilize a thoracic fracture. The antero-posterior radiograph and CT scan show medial perforation of a screw put into the right pedicle of T8. The patient was paraplegic after the operation. (c) The pedicle screw penetrates the anterior cortex on the lateral radiograph. The screw tip is in close proximity to the aorta (Ao) on the CT scan.

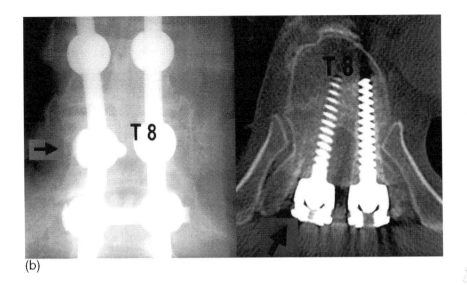

(b)

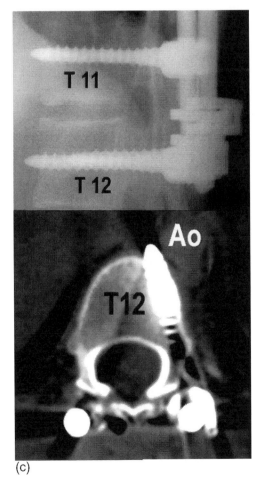

(c)

Figure 1 (*continued*)

87% of the thoracic screws in their study were correctly inserted and found a medial wall perforation rate of only 1%.

In idiopathic scoliosis, Halm et al. (18) found 19 of 104 screws (18.3%) to be misplaced but encountered no neurological complications. Liljenqvist et al. (5) observed that 30 of 120 thoracic pedicle screws (25%) penetrated the pedicle cortex or the anterior cortex of the vertebral body using computed tomography. Suk et al. (19) found 67 of 4604 thoracic pedicle screws to be malpositioned (1.5%) when used for various types of deformities. The direction of penetration was inferior in 33, lateral in 18, superior in 12, and medial in 4 pedicles.

Although the incidence of pedicle screw misplacement is significant, the rate of neurological consequences is fortunately much lower. Surgeon's experience and mastery of the surgical technique seems to be one of the most important variables in reducing the incidence of pedicle screw misplacement.

B. Neurological Complications

Neurological injury is the most feared complication of pedicle screw usage (Fig. 1b). Neurological sequelae can range from minor discomfort or paresthesia to total paralysis. Reported incidences of screw-related neurological complications in the lumbar spine vary from 0 to 41%. Castro (20) reported 5 root injuries among 12 patients receiving pedicle screws for an injury rate of 41.6%. In contrast, Roy-Camille et al. (14) observed only 12 neurological injuries among 227 patients receiving screws for a 5% incidence of neurological injury. Esses et al. (21) found transient neuropraxia in 2.4% and permanent nerve root injury in 2.3% of 617 patients reviewed by an American Back Society questionnaire. Schulze (22) noted only one patient (0.5%) with radicular irritation due to a screw, which was placed more than 6 mm medial to the pedicle wall despite the fact that 41% (100 of 244) of screws in this study had a medial wall breech. Lonstein et al. (15) found a 0.2% incidence of nerve root irritation in 4790 pedicle screws and concluded that there are few problems associated with the insertion of screws, assuming they are placed by an experienced surgeon who adheres to the principles of the operative technique. Brown et al. (23) noted a 2.2% incidence of transient radicular complaints following screw placement but found no residual sequelae among 759 pediatric thoracolumbar and lumbar pedicle screws used in the treatment of various pediatric spinal disorders.

Compared to the rate of developing a neurological symptom in the lumbar spine, the incidence of neurological complications in the thoracic spine is surprisingly low, ranging from 0 to 6% for thoracic pedicle screws used in the treatment of spinal deformities. This low incidence of neurological complication may be attributed to anatomical characteristics or the fact that root injuries in the thoracic level are inconspicuous and may rarely be detected. Belmont et al. (16) reported no neurological complications in the placement of 279 titanium thoracic pedicle screws of various diameters (4.5–6.5 mm). Liljenqvist et al. (5) also reported no neurological complications among 120 thoracic pedicle screws in idiopathic scoliosis. Gertzbein and Robbins (4) reviewed two "minor" neurological injuries among 71 thoracic screws (T8–T12) despite a 26% incidence of medial cortical penetration of up to 8 mm. This led them to hypothesize the 4 mm "safe zone" of medial encroachment mentioned above. Suk et al. (19) reported one screw-related neurological complication in 462 patients recieving 4604 (0.2%) thoracic pedicle screws for the treatment of a spinal deformity. The one neurological complication resulted in a transient paraparesis.

C. Dural Lacerations

Dural lacerations are more commonly encountered during drill or probe use as the pilot hole is prepared than during pedicle screw insertion. Though the dural tear is easily detected by the presence of spinal fluid, it is difficult to repair without a wide decompression of the surrounding neural elements. Fortunately, packing the pilot hole with gelfoam has been a successful alternative method of treatment for dural lacerations due to preparation of the pilot hole. Early reports by Greenfield (13%) (24), Steffee (6%) (25), and Whitecloud (5%) (26) demonstrated relative high rates of dural laceration. More recently, West et al. (27) reported a dural laceration rate of 5.6%, but Faraj and Webb (28) found only two cerebrospinal fluid leaks during the placement of 648 pedicle screws for an incidence of 0.3%. Lonstein et al. (15) also reported a very low rate of dural laceration of 0.1% (4 of 4790 screws). Suk et al. (19) encountered three dural tears in 462 patients receiving 4604 thoracic pedicle screws for an incidence of 0.6%.

D. Delayed Epidural Hematoma

Delayed epidural hematoma may result in a severe neurological complication several days after an operation. Horowitz (29) reported an epidural hematoma causing cauda equina syndrome as a consequence of pedicle screw placement. Suk et al. (19) also experienced one delayed epidural hematoma in a case of a neurofibromatosis causing thoracic scoliosis. The patient in this case developed transient paraparesis a week after the surgery due to medial perforation of the pedicle by a pedicle screw.

E. Vascular Injury Due to Overpenetration

Major visceral injuries, especially vascular injuries, caused by overpenetration of pedicle screw are rare but have been reported (Fig. 1c). Heini (30) reported a case of fatal cardiac tamponade caused by a guidewire that penetrated the right coronary artery. Considering the close proximity of the major vessels to the anterior surface of the thoracic vertebra and the presence of the parietal pleura just lateral to the vertebral body, the placement of thoracic pedicle screws should be done with the utmost care. Liljenqvist et al. (5) reported three anterior vertebral cortex penetrations in 120 thoracic pedicle screws (2.5%) placed for idiopathic scoliosis. One of these three screws was replaced because of its direct proximity to the thoracic aorta.

In the lumbar spine, Lonstein et al. (15) reported that 2.8% of screws had perforated the anterior cortex among 4790 pedicle screws placed (2.4% incidence of perforation in sacrum). None of these anterior perforations resulted in major complications. Esses et al. (21) reported a 0.16% incidence of anterior perforation, whereas Belmont et al. (16) reported a 6.1% incidence of anterior vertebral cortex penetration but no vascular complications.

F. Pedicle Fractures / Vertebral Body Fractures

Intraoperative fracture of the pedicle can be caused by the gross discrepancy between the diameters of the pedicle and the screws inserted or because of penetration and weakening of the pedicle wall during screw site preparatation. Another less common cause of pedicle fracture can be due to placement of torque on a rod construct during final tightening, and therefore it is imperative to use an appropriate antitorque device during final tightening.

Blumenthal (31) reported a 0.4% incidence of pedicle fracture among 470 patients undergoing pedicle fixation. Esses et al. (21) found a 2.7% incidence in 617 patients based on the American Back Society survey. Faraj and Webb (28) reported a 0.3% incidence during the placement of 648 pedicle screws. Suk et al. (19) found a 0.2% incidence (11 pedicle fractures in 4604 thoracic pedicle screws placed) in his series. In the osteoporotic bone, the rate of pedicle fracture is higher due to the thinner cortex, which is more easily broken by an overly large screw.

G. Intraoperative Screw Loosening, Screw Breakage, and Other Complications

Intraoperative screw loosening ranges from 0 to 4%. Yuan (32) reported a 1.7% incidence of screw loosening; Greenfield (24), reported a 3% incidence, and Faraj and Webb (28) reported a 0.3% incidence of screw loosening. Intraoperative screw loosening may be caused either by use of an overly small screw relative to the pedicle, especially in an osteoporotic spine, or by placement of the screw at a slightly different angle than that of the prepared hole in the pedicle. If screw loosening is recognized and the pedicle is intact, placement of a larger diameter screw is recommended.

Yuan (32) reported a screw breakage incidence of 0.2%, while Esses et al. (21) found a screw breakage rate of 2.9%. Lonstein et al. (15) reported that screw breakage occurred with an incidence of 0.5% with early screw designs in a series of 4790 screws. Screw breakage is most commonly found in conjunction with one or more of the following three factors: a poorly designed screw, the presence of a pseudarthrosis, and use of short pedicle screw constructs in situations with poor anterior column support (burst fractures). Screw breakage most often results in no clinical problems when the screw is positioned correctly. However, if the broken screw is placing any neurovascular structure at risk, it should be removed. Specific removal instruments, deep pedicular dissection, or a posterior pedicular osteotomy may be required to retrieve a broken screw. If a broken screw has migrated anteriorly to the vertebral body, an anterior approach is generally required. Steffee (25) reported one screw migration among 120 cases, with an incidence of 0.8%. Faraj and Webb (28) reported a 0.2% incidence of rod-screw disconnection in 648 pedicle screws placed.

H. Infection

Although infection is not a complication specific to the use of pedicle fixation, any spinal case in which implants are placed and in which the skin is open for a prolonged period of time is at a higher than average risk for deep wound infection. The overall rate of infection for spinal procedures has been reported to range from 0.3 to 13%. Roy-Camille et al. (14) noted a 5.7% incidence of deep infection, while Louis (33) reported a 1% incidence. Whitecloud (26) observed a 7.5% infection rate, Esses et al. (21) noted a 4.2% infection rate, and Faraj and Webb (28) reported a 5.4% infection rate. Brown (34) found only 0.3% deep infections among his patients, and Suk et al. (19) found a rate of deep infections of 1.9% when treating spinal deformities.

IV. METHODS OF PREVENTING COMPLICATIONS

A. Screw Misplacement

Pedicle screw misplacement can be prevented by adherence to strict pedicle insertion technique and careful confirmation of the pilot hole prior to insertion of the pedicle screws. There are several methods of pedicle screw insertion besides the conventional radiographic-guided method, including computer-assisted image guidance software systems and the laminotomy method, to allow direct pedicle wall palpation. In addition, intraoperative elicited EMG may be used to increase the sensitivity of detecting perforations of the pedicular cortex. Other methods of detecting pedicle wall penetrations, including intraosseous endoscopy, pedicle impedance testing, or the saline challenge test, have been investigated. Although none of these newer techniques have been used as widely as traditional techniques based on spinal topography, they appear promising and may be useful adjuvants in the future. Whatever method a surgeon uses to prepare the pedicle, most important is to adhere to a technique based on an accurate under-standing of the local anatomy and to confirm the integrity of the pilot hole before the insertion of a screw.

1. Sound Pedicle Insertion Technique

Besides identification of the appropriate anatomical landmarks, intraoperative plain radiographs (lateral and postero-anterior radiographs), C-arm fluoroscopy, or image-guided surgery systems (IGSS) are currently used to improve the accuracy of pedicle screw insertion.

Conventional Method (Anatomical Landmarks with Plain Radiographs or Fluoro-scopy). The time-honored method of assessing a pedicle screw pilot hole is through the use of intraoperative radiographs using Kirshner wires in the pedicle hole to determine the accuracy of hole placement in the coronal and sagittal planes (Fig. 2). This conventional method is easily reproduced with standard equipment available in most operating theaters. It is a more cost-effective image than image-guided technology (IGSS) and avoids the need for preoperative and intraoperative image registration. Unfortunately, many

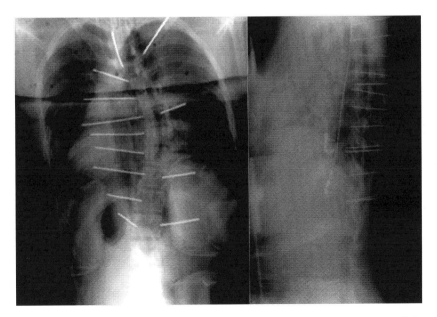

Figure 2 The K-wires on intraoperative radiographs guide the ideal pedicle entry point and screw-insertion angle both in the coronal and sagittal planes.

studies have shown that plain radiographs alone cannot completely rule out pedicle wall perforation. The conventional radiographic technique is especially difficult to use in severe spinal deformities due to spinal rotation and curvature, which make film interpretation difficult and in certain regions of the spine, such as the upper thoracic region where the presence of the shoulders, make the lateral radiograph difficult to obtain. Obtaining acceptable radiographs in markedly obese patients is also challenging.

Steinmann et al. (35) found that 3 of 90 screws (3.3%) placed with intraoperative postero-anterior fluoroscopy were found to be malpositioned. In contrast, Boachie-Adjei et al. (36) reported a 3% incidence (9 of the 282 screws) of pedicle screw misplacement (none causing clinical sequelae) using a pedicle-probing technique alone and concluded that a "free-hand technique" was safe and cost-effective for pedicular screw placement during adult spinal deformity surgery. Unfortunately, a false-negative appreciation of a pedicle breech with a sounding probe may be as high as 14% in deformity cases. Weinstein et al. (37) emphasized a combination of visual/tactile clues in placing pedicle screws. Suk et al. (10,19) used conventional intraoperative postero-anterior and lateral radiographs with Kirshner wires during the placement of 4604 thoracic pedicle screws. In their studies, 67 malpositioned screws (1.5%) were encountered.

IGSS or Fluoroscopic Navigation. Computer-assisted guidance systems may be helpful in determining the entry points and pilot hole direction during pedicle screw placement (Fig. 3). This "high-tech" method has the advantage that preoperative surgical planning can be carried out using a three-dimensional imaging study such as a CT or MRI scan. By tracking the instruments used to prepare the pedicle in real time, the surgeon may have increased confidence in pedicle preparation and the anatomical dimensions of the pedicle.

A wide range of accuracy has been reported with the use of image-guidance techniques, ranging from 0 to 38% pedicle breeches. Glossop (38) studied an image guidance technique, placing guidewires into pedicles. In this study, the average distance

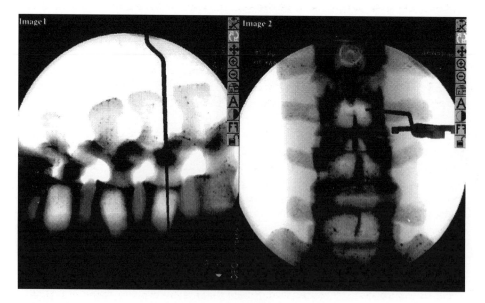

Figure 3 Computer-assisted pedicle screw guidance systems may be helpful in determining the entry points and pilot hole direction when inserting pedicle screws.

between the planned and actual wire entry point was 1.2 mm, and the average difference between the planned and resulting pilot hole trajectory was 6.0 degrees. Kim (39) documented a learning curve for mastery of image guidance with a pedicle perforation rate of 37.5% in the first cadaver, which decreased to 4.2% in the last two cadavers. Laine et al. (40) found computer-assisted screw application to be more accurate than conventional fluoroscopic techniques, with a perforation rate of 4.6% compared to 13.4% in the fluoroscopic technique. Amiot et al. (17) reported a 95% success rate with computer-assisted pedicle screw insertion compared to an 85% success rate with conventional methods. Other authors have documented a range of screw misplacement using IGSS of 0–4.6% in nondeformity cases but rates of up to 20% in scoliosis surgery.

Despite better results claimed by IGSS advocates, IGSS using currently available systems is more cumbersome and time-consuming compared with conventional techniques. This seems to be due to the multiple steps required for registration and navigation with current generation systems. However, technology in this area is advancing rapidly, and the time required to use image guidance seems to be decreasing. Another complaint regarding the use of IGSS is the accuracy of these systems, which depends on the slice thickness of the preoperative study as well as the position and rigidity of the attached reference array. As the surgeon navigates further from the reference array, the accuracy falls off due to subtle changes in the position of the spine relative to the position in the preoperative CT scan. Applying pressure to the spine, such as during insertion of a pedicle probe, can move spinal joints, changing the position of spinal segments relative to the registration, and lead to subtle inaccuracies. In the thoracic spine, where the pedicle anatomy is small, minor changes in direction can have a large affect on accuracy. Finally, the added cost of obtaining preoperative imaging studies and the capital cost of the IGSS equipment add significantly to the cost of providing care for the patient and must be considered. Therefore, the surgeon must weigh the added cost and time to use CT-based IGSS against the potential increased accuracy in determining whether the use of the technology makes sense.

Fluoroscopy-based surgical navigation is an alternative to CT-based computer navigation. This technique uses intraoperative fluoroscopy images rather than a preoperative CT scan and thus is generally less expensive to use. It allows tracking of reference instruments in real time relative to the fluoroscopic images. Fluoroscopic navigation has been shown to reduce radiation exposure and operating time in certain situations. The limitation of fluoroscopic navigation is that only two-dimensional views of the spine are used and thus the position of the instruments in the axial plane is not visualized as in IGSS based on either CT or MRI.

For the time being, conventional methods are still more commonly used for thoracic pedicle screw insertion. With advances in technology, IGSS and fluoroscopic navigation may play larger roles in screw insertion in the future. In addition, other methods of screw insertion, such as the open laminoforaminotomy technique (41) to directly visualize the medial border of the pedicle, can be helpful in certain situations and should be kept in the mind for difficult anatomical situations.

2. Confirmation of Pilot Hole Placement

Conventional Method. After the pilot hole is made, confirmation of intact pedicle walls is critical to ensure safe screw insertion. Suk et al. (19) advocated the use of a small probe to make the pilot hole. Following this, the boundaries of the pedicle pilot hole are carefully palpated with a sounding probe to ensure that the walls are intact. With this technique, gross pedicle wall violation is usually obvious, but subtle breaks in the pedicle wall may fail to be detected. A radiographic check is also advocated using intraoperative radiographs or fluoroscopy to ensure that a pedicle marker appears to be placed correctly within the pedicle. If a laminectomy is performed for decompression, direct visualization or palpation of the pedicle wall is an effective method to ensure that the pedicle wall is not breeched. When the pedicle has been tapped, the wall should again be palpated. It is often easier to feel the "ridges" along an intact pedicle wall following tapping. During screw placement, the insertion torque can give some information about an intact wall as a firm feel to insertion should be present. The screw may be gently "wiggled" within the pedicle, and the entire vertebral segment should gently move as a unit. The surgeon should pay close attention to the trajectory of screw insertion. If the screw trajectory changes during insertion, it usually means that the screw has exited laterally and is riding along the lateral aspect of the vertebral body causing the screw to obtain a more vertical direction during insertion. Postoperatively, plain antero-posterior (AP) and lateral radiographs should be obtained and may offer further information about the position of the screws. It should be recognized, however, that plain radiographs are notoriously inaccurate for detecting subtle pedicle breeches (37). Postoperative CT scan is the gold standard for defining the position of pedicle screws and should be used in cases where the accuracy of implant placement is in question.

Electrically Elicited EMG.   Intraoperative-evoked potentials (SSEP or MEP) have become a standard method of monitoring spinal cord function during spinal deformity surgery. Spinal cord monitoring enables the surgeon to detect changes in the functional integrity of the spinal cord throughout surgery, especially when deformity correction is planned. In addition to monitoring cord function, electrical monitoring can be used to determine the accuracy of pedicle screw implant placement. For this purpose elicited or stimulus evoked EMG is used. The principle of stimulus-evoked EMG relies on creating a simple circuit between the pedicle implant and a distant site. Because intact cortical bone is an excellent insulator to the flow of electricity, minimal current will travel between an electrical lead attached to the pedicle implant and the distant site. When adequate voltage is applied to the circuit in the setting of a pedicle breech, current flows between the pedicle implant and the distant site, which can be detected by depolarization potentials detected on EMG of the muscles supplied by the adjacent nerve roots. Although stimulus-evoked EMG has become standard in some centers with lumbar pedicle screws, monitoring of thoracic screws is somewhat more difficult in that the segmental intercostals and abdominal muscles must be monitored. EMG monitoring of thoracic pedicle screws is under investigation in some centers. Calancie et al. were the first to popularize the use of stimulus-evoked EMG for lumbar pedicle screw placement (42). Lenke et al. (43) reported that a threshold for EMG stimulation of greater than 8 mA was associated with an intact pedicle, while a threshold value of less than 4 mA was associated with a strong likelihood of a significant pedicle wall defect in the lumbar spine. Lewis et al. (44) reported that stimulus-evoked EMG thresholds in the thoracic spine were difficult to define due to small electrical threshold differences between the intact and breeched pedicle. Despite this, others have reported successful use of stimulus-evoked monitoring in the thoracic spine. In the thoracic region, the use of EMG monitoring techniques remains an issue of active investigation at the time of this writing.

Other Tests for Confirmation of Pedicle Screw Accuracy.   Other tests, such as pedicle impedance testing (45) or intraosseous endoscopy (46) have been suggested to monitor pilot hole accuracy. The saline challenge test, described by An (47), has been suggested as a means to define intact pedicle walls. Unfortunately, an 18% false-negative rate has been reported with this technique. Kosay et al. (48) has suggested that the outflow of blood and fatty particles immediately after drilling or probing the pedicle lumen is a simple and reliable means of determining pedicle accuracy. However, the role of this procedure in thoracic screw placement has not been studied.

B. Neurological Complications

Neurological complications following pedicle screw instrumentation can be due to multiple factors, including direct injury of the neurological structures with a pedicle preparation instrument or implant, postoperative hematoma, overdistraction of the spine, or other causes. It is important to rapidly detect any neurological injury and perform a comprehensive evaluation to define correctable etiologies of the injury. In some cases the deficit may be noted intraoperatively due to changes in monitoring or a deficit noted on a Stagnara wake-up test. When a deficit is noted, timely imaging of the spine should be obtained and can include CT, CT myelography, or MRI depending on the suspected cause of the deficit. In some cases the exact location or screw path may be difficult to define due to imaging artifacts. Although plain CT is excellent for determining the location of pedicle implants relative to the bone or the pedicle, the position of the neural elements is better defined with myelographic contrast or MRI. Although titanium screws allow better postoperative MRI imaging than stainless steel, subtle detection of neural tissues immediately adjacent to implants remains a challenge. Any misplaced screw that appears to be adjacent to the spinal cord should be removed immediately.

C. Screw Overpenetration

Screw overpenetration may be prevented by careful preservation of the anterior vertebral cortex during the preparation of the pedicle hole and by selection of an appropriately sized pedicle implant. When preparing the pedicle pilot hole, the surgeon should attempt to limit the depth of drilling or probing to a distance sufficient to pass beyond the pedicle into the vertebral body. Imaging and palpation can both be useful in helping to define the depth of pedicle hole preparation. When a screw is inserted, the depth should not exceed 80% of the apparent anteroposterior distance of the vertebral body on lateral radiograph to decrease the risk of inadvertent anterior cortical penetration. Because the majority of the holding power of a pedicle screw comes from purchase of the pedicle and not the vertebral body, an excessively long screw is generally not warranted on the basis of biomechanical considerations. If overpenetration of the vertebral body is noted and the screw is adjacent to any vascular structure, immediate screw removal should be performed.

D. Pedicle Fracture

Pedicle fractures are mostly attributed to drilling an excessively large pilot hole or use of an overly large pedicle implant. To avoid this, the pedicle size should be carefully evaluated on preoperative imaging studies. Generally small drills or probes should be used to prepare the pilot hole. In some cases the size of the pilot hole can be gradually dilated up to an ideal size by sequentially tapping of the pedicle with taps of increasing size. The selected implant in adults should not have a major diameter exceeding the inner cortical diameter of the pedicle. To avoid excessive insertional torques, the prepared pedicle pilot hole should approximate the minor diameter of the selected pedicle screw.

In the pediatric spine, a pedicle screw with a diameter up to 115% larger than the diameter of the pedicle can be used due to plastic deformation of the immature pedicle (49). Use of pedicle implants in very small patients, however, is associated with a higher rate of fractures. When treating pediatric patients, small pedicle implants should be available. In some cases, adequate mechanical purchase case be obtained even with a cracked pedicle, and therefore an implant that is in an otherwise good position may be retained and incorporated into a spinal construct.

E. Vertebral Body Fracture

Intraoperative vertebral body fractures sometimes occur when excessive forces are applied to a pedicular implant while connecting the implant to a construct or performing a corrective maneuver. To avoid this one should introduce the rods carefully into the pedicle screw utilizing appropriate instruments (i.e., reduction screws or rod introducers). In some cases reinforcement of a distal pedicle screw with an infralaminar hook may be effective in preventing screw pullout (50).

F. Infection

Major instrumented spinal procedures are associated with a significant rate of deep soft tissue infection. Careful soft tissue handling during surgery, minimizing the length of surgery, intermittent retractor release, and irrigation are all important to minimize the risk of infection. The use of prophylactic antibiotics has become standard to lessen the risk of infection in the perioperative period.

V. AUTHOR'S PREFERRED METHOD OF PEDICLE SCREW INSERTION

Suk has been using pedicle screws for the management of spinal deformities since 1988. Thoracic pedicle screw fixation for spinal deformities became routine only after extensive experience with lumbar pedicle screw fixation had been gained. Initially, thoracic screws were used in the thoracolumbar spine where the pedicles were large and well visualized. As experience was gained, pedicle screws were gradually used in more proximal levels. Good results were obtained due to the superior intraoperative control in major spinal deformities. As a result, other means of spinal fixation were abandoned in favor of pedicle screw construct since 1992. Initially, the screws were placed in the typical hook deformity pattern recommended by the CD group. However, although screw fixation did offer superior-fixation to that of hooks (49), true segmental control of the spinal deformity was not achieved with this pattern. By adding more screws, a true segmental construct was achieved that dispersed the stresses over the curve and allowed earlier mobilization of patients.

A. Determination of Accurate Pedicle Entry Point

Guide pins, about 15 cm long and made from K-wires, are inserted shallowly in all segments at the presumed pedicle entry point before making a pilot hole. The ideal entry point in the thoracic spine is at the junction of the upper margin of the transverse process, just lateral to the facet joint (Fig. 4). In the lumbar spine, the pedicle entry point is determined by a line drawn through the middle of the transverse process in the horizontal plane and a vertical line along the lateral margin of the facet joint (Weinstein technique). With the guide pins placed in the presumed entry points, intraoperative PA and lateral

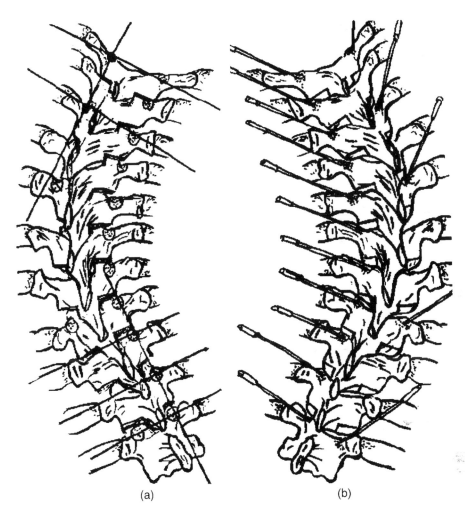

(a)   (b)

Figure 4 Determination of accurate pedicle entry point. (a) Decortication is performed at the presumed pedicle entry points. In the thoracic spine, it is located at the junction of the superior margin of the transverse process and the lamina. (b) Guide pins are inserted at the presumed entry site. They are inserted shallowly, just enough to hold in the exposed cancellous bone.

roentgenogram are taken to determine the relationship between the selected points and the ideal pedicle entry point and the trajectory of each pedicle. The angle of the pedicle is considered on preoperative imaging study. In the case of spinal deformities, the rotation of the vertebrae is considered to allow correct angulation in the transverse plane. The ideal entry point on the convex side in scoliosis moves more medially and the trajectory is directed less medially than in the undeformed spine. On the concave side of the spine, the entry point is slightly more laterally and the trajectory is directly more medially than in the undeformed spine (Fig. 5).

B. Pilot Hole Preparation (Pedicle Entry)

After determining the ideal pedicle entry point and the direction relative to the guide pin, the pedicle is entered with an awl, a curette, or small-diameter drill, considering the normal

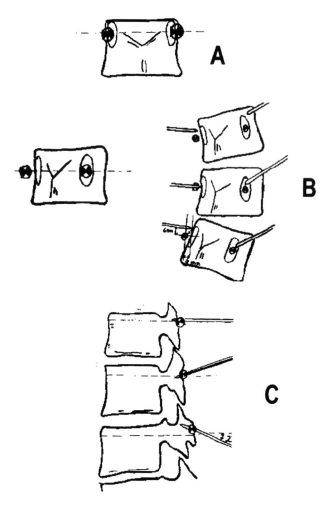

Figure 5 Ideal pedicle entry point (IPEP). (a) For a neutrally rotated vertebra, the ideal pedicle entry point is at the junction of the line parallel to the end plate at the level of the pedicle and the lateral margin of the pedicle ring shadow. (b) In a rotated vertebra, the ideal pedicle entry point moves medially on the rotation (convex) side and more laterally on the opposite (concave) side. (c) On the lateral view, the ideal pedicle entry point is situated at the junction of the line passing through the axis of the pedicles and the junction of the posterior border of the facet joints.

transverse pedicle angle and spinal rotation. Use of low-speed hand drills or probes can reduce the chances of medial cortical perforation. Excessive force in preparing the pedicle pilot hole should be avoided; cancellous bone in the central region of isthmus of the pedicle should offer little resistance. If excessive force is required, the trajectory of the pedicle-preparing instrument should be questioned. Once a small entry hole is made with a small probe, a pedicle path is drilled with a bit similar in diameter to the minor diameter of the screw to be used. To achieve the greatest pull-out strength, the prepared pedicle hole is approximately 60% of the pedicular isthmus outer diameter.

In the scoliotic thoracic spine, due to vertebral rotation the spinal cord is shifted towards the concave side, leaving extra space on the convex side of the spine (Fig. 6). This makes pedicle instrumentation safer on the convex side even if slight medial penetration

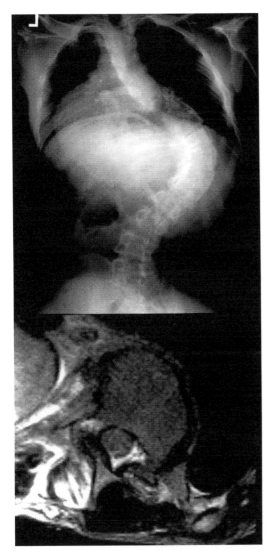

Figure 6 Idipoathic scoliosis with a right thoracic curve. In the scoliotic thoracic spine, the vertebra is rotated towards the convex side with the cord shifted to the concave side leaving a spacious canal on the convex side. The left shift of the cord is well demonstrated on the T2 weighted axial MRI.

occurs. By understanding the angle of the pedicle in spinal deformities, pedicle screw fixation in a scoliotic deformity can be performed safely with experience.

C. Confirming the Pilot Hole and Screw Insertion

The pedicle screw is inserted after confirming bony containment of the drilled pilot hole with a probe. Safe entry is confirmed with a probe that feels cancellous bone at the probe tip with bone globally surrounding the instrument in all directions. When starting screw insertion, the screw should be turned gently to ensure that it follows the prepared path

(Fig. 7). A screw that fails to gain firm purchase at the end of insertion generally indicates that it is misplaced. Either a misplaced screw can be corrected by following all steps, as in a virgin pedicle, or the screw site may be skipped.

D. Screw Size, Length and Instrumentation

In a non-destructive study using young porcine vertebrae, Suk found that the use of a drill diameter 60% the size of the pedicle diameter and a screw diameter 80% of the pedicle diameter offers maximal holding strength (49). Therefore, we advocate the use of 4 mm diameter screws above T5, 4.5 mm diameter screws above T9, 5.5 mm diameter

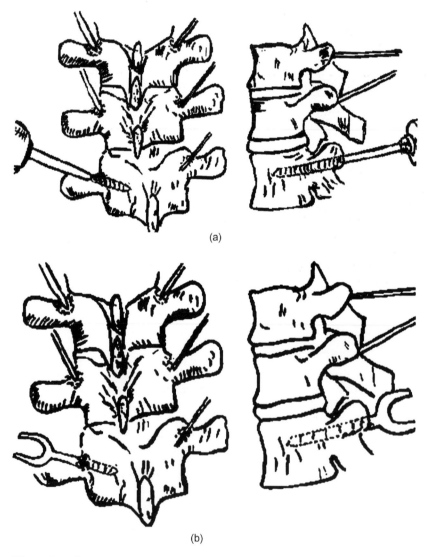

(a)

(b)

Figure 7   Pilot hole preparation and screw insertion. (a) Deep drilling is performed. For maximum holding power, the diameter of the drill should be equal to that of the minor diameter of the screw inserted. (b) Screw is inserted gently into the prepared hole.

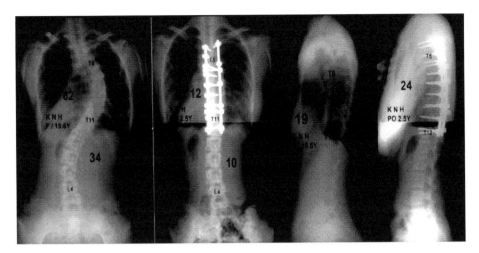

Figure 8 In rigid scoliosis, it is preferable to insert screws in every segments on the correction side (concave in thoracic and convex in lumbar) and every other or third vertebra on the support sides.

screws in lower thoracic, and 6.5 mm diameter screws in the lumbar spine. In the pediatric population screws up to 115% of the outer pedicle diameter may be inserted without resulting in a pedicle fracture due to the plasticity of the cortical bone. The depth of screw insertion does not significantly affect the pull-out strength when it passes deeper than the posterior half of the vertebral body. Screws that penetrate 60–70% of the AP vertebral diameter are generally used—i.e., 40 mm in the lower lumbar spine (L3 and below), 35 mm at the thoracolumbar junction and upper lumbar spine (T10–12), 30 mm in the midthoracic (T5–T9) region and 25 mm in the upper thoracic spine (T1–T4). Bilateral pedicle screw instrumentation is commonly used to enhance resistance to torsional forces. In rigid scoliosis, screws are generally used in all segments on the correction side (concave in thoracic and convex in lumbar) and every second or third vertebra on the support sides (Fig. 8).

REFERENCES

1. Zindrick MR, Wiltse LL, Doornik A, Widell EH, Knight GW, Patwardhan AG, Thomas JC, Rothman SL, Fields BT. Analysis of the morphometric characteristics of the thoracic and lumbar pedicles. Spine 1987; 12(2):160–166.
2. Cinotti G, Gumina S, Ripani M, Postacchini F. Pedicle instrumentation in the thoracic spine. A morphometric and cadaveric study for placement of screws. Spine 1999; 24(2):114–119.
3. Reynolds AF Jr., Roberts PA, Pollay M, Stratemeier PH. Quantitative anatomy of the thoracolumbar epidural space. Neurosurgery 1985; 17(6):905–907.
4. Gertzbein SD, Robbins SE. Accuracy of pedicular screw placement in vivo. Spine 1990; 15(1):11–14.
5. Liljenqvist UR, Halm HF, Link TM. Pedicle screw instrumentation of the thoracic spine in idiopathic scoliosis. Spine 1997; 22(19):2239–2245.
6. Liljenqvist UR, Link TM, Halm HF. Morphometric analysis of thoracic and lumbar vertebrae in idiopathic scoliosis. Spine 2000; 25(10):1247–1253.
7. O'Brien MF, Lenke LG, Mardjetko S, Lowe TG, Kong Y, Eck K, Smith D. Pedicle morphology in thoracic adolescent idiopathic scoliosis: is pedicle fixation an anatomically viable technique? Spine 2000; 25(18):2285–2293.

8. Ferree BA. Morphometric characteristics of pedicles of the immature spine. Spine 1992; 17(8):887–891.

9. Maat GJ, Matricali B, van Persijn van Meerten EL. Postnatal development and structure of the neurocentral junction. Its relevance for spinal surgery. Spine 1996 Mar 15; 21(6): 661–666.

10. Suk SI, Lee CK, Kim WJ, Chung YJ, Park YB. Segmental pedicle screw fixation in the treatment of thoracic idiopathic scoliosis. Spine 1995; 20(12):1399–1405.

11. Zindrick MR, Knight GW, Sartori MJ, Carnevale TJ, Patwardhan AG, Lorenz MA. Pedicle morphology of the immature thoracolumbar spine. Spine 2000; 25(21):2726–2735.

12. Vaccaro AR, Rizzolo SJ, Allardyce TJ, Ramsey M, Salvo J, Balderston RA, Cotler JM. Placement of pedicle screws in the thoracic spine. Part I: morphometric analysis of the thoracic vertebrae. J Bone Joint Surg Am 1995; 77(8):1193–1199.

13. Vaccaro AR, Rizzolo SJ, Balderston RA, Allardyce TJ, Garfin SR, Dolinskas C, An HS. Placement of pedicle screws in the thoracic spine. Part II: an anatomical and radiographic assessment. J Bone Joint Surg Am 1995; 77(8):1200–1206.

14. Roy-Camille R, Saillant G, Mazel C. Internal fixation of the lumbar spine with pedicle screw plating. Clin Orthop 1986; 203:7–17.

15. Lonstein JE, Denis F, Perra JH, Pinto MR, Smith MD, Winter RB. Complications associated with pedicle screws. J Bone Joint Surg Am 1999; 81(11):1519–1528. (Comment in J Bone Joint Surg Am 2000; 82-A(10):1515.)

16. Belmont PJ Jr, Klemme WR, Dhawan A, Polly DW Jr. In vivo accuracy of thoracic pedicle screws. Spine 2001; 26(21):2340–2346.

17. Amiot LP, Lang K, Putzier M, Zippel H, Labelle H. Comparative results between conventional and computer-assisted pedicle screw installation in the thoracic, lumbar, and sacral spine. Spine 2000; Mar 1; 25(5):606–614.

18. Halm H, Niemeyer T, Link T, Liljenqvist U. Segmental pedicle screw instrumentation in idiopathic thoracolumbar and lumbar scoliosis. Eur Spine J 2000; 9(3):191–197.

19. Suk SI, Kim WJ, Lee SM, Kim JH, Chung ER. Thoracic pedicle screw fixation in spinal deformities: are they really safe? Spine 2001; 26(18):2049–2057.

20. Castro WH, Halm H, Jerosch J, Malms J, Steinbeck J, Blasius S. Accuracy of pedicle screw placement in lumbar vertebrae. Spine 1996; 21(11):1320–1324.

21. Esses SI, Sachs BL, Dreyzin V. Complications associated with the technique of pedicle screw fixation. A selected survey of ABS members. Spine 1993; 18(15):2231–2239.

22. Schulze CJ, Munzinger E, Weber U. Clinical relevance of accuracy of pedicle screw placement. A computed tomographic-supported analysis. Spine 1998; 23(20):2215–2220.

23. Brown CA, Lenke LG, Bridwell KH, Geideman WM, Hasan SA, Blanke K. Complications of pediatric thoracolumbar and lumbar pedicle screws. Spine 1998; 23(14):1566–1571.

24. Greenfield RT 3rd, Grant RE, Bryant D. Pedicle screw fixation in the management of unstable thoracolumbar spine injuries. Orthop Rev 1992; 21(6):701–706.

25. Steffee AD, Sitkowski DJ. Posterior lumbar interbody fusion and plates. Clin Orthop 1988; 227:82–89.

26. Whitecloud TS 3rd, Butler JC, Cohen JL, Candelora PD. Complications with the variable spinal plating system. Spine 1989; 14(4):472–476.

27. West JL 3rd, Ogilvie JW, Bradford DS. Complications of the variable screw plate pedicle screw fixation. Spine 1991; 16(5):576–579.

28. Faraj AA, Webb JK. Early complications of spinal pedicle screw. Eur Spine J 1997; 6(5): 324–326.

29. Horowitch A, Peek RD, Thomas Jr JC, et al. The Wiltse pedicle screw fixation system: early clinical results. Spine 1989; 14:461–467.

30. Heini P, Scholl E, Wyler D, Eggli S. Fatal cardiac tamponade associated with posterior spinal instrumentation. A case report. Spine 1998; 23(20):2226–2230.

31. Blumenthal S, Gill K. Complications of the Wiltse Pedicle Screw Fixation System. Spine 1993; 18(13):1867–1871.

32. Yuan HA, Garlin SR, Dickman CA, Mardjetko SM. A historical cohort study of pedicle screw fixation in thoracic, lumbar, and sacral spinal fusions. Spine 1994; 19S:2279–2296.
33. Louis R. Fusion of the lumbar and sacral spine by internal fixation with screw plates. Clin Orthop 1986; 203:18–33.
34. Brown CA, Lenke LG, Bridwell KH, Geideman WM, Hasan SA, Blanke K. Complications of pediatric thoracolumbar and lumbar pedicle screws. Spine 1998; 23(14):1566–1571.
35. Steinmann JC, Herkowitz HN, el-Kommos H, Wesolowski DP. Spinal pedicle fixation. Confirmation of an image-based technique for screw placement. Spine 1993; 18(13):1856–1861.
36. Boachie-Adjei O, Girardi FP, Bansal M, Rawlins BA. Safety and efficacy of pedicle screw placement for adult spinal deformity with a pedicle-probing conventional anatomic technique. J Spinal Disord 2000; 13(6):496–500.
37. Weinstein JN, Spratt KF, Spengler D, Brick C, Reid S. Spinal pedicle fixation: reliability and validity of roentgenogram-based assessment and surgical factors on successful screw placement. Spine 1988; 13(9):1012–1018. (Comment in Spine 1990; 15(3):251.)
38. Glossop ND, Hu RW, Randle JA. Computer-aided pedicle screw placement using frameless stereotaxis. Spine 1996; 21(17):2026–2034.
39. Kim KD, Patrick Johnson J, Bloch BS O, Masciopinto JE. Computer-assisted thoracic pedicle screw placement: an in vitro feasibility study. Spine 2001; 26(4):360–364.
40. Laine T, Lund T, Ylikoski M, Lohikoski J, Schlenzka D. Accuracy of pedicle screw insertion with and without computer assistance: a randomised controlled clinical study in 100 consecutive patients. Eur Spine J 2000; 9(3):235–241.
41. Xu R, Ebraheim NA, Shepherd ME, Yeasting RA. Thoracic pedicle screw placement guided by computed tomographic measurements. J Spinal Disord 1999; 12(3):222–226.
42. Calancie B, Madsen P, Lebwohl N. Stimulus-evoked EMG monitoring during transpedicular lumbosacral spine instrumentation. Initial clinical results. Spine 1994; 19(24):2780–2786.
43. Lenke LG, Padberg AM, Russo MH, Bridwell KH, Gelb DE. Triggered electromyographic threshold for accuracy of pedicle screw placement. An animal model and clinical correlation. Spine 1995; 20(14):1585–1591.
44. Lewis SJ, Lenke LG, Raynor B, Long J, Bridwell KH, Padberg A. Triggered electromyographic threshold for accuracy of thoracic pedicle screw placement in a porcine model. Spine 2001; 26(22):2485–2490.
45. Myers BS, Hasty CC, Floberg DR, Hoffman RD, Leone BJ, Richardson WJ. Measurement of vertebral cortical integrity during pedicle exploration for intrapedicular fixation. Spine 1995; 20(2):144–148.
46. Stauber MH, Bassett GS. Pedicle screw placement with intraosseous endoscopy. Spine 1994; 19(1):57–61.
47. An HS, Benoit PR. Saline injection technique to confirm pedicle screw path: a cadaveric study. Am J Orthop 1998; 27(5):362–365.
48. Kosay C, Akcali O, Berk RH, Erbil G, Alici E. A new method for detecting pedicular wall perforation during pedicle screw insertion. Spine 2001; 26(13):1477–1481.
49. Suk SI, Cha SI, Lee CK, Kim WJ. A study on the pull-out strength of pedicle screws in relation to the size of the drill holes and inserted screws. 30th Annual Meeting of the Scoliosis Research Society, Asheville, NC Sept. 13–16, 1995.
50. Yerby SA, Ehteshami JR, McLain RF. Loading of pedicle screws within the vertebra. J Biomech 1997; 30(9):951–954.

27

Complications of Anterior Thoracolumbar Plating

Robert A. McGuire
University of Mississippi Medical Center, Jackson, Mississippi, U.S.A.

Classically, spinal problems involving both the anterior and posterior column of the spine required a two-incision approach (1). The first required an anterior approach to accomplish decompression of the neural elements and reconstruction of the anterior column, and afterward a second posterior approach was necessary for posterior spinal stabilization (2).

With the development of better materials and implant designs, the ability to address spinal problems from the anterior approach alone has improved (3–5). Not only can decompression of neural elements be accomplished, but reconstruction and stabilization of the spine can be performed through the same incision with less morbidity to the patient (6,7).

With the increased use of anterior plate fixation to the spine, there has arisen a unique set of related complications. Complications as a result of anterior plating can be divided into (a) those related to surrounding soft tissues, including viscus, vessel, and nerves, (b) those related to loss of spinal correction or reduction, (c) those related to implant failure, and (d) those related to inappropriate use of the implant.

I. SOFT TISSUE COMPLICATIONS

When addressing the thoracolumbar region, multiple soft tissue structures can be potentially problematic. With this approach the diaphragm must often be taken down to gain the full approach to the thoracolumbar spine. Since the diaphragm is innervated from central to peripheral, should the incision be made too far centrally, denervation can occur, leading to diaphragm paralysis, which can lead to loss of lung volume. If it is incised too far laterally, there may not be enough of a cuff left to reattach the diaphragm, leading to a hernia in which the abdominal contents will displace into the chest cavity (8).

The retroperitoneal approach on the left side puts both the kidney and spleen at risk if retractors are placed incorrectly or too much force applied. It is critical to visualize the ureter during this approach to prevent injury to this structure. In repeat approaches, the ureter can be lost in the scar and transected, therefore, one may want to have a consulting urologist place a stent prior to surgery to better identify this structure. The stent allows the ureter to be palpated during the approach, minimizing the potential for injury. It is also important during this approach to make sure to remain anterior to the psoas, as dissection posterior to this muscle can lead to avulsion of the nerve roots. The sympathetic chain must also be identified and protected on its course over the anterior aspect of the muscle. Injury to this structure leads to a temperature differential in the lower extremities and can be quite uncomfortable and disconcerting to the patient (9).

When working in the thoracic cavity, the thoracic duct can be injured with approaches to the anterior aspect of the spine. The path of this structure is cephalad from the cisterna chyli at the L2 level, crossing the intercostal arteries and ending in the left subclavian vein, with its main function to collect and return the lymph fluid to the vascular system. If this structure is cut and not addressed, the fluid can collect in the chest cavity, leading to a chylothorax, which may require reexploration of the surgical site or prolonged use of a chest tube (10). Working in the thoracic cavity can lead to potential injury to the lung itself from overvigorous retraction or laceration from instrumentation. This can lead to prolonged air leaks from parenchymal damage. Most of the time these will heal without further intervention, but occasionally sclerosing agents may need to be introduced to facilitate scarring, which stops the leak itself.

Mobilization of the vessels in the thoracic and lumbar spine can be a source of potential complication in anterior surgery (11). In order to obtain access to the spine, the segmental vessels must occasionally be isolated, ligated, and transected in order to mobilize the vessels anteriorly to expose the spine. If the vessels are ligated too close to the trunk of the aorta, the ligature does not have enough vessel stump to gain a good purchase and can loosen. This can lead to gross hemorrhage that requires reexploration and oversewing the side wall of the vessel. If the vessel is ligated too close to the foramen and the vessel is a major feeder to the conus (artery of Adamkiewicz), potential infarction of the cord could occur, leading to neurological compromise (12). Excessive manipulation of the venous structures during the exposure can lead to damage to the intima of the vessels and increase the risk of internal clot formation and subsequent emboli or deep venous thrombosis (13).

II. LOSS OF REDUCTION/CORRECTION

The objectives for performing anterior reconstructive surgery are to reestablish the anterior column's weight-bearing capability and correction of the malalignment of the thoracolumbar segment in the axial and coronal planes. The normal alignment of the thoracolumbar junction is one of neutrality, as it functions as a transitional zone between the normal thoracic kyphosis and lumbar lordotic segment (14). This neutral alignment provides for normal muscle balance with minimal energy expenditure to maintain postural mechanics. Deviation from this normal alignment can stress the adjacent segments, potentially increasing the rate of degenerative changes in both the facets and disk complex (15). It can also lead to muscle fatigue, which occurs as the result of a change in the mechanical advantage by the muscle being effectively lengthened or shortened due to the abnormal angulation of the spinal column. This change in Blick's curve therefore weakens the musculature, leading to this decrease in stamina.

III. LOSS OF CORRECTION

Loss of correction or reduction can occur as a result of biologic failure, incomplete reduction of the deformity or failure to adequately protect the reconstructed anterior column from deforming forces.

Biological failure usually occurs when materials of a higher modulus of elasticity than bone are used for anterior column reconstruction. In patients with osteoporosis, the use of allograft bone or reconstruction cages or struts will often overpower the endplate strength of the host bone, causing fracture of the endplate and resulting in subsidence into the vertebral body with loss of correction (16) (Fig. 1).

Similar loss of reduction can occur if the biological graft is not strong enough to support the weight of the anterior column. An example of this would be using a single rib strut for interbody reconstruction. Failure occurs as a result of either fracture of the rib or piercing of the endplate due to high stresses over the small contract area of the rib tip with migration of the rib into the vertebral body.

The relationship of the vertebral body and the placement of the graft or constructive cage is also important. Studies reveal the major portion of weight-bearing capability to be on the outer third of the vertebral end plate circumferentially (17). The reconstructive material must be of sufficient width to effectively distribute the weight-bearing forces over this larger surface area. This can be done by packing the cages completely with bone graft and placing a weight-bearing cap on the device or cutting a large enough iliac crest strut or allograft to effectively span this distance.

Fracture of the endplate with loss of reduction can also occur by trying to fit too large a graft or cage into the corpectomy space using excessive force to tamp the

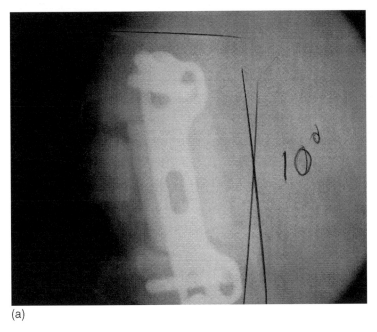

(a)

Figure 1 (a) The anterior column for this patient with a posttraumatic kyphosis was reconstructed with an allograft tibia. (b) The tibia allograft is noted to have subsided into the cephalad vertebral body as a result of endplate fracture.

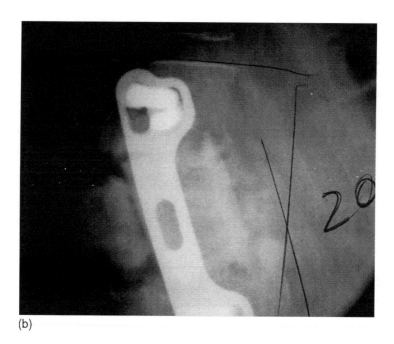

(b)

Figure 1 (*continued*)

reconstructive material into position or applying too much force on the endplate with a
mechanical spreader in an attempt to gain correction of the deformity. Biological failure
can also occur as a result of incomplete healing of the construct leading to a pseudarthrosis
(18). Many factors can account for this, such as nonsteroidal anti-inflammatory drug
(NSAID) and tobacco use, overall patient nutritional status, endplate preparation, and
graft/construct stability. The use of tobacco products inhibits early neovascularization,
which is required for bone healing. The inflammatory phase of bone healing, which
is required, can be affected by nonsteroidal anti-inflammatory medication, leading to nonunion. Poor nutritional status can lead to a catabolic state in which the patient has little or
no reserve left to assist in the healing of the interbody reconstruction. Incomplete removal
of the cartilaginous portion of the endplate will prevent the bone/graft interface from
healing, again by preventing the normal neovascularization from occurring. Penetration
of the cortical endplate can compromise the weight-bearing capabilities of the bone,
leading to graft subsidence, loss of reduction, and subsequent pseudarthrosis as a result
of the loss of graft stability. Graft stability can also be effected by placing a cage or strut
that is too short to fill the defect or placing it at an abnormal angle, causing concentrated
areas of abnormal force on the endplate and leading to failure and loss of reduction. Loss
of correction can also occur as a result of incomplete reduction of the deformity, which
concentrates abnormal bending forces at the graft/endplate interface, resulting in
fracture of the cephalad or caudal vertebrae and loss of correction and return of the
deformity.

Once the reconstructive device or graft is placed, it must be adequately protected.
Choosing a stabilization device that does not adequately control flexion, extension, and
rotatory movements of the reconstructed segment can lead to dislodgement or subsidence
of the graft and ultimate failure or nonunion (3).

IV. HARDWARE FAILURE AND INAPPROPRIATE IMPLANT USE

Complications regarding thoracolumbar instrument failure can be categorized into inappropriate selection of the device for the pathological process being treated, poor technical application of the device, and instrumentation that overpowers the biological system in which it is applied.

Selection of the correct implant depends upon the desired amount of stability needed for the specific problem being treated. Pathological processes involving fractures often require more rigid fixation and stabilization than those involving degenerative and neoplastic processes. The device must be able to negate flexion, extension, and rotational forces in grossly unstable situations. The stability of the constructs is highly dependent upon good carpentry, with reconstruction of the interbody defect allowing compression to be applied, enhancing stability. These implants, although extremely strong, do not provide enough stability themselves long term without fusion to maintain spinal integrity.

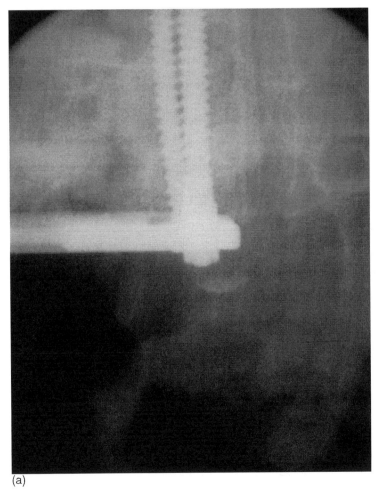

(a)

Figure 2 (a) This radiograph reveals appropriate placement of the anterior plate following reconstruction. (b) The locking nut has loosened on the posterior bolt causing loss of reduction.

Lack of bone union can also lead to late failure of the implant. If devices are selected that do not adequately control rotational forces and the fracture is of the type involving gross rotational instability, the plate or fixation device will be doomed to failure from the start. Correct selection is a must and is highly dependent on the type of stability needed for the specific spinal pathology being treated.

Poor implant application is also a reason for failure of anterior plating. Excellent carpentry or good fitting of the interbody device or graft and endplate has already been addressed. One cannot expect the implant to make up for poor grafting or reconstruction skills. If the interbody grafts or devices do not provide load-sharing capability due to poor fitting and the implant is left to be load bearing, it will fail due to fatigue. This failure will usually occur at the screw/plate interface. Inappropriate torque of the locking nuts or screws can lead to loosening and subsequent failure of the system (Fig. 2). Inappropriate application of the device position on the spine can lead to neurological and vascular compromise. Devices designed for lateral application on the spine that are then placed too anteriorly can lead to bolts or screws being placed into the spinal canal leading to neurological injury. Bolts and screws that are too long when gaining bicortical vertebral body fixation can potentially lead to vascular compromise in the lower thoracic region by

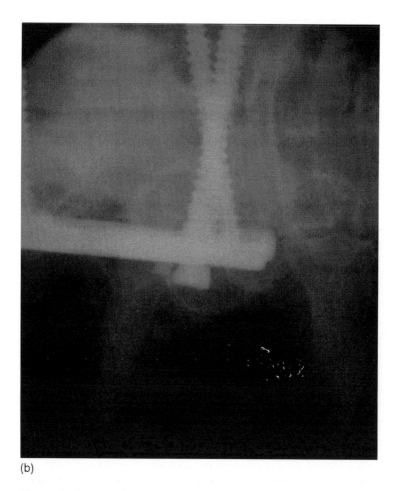

(b)

Figure 2 (*continued*)

impinging on the aorta and venal cava. Further vascular compromise can also occur should these devices, which are designed to be placed laterally on the spine, be used to cross the lumbosacral junction. Injury to the iliac artery and vein as well as loss of fixation can occur due to inappropriate use of the device in this area.

Not placing the construct under compression, can lead to pseudarthrosis and failure. Resorption of the bone at either end of the construct will lead to failure in the same manner as inappropriate graft fitting. The bone/screw interface can also be compromised if overloading occurs with excessive distraction during reduction maneuvers or compression during plate application without good graft fitting. This can lead to toggling of the screw in the bone with further weakening of the construct and ultimate failure as the patient mobilizes (19).

V. CONCLUSION

The use of anterior thoracolumbar plating can be successful in treating unstable fractures and kyphotic deformity if strict attention to detail is maintained. Good carpentry and technical skills in the application of the device is a must to minimize potential complications. A thorough understanding of the pathological process is required to determine the correct implant selection for stabilization of the segment with minimization of potential complications in order to achieve a good expected outcome.

REFERENCES

1. Dimar JR 2nd, Wilde PH, Glassman SD, Puno RM, Johnson JR. Thoracolumbar burst fractures treated with combined anterior and posterior surgery. Am J Orthop 1996; 25(2):159–165.
2. Gurr KR, McAfee PC, Shih CM. Biomechanical analysis of anterior and posterior instrumentation systems after corpectomy. J Bone Joint Surg AM 1988; 70:1182–1191.
3. An HS, Lim TH, You JW, Hong JH, Eck J, McGrady L. Biomechanical evaluation of anterior thoracolumbar spinal instrumentation. Spine 1995; 18:1979–1983.
4. Kaneda K, Taneichi H, Abumi K, Hashimoto T, Satoh S, Fujiya M. Anterior decompression and stabilization with the Kaneda device for thoracolumbar burst fractures associated with neurological deficits. J Bone Joint Surg AM 1997; 79(1):69–83.
5. Stambough JL, El Khatib F, Genaidy AM, Huston RL. Strength and fatigue resistance of thoracolumbar spine implants: an experimental study of selected clinical devices. J Spinal Disord 1999; 12(5):410–414.
6. McGuire RA Jr. The role of anterior surgery in the treatment of thoracolumbar fractures. Orthopedics 1997; 20(10):959–962.
7. Ghanayem AJ, Zdeblick TA. Anterior instrumentation in the management of thoracolumbar burst fractures. Clin Orthop 1997; 335:89–100.
8. McDonnell MF, Glassman SD, Dimar JR 2nd, Puno RM, Johnson JR. Perioperative complications of anterior procedures on the spine. J Bone Surg Am 1996; 78(6):839–847.
9. McAfee PC. Complications of anterior approaches to the thoracolumbar spine. Emphasis on Kaneda instrumentation. Clin Orthop 1994; 306:110–119.
10. Nagai H, Shimizu K, Shikata J, Iida H, Matsushita M, Ido K, Nakamura T. Chylous leakage after circumferential thoracolumbar fusion for correction of kyphosis resulting from fracture. Report of three cases. Spine 1997; 22(23):2766–2769.
11. Coimbra R, Yang J, Hoyt DB. Injuries of the abdominal aorta and inferior vena cava in association with thoracolumbar fractures; a lethal combination. J Trauma 1996; 41(3):533–535.
12. Lu J, Ebraheim NA, Biyani A, Brown JA, Yeasting RA. Vulnerability of great medullary artery. Spine 1996; 21(16):1852–1855.

13. Birch BD, Desai RD, McCormick PC. Surgical approaches to the thoracolumbar spine. Neurosurg Clin North Am 1997; 8(4):471–485.
14. Ching RP, Tencer AF, Anderson PA, Daly CH. Comparison of residual stability in thoracolumbar spine fractures using neutral zone measurements. J Orthop Res 1995; 13(4):533–541.
15. Oner FC, van der Rijt RR, Ramos LM, Dhert WJ, Verbout AJ. Changes in the disc space after fractures of the thoracolumbar spine. J Bone Joint Surg Br 1998; 80(5):833–839.
16. Edmondston SJ, Singer KP, Day RE, Price RI, Breidahl PD. Ex vivo estimation of thoracolumbar vertebral body compressive strength: the relative contributions of bone densitometry and vertebral morphometry. Oseoporos Int 1997; 7(2):142–148.
17. Heggeness MH, Doherty BJ. The trabecular anatomy of thoracolumbar vertebrae: implications for burst fractures. J Anat 1997; 191(2):309–312.
18. Finkelstein JA, Chapman JR, Mirza S. Anterior cortical allograft in thoracolumbar fractures. J Spinal Disord 1999; 12(5):424–429.
19. Sweet FA, Lenka LG, Bridwell KH, Blanke KM, Whorton J. Prospective radiographic and clinical outcomes and complications of single solid rod instrumented anterior spinal fusion in adolescent idiopathic scoliosis. Spine 2001; 26(18):1956–1965.

28

Complications of Interbody Fusion Cages

Ben B. Pradhan* and Jeffrey C. Wang
UCLA School of Medicine, Los Angeles, California, U.S.A.

I. INTRODUCTION

Since the Bagby and Kuslich cage (BAK cage, Spine-Tech, Minneapolis, MN) received FDA approval for lumbar interbody spinal fusion in 1996, interbody cage usage by spine surgeons has grown significantly. In the last 5 years, more than 80,000 lumbar interbody fusion cages have been placed, and in the United States over 5000 cages are surgically placed each month (1). The initial prospective multicenter clinical trial of the BAK interbody fusion system by Kuslich et al. claimed promising results: 98.3% fusion at 36 months, 91% return-to-work at 36 months, 85% pain improvement at 24 months, and 90.7% functional improvement at 24 months (2). To quote the authors verbatim, who incidentally were also involved in the innovation of the BAK cage, "carefully selected middle-aged patients with chronic low back pain secondary to degenerative disk disease can be treated effectively and safely by skilled surgeons using the BAK device for one- and two-level interbody fusion." However, there were some basic design flaws with the study, including a follow-up of only 25% of the original group who underwent the procedure. Needless to say, not everyone has been able to reproduce these results. O'Dowd et al. reported an overall failure rate requiring revision of 31% of the cages due to clinical failures at a mean period of 15 months (3). Elias et al. reported a radiographic failure rate of 28% and additonal surgery rate of 21% (4).

The ideal interbody graft should be able to withstand the compressive, shear, and torsional loads across the disk space and at the same time be able to provide a matrix with osteoconductive, osteoinductive, and osteogenic properties. The gold standard for this matrix is autogenous corticocancellous bone graft, which, however, has less than ideal mechanical strength. It was using this premise that the threaded interbody fusion cage was designed. It is metallic but hollow to accommodate autogenous iliac crest cancellous bone graft and fenestrated to allow fusion bone mass to interdigitate with the cage. This construct combines the mechanical strength of the cage to counter disk space compressive, shear, and torsional forces, with the favorable biological properties of the autogenous cancellous bone to encourage fusion mass formation. Unlike allograft bone dowels,

---

*Current affiliation: The Spine Institute, Saint John's Health Center, Santa Monica, California, U.S.A.

titanium interbody cages are not subject to supply shortages and processing problems (i.e., compromise of biomechanical properties, disease transmission, etc).

Since Kuslich's initial modification of the "Bagby basket" (an interbody device used for cervical spine instability in horses) for use in the human lumbar spine, interbody fusion cages have undergone several design advancements with the help of spine surgeons (5). As a result, there exist several versions of the latest generation of the cage. Examples include the BAK cage, the Ray TFC (Surgical Dynamics, Norwalk, CT), the LT cage (Medtronic Sofamor Danek, Memphis, TN), and the INTER FIX cage (Medtronic Sofamor Danek, Memphis, TN). These devices have been designed to improve on the older models with regard to restoration of intervertebral height while promoting fusion. The operative insertion techniques and tools have also been improved and simplified for the surgeon.

II. CAGE DESIGN CONSIDERATIONS

Despite the improvements in design of the interbody fusion cage, there remain some fundamental issues with its basic construct. The metallic cage itself can withstand tremendous loads before failure. However, it is a stiff object and prevents the bone graft inside from experiencing any significant biomechanical load. This may reduce the quality and quantity of bone interdigitating through the cage. A partial solution has been to pack bone graft around and between the cages to expose them to some physiological biomechanical loads. However, a very stiff cage will prevent physiological load transmission across the rest of the intervertebral space as well.

Another issue is the limited surface area of fenestrations through which bone graft can grow. There is an obvious compromise between cage mechanical strength and size or number of fenestrations. As mentioned above, packing bone graft around and between the cages helps alleviate this problem as well, increasing the surface area of the vertebral endplates exposed to bone graft while simultaneously helping seal the cage in the fusion mass. Another solution has been to use stronger materials to construct the cage, allowing larger or more fenestrations. However, on the flip side, a stronger but stiffer cage is less advantageous due to stress shielding as explained above.

Another problem is that the cages do not cover the entire cross-sectional area of the intervertebral space, even when two are used at a level. Compared to ringed (such as the femoral ring allograft) or boxed structures, the cross-sectional area presented by a cylinder is smaller. Calculations have shown that the maximum interface area between a cylindrical cage surface and endplate is only about 10% of the total endplate surface area (6). A smaller graft area means higher peak stresses, increasing the risk of graft or endplate collapse and disk space subsidence. Closkey et al. concluded that the interbody bone graft area should be significantly greater than 30% of the total endplate area to prevent failure (7). However, in the case of a cylinder, to expose more surface area for fusion, additional endplate and subchondral vertebral bone will have to be cored out. This means that more of the cylinder will lie inside the vertebral bodies. Not only will this risk subsidence due to removal of the mechanically stronger subchondral bone, but less diameter of the cylinder is available to distract the intervertebral space.

If only a cylindrical channel of disk material and endplate is removed for each cage, a significant amount of disk material and endplate is left untouched, limiting the fusion area. The obvious solution is to remove as much disk material as possible, prepare the endplates, and apply autogenous cancellous bone graft throughout as much of the disk space as possible. This technique has been shown by McAfee et al. (8) to significantly improve

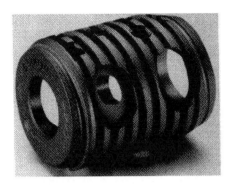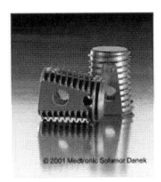

Figure 1 Standard cylindrical cage (left, BAK Cage Spine-Tech, Minneapolis, MN) and cages with flattened sides for closer placement and taper for recreating lumbar lordosis (right, LT Cage, Medtronic Sofamor Danek, Memphis, TN).

fusion rates. However, this reveals a major weakness of the cage fusion technique, which was originally designed to be a quicker and easier procedure than formal endplate preparation and bone grafting. Obviously, adding this step entails additional morbidity and surgical time. This is especially true in laparoscopic cage insertion.

Yet another problem with the cage is that to attain more disk space distraction, the diameter has to be increased. In the case of a cylinder, an increase in diameter also increases width. This makes it more difficult to accurately place two cages symmetrically and centered within the disk space. This can result in the second cage being placed too far lateral, compromising its stability or causing posterior impingement. A solution has been to flatten two sides of the cylinder so that the pair of them can be placed closer together. In their final positions, the threaded portions bite the superior and inferior endplates and the flattened sides are adjacent. The LT cage is an example of this modification (Fig. 1). Fortunately, well-placed cages have been shown by Sandhu et al. (9) to maintain intervertebral space distraction better than bone dowels, so cages larger than those that fit easily inside the disk space are not usually necessary.

Another issue with the cage's shape has been the difficulty in recreating the lumbar lordosis accurately with cylinders. The disk spaces are responsible for most lordosis in a normal lumbar spine. Cylindrical cages placed in such disk spaces are uneven in terms of their bony purchase and suffer either little endplate purchase anteriorly or excessive subchondral bone removal posteriorly. Such cages have increased risk of migration or subsidence with lumbar motion and loading. However, there are now tapered cages in the market that have greater height anteriorly and that use tapered reamers to prepare the disk space. Again, the LT cage incorporates this design modification as well.

III. NEED FOR ADDITIONAL STABILIZATION

Although originally designed for specific indications as stand-alone devices, there are certain other scenarios where threaded cylindrical interbody cages are being used but for which their use without additional posterior stabilization may not be appropriate. Authors who have not had great success with cages alone have in fact recommended routine posterior adjunctive stabilization for most indications. Biomechanically, the most compelling indication for posterior instrumentation of an interbody cage approach is spondylolisthesis and any significant instability, especially when the cage is inserted through a posterior approach (5). Tsantrizos et al. performed biomechanical comparisons of posteriorly placed interbody cylindrical cages, box-like cages, and trapezoidal allografts, and found that posterior (pedicle screw) instrumentation is needed in all three constructs to confer adequate initial stability (10). Dimar et al. found that posteriorly placed interbody cages did not increase spine stiffness significantly in any tested range of motion in a human cadaveric model (11). Supplemental posterior pedicular screw/rod instrumentation, however, significantly increased stiffness. Cagli et al. evaluated the biomechanics of lumbar cages and pedicle screws for treating spondylolisthesis in a human cadaveric model (12). They concluded that biomechanically, cages or dowels alone were suboptimal for treating lumbar spondylolisthesis, especially when compared to pedicle screws and rods. Threaded cages or dowels used together with pedicle screws and rods created the most stable construct.

A less invasive method of posterior lumbar spine stabilization in conjunction with interbody cage fusion is translaminar facet screw fixation. This method, devised by Magerl (13), has demonstrated success with few complications in several studies. Heggeness and Esses showed increased lumbar and lumbosacral spine stiffness after translaminar facet screw fixation (14). This was corroborated by Vanden Berghe et al., who conducted biomechanical studies to show significantly increased stability in flexion, extension, and rotation with translaminar facet screws (15). Zhao et al. showed that even in a posterior lumbar interbody fusion with a single cage (unilateral facetectomy), translaminar screw fixation of the remaining facet added significant stability in all directions (16). This study also showed that posterior two-cage placement with bilateral facetectomy was the least stable construct, driving home the points that PLIF procedures are most likely to benefit from additional posterior stabilization and that translaminar facet screws are sufficient for this.

As far as number of levels is concerned, authors have reported acceptable results of cage fusions for one- or two-level degenerative disk disease, but outcomes may be less than optimal for more than two levels of fusion and may require posterior stabilization as well. The original clinical trials for BAK cages specifically recommended their use for one or two levels (2).

IV. COMPLICATIONS

Complications are associated with interbody fusion cage application and can be divided into two main categories: approach related and cage related. Interestingly, the majority of complications are still approach related (2,17,18). Although complications exist with both anterior and posterior approaches, there are many theoretical advantages to an anterior approach for an experienced surgeon, such as (a) ease and duration of dissection, (b) reduced operative time and blood loss (19,20), (c) avoidance of inciting posterior element pain generators (e.g., facet joints), (d) direct removal of the anterior discogenic pain source, (e) avoidance of dissecting and injuring the posterior muscles, (f) avoidance of retracting the spinal cord or nerve root, and (g) avoidance of scarring in the spinal canal. Approach-related complications are discussed in more detail in other chapters in this book, so we will focus on cage-related issues here.

It is most important to mention that overlying all possible complications in interbody fusion using cylindrical cages is the importance of proper decision making, especially in patient selection. As with any surgical treatment, the patient's psychology, issues of secondary gain, and third-party claims should be appropriately investigated. Diagnostic tests used to determine the need for surgery should be proven and reliable, and the use of stand-alone cages for disorders other than that recommended by the designers and manufacturers should be avoided (e.g., for multilevel disease and/or instability).

A. Approach-Related Complications

1. Complications Associated with the Anterior Approach

Complications associated with the anterior approach include superficial or deep wound infection, wound dehiscence, incisional hernia (21), ileus, bowel obstruction (22), hematoma, seroma, retrograde ejaculation, major vessel damage (23,24), thrombosis (25), thrombophlebitis, atelectasis, pneumonia, urological complications (ureteral damage, testicular swelling, prostatitis, epididymitis, etc.) (26), and others (gastrointestinal bleeding, drainage, anemia, etc.) (2). These are discussed in a separate chapter in this book.

2. Complications Associated with the Posterior Approach

Complications associated with the posterior approach include superficial or deep wound infection, ileus, hematoma, seroma, bleeding, thrombosis, thrombophlebitis, dural tears, neurological injury, and others (anemia, drainage, etc.) (2). Extended rehabilitation time due to posterior muscular dissection injury is expected (19,20). Violation of the integrity of certain posterior elements may theoretically produce pain generators (e.g., facet joints). Again, these approach-related complications are discussed in a separate chapter.

3. Complications Associated with the Laparoscopic Anterior Approach

The laparoscopic approach has an inherently higher complication rate compared to open surgery, especially during a surgeon's learning curve for the technique. With a laparoscopic approach, it is easier to simply ream and place two cages in a disk space than to perform a complete discectomy, endplate preparation, and bone grafting, which often improves the chance of fusion as suggested by McAfee et al. (8). However, with proficiency comes the potential to substantially reduce perioperative morbidity by reducing blood loss, ileus, rehabilitation time, etc. Regan et al. have shown that this is a promising technique (18,27). Zdeblick and David found no significant difference in operative time, blood loss, or length of stay using the laparoscopic technique compared to the mini-ALIF (anterior lumbar interbody fusion) approach, but did find a significantly increased complication rate (20% vs. 4%) (28).

B. Cage-Related Complications

Complications associated with interbody fusion cages are usually due to one of three reasons: error in placement, failure of fixation, or failure of healing. (Note that these are most often due to surgeon errors and/or patient biology, and not due to any intrinsic flaw of the cages themselves.). These result in implant malposition, migration, or pseudarthrosis and other associated problems. Unlike corticocancellous grafts, however, there have been no reported case of structural failures of the cages themselves.

1. Cage Malposition

The recommended interbody fusion configuration is two parallel cylindrical cages oriented parasagittally across the disk space, symmetrical on each side of the midline. Studies have shown that cages in this configuration impart increased interbody distraction and stiffness as compared to the intact spine (9,29–32) and are able to withstand physiological lumbar spinal loading forces (2,29,33,34). Since the anteroposterior diameter of the interbody disk space is largest at midline, it is desirable to position the cages close to center, while maintaining a reasonably wide base of support for the spinal column. The reasoning is twofold: to get more bony purchase by using longer cages and to avoid cage prominence outside the disk space.

In one of the few published studies on revision surgery strategies after cage implantation, the most common revision procedure performed was posterior exploration of a symptomatic nerve root with foraminotomy for unrecognized lateral recess stenosis (35). Iatrogenic spinal stenosis secondary to cages backing out into the canal, either during insertion or later due to migration, can also occur.

In anterior approaches, excessively laterally directed titanium cages or threaded cortical bone dowels can cause direct foraminal nerve root compression and radiculopathy (8,17,36). This often can be a result of the surgeon failing to accurately identify the anterior vertebral anatomical midline prior to inserting the paired interbody devices. A centering pin can be used to mark what the surgeon believes to be the middle of the disk space in the coronal plane. The pin can be checked with fluoroscopy and adjusted as needed. Once central placement is confirmed, marks can be made on the vertebral bodies both above and below to indicate the midpoint. A longer shaft can then be attached to the pin to give the surgeon a sense of the direction in which the cages should point to avoid lateral divergence and foraminal encroachment. Taylor et al. concluded that the "safe zone" for centering the cages extends approximately 5 mm on either side of midline (37).

Laterally placed cages inserted through the lateral decubitus approach can also cause disk herniations due to retropulsion of disk material into the spinal canal. This has been reported with cages inserted through the anterior approach directed straight posteriorly and parallel to each other. If the starting point is too far lateral, iatrogenic disk herniation can also result. This usually causes compression of the exiting root in the manner of a "far lateral" disk herniation. This is because reaming or inserting the cage in this lateral position risks pushing disk contents posterolaterally through an area that lacks the protective posterior longitudinal ligament expansion—an area that is naturally prone to disk herniations.

Spinal cord or dural injuries associated with the anterior placement of threaded interbody devices have not been reported, although they are well-recognized complications with posterior approaches and cage placements (see complications associated with posterior approaches) (2,17,38). At least one large study found that the posterior lumbar interbody fusion technique, by the very nature of its dorsal approach, is associated with a 10% incidence of dural injury and can lead to paresthesias from prolonged or excessive nerve root retraction (2).

2. Cage Migration or Subsidence

Interbody cage migration has been reported in about 2% of patients, with slightly over 1% of the total requiring reoperation (2). The cause for implant migration is a lack of tight fixation due to cage malposition, undersizing of the implant, oversizing of the implant, or weakened bonecage interface.

Cage malposition can compromise fixation by reducing contact area between the cylinder and vertebral bone. The optimal position for fixation is near the midline where a longer cylinder can be used because of the larger anteroposterior disk diameter. The larger the cages needed (for adequate distraction of disk space), the further apart (and thus more lateral) they have to be. To minimize this compromise, a new design change has been to flatten two sides of the cylinder. This allows placement of the cages closer to each other near the midline when the flat edges are aligned next to each other (Fig. 1).

Intuitively, a cage that is too small will be unstable. Using an undersized cage reduces contact area with the vertebral bone and by decreasing distraction will impart less stabilizing load to the cage. Stability with distraction occurs because of tensioning of the surrounding anulus in the disk space. A narrow cage results in "looser" cage-vertebrae contact due to inadequate soft tissue tension, increasing the risk of cage slip during lumbar spine motion.

An oversized cage may experience large peak forces because of excessive distraction, causing the threadbone interface to fail catastrophically and the cage to be thrust out during lumbar spine motion. This is compounded by the fact that large cages may make the entire motion segment more unstable. Several biomechanical studies have shown that anterior interbody devices improve overall spine stiffness, but are least rigid in extension and axial rotation (35,39,40). This was initially thought to be due to the sectioning of the anterior longitudinal ligament. However, Lund et al. showed that extension instability occurred with posteriorly placed interbody cages as well (41). Oxland et al. concluded that this lack of rigidity was due to excessive distraction of the facet joints after interbody cage placement (39).

A weakened bonecage interface refers mainly to the quality of bone at the bone surface interface rather than any deficiencies with the cage itself. Structural failure of the cage itself has not been widely reported. The thread dimensions on a cage affect pullout strength, but mechanical failure almost always occurs in the vertebral bodies adjacent to the cage implant. Assuming a uniform thread design, the bone quality is the main variable in this problem.

The strongest bone in the vertebral body lies in the subchondral region of the cortical endplate. However, it is necessary to ream this vertebral endplate to prepare the pair of adjacent circular holes for the cages, exposing the weak but vascular cancellous bone, especially at the apex of the cavity. Excessive tightening of the threaded cage can easily result in stripping of the bonecage interface at this level, which can be a set-up for implant migration.

To optimally utilize the endplate, the surgeon can perform minimal shaving of the endplate and use a precisely conforming bone graft or implant to share the load evenly over more of the endplate surface. This allows a greater surface of contact between the graft and vertebral body. Wang et al. showed that these steps reduce peak stresses in the graft (42,43). Unfortunately, this is not possible using cylindrical threaded cages.

3. Pseudarthrosis

There are few large studies documenting rates of fusion using interbody cages. In one of the original large studies, Kuslich et al. claimed a fusion rate of over 98% (2). Blumenthal et al. also found a low overall revision rate of about 3% (44). However, not all surgeons have enjoyed that kind of success, and several studies with smaller patient pools have reported higher rates of pseudarthroses (3,4,35).

Failure of fusion may be a long-term consequence of any of the above-named cage-related complications. Moreover, pseudarthrosis can occur without any evidence of cage-related complications, or fusion may very well occur despite obvious evidence of less than ideal cage placement. This is because fusion can be described as a race between bony healing and implant loosening or failure. The patient's biology plays a big role in the ultimate effect of cage malposition, migration, or settling on spinal fusion. Thus the patient's general health and nutrition, medications, any history of irradiation, or smoking should be explored thoroughly, as they can significantly affect healing.

Infection can also cause loosening and pseudarthrosis, especially in the setting of previous or current infection at or near the operative site. The inherent stability of the spine plays another big role. Cages are not indicated as stand-alone devices for multilevel disease or significant spinal instability. In such cases, additional posterior stabilization may be helpful and is recommended (10,11,45–48).

V. MANAGEMENT OF CAGE COMPLICATIONS

A. General Cage Revision Concepts

There is a dearth of literature on revision strategies for failed interbody fusion with cylindrical cages. McAfee et al. identified several cage-related complications that could benefit from revision surgery (35):

> Undersized cages
> Malpositioned cages
> Migrating cages
> Spinal canal stenosis
> Disk herniation with neural impingement
> Pseudarthrosis

Of course these complications must lead to symptoms before the patient is subjected to any revision surgery. Symptoms may manifest as residual back pain, new back pain, residual radiculopathy, or new radiculopathy. If the symptoms are significant or do not improve with nonoperative management, a work-up must be initiated to identify whether the problems listed above are responsible.

Radiographs that show inadequate distraction across the disk space are diagnostic for undersized cages. This may be seen immediately postoperatively or later with progressive settling of the vertebrae around the cages. MRI or CT-myelogram may show neural impingement across the foramina due to inadequate distraction. Similarly, malpositioned and migrating cages can be diagnosed by plain radiographs. Patient symptoms may be explained by CT scans (with or without contrast) showing implant migration into the spinal canal or foramina. A disk herniation can be seen with an MRI or CT-myelogram as well.

A history of a pain-free interval is probably the most sensitive indicator of possible pseudarthrosis (1). The next step is to obtain plain A-P and lateral flexion-extension radiographs. These can be difficult to interpret. Pseudarthrosis can be presumed based on motion of the cages on lateral flexion-extension views, lucencies around the entire implant, or late and/or progressive migration of the cages (17,49,50) (Fig. 2). However, the radiographic thresholds to diagnose fusion or lack thereof are very controversial. Allowable motion differs from 1 to 5° in various studies (2,8,17,38,51,52). A false diagnosis of fusion can be made as often as 20% of the time based entirely on flexion-extension films alone versus including other criteria such as peri-implant lucencies (17,53).

Some authors suggest that the best indication of fusion with threaded interbody implants is the presence of a "sentinel sign"—radiographically evident bridging trabecular bone anterior to the interbody device (17,35). In order to improve clinical results and assist in fusion determination, the concept of "ream long, fuse short" has been proposed.

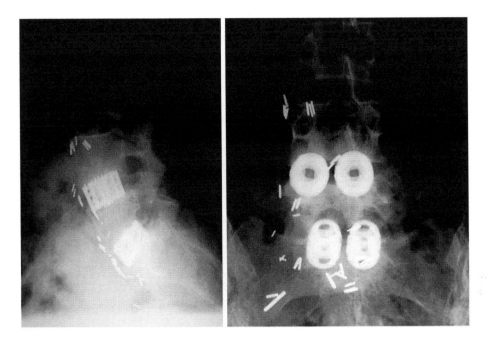

Figure 2 Radiographs of two-level anterior cage interbody fusion with obvious pseudarthrosis at the lower level with radiolucency visible surrounding both cages.

The threaded cylindrical interbody device is placed at the far posterior portion of the reamed and tapped channel, allowing room in the interspace anterior to the device for the packing of cancellous bone graft. This allows for a large sentinel sign to be visible in radiographs later on if fusion is successful (Fig. 3). However, it must be borne in mind

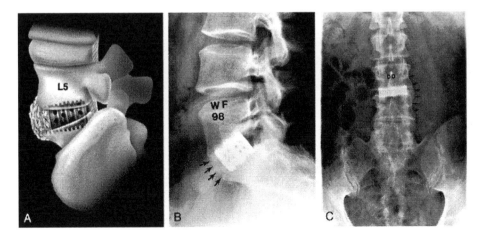

Figure 3 (A) The principle of "ream long and cage short" in more than 200 Bagby and Kuslich (BAK) fusion cage procedures was the most reliable assurance of a solid arthrodesis documented by solid trabecular bony bridging anterior to the cage. (B) Solid bone incorporated anterior to an L5–S1 BAK procedure. (C) Continuous bone in continuity bridging L3 to L4, a sentinel sign of fusion after a laterally inserted BAK device. (From Ref. 17.)

that such placement may increase the risk of settling since the interbody implant is not resting on the anterior cortical margin, but on the softer cancellous endplate.

CT scans can add detail to radiographs in assessing fusion across cages, although they are occasionally more difficult to interpret because of metal artifact (in contrast with the use of bone dowels). A lack of viable bone extending through the cage into the vertebral marrow on reconstructed thin-section, high-resolution CT suggests lack of fusion. Despite this, studies have shown that CT scans are not completely reliable in diagnosing fusion across cages (6,8,49,54). Even when bridging bone is seen entering the cage through its fenestrations on a CT scan, histological analyses of retrieved cages have shown that the quality of the bone can be suboptimal and their structure noncontinuous (35,49,54).

B. Specific Cage Complications and Their Management

Early postoperative cage removal is simpler because of the lack of scar and bony ingrowth. Although it is preferable to use the previous incision for significant malposition or migration of the implant, the surgeon may have to use a new approach. Late cage removal can be more difficult because of scar and bony overgrowth. Specific cage revision tool sets have been developed to remove implant interbody cages. Some of the basic tools that are very effective in extracting well-fixed cages include (Figs. 4–6):

> Curved or angled osteotomes
> Hollow reamers
> Rongeurs
> Burrs
> Disk space distractors
> Awls
> Implant graspers

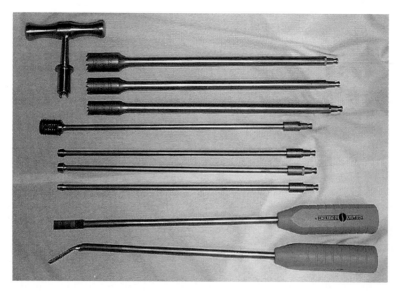

Figure 4 Hollow reamers, angled osteotomes, and threaded cage drivers designed to remove surrounding bone or scar tissue and extract the cage. (From J. S. Thalgott M.D., International Spinal Development & Research Foundation, Las Vegas, NV.)

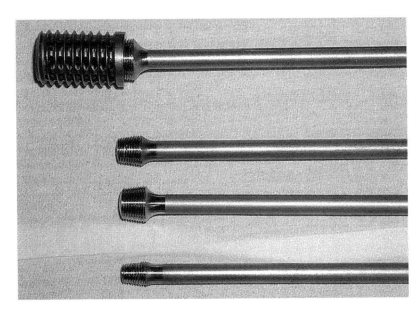

Figure 5 Threaded cage drivers that can be inserted inside the cage and then used to twist it out. (From J. S. Thalgott M.D., International Spinal Development & Research Foundation, Las Vegas, NV.)

1. Undersized, Malpositioned, or Migrating Cages

Cages are usually more easily removed anteriorly, regardless of the original approach, because of the risk of damage to neural tissues with posterior extraction of a malpositioned device. However, when deciding on an approach, consideration must also be given to the fact that threaded extraction devices may only be able to fit into one side of the cage. If a threaded device cannot be used to grip the cage from inside, an inordinate amount of bone may have to be removed from around it. If the cage is completely or significantly extruded posteriorly, it may be necessary to remove it with a posterior approach and decompress the nerve(s) or spinal cord. A posterior approach may also be chosen if only part of a well-fixed cage is causing impingement, in which case it may be possible to simply burr it down. A key technical point in removing cages through a posterior approach is to translate the cage laterally within the disk space before extracting it posteriorly through the spinal canal (35). This may require clearing off more disk or bone around the lateral aspect of the cage before pulling it out. Minimizing nerve root

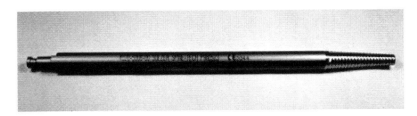

Figure 6 For cages suboptimally placed or compressing neurologic structures, a T-shaped awl is a useful extraction device. The awl atraumatically unscrews the cage and breaks up fibrous adhesions. (From Ref. 17.)

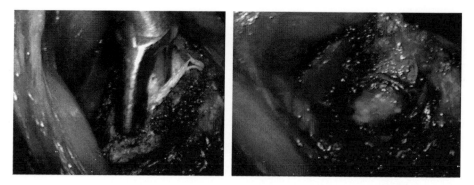

Figure 7   After the disk space is approached, a rongeur is used to remove overlying scar tissue and expose the face of the cage. (From J. S. Thalgott M.D., International Spinal Development & Research Foundation, Las Vegas, NV.)

mobilization is obviously much more difficult in a repeat posterior approach compared to the original procedure because of epidural fibrosis.

Osteotomes or hollow reamers are needed to remove well-fixed cages from surrounding bone or well-healed scar tissue. To avoid removal of excessive bone, curved osteotomes of various radii of curvature are available to fit around cages of different sizes. Once the overgrown bone and adherent scar tissue are released from the cage surface (Fig. 7), an awl or a grasper may be used to remove the cage. If the exposure is end-on to the cage end-face, it can be spun out with the threaded awl (Fig. 8). This awl is a specialized tool that has a tapered end with reverse threads, which inserts into the open end of the cage and progressively grips it tighter as it is twisted in a counter-clockwise direction, while at the same time unscrewing the cage from its bed. However, if the cage cannot be turned so its end-face is visible, substantially more bony excavation and disk-space distraction may be needed.

If a malpositioned cage is intruding into the canal or foraminal space and it is well fixed, a partial vertebrectomy may have to be performed to remove the cage (55). If the offending segment of the cage is within reach, but it is still difficult to remove the entire cage, a burr may be used to smooth down that segment. If the entire cage is

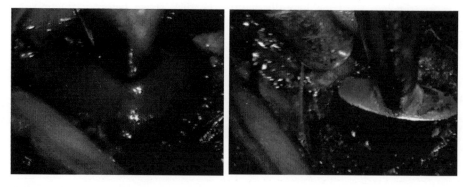

Figure 8   A well-fitting threaded awl or cage driver can then be inserted and used to unscrew the cage from the disk space. (From J. S. Thalgott M.D., International Spinal Development & Research Foundation, Las Vegas, NV.)

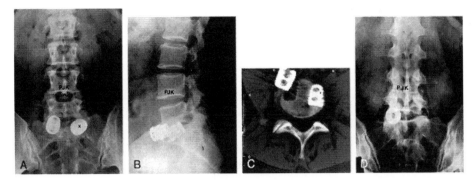

Figure 9 A 45-year-old woman had undergone laparoscopic L5–S1 fusion and instrumentation with two Bagby and Kuslich (BAK) devices. The (A) anteroposterior and (B) lateral radiographs obtained 6 weeks later show that one cage had dislodged anterior to the L5-S1 disk space. A computed tomographic scan through the L5 vertebral body (C) shows that the right cage is completely out and the original seating was too far lateral with a lateral bony bridge insufficient to anchor the cage. The dislodged cage was removed laparoscopically. (D) At long-term follow-up, the patient had a successful clinical result and arthrodesis. (From Ref. 17.)

removed, there is no consensus on what to do next. The surgeon must decide whether to end the procedure, add bone graft (cancellous versus structural), reorient the cage, use a bigger cage, or use a different structural device altogether if needed. The decision is obviously case dependent (35) (Fig. 9).

Removal of a migrating cage is often less complicated than removing a poorly placed cage due to its inherent looseness. To remove a loose cage, the intervertebral space is exposed and a grasping tool is used to attach to the cage. In some cases a threaded awl may be placed within a circular cage and removed in a reverse direction of the cage threads. Distraction of the intervertebral space may be needed to ease cage extraction. Extraction of progressively migrating cages that are easily accessible may be possible through laparoscopic techniques (35). Occasionally, if not discovered early enough, the migrated cages may become fixed in their new position, requiring techniques of fixed-cage extraction described above.

2. Spinal Canal Stenosis or Disk Herniation with Neural Impingement

A patient with symptomatic canal or foraminal impingement by a cage or disk herniation caused during cage placement may require surgical decompression. A symptomatic disk herniation may be treated with a posterior decompression. Neural impingement by the cage itself can be addressed by removing the cage, especially in the early postoperative period, with the techniques mentioned above. If the cage is well fixed, simply burring down the offending part posteriorly may be sufficient (Fig. 10).

3. Pseudarthrosis and/or Loose Implant

Symptomatic pseudarthrosis after cage interbody fusion is usually treated with a posterior instrumented fusion using pedicle screws (Fig. 11). If the cages are in a non-offending position (i.e., still inside the disk space), they do not need to be removed. However, if the cages have grossly migrated out of the disk space and there is significant loss of bone or height in the motion segment, it may not be enough to revise the construct

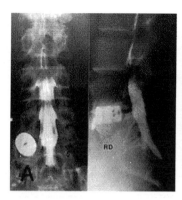
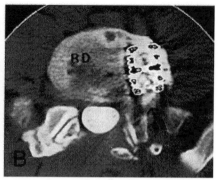

Figure 10 A 45-year-old man had undergone laparoscopic cage placement at L4-L5 and had left-side leg pain 4 days after the procedure. Only one cage had been placed because of technical difficulties in mobilizing the vessels during the procedure. (A) An anteroposterior and lateral myelogram was largely normal, because the nerve root compression was farther lateral than the myelographic dye filling of the nerve root. (B) A computed tomographic scan shows narrowing of the foramen blocking the left L4 nerve root. Patient underwent posterior decompression with resolution of symptoms. (From Ref. 17.)

with posterior instrumented fusion alone (1). Such situations may require cage removal and anterior column reconstruction to obtain a solid fusion and pain relief. The reconstruction may involve using structural bone graft or a larger noncylindrical cage with bone graft. Anterior reconstruction techniques are discussed in a separate chapter in this textbook.

4. Infection

Infection can result in implant loosening and pseudarthrosis through osteolysis. Although there are other factors that can lead to infection and pseudarthrosis, patients with diabetes are at a higher risk for development of these complications (56). There are no reports in the

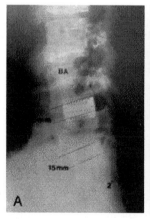
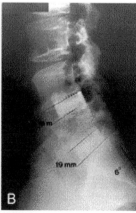
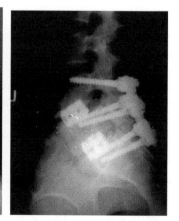

Figure 11 Lateral flexion and extension radiographs show motion at the L4-L5 interspace at 9 mm with flexion and 15 mm with extension, demonstrating pseudarthrosis with cages in acceptable position. This can be treated with posterior instrumented fusion, as shown. (From Ref. 17.)

literature on the management of infected cages other than anecdotal accounts. It only makes sense that an infected and loose cage will need to be removed, since it will not provide any stability to the spine and as a foreign body will only make it difficult to eradicate the microorganism. The other cage may be left in place if not loose, because it may provide enough stability to forgo a posterior stabilizing procedure. If both cages are grossly infected and unstable, removal of both devices and a complete debridement may be necessary, followed by anterior reconstruction with bone graft. McAfee et al. described their treatment of a patient who developed back and leg pain and a deep wound methicillin-resistant *Staphylococcus aureus* infection (35). One of the cages had subsequently loosened and retropulsed into the spinal canal. The patient was managed with a surgical debridement, extraction of only the migrated cage, 6 weeks of intravenous antibiotics, and two reconstructive procedures. Ultimately a solid arthrodesis was achieved with resolution of the spinal infection.

VI. CONCLUSIONS

Most complications related to lumbar interbody fusion cages are failure of surgical technique or poor patient selection rather than an intrinsic defect in fusion cage technology (1,35). The optimal candidate is a patient with symptomatic degenerative disk disease at a single level with decreased disk height. The major factors associated with failure of the original insertion procedure include failure to achieve adequate distraction of the anulus fibrosis; use of undersized cages, especially in the PLIF approach; cerebrospinal fluid leakage or pseudomeningocele; presence of type 2 diabetes mellitus; use of local bone graft rather than iliac crest bone graft inside the cage; an ALIF approach with insertion in a position too lateral resulting in symptoms similar to a far lateral disk herniation; and failure to identify the vertebral midline. Salvaging failed cages consists of removing the offending cages and/or adding stabilization with instrumentation and bone graft. In the future, cages may be inserted using minimally invasive posterior stabilization techniques, thereby decreasing patient morbidity and length of acute hospital stay.

REFERENCES

1. Vacarro AR. Complications of cages and dowels: treatment principles. DePuy Acromed Spine Symposium, Los Angeles, August 21–22, 2002.
2. Kuslich SD, Ulstrom CL, Griffith SL, Ahern JW, Dowdle JD. The Bagby and Kuslich method of lumbar interbody fusion. History, techniques, and 2-year follow-up results of a United States prospective, multicenter trial. Spine 1998; 23(11):1267–1279.
3. O'Dowd JK, Lam K, Mulholland RC, et al. BAK cage—Nottingham results. 13th Annual Meeting, North American Spine Society, San Francisco, Oct. 28–31, 1998.
4. Elias WJ, Simmons NE, Kaptain GJ, Chadduck JB, Whitehill R. Complications of posterior lumbar interbody fusion when using a titanium threaded cage device. J Neurosurg 2000; 93(1 suppl):45–52.
5. Sasso RC. Screw, cages or both? In: resources/surgical treatment/cages. WWW.Spineuniverse. com, Oct. 2002.
6. Weiner BK, Fraser RD. Spine update lumbar interbody cages. Spine 1998; 23(5):634–640.
7. Closkey RF, Parsons JR, Lee CK, Blacksin MF, Zimmerman MC. Mechanics of interbody spinal fusion. Analysis of critical bone graft area. Spine 1993; 18(8):1011–1015.
8. McAfee PC, Lee GA, Fedder IL, Cunningham BW. Anterior BAK instrumentation and fusion: complete versus partial discectomy. Clin Orthop. 2002; 394:55–63.

9. Sandhu HS, Turner S, Kabo JM, Kanim LE, Liu D, Nourparvar A, Delamarter RB, Dawson EG. Distractive properties of a threaded interbody fusion device. An in vivo model. Spine 1996; 21(10):1201–1210.

10. Tsantrizos A, Baramki HG, Zeidman S, Steffen T. Segmental stability and compressive strength of posterior lumbar interbody fusion implants. Spine 2000; 25(15):1899–1907.

11. Dimar JR, Wang M, Beck DJ, Glassman SD, Voor MJ. Posterior lumbar interbody cages do not augment segmental biomechanical instability. Posterior lumbar interbody cages do not augment segmental biomechanical stability. Am J Orthop 2001; 30(8):636–639.

12. Cagli S, Crawford NR, Sonntag VK, Dickman CA. Biomechanics of grade I degenerative lumbar spondylolisthesis. Part 2: treatment with threaded interbody cages/dowels and pedicle screws. J Neurosurg 2001; 94(1 suppl):51–60.

13. Magerl FP. Stabilization of the lower thoracic and lumbar spine with external skeletal fixation. Clin Orthop. 1984; 189:125–141.

14. Heggeness MH, Esses SI. Translaminar facet joint screw fixation for lumbar and lumbosacral fusion. A clinical and biomechanical study. Spine 1991; 16(6 suppl):S266–S269.

15. Vanden Berghe L, Mehdian H, Lee AJ, Weatherley CR. Stability of the lumbar spine and method of instrumentation. Acta Orthop Belg 1993; 59(2):175–180.

16. Zhao J, Hai Y, Ordway NR, Park CK, Yuan HA. Posterior lumbar interbody fusion using posterolateral placement of a single cylindrical threaded cage. Spine 2000; 25(4):425–430.

17. McAfee PC. Interbody fusion cages in reconstructive operations on the spine. J Bone Joint Surg Am 1999; 81(6):859–880.

18. Regan JJ, Yuan H, McAfee PC. Laparoscopic fusion of the lumbar spine: minimally invasive spine surgery. A prospective multicenter study evaluating open and laparoscopic lumbar fusion. Spine 1999; 24(4):402–411.

19. Scaduto AA, Wang JC, Yu WD, Huang J, Delamarter RB. Perioperative complications of lumbar interbody cage fusion: anterior versus posterior approach. 14th Annual Meeting, North American Spine Society, Chicago, Oct. 20–23, 1999.

20. Pradhan BB, Nassar JA, Delamarter RB, Wang JC. Single-level lumbar spine fusion: a comparison of anterior and posterior approaches. J Spinal Disord Tech. 2002; 15(5): 355–361.

21. Inoue S, Watanabe T, Hirose A, Tanaka T, Matsui N, Saegusa O, Sho E. Anterior discectomy and interbody fusion for lumbar disk herniation. A review of 350 cases. Clin Orthop. 1984; 183:22–31.

22. Humphries AW, Hawk WA, Berndt AL. Anterior interbody fusion of lumbar vertebrae. Surg Clin North Am 1961; 41:1685–1700.

23. Kozak JA, Heilman AE, O'Brien JP. Anterior lumbar fusion options: technique and graft materials. Clin Orthop 1994; 300:45–51.

24. Baker JK, Reardon PR, Reardon MJ, Heggeness MH. Vascular injury in anterior lumbar surgery. Spine 1993; 18(15):2227–2230.

25. Chow SP, Leong JC, Ma A, Yau AC. Anterior spinal fusion or deranged lumbar intervertebral disk. Spine 1980; 5(5):452–458.

26. Stauffer RN, Coventry MB. Anterior interbody lumbar spine fusion. Analysis of Mayo clinic series. J Bone Joint Surg 1972; 54A:756–768.

27. Regan JJ, Aronoff RJ, Ohnmeiss DD, Sengupta DK. Laparoscopic approach to L4-L5 for interbody fusion using BAK cages: experience in the first 58 cases. Spine 1999; 24(20):2171–2174.

28. Zdeblick TA, David SM. A prospective comparison of surgical approach for anterior L4-L5 fusion: laparoscopic versus mini anterior lumbar interbody fusion. Spine 2000; 25(20):2682–2687.

29. Tencer AF, Hampton D, Eddy S. Biomechanical properties of threaded inserts for lumbar interbody spinal fusion. Spine 1995; 20(22):2408–2414.

30. Brodke DS, Dick JC, Kunz DN, McCabe R, Zdeblick TA. Posterior lumbar interbody fusion. A biomechanical comparison, including a new threaded cage. Spine 1997; 22(1):26–31.

31. Glazer PA, Colliou O, Klisch SM. Biomechanical analysis of multilevel fixation methods in the lumbar spine. Spine 1997; 22(2):171–182.

32. Glazer PA, Colliou O, Lotz JC, Bradford DS. Biomechanical analysis of lumbosacral fixation. Spine 1996; 21(10):1211–1222.

33. Rapoff AJ, Ghanayem AJ, Zdeblick TA. Biomechanical comparison of posterior lumbar interbody fusion cages. Spine 1997; 22(20):2375–2379.

34. Jost B, Cripton PA, Lund T, Oxland TR, Lippuner K, Jaeger P, Nolte LP. Compressive strength of interbody cages in the lumbar spine: the effect of cage shape, posterior instrumentation and bone density. Eur Spine J 1998; 7(2):132–141.

35. McAfee PC, Cunningham BW, Lee GA, Orbegoso CM, Haggerty CJ, Fedder IL, Griffith SL. Revision strategies for salvaging or improving failed cylindrical cages. Spine 1999; 24(20):2147–2153.

36. Hacker RJ. Comparison of interbody fusion approaches for disabling low back pain. Spine 1997; 22:660–666.

37. Taylor BA, Vaccaro AR, Hilibrand AS, Zlotolow DA, Albert TJ. The risk of foraminal violation and nerve root impingement after anterior placement of lumbar interbody fusion cages. Spine 2001; 26(1):100–104.

38. Ray CD. Threaded titanium cages for lumbar interbody fusions. Spine 1997; 22:667–680.

39. Oxland TR, Hoffer Z, Nydegger T. Comparative biomechanical investigation of anterior lumbar interbody cages: central and bilateral insertion. Orthop Trans 1999; 22:728–729.

40. Rathonyi GC, Oxland TR, Gerich U, Grassmann S, Nolte LP. The role of supplemental translaminar screws in anterior lumbar interbody fixation: a biomechanical study. Eur Spine J 1998; 7(5):400–407.

41. Lund T, Oxland TR, Jost B, Cripton P, Grassmann S, Etter C, Nolte LP. Interbody cage stabilisation in the lumbar spine: biomechanical evaluation of cage design, posterior instrumentation and bone density. J Bone Joint Surg Br 1998; 80(2):351–359.

42. Wang JC, Zou D, Yuan H, Yoo J. A biomechanical evaluation of graft loading characteristics for anterior cervical discectomy and fusion. A comparison of traditional and reverse grafting techniques. Spine 1998; 23(22):2450–2454.

43. Pradhan BB, Wang JC. Loading characteristics of femoral ring interbody allografts— a biomechanical study. 37th Annual Meeting, Scoliosis Research Society, Seattle, WA, Sept. 19–21, 2002.

44. Blumenthal, SL, Regan JJ, Hisey MS, et al. Can threaded fusion cages be used effectively as stand-alone devices? 14th Annual Meeting, North American Spine Society, Chicago, Oct. 20–23, 1999.

45. Rathonyi GC, Oxland TR, Gerich U, Grassmann S, Nolte LP. The role of supplemental translaminar screws in anterior lumbar interbody fixation: a biomechanical study. Eur Spine J 1998; 7(5):400–407.

46. Volkman T, Horton WC, Hutton WC. Transfacet screws with lumbar interbody reconstruction: biomechanical study of motion segment stiffness. J Spinal Disord 1996; 9(5):425–432.

47. Cagli S, Vrawford NR, Sonntag VKH, Dickman CA. Biomechanics of grade I degenerative lumbar spondylolisthesis Part 2: treatment with threaded interbody cages/dowels and pedicle screws. J Neurosurg 2001; 94(1 suppl):51–60.

48. Vamvanij V, Fredrickson BE, Thorpe JM, Stadnick ME, Yuan HA. Surgical treatment of internal disk disruption: an outcome study of four fusion techniques. J Spinal Disord 1998; 11(5):375–382.

49. Cizek GR, Boyd LM. Imaging pitfalls of interbody spinal implants. Spine 2000; 25(20):2633–2636.

50. Fraser RD. Interbody, posterior, and combined lumbar fusions. Spine 1995; 20:167S–177S.

51. Kumar A, Kozak JA, Doherty BJ, Dickson JH. Interspace distraction and graft subsidence after anterior lumbar fusion with femoral strut allograft. Spine 1993; 18(16):2393–2400.

52. Zdeblick TA. A prospective randomized study of lumbar fusion: preliminary results. Spine 1993; 18:983–991.

53. Hacker RJ. Comparison of interbody fusion approaches for disabling low back pain. Spine 1997; 22:660–666.

54. Heithoff KB, Mullin JW, Holte D, et al. Failure of radiographic detection of pseudarthrosis in patients with titanium lumbar interbody fusion cages. 14th Annual Meeting, North American Spine Society, Chicago, Oct. 20–23, 1999.

55. Glassman SD, Johnson JR, Raque G, Puno RM, Dimar JR. Management of iatrogenic spinal stenosis complicating placement of a fusion cage. A case report. Spine 1996; 21(20): 2383–2386.

56. Brown CA, Eismont FJ. Complications in spinal fusion. Orthop Clin North Am 1998; 29(4):679–699.

29

Posttraumatic Thoracolumbar Kyphosis

Jeff S. Silber
Long Island Jewish Medical Center, New Hyde Park, New York, U.S.A.

Alexander R. Vaccaro
Thomas Jefferson University and the Rothman Institute, Philadelphia, Pennsylvania, U.S.A.

I. INTRODUCTION

Trauma to the spinal cord and column is a devastating injury that often results in an abrupt change in the quality of the patient's life and for the immediate family. Each year in the United States there are more than 1 million acute injuries to the spine, with approximately 50,000 of these resulting in fractures to the bony spinal column, many of which involve the thoracolumbar region (8). Although there are between 7,000 and 10,000 new cases of spinal cord injury each year, the majority of spinal injuries are minor and without long-term consequence (19). The majority of spinal injuries involve only the paraspinal soft tissue structures and are successfully managed conservatively and do not require surgical stabilization or prolonged orthotic immobilization.

The mechanism producing a thoracolumbar burst fracture or associated middle column injury has been shown to result from stress concentration noted at the pedicle and the adjacent posterosuperior part of the vertebral body (10). Functional outcomes following thoracolumbar burst fractures managed nonoperatively with early ambulation and an orthosis has produced satisfactory results even with a degree of progressive kyphosis (4). Weinstein et al. (27) evaluated 42 patients with thoracolumbar burst fractures treated non-operatively at an average follow-up of 20.2 years (range 11–55 years). At final follow-up, the authors calculated an average focal kyphosis angle of 26.4° and found that the degree of posttraumatic kyphosis did not correlate with post injury pain or function. Furthermore, no patient experienced a decrease in neurological function.

Aside from the obvious initial loss of function and ability to interact with one's environment, several chronic complications may develop over time in patients with a thoracolumbar spine injury. These complications can further impede functional as well as emotional rehabilitation. One of these complications following the initial management of thoracolumbar compression/burst fractures is posttraumatic kyphotic deformity of the spinal column.

The vast majority of unstable thoracolumbar spinal injuries are recognized early and managed with either prolonged immobilization or surgical stabilization. Rarely, the initial treatment may be inadequate, resulting in late progressive instability leading to increasing kyphotic deformity associated with pain and, in severe cases, loss of neurological function. In less obvious injuries, initially less aggressive immobilization techniques may have been chosen, but due to the unrecognized occult instability and repeated exposure to chronic physiological stresses (flexion and axial loading), a gradual kyphotic deformity may become apparent (9,16). In rare cases requiring surgery, the operative management may have been inadequate in achieving adequate spinal stability. This may result in inadequate biomechanical stability and, in the face of continued physiological stresses, may result in a gradual posttraumatic kyphotic deformity. This may further impede the functional and emotional recovery in this group of patients.

On physical examination, global sagittal balance is present when the head is positioned directly over the pelvis. On plain full-length radiographic evaluation, a plumb line dropped from the external auditory meatus should drop posterior to the hip joint and approximately through the anterior aspect of the S1-S2 sacral segment (21). An increase in the normal thoracic kyphosis, as is often seen in thoracolumbar fractures, results in an altered sagittal alignment and causes a compensatory hyperextension of adjacent spinal segments. This abnormal relationship between spinal motion segments results in several pathological changes. These include increased intervertebral shear and altered facet joint motion leading ultimately to segmental instability and the acceleration of potential degenerative changes (4,5,21).

Many authors agree that in patients with a localized kyphotic deformity of more than 30° there is an increased risk for continued chronic discomfort at the thoracolumbar kyphotic segment with a potential risk for progressive deformity. Surgical intervention is often considered in this setting or in the presence of radiographically identified kyphotic spinal deformity progression (11,15,22). The relative considerations for late surgical intervention include patients with an unacceptable cosmetic appearance associated with pain.

The management of posttraumatic kyphotic deformity of the thoracolumbar spine can be extremely challenging. A careful history and examination of all initial and subsequent imaging studies is necessary to determine the mechanism and extent of the initial injury. It should be determined if the index surgical procedure or bracing regiment was biomechanically sufficient as a treatment method. These imaging studies should be compared to more recent studies to get an understanding of the patient's global sagittal and coronal balance. Dynamic plain radiographs are also obtained to evaluate for any objective evidence of instability.

II. CONSEQUENCES OF THORACOLUMBAR KYPHOSIS

A. Thoracolumbar Pain

The most common complaint following progressive thoracolumbar kyphotic deformity managed either nonoperatively or operatively is pain. This is due to spinal imbalance in the coronal and/or sagittal plane from progressive deformity. This may be seen following nonoperative management or surgical complications leading to a progressive deformity including failed instrumentation, or from a symptomatic pseudoarthrosis. The pathophysiology of this pain is due to spinal column imbalance and resultant abnormal forces placed on the soft tissue structures leading to gradual soft tissue fatigue and pain. Furthermore, pain may also be a consequence of premature degenerative changes associated with the spinal deformity. Patients typically complain of a constant aching discomfort located in the apical segment of the deformity. Occasionally, either the patient or the patient's relatives may notice an obvious postural deformity or instrumentation prominence. Pain may become exacerbated with activities such as bending, walking, lifting, and twisting. At times pain can also be aggravated with either prolonged sitting or standing (15).

B. Neurological Sequela

Fortunately, only a minority of patients developing a posttraumatic spinal deformity with progressive thoracolumbar kyphosis may manifest symptoms of neurological deterioration (Fig. 1). It has been reported that patients developing less than 15° of a posttraumatic kyphosis or canal stenosis of less than 25% had a 50% less likely chance of developing

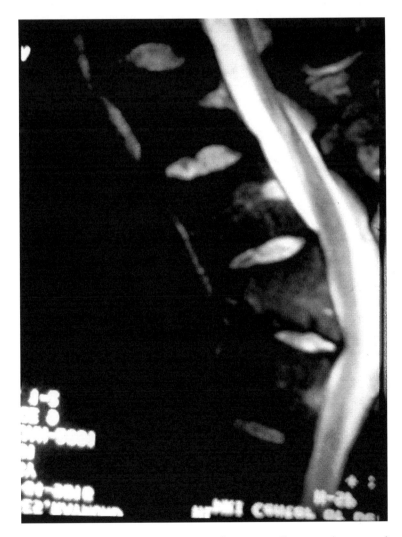

Figure 1 Sagittal magnetic resonance image revealing neural compression resulting in increasing neural deficit.

spinal cord cystic change which has been shown to develop in patients developing a greater deformity (1). Furthermore, Mohanty and Venkatram showed that in patients suffering a thoracolumbar burst fracture, there was no correlation between the neurological deficit and subsequent recovery with the initial extent of spinal canal compromise (17). Neurological dysfunction has been shown to result from several posttraumatic developments including progressive kyphosis, canal stenosis, spinal instability, arachnoiditis, and spinal cord tethering (1). Due to the potential for late-onset pain and neurological dysfunction, the treating physician must practice heightened vigilance in preventing the occurrence of a significant progressive spinal kyphotic deformity via continued brace treatment or with surgical intervention. Close follow-up with repeat physical and radiographic examinations is important to identify any changes in spinal alignment in the posttraumatic or postsurgical period. Even in the setting of a static long-term kyphotic deformity, it is important not to underestimate the potential for a progressive myelopathy to develop. This development may manifest itself with neurological dysfunction only with activity. In this scenario, patients may present with no obvious neurological findings on physical examination, but a history of the patient's symptoms including lower extremity weakness, incoordination, and loss of balance with ambulation may be significant. These dynamic symptoms are attributed to tethering of the scarred neural elements of the spinal cord draped over the prominent vertebral fracture fragment or deformity during ambulation. Additionally, neurological worsening following an initial period of improvement or plateauing may be secondary to intramedullary spinal cord cyst or cavity development. This pathological development, known as either a posttraumatic syringomyelia or progressive posttraumatic cystic myelopathy, has a reported prevalence between 3.2 and 40% (9,14). These processes can be recognized and diagnosed early in patients with complaints of neurological deterioration with widely available advanced imaging studies such as magnetic resonance imaging.

The most common causes of spinal cord cyst or cavity development include progressive deformity from spinal column instability resulting in spinal cord compression and spinal cord tethering resulting in microcystic cord degeneration. The pathoanatomy of posttraumatic syringomyelia consists of a confluent cyst within the spinal cord parenchyma. When numerous microcysts exist in the absence of a large cyst, it is referred to as posttraumatic myelomalacic myelopathy (14). Unfortunately, shunting of the cyst alone has resulted in disappointing long-term improvement, with shunt revisions frequently needed (3). More recently, surgical intervention for this syndrome consists of cyst shunting or fenestration as well as releasing any existing tether.

III. RADIOGRAPHIC EVALUATION

A. Plain Radiographs

When measuring a focal kyphotic deformity, it has been shown that direct measurement of the fractured vertebrae is fraught with significant observer variation (20). Therefore, measurement of the focal kyphotic deformity is best obtained when comparisons are made between the superior and inferior endplates of the vertebral bodies above and below the segment of injury (21). Initial plain radiographs, including full-length antero-posterior and lateral views, are obtained and are used to evaluate the following:

1. Coronal and sagittal alignment
2. Bone quality

3. If applicable, the integrity of the existing spinal implants
4. The presence or absence of fusion healing.

Lateral flexion and extension as well as anteroposterior side bending views are also important in assessing the status of the flexibility of the existing deformity, the status of the fusion, if present, and to help identify subtle loose hardware. When surgical intervention is necessary due to progressive deformity, the degree of presurgical deformity flexibility aids in predicting the expected deformity correction. It also helps determine the mapping of spinal implants and the location of osteotomies when necessary. The comparison of follow-up imaging studies with prior films to help assess and document the extent of spinal deformity progression and rate of hardware migration or failure is of utmost importance (6).

B. Computed Tomography

Computed tomography (CT) is the imaging modality of choice to assess detailed evaluation of the spinal bony architecture and the position of spinal implants. Through the use of 3 mm axial images, sagittal and coronal reconstructions may be reformatted, allowing visualization of subtle changes in the structural integrity of the bony spinal architecture. CT scanning is ideal in the assessment of fusion integrity, the presence of a pseudoarthrosis, and subtle instrumentation loosening. Additionally, when magnetic resonance imaging (MRI) is not available or is not helpful in the setting of ferromagnetic implants, CT myelography can be useful in demonstrating neural compromise, especially in patients with new-onset or progressive neural deficits.

C. Magnetic Resonance Imaging

In the setting of symptomatic neural compression, MRI is the imaging modality of choice. It offers detailed visualization of spinal neural structures such as the spinal cord and cauda equina. When ferromagnetic spinal implants are present, degradation of imaging resolution may be present. Information of the neural structures based on the MRI is extremely important if corrective surgical intervention involves spinal column manipulation with the potential for additional neural stretching or compression.

D. Ultrasound

Ultrasound has recently been shown to be an excellent diagnostic adjunct in detecting injuries to the posterior spinal ligament complex including the supraspinaous and inter-spinous ligaments. Although the sensitivity was shown to be less than with MRI, this modality is especially useful in settings where patients are unable to undergo magnetic resonance imaging or where it is unavailable (18).

IV. POSTSURGICAL PROGRESSIVE KYPHOSIS

A. Inadequate Mechanical Stability

This cause of surgical failure is closely related to the causes of instrumentation failure. Postsurgical thoracolumbar deformity progression may occur in the setting of inadequate restoration of spinal stability. This is more commonly seen following either anterior- or posterior-alone procedures in which significant incompetence still exists in the nonsurgically addressed spinal columns. Furthermore, it has been reported that fusion procedures of inadequate length may not adequately stabilize a spinal injury, especially if all three columns are involved leading to a gradual progression in spinal deformity. Keene et al. (12) reported on 106 patients who underwent operative stabilization for unstable thoracolumbar fractures. Due to chronic instability and a progressive kyphotic deformity progression, 16 patients (15%) eventually required additional surgery 4 months to 16 years after the index procedure. Furthermore, the authors concluded that the most common risk factors responsible for posttraumatic postsurgical kyphotic progression included the presence of a laminectomy and/or a short fusion segment (Fig. 2). Additionally, long-term spinal alignment without significant progression of a kyphotic deformity was observed when five or more spinal levels were incorporated into the fusion segment posteriorly or when a posterior laminectomy was not performed at the initial surgery (12) (Fig. 3). Shen et al. (23) compared operative versus non-operative

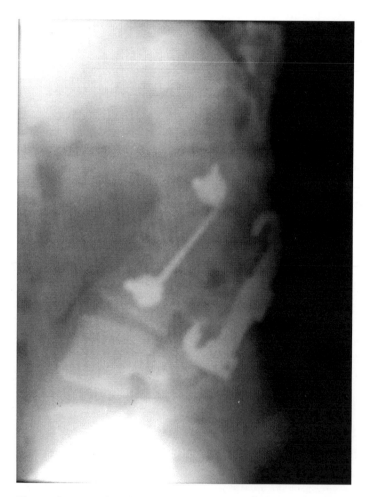

Figure 2 Lateral radiograph 12 months following an L1 burst fracture managed with a short-segment anterior/posterior procedure. A focal kyphotic deformity developed, producing increased pain and neural dysfunction.

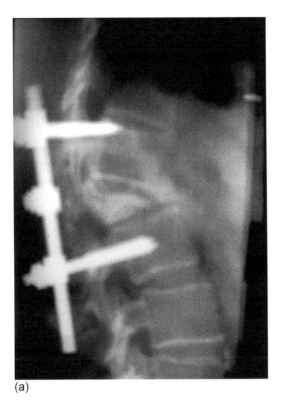

(a)

Figure 3 (a) Lateral radiograph showing a failed short-segment posterior instrumented fusion in the management of an L1 burst fracture. The patient developed an increased kyphotic deformity with posterior skin breakdown. (b) Postoperative lateral radiograph demonstrating the reestablishment of sagittal plane alignment. This was accomplished following an anterior decompression and reconstruction along with a long segmental posterior instrumented fusion.

management in 80 neurologically intact patients following a single-level burst fracture from T11–L2 regardless of kyphosis. Their study showed that the operative group fixed with a short-segment construct reported less pain at 3 and 6 months, but the outcome was similar afterwards. At 2-year follow-up in the nonoperative group, the kyphosis worsened an average of 4° and canal retropulsion decreased from 34 to 15% compared to an initial improvement of kyphosis of 17% in the operative group with gradual loss of correction. The authors concluded that short-segment posterior fixation provides partial kyphosis correction and earlier pain relief, but long-term functional outcome is similar to nonoperative management (23).

B. Pseudoarthrosis

A postoperative pseudoarthrosis or nonunion may result in a progressive spinal deformity. This is more common in the setting of inadequate fusion level selection and/or inadequate instrumentation, but may occur in the presence of a previously adequately performed spinal reconstructive procedure. Patients with a symptomatic pseudoarthrosis often present with increasing pain, with or without activity, localized to the nonunion site. Pain intensity is usually most severe within the first year following the index procedure.

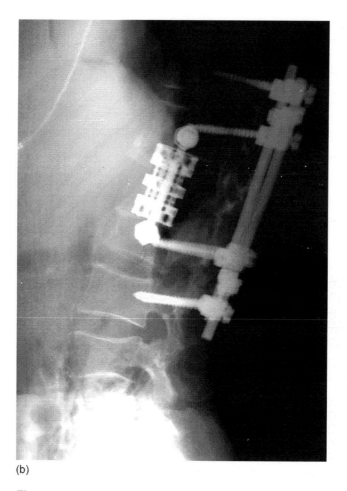

(b)

Figure 3 (*continued*)

The pain may plateau or worsen gradually, depending on the integrity of the spinal instrumentation. As the deformity worsens, a change in posture may also be noticed over time. It is imperative to exclude the possibility of an occult deep infection when a symptomatic nonunion is identified. Fortunately, the vast majority of nonunions following spinal fusions are asymptomatic and do not result in a progressive spinal deformity. Radiographic examination may reveal evidence of instrumentation loosening or failure and, although difficult to assess at times, an obvious pseudoarthrosis.

C. Instrumentation Failure

Spinal implant loosening or failure may be the cause of or result in a pseudoarthrosis and kyphotic deformity progression and is the most common reported complication resulting in a posttraumatic deformity. It has been reported in up to 16% of patients following a posterior instrumented–alone fusion procedure. Selecting inappropriate fusion levels or the length of stabilization is a common error resulting in fusion failure and the potential for deformity. Instrumentation failure in this setting eventually results from excessive axial forces at the implant bone junction leading to implant migration, displacement, or breakage. Revision stabilization is often required when early failure of instrumentation occurs.

Charcot spine is a rare developement that may result in a neuropathic spinal deformity. It often leads to a significant posttraumatic deformity in active young patients following a complete spinal cord injury treated nonoperatively or operatively. The spinal deformity that develops is a consequence of the insensate proprioceptive environment of the vertebral elements below the level of spinal cord injury. This type of deformity has been reported to occur even decades after the initial injury (16,26). The pathophysiology involves abnormal motion between vertebrae of the neuropathic segments, resulting in loss of integrity with cartilage and ligament breakdown. This results in vertebral endplate fracture and failure of subchondral bone, ultimately leading to vertebral collapse. The end stage of this insensate destructive process is a massive pseudoarthrosis. Although this process is initiated in the environment of insensate vertebral segments, patients commonly complain of worsening back pain. Other developments may involve increased lower extremity spasticity and a palpable and audible crepitus with increased motion at the Charcot segment. A progressive kyphotic gibbus formation may result in loss of sitting balance (6,26). Similar to Charcot joints in other areas of the body, radiographic examination in the early stages demonstrates hypertrophic bone formation seen in the adjacent vertebral segments below the level of the spinal cord lesion. When treated operatively, this hypertrophic bone formation may also develop immediately below a fusion segment (6,16). Later stages of the process result in fragmentation of the intervertebral disk space and vertebral endplates, leading to the final stages of massive hypertrophic bone formation and pseudoarthrosis resulting in audible and palpable crepitus with spinal motion (16). Early detection through repeated physical and radiographic evaluation is necessary in order to prevent the development of a rapid spinal deformity occasionally seen with this disorder (7,25). When necessary, operative treatment consisting of partial resection of the Charcot joint (pseudoarthrosis) with structural bone grafting followed by a posterior segmental instrumented fusion has been reported to produce good long-term results in maintaining deformity correction (16). Unfortunately, secondary Charcot spinal segments have been reported to occur below a previously successful fusion for this disorder (7).

V. SURGICAL CONSIDERATIONS

All imaging data along with a history defining the impact of the present deformity on the functional status of the patient will determine if surgical intervention is recommended. Surgical intervention may be considered if the spinal deformity is progressive, the deformity is considered responsible for the patient's unrelenting back pain or functional disability and/or if there is a static or progressive neurological deficit.

Many surgical strategies are available in the setting of a radiographically identified spinal deformity. The main goals of surgical intervention include correction of spinal deformity with the relief of symptomatic neurological compression and hopefully the alleviation of pain. The surgical approach may include either a posterior- or anterior-only approach or any variation of a combined anterior and posterior procedure.

It has been shown that a posterior-only primary or revision approach is often inadequate for optimal deformity correction in the setting of a posttraumatic thoracolumbar kyphosis unless an adequate posterior column shortening osteotomy is performed. A posterior-only fusion in the presence of an existing kyphotic deformity results in an obvious biomechanical disadvantage. This is due to the considerable tension forces placed on the posterior instrumentation. These constant stresses often exist regardless of the adequacy of sagittal plane correction provided with instrumentation. If a posterior-only approach is selected, then one should consider the use of an osteotomy to obtain the desired sagittal correction required to balance the C7 vertebral body over the sacral elements. This will improve the biomechanical integrity of a posterior-only procedure and alleviate some of the tensile forces placed on the construct.

An alternative strategy is a combined anterior and posterior approach, which has proven to provide long-term stability in the setting of pronounced sagittal plane deformities. This involves either an initial anterior release or decompressive procedure and grafting followed by a posterior segmental instrumented stabilization procedure. This combined approach provides a superior biomechanical environment, allowing significant manipulation and restoration of spinal sagittal alignment as well as providing improved fusion success. In the setting of a stable posterior spinal column, an anterior-alone approach has been shown to provide good long-term stability with maintained sagittal plane deformity correction (22).

In less mobile deformities, in order to establish spinal mobility for adequate sagittal reconstruction, osteotomies may have to be performed. Kostuik et al. (13) reported on 54 patients managed with a combined anterior opening wedge osteotomy and instrumentation followed by a posterior closing extension osteotomy with instrumentation in order to establish sagittal spinal balance in the thoracolumbar and lumbar spine. They reported significant postoperative pain reduction in over 90% of the patients. In the setting of a previously failed instrumented posterior only procedure, Shufflebarger popularized the back-front-back procedure. This consisted of an initial posterior release with removal of existing instrumentation and the performance of osteotomies and facetectomies when necessary. This was followed by an anterior release and reconstruction and, lastly, posterior placement of instrumentation to create a posterior tension band (24).

It has been reported that the long-term outcome following surgical management for progressive thoracolumbar kyphosis has been satisfactory. It is intuitive that the earlier the surgical intervention is provided to the patient, the better the overall long-term outcome. Since surgical intervention to address this deformity often requires a combined anterior/ posterior approach, an increased risk of operative complications is seen in this difficult group of patients. These include wound breakdown with or without infection, neurological worsening, and pseudarthrosis with possible implant failure. Neurological worsening is the most feared complication and is often the consequence of the existing kyphotic spinal deformity. This results in the draping, scarring, or tethering of the spinal cord and cauda equina over the posterior aspect of the vertebral bodies. Often the patient in this setting has a baseline neurological deficit, and surgical deformity correction with neural manipulation may result in a subtle tension force resulting in progressive neural dysfunction.

VI. NEUROLOGICAL COMPLICATIONS

The potential for neurological injury in the late surgical management of a progressive posttraumatic thoracolumbar kyphosis may exist due to the complexity of the deformity, resulting in anterior draping of the scarred neural elements over the posterior aspects of the anterior located vertebral bodies. Furthermore, the incidence is significantly higher in the surgical management of a previously failed surgical procedure. In the setting of a preexisting spinal cord injury, often associated with spinal cord tethering, neural element scarring, and vascular ischemia, the neural elements may be more vulnerable to the potential for stretch injury from manipulation following deformity correction. Fortunately, new-onset or progressive neurological injury has been reported to be approximately 1% following all spinal surgery. The increased usage of intraoperative spinal cord monitoring should reduce the incidence of neurological deterioration even further. The use of spinal cord monitoring cannot be overemphasized as it aids in the detection of early changes in neurological function both during surgical manipulation and with the placement of instrumentation (8). The decision to release the correction and/or the removal of hardware must be seriously considered if neurological changes are detected during deformity correction or hardware placement.

VII. SUMMARY

Trauma to the thoracolumbar spinal column and spinal cord is a devastating injury that may be fraught with many complications, including posttraumatic deformity. Certainly the best treatment is prevention of initial spinal deformity through strict adherence to the principles of fracture care involving close follow-up, brace immobilization, and, when necessary, early surgical intervention. Once failure of the index management presents itself, treatment of the posttraumatic deformity follows basic principles. These include protection of the neural elements or improvement of neurological function and stabilization or reestablishment of the integrity of the compromised spinal columns and spinal balance. To accomplish this, surgery may be indicated and may involve an anterior, posterior, or combined surgical approach with or without spinal osteotomies. One must be extremely cautious when manipulating the sagittal profile of the spinal column so as not to overlengthen the neural elements. This development is poorly tolerated by the neural elements, especially in the setting of a preexisting spinal cord injury.

The long-term outcome following the surgical management of posttraumatic thoracolumbar kyphosis is predicated on several factors. These include the patient's age and medical status, the type, severity, and mechanism of the initial injury, the time period between the initial injury and surgical deformity correction, bone quality, and the experience of the surgical team.

The surgical management of posttraumatic thoracolumbar kyphosis is a challenging problem. The treating physician must pay strict attention to the biomechanics of the entire spinal column and be cognizant of the response of the neural elements to any form of manipulation. These basic principles will hopefully provide a successful long-term functional outcome to the patient with such a deformity.

REFERENCES

1. Abel R, Gerner HJ, Smit C, Meiners T. Residual deformity of the spinal canal in patients with traumatic paraplegia and secondary changes of the spinal cord. Spinal Cord 1999; 37:14–19.
2. Aligizakis A, Katonis P, Stergiopoulos K, Galanakis I, Karabekios S, Hadjipavlou A. Functional outcome of burst fractures of the thoracolumbar spine managed non-operatively, with early ambulation, evaluated using the load sharing classification. Acta Orthop Belg 2002; 68:279–287.
3. Batzdorf U, Klekamp J, Johnson JP. A critical appraisal of syrinx cavity shunting procedures. J Neurosurg 1998; 89:382–388.

4. Bohlman HH. Treatment of fractures and dislocations of the thoracic and lumbar spine. J Bone Joint Surg 1985; 67A:165–169.

5. Bohlman HH, Freehafer A, Dejak J. The results of treatment of acute injuries of the upper thoracic spine with paralysis. J Bone Joint Surg 1985; 67A:360–369.

6. Bolesta MJ, Bohlman HH. Late sequelae of thoracolumbar fractures and fracture-dislocations: surgical treatment. In: Frymoyer JW, ed. The Adult Spine: Principles and Practice 2nd ed. Philadelphia: Lippincott-Raven Publishers, 1997:1513–1533.

7. Brown CW, Jones B, Donaldson DH, Akmakjian J, Brugman JL. Neuropathic (charcot) arthropathy of the spine after traumatic spinal paraplegia. Spine 1992; 6:S103–S108.

8. Connelly PJ, Abitbol JJ, Martin RJ, Yuan HA. Spine: trauma. In: Garfin SR, Vaccaro AR, eds. Orthopaedic Knowledge Update: Spine. Rosemont, IL: American Academy of Orthopaedic Surgeons, 1997:197–217.

9. Curati WL, Kingsley DPE, Moseley IF. MRI in chronic spinal trauma. Neurorad 1992; 35:30–35.

10. Dai L. Mechanism of thoracolumbar burst fractures: a biomechanical study. Chin Med J 2002; 115:336–338.

11. Gertzbein SD. Scoliosis Research Soceity. Multicenter spine fracture study. Spine 1992; 17:528–540.

12. Keene JS, Lash EG, Kling TF Jr. Undetected posttraumatic instability of "stable" thoracolumbar fractures. J Orthop Trauma 1988; 2:202–211.

13. Kostuik JP, Gilles RM, Richardson WJ, Okajima Y. Combined single stage anterior and posterior osteotomy for correction of iatrogenic lumbar kyphosis. Spine 1988; 13:257–266.

14. Lee TT, Alameda GJ, Gromelski EB, Green BA. Outcome after surgical treatment of progressive posttraumatic cystic myelopathy. J Neurosurg 2000; 92:149–154.

15. Malcolm BW, Bradford DS, Winter RB, Chou SN. Posttraumatic kyphosis. A review of forty-eight surgically treated patients. J Bone Joint Surg 1981; 63A:891–899.

16. McBride GG, Greenberg D. Treatment of charcot spinal arthropathy following traumatic paraplegia. J Spinal Disord 1991; 2:212–220.

17. Mohanty SP, Venkatram N. Does neurological recovery in thoracolumbar and lumbar burst fractures depend on the extent of canal compromise? Spinal Cord 2002; 40:295–299.

18. Moon SH, Park MS, Suk KS, Suh JS, Lee SH, Kim NH, Lee HM. Feasibility of ultrasound examination in posterior ligament injury of thoracolumbar spine fracture. Spine 2002; 27:2154–2158.

19. National Spinal Cord Injury Statistical Center. Spinal Cord Injury Facts and Figures at a Glance. Birmingham: University of Alabama, 1999.

20. Oda I, Cunningham BW, Buckley RA, et al. Does spinal kyphotic deformity influence the biomechanical characteristics of the adjacent motion segments? An in vivo animal model Spine 1999; 24:2139–2146.

21. Polly DW Jr, Klemme WR, Shawen S Management options for the treatment of posttraumatic thoracic kyphosis. Spine 1985; 10:307–312.

22. Roberson JR, Whitesides TE Jr. Surgical reconstruction of late post-traumatic thoracolumbar kyphosis. Spine 1985; 10:307–312.

23. Shen WJ, Liu TJ, Shen YS. Nonoperative treatment versus posterior fixation for thoracolumbar junction burst fractures without neurologic deficit. Spine 2001; 26:1038–1045.

24. Shufflebarger HL, Clark CE. Thoracolumbar osteotomy for postsurgical sagittal imbalance. Spine 1992; 17:S287–S290.

25. Sobel JW, Bohlman HH, Freehafer AA. Charcot's arthropathy of the spine following spinal cord injury. J Bone Joint Surg 1985; 67A:771–776.

26. Standaert C, Cardenas DD, Anderson P. Charcot spine as a late complication of traumatic spinal cord injury. Arch Phys Med Rehabil 1997; 2:221–225.

27. Weinstein JN, Collata P, Lehmann TR. Thoracolumbar "burst" fractures treated conservatively: a long-term follow-up. Spine 1988; 13:33–38.

30

Complications in Thoracolumbar Deformity Surgery

Sigurd Berven and David S. Bradford
University of California–San Francisco, San Francisco, California, U.S.A.

> ...complications will occur in spite of the best care. A poor result does not mean that there has been negligence or malpractice.
>
> Charles H. Epps, Jr., M.D.

I. INTRODUCTION

The surgical management of spinal deformity is challenging, and numerous adverse outcomes may result from the surgical approach and correction of spinal deformity in the adolescent and adult patient. The goals of surgery for deformity of the spine include the treatment of present pain and disability and the prevention of future consequences of progressive deformity. Surgical correction of spinal deformity introduces the risk of both perioperative and long-term complications (1,2). Knowledge of these complications is important and valuable for both the patient and the surgeon. The patient benefits by gaining information on potential adverse outcomes and being empowered to make an informed choice regarding the benefits and risks of surgery (3). The surgeon treating the spinal deformity benefits from recognition of these potential complications and being informed as to the choice of surgical strategies and implant options that optimize the ability to effectively realign the spinal column while minimizing the risks of complications. Recognition of potential complications may lead to prevention of adverse outcomes in practice (4). The purpose of this chapter is to identify the major complications of deformity correction in the thoracic and lumbar spine and to suggest strategies for avoiding these complications.

II. DEFORMITY CORRECTION: NEURAL RISKS

Neural injury is among the most devastating complications in spinal deformity surgery and an important concern for both the surgeon and patient (5). Neural structures may be at risk in the unstable spine or in the spine with progressive deformity, and in these cases an important goal of surgery is to prevent the consequence of neural deterioration with nonoperative management. The risk of neural compromise in the natural history of deformity progression has been reported with significant variation in the literature and is generally a significant concern in severe congenital and early-onset deformities and not a usual part of the natural history of adolescent or adult idiopathic scoliosis (6–8). Understanding that paraplegia is not usually expected in the natural history of idiopathic spinal deformity, the risk of paraplegia as a result of spinal surgery is introduced by the choice of surgery for correction of deformity.

Neural injury in spinal deformity surgery may result from direct trauma or compression of the neural elements by instrumentation or by bone and soft tissue displaced during deformity correction. Neural injury may also be caused indirectly, as a result of vascular compromise or elongation of the spinal cord. Cusick et al. (9) demonstrated that distraction and elongation of the monkey spinal cord resulted in a demonstrable reduction in the amplitude of evoked potentials from multiple locations. Using evoked potential monitoring combined with a radioactive microspherical technique to monitor spinal cord perfusion, the authors demonstrated that early compromise of spinal cord function was related to traction on the neural elements directly, and sustained traction resulted in injury from both a direct effect on the spinal cord and an effect of ischemia due to distraction-induced compromise of circulation to the spinal cord. Others have demonstrated a similar effect of traction-induced hypoperfusion of the spinal cord, with neurological function being directly related to spinal cord blood flow (10,11). Direct pressure on the spinal cord has an additive effect with ischemia in the etiology of spinal cord injury (12). Many deformity correction maneuvers including anterior instrumentation with cages and posterior instrumentation with curve correction result indirectly in an elongation of the spinal canal and may place the neural elements under traction (13). The knowledge of this basic pathophysiology is important in the assessment of risk in correction of spinal deformity, in the use of instrumentation that may compromise the space of the neural elements, and in the judicious use of controlled intraoperative hypotension.

The prevalence of neurological injury in spinal deformity surgery is unknown, and existing data from individual centers are likely to underrepresent the problem at a more generalizable level. Using Harrington rod distraction instrumentation, MacEwen et al. (14) reported an incidence of neural injury of 0.72%. This series was based upon a survey of the Scoliosis Research Society and did not represent a consecutive series or a comprehensive collection from all members. The results of the survey revealed 74 complications involving the spinal cord, with 41 involving complete paralysis and 33 incomplete lesions. The authors identified risk factors for neural injury including congenital scoliosis, nonidiopathic scoliosis, severe kyphosis distraction instrumentation without preoperative traction, and failure of the surgeon to identify insufficiency of the posterior elements. With the advent of segmental instrumentation systems, multiple sublaminar and intrapedicular fixation sites, and the improvement of capacity to correct deformity, one might expect the risk of neural injury in deformity surgery to increase significantly. However, in subsequent surveys of the Scoliosis Research Society, no overall increase in the prevalence of spinal cord injury has been observed (15). The report of neural complications from the experience of individual surgeons and surgical centers may represent a more consecutive series and complete assessment, and such reports have demonstrated complete or partial cord deficits in up to 16% of patients undergoing correction with a combination of sublaminar wiring and distraction instrumentation (16–18). In a comprehensive review of over 11 years of experience using posterior and/or anterior spinal segmental instrumentation, Bridwell et al. (19) reported four cases of major neural injury out of 1090 surgeries. All four cases involved a combined anterior and posterior approach to the spine, with harvesting of the convex segmental vessels. Risk factors for neural injury were identified as hyperkyphosis and combined anterior and posterior surgery.

The type of instrumentation used for gaining correction of deformity is an important factor in determining the risk of neural injury, both as a result of direct injury to the neural elements and as a result of the corrective potential of the instrumentation. Historically, the addition of sublaminar wires to distraction instrumentation measurably increased the prevalence of spinal cord injury (20). Sublaminar wires and hooks necessarily occupy space within the spinal canal, and neural injury may result from placement of the instrumentation or from the space-occupying effect of the instrumentation. Similarly, pedicle screws and vertebral body screws that are malpositioned may injure the neural elements either directly or as a space-occupying lesion (Fig. 1). The use of transpedicular fixation in the management of spinal deformity introduces the ability to gain significantly improved deformity correction in adult and pediatric deformity. Barr et al. (21) and Hamill et al. (22) independently demonstrated that lumbar pedicle screws in double major curves in adolescent idiopathic scoliosis resulted in greater lumbar curve correction, better maintenance of correction, and greater correction of the uninstrumented segments of the spine, without introducing an increased risk of neural injury. In the thoracic spine, Liljenqvist et al. (23) demonstrated improved primary and secondary curve correction and a shorter fusion length in idiopathic thoracic scoliosis with the use of thoracic screws rather than a combination of hooks and screws, with no difference in neurological complications. The accuracy of pedicle screw placement in the thoracic spine has been reported by Belmont et al. (24) using postoperative computed tomography on a consecutive series of patients. The authors demonstrated that only 57% of screws were confined totally within the pedicle. However, only 2 of 279 screws (<1%) penetrated more than 2 mm medial to the pedicle, and there were no postoperative neural deficits. In patients with coronal plane deformity, penetration of the anterior vertebral cortex is more common than in patients without deformity (25). In a larger series involving 4604 thoracic pedicle screws in 462 patients, screw malposition was determined by plain films and selective computed tomography, demonstrating malposition in 1.5% of cases, affecting 10.4% of patients (26). Neural injury related to screw malposition occurred in four patients (0.8%), with one case of transient paresis and three dural tears. Overall, the use of contemporary instrumentation systems including pedicle fixation has led to improved deformity correction without evidence of increased risk to the neural elements.

III. PREVENTION OF NEURAL INJURY: PREOPERATIVE IDENTIFICATION AND INTRAOPERATIVE RECOGNITION

Two important methods for minimizing the risk of neural injury in deformity surgery are preoperative evaluation of the patient and intraoperative neural monitoring (27). Preoperative evaluation of the patient enables the surgeon to identify the high-risk case and to make appropriate adjustments in the preoperative plan. Congenital deformity (both scoliosis and kyphosis), skeletal dysplasia, neurofibromatosis, severe rigid deformities, and hyperkyphosis are associated with a high risk of neurological deterioration and paraplegia after corrective surgery (28). Congenital spinal deformities have an increased risk of intraspinal anomalies including tethering of the spinal cord,

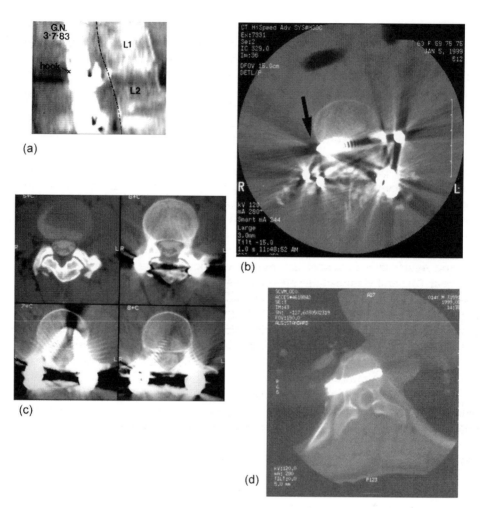

Figure 1 Examples of implant placement in patients with postoperative neural deficits. a) Sublaminar hook at L1; b) anterior vertebral body screw placed in open surgery; c) posterior pedicle screw at L2; d) thoracoscopic screw at T9.

syringomyelia, and diastematomyelia. Bradford et al. (29) studied 42 patients with congenital deformity of the spine with magnetic resonance imaging (MRI), demonstrating a prevalence of intraspinal anomalies including 38% of patients with a tethered cord, 9% with diastematomyelia, and 9% with syringomyelia. Patients with intraspinal anomalies may experience spontaneous neurological deterioration as an effect of growth alone, and surgical correction and sudden straightening of the spine is an important cause of postoperative paraplegia in this patient group (30,31). While a detailed neurological exam may elicit signs of intraspinal anomalies, a preoperative MRI scan is a sensitive tool for the detection of occult intraspinal anomalies and is necessary before surgery on patients with congenital scoliosis (32–34). Patients with left thoracic scoliosis, abnormal findings on neurological examination, and painful scoliosis may also be considered for MRI evaluation prior to surgical correction in order to rule out intraspinal anomalies associated with these findings (35–37). Other organ anomalies including cardiac and renal anomalies are associated with congenital scoliosis (38). Basu et al. (38) reported that 50% of patients with cardiac anomalies required medical or surgical care before deformity correction. In a review of 43 cases of neural injury after deformity correction surgery, Lonstein et al. (39) identified kyphosis as an important risk factor for postoperative paraplegia, and the authors made a plea for early recognition and correction of this deformity. Syndromes involving hyperkyphosis, including achondroplasia, Kniest syndrome and other skeletal dysplasias, myelodysplasia, mucopolysaccharidoses, and Ehlers-Danlos syndrome may be at increased risk of neural compromise with attempted deformity correction due to the elongation of the spinal canal and vascular compromise (40,41). The specific problem of neurological injury following correction of sagittal kyphosis in Scheuermann disease may be more common than neural injury after correction of idiopathic scoliosis, and preoperative evaluation with MRI may be useful in these cases to rule out concurrent stenosis in the thoracic spine (42). In patients with deficient posterior elements, including those with myelodysplasia, spondylolisthesis, Marfan syndrome and neurofibromatosis, direct injury to the neural elements may result from exposure, again supporting the need for preoperative recognition and appropriate imaging.

Neural injury as a result of spinal deformity instrumentation and correction is most commonly an early effect of direct or indirect compromise of the spinal cord or nerve roots as described above. Therefore, intraoperative assessment of neural function is useful for the early detection of neural injury and for the reversal of traction or compression that may be etiological. An intraoperative assessment of neural function may be made directly by awakening the patient after instrumentation and deformity correction and demonstrating intact corticospinal tracts by having the patient move the lower extremities voluntarily. The Stagnara wake-up test provides a functional assessment of spinal cord integrity and remains a useful tool, especially in the event of a change in monitored evoked potentials (43,44). Continuous intraoperative neurological monitoring is available with the use of evoked potentials. Somatosensory-evoked potentials (SSEP) measure conduction from the extremities through the dorsal column medial-lemniscal pathways (45). SSEP monitoring has led to a significant reduction in the incidence of postoperative neural deficits in scoliosis surgery and in surgery of the spine in general when compared to historical controls (46). A total of 282 neurological deficits were detected in 51,263 procedures. Of these, 18 were delayed in onset. The false-negative rate was 0.13%, and the false-positive rate was only 1.5%. However, in a separately published survey of the Scoliosis Research Society and the European Spinal Deformity Society, an estimated 28% of cases of postoperative neural injury were not detected by the use of SSEP alone (47). Injury to the anterior spinal cord without detection by SSEP monitoring has been reported in several cases (48–51). Direct monitoring of the corticospinal tract is accomplished by motor-evoked potentials (MEP). The combination of motor- and somatosensory-evoked potential monitoring improves the sensitivity and the predictive value of intraoperative changes in amplitude and latency (52).

The utility of intraoperative monitoring is based upon the hypothesis that early detection of dysfunction in neural structures will lead to a change in mechanical or physiological stresses on the spinal cord, permitting reversal of the injury. In their series defining a new universal instrumentation system for spine surgery, Cotrel et al. described two cases of postoperative paraplegia related to hook placement, both of which resolved with early implant removal (53). Winter reported a case of immediate improvement of neural function after removal of a sublaminar hook, and removal of instrumentation remains accepted as the initial approach to the management of a post-operative paraplegia or paraparesis (54,55). However, Been et al. (56) reported that even prompt recognition and removal of laminar hooks may not reliably restore neural integrity. Mooney et al.

(57) reviewed the management of neural dysfunction detected intraoperatively and postoperatively. The authors recommended immediate optimization of blood pressure (mean arterial pressure > 70 mmHG) and improved oxygenation. Hypotension and poor oxygenation can cause changes in neural monitoring and may cause further damage to a compromised spinal cord (58–60). If the patient fails the wake-up test, tension of instrumentation should be reduced, and if neural function does not recover, instrumentation should be removed unless removal would significantly compromise the stability of the spine and risk further neural injury.

Neural injury is generally recognizable intraoperatively, or immediately after surgery. However, the onset of paraplegia may be delayed up to 72 hours after surgery (61,62). The mechanism of delayed-onset paraplegia is most likely related to hypoperfusion of the spinal cord, and dysfunction may be reversed by improving fluid volume status and oxygenation (63). Neural injury related to instrumentation may also be a late complication, presenting months to years after surgery. Cases of neural dysfunction with late onset are due to the space-occupying effect of instrumentation and superimposed degenerative changes or adjacent segment changes (64–67). Case 1 demonstrates a cauda equina syndrome arising 8 years after posterior instrumented fusion for degenerative spondylolisthesis. The patient presented with a subacute onset of bowel and bladder dysfunction, and a myelogram demonstrated a complete block due to adjacent segment spondylolisthesis.

Injury to peripheral nerves and cranial nerves are also important considerations in spinal deformity surgery. Operations for the correction of spinal deformity are lengthy, and the patient may often be in a dependent position with direct pressure on peripheral

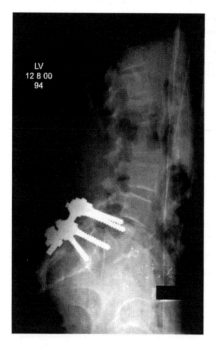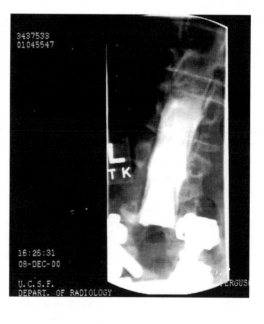

Case 1 Plain film of the lumbar spine and myelogram in a 94 yo female with spondylolisthesis adjacent to a previously instrumented fusion at L5-S1. The patient presented with symptoms of a subacute cauda equina syndrome. The myelogram demonstrates a complete myelographic block above a prior instrumented fusion.

nerves for several hours. Injury to peripheral nerves and functional recovery is related to the magnitude and duration of compression (68). Injuries to peripheral nerves of the brachial plexus, the ulnar nerve at the elbow, the lateral femoral cutaneous nerve at the anterior superior iliac spine, and the peroneal nerve at the fibular head have been reported as complications of positioning during spine surgery and during surgery in general (69–74). Mirovsky and Neuwirth (75) reported a 20% prevalence of injury to the lateral femoral cutaneous nerve in spine surgery, most commonly from direct compression, but also due to anterior exposure and bone grafting from the anterior iliac crest. Care during patient positioning is the most effective way to prevent injury to the peripheral nerves during spinal deformity surgery. Specifically, avoiding more than 70 degrees of shoulder abduction and padding the anterior superior iliac spine and area around the fibular head in the prone patient, maintaining forearm supination in the supine patient, and using an axillary role and fibular pad in the patient in the lateral position may prevent many peripheral nerve injuries during deformity surgery.

Visual loss as a complication of spine surgery is most commonly caused by ischemic optic neuropathy, retinal artery occlusion, or cerebral ischemia. In a survey of the members of the Scoliosis Research Society, Myers et al. reported 37 patients who experienced visual loss after spine surgery, 11 of which were bilateral, and 15 of which involved complete loss of sight in at least one eye (76). Most cases were associated with prolonged surgery [average length 410 minutes, with significant intraoperative blood loss (3500 cc)] and intraoperative hypotension. In a smaller series by Stevens et al., (77) the authors reported that most cases of visual loss were due to ischemic optic neuropathy. They hypothesized that the optic nerve was ischemic due to a combination of hypotension, reducing the perfusion pressure of the posterior ciliary arteries, and increased intraocular pressure due to prone positioning. Prevention of high intraocular pressure and early detection with optimization of perfusion pressure were recommended to prevent the complication of vision loss.

IV. DEFORMITY CORRECTION: VASCULAR RISKS

The great vessels are intimately opposed to the thoracic and lumbar spine. The surgical approach to deformity correction and the correction of deformity places the aorta and vena cava at risk of direct and indirect injury. The risk of vascular injury during scoliosis surgery can be minimized by a working knowledge of vascular anatomy and its variance combined with meticulous surgical technique.

Vascular structures are directly at risk during the anterior approach to the thoracic, lumbar, and sacral spine. The choice of surgical approach may minimize the risk of vascular injury, and effect the ability to repair bleeding vessels. In separate publications within one year, McAfee reported on complications of the open anterior approach to the thoracolumbar spine and the endoscopic approach for thoracolumbar spinal reconstruction (78,79). Vascular complication occurred only in one laparoscopic case, and this was repaired with an open approach. Other series have reported a rate of up to 18% significant vascular injury resulting from the anterior approach to the spine (80–85).Vascular injury from the posterior approach to the spine is less common, but can result in devastating complications (86). Papadoulas et al. (87) identified a prevalence of injury to the major anterior vessels in 1–5 cases/10,000 following a posterior lumbar disk excision. Presentations included acute hemorrhage and shock and late presentations of pseudoaneurysm and arteriovenous fistula. Vascular injury may also result from thromboembolism to the aorta, iliac, or femoral arteries as a result of manipulation (88). Kulkarni et al. (89) reported eight cases of vascular insufficiency to the lower extremity after an anterior approach to the L4-5 level. Five cases involved thrombosis to the common iliac or femoral arteries, two cases involved functional vasospasm, and one involved an intimal tear. The authors recommended intraoperative monitoring with pulse oximetry to the toes to assist in early detection of patients at risk. Case 2 was a 70-year-old female who had undergone multiple prior spine surgeries and presented with a symptomatic pseudarthrosis and progressive lumbar kyphosis. She had a postoperative thrombosis of the common iliac vein after an anterior reconstruction of the spine and was treated with a femoral-femoral bypass surgery.

Spinal instrumentation may present important risks to vascular structures when implanted from the anterior or posterior approach. Metallic implants opposed to pulsatile vessels including the aorta and iliac arteries may cause erosion into the tunica externa of the vessels and late perforation, pseudoaneurysm, or arteriovenous fistula formation. Choi et al. (90) reported a case of pseudoaneurysm with an aorto-chest wall fistula in a patient with a T6 pedicle screw in contact with the thoracic aorta. The risk of vascular injury with spinal instrumentation adjacent to pulsatile vessels has not been determined. In a CT analysis of screw placement using thoracoscopic anterior spinal instrumentation in adolescent idiopathic scoliosis, Kassah et al. (91) reported that 14% of screws were adjacent to the aorta, and 12% were causing a contour defect in the aorta. The proximity of the screw tips to the aorta appears to be due to displacement of the aorta leftward in right-sided thoracic curves. No cases of vascular complications associated with anterior thoracic instrumentation have been reported (92). Case 3 demonstrated a thoracic pedicle screw in T8 that is in contact with the thoracic aorta. This screw was removed because of concern for possible vascular injury. This risk of vascular injury is unknown.

V.   DEFORMITY SURGERY AND VISCERAL ORGAN COMPLICATIONS

Spinal deformity surgery may compromise visceral organs as a result of the surgical approach, or indirectly as an effect of spinal deformity correction. Visceral structures at risk include gastrointestinal and genitourinary.

A postoperative ileus is the most common gastrointestinal complication of spine surgery and has been reported as a complication in 3.5–6% of anterior spine surgeries (93,94). Postoperative ileus may be related to handling the peritoneum during the anterior approach, narcotic analgesics, or distraction of the posterior peritoneum during the posterior approach to deformity correction, and is usually self-limited and without long-term sequelae (95). Superior mesenteric artery (SMA) syndrome, or cast syndrome, may present with similar findings to postoperative ileus, but recognition of SMA syndrome is important for avoidance of potentially significant bowel ischemia and death (96). Obstruction of the third portion of the duodenum by the descending superior mesenteric artery may result from the surgical correction of thoracolumbar deformity, resulting in a superior displacement of the origin of the SMA from the aorta and consequent reduction of the angle between the descending SMA and the aorta. This effect may directly compress the third portion of the duodenum between the aorta and SMA, resulting is upper small bowel obstruction (97). The "duodenal ileus" was reported by Wilkie in 1921 in a description of a patient with intractable vomiting after application of a plaster cast for management of scoliosis (98). The observation of upper intestinal

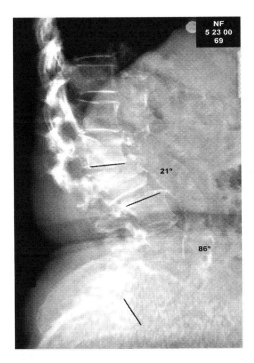

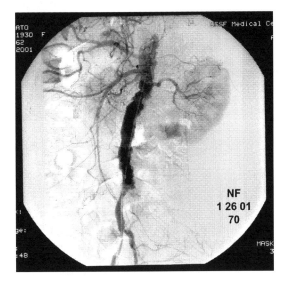

Case 2 Preoperative lateral view of the lumbar spine, with a postoperative angiogram. The patient is a 70 yo female with post-laminectomy scoliosis and kyphosis, and progressive pain and deformity. After the anterior approach to her thoracolumbar spine she was noted to have a pulseless foot on the left side, and an intraoperative myelogram demonstrated a complete occusion of the common iliac artery on the left side.

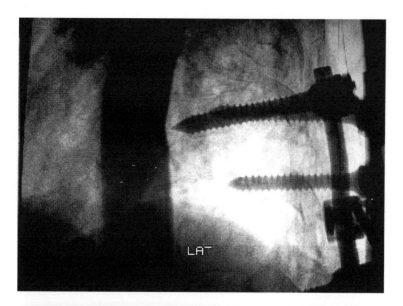

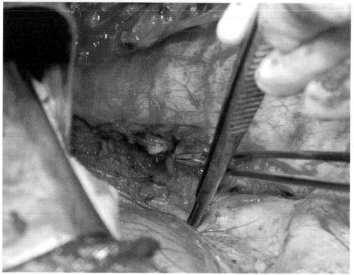

Case 3 Angiogram demonstrating a T8 pedicle screw displacing the descending thoracic aorta, and an intraoperative photo demonstrating the tip of the screw anterior to the vertebral body at T8. The patient is a 36 yo male who presented with complaints of chest and back pain. He was found to have a pseudarthrosis on revision surgery.

obstruction after cast-induced correction of deformity led to the introduction of the term "cast-syndrome" by Dorph in 1950 (99). With the introduction of segmental instrumentation systems and the consequent improved correction of deformity, one might expect that the incidence of superior mesenteric artery syndrome would increase proportionally to the improvement of curve correction. However, reports of superior mesenteric artery syndrome remain rare with segmental instrumentation systems, and this may be due to the relative preservation of thoracic kyphosis with segmental instrumentation systems (100).

The transperitoneal approach to the lumbar spine may place the superior hypogastric plexus of the sympathetic nervous system at risk of injury. The results may be a disturbance of urogenital function with retrograde ejaculation or sterility in males. Injury to the superior hypogastric plexus may be minimized by the retroperitoneal approach to the lumbosacral spine with minimal dissection to the iliac vessels. In a survey of 20 surgeons and an estimated 4500 cases involving deformity in prepubertal and adolescent males, retrograde ejaculation was reported in 0.42% and impotence in 0.44% (101). However, subsequent studies with more rigorous follow-up assessment have reported significantly higher rates of sexual dysfunction after an anterior approach to the lumbosacral spine in males (102). In a series comparing complications in video-assisted and open anterior approaches for lumbar fusion, Escobar et al. (103) reported retrograde ejaculation in 3 of 12 men (75%) treated with a transperitoneal video-assisted approach to L4-5 and L5-S1, and in only one of 51 patients (2%) treated with a mini-open approach. Injuries to the ureter occurred in 1.5% of patients, with a similar incidence in the open and endoscopic groups.

VI. CONSEQUENCES OF SURGERY

A. Reoperation

The avoidance of the consequences of deformity is an important goal in surgery for deformity correction in the child or adolescent. Unfortunately, arthrodesis of the spine introduces potential consequences that may lead to impairment and the need for revision surgery. In a review of all spine surgeries in the province of Ontario, Hu et al. (104) reported that in less than 4 years of follow-up the rate of reoperation was 9.5%. In degenerative conditions of the spine and spondylolisthesis, Malter et al. (105) observed a reoperation rate of 18.2% after fusion surgery at 5 years follow-up, and complications were recorded for 18% of cases involving spinal fusion. In idiopathic scoliosis, reoperation rates have been reported at even higher rates. Cook et al. (106) determined a frequency of reoperation after dorsal instrumentation for treatment of idiopathic scoliosis of up to 21% at 6-year follow-up in a mixed population of children and adults. The authors identified factors leading to reoperation in order of frequency: late operative site pain (8%), pseudarthrosis (4%), implant prominence (2%), adjacent segment disorder (2%), periadjacent segment disorder (0.5%), and malalignment requiring further surgery (0.5%). Other important causes for reoperation include neurologic injury, infection, implant dislodgement or breakage, and scar revision (107–111).

B. Pseudarthrosis

Pseudarthrosis is an important cause of failed lumbar surgery and is a contributing factor in up 80% of patients who require reoperation (112–116). Pseudarthrosis, meaning false joint, is diagnosed when the spine has failed to achieve solid bony union at one year after an attempted arthrodesis (117). The reported rates of Pseudarthrosis are highly variable, and an important cause of observed variability in published rates is the difficulty of making a radiographic diagnosis of pseudarthrosis (118,119). In a study correlating radiographic findings with intraoperative findings, Dawson et al. reported that anteroposterior tomography was the most accurate method for identifying pseudarthrosis, with a 96% correlation with findings at surgery (120). Deckey et al. reported a finding of progressive deformity in 4 of 14 patients who underwent a removal of instrumentation with an apparently solid fusion (121). This finding calls into question the accuracy of even second-look surgery. DePalma and Rothman (122) reported that the condition of pseudarthrosis is iatrogenic and that its responsibility lies entirely within the hands of the surgeon. Although surgical technique is an important consideration in the generation of a successful arthrodesis, factors including the region of the spine fused, surgical approach, underlying diagnosis, implant stiffness, local conditions for bone formation, smoking, infection, and bone graft choices have an important influence on the occurrence of nonunion in the spine (123–130).

Rates of pseudarthrosis may be reduced with the use of combined anterior and posterior surgery (131–133). However, complication rates for combined anterior and posterior surgery are clearly higher than for posterior-only surgery (134–136). Using Luque-Galveston instrumentation, Boachie-Adjei et al. (137) reported an overall complication rate of 82% in a series of adults undergoing combined anterior and posterior surgery for correction of deformity. Lapp et al. (138) reported on long-term complications in adults undergoing combined surgery and demonstrated a 44% overall complication rate in primary surgeries and 35% in revision surgeries. In a series of 25 adults undergoing combined anterior and posterior surgery for the management of fixed sagittal plane deformity, Berven et al. (139) reported 8 patients (32%) with early perioperative complications, including wound infection, dural tear, and pneumonia. Late complications requiring revision surgery occurred in 10 patients (40%), including pseudarthrosis at segments not fused circumferentially, and iliac screw prominence. In adolescents undergoing combined surgery for scoliosis, major complications have been reported at a lower rate (140). However, in the series by Weis et al. (140), minor complications (defined as those necessitating a prolonged hospitalization, a second minor surgery, or significant temporary hardship or permanent minor problem) were recorded in 46% of adolescents undergoing anterior only or combined anterior and posterior surgery. Factors that are important in predicting complications in combined anterior and posterior surgery for deformity include perioperative nutrition and staging of surgery. Hu et al. (141) demonstrated a measurable depletion of nutritional parameters of albumin and prealbumin in patients undergoing combined anterior and posterior surgery, and this negative effect could be minimized by the use of total parenteral nutrition between stages. Understanding the reported complications of combined anterior and posterior surgery influences informed choice for both the physician and the patient. Several studies have concluded that same-day anterior and posterior surgery results in fewer complications, less blood loss, less operative time, shorter hospital stay and reduced costs compared with delayed two-stage surgery (142–144). However, all of these studies are retrospective and do not control for the complexity of surgery. We recommend same-day surgery when the estimated blood loss from the anterior procedure is less than 1500 cc and the estimated time for the entire procedure is less than 12 hours.

C. Crankshaft Phenomenon

In the presence of a solid fusion and effective arthrodesis of the affected segments in spinal deformity, progressive deformity may arise from continued growth of the spine within the fused segments or from curve progression or degenerative changes at adjacent segments. In children with spinal deformity, progressive curvature, vertebral rotation, and rib prominence after a posterior fusion may be due to continued anterior column growth of the spine despite a solid posterior arthrodesis. This pattern of deformity progression was first identified by Hefti and McMaster (145). Duboisset et al. (145a) introduced the term "crankshaft phenomenon" as a descriptive term for this type of progressive deformity, making the analogy with an automotive crankshaft rotating around a center arm. Patients with significant anterior growth remaining at the time of a posterior spine fusion are at risk of postoperative deformity progression, and incidences of 37–43% have been reported in patients who are Risser 0 and have open triradiate cartilages at the time of posterior fusion (146,147). A more accurate radiographic parameter for predicting the risk of the crankshaft phenomenon after posterior surgery may be the assessment of peak height velocity. Saunders et al. (148) reported a high incidence (8/8) of crankshaft phenomenon in patients fused before reaching peak height velocity and a rare incidence (2/15) in patients fused after reaching peak height velocity. The risk of crankshaft phenomenon causing progressive deformity in children may be limited in the setting of contemporary rigid segmental instrumentation systems. Burton et al. (149) reported only one case of progressive deformity after posterior-only surgery in a cohort of immature patients, suggesting that anterior surgery may be unnecessary to prevent crankshaft deformity. In a corollary to the crankshaft phenomenon, D'Andrea et al. (150) observed progressive kyphotic deformity in skeletally immature patients undergoing anterior-only surgery for the correction of deformity. The authors recommend preserving sagittal profile with intervertebral spacers and rigid rods to prevent this form of postoperative decompensation in children.

D. Flatback Syndrome

Spinal decompensation refers to a malalignment of the occiput, trunk, and pelvis in the coronal and/or sagittal plane. Spinal decompensation may result from progressive deformity adjacent to a solid arthrodesis, or may be the result of arthrodesis of the spine in a malaligned position. The avoidance of spinal decompensation after surgical arthrodesis is an important goal of the deformity surgeon, and this complication may be avoided with an understanding of the goals of deformity correction in all three planes. An important cause of spinal decompensation is the loss of sagittal balance of the spine caused by distraction instrumentation for the treatment of scoliosis. Flatback deformity was initially recognized by Doherty in 1973 (151). The transition from Harrington distraction instrumentation to segmental fixation has limited the generation of sagittal decompensation with distraction of a coronal plane curve. However, kyphotic decompensation after segmental instrumentation remains an important and significant iatrogenic etiology of postoperative sagittal deformity (152). Attention to restoration of regional as well as global balance to the spine is important in surgical planning and execution in deformity surgery. Case 4 illustrates a case of sagittal decompensation after circumferential arthrodesis of the spine. This deformity was corrected with a transpedicular wedge resection osteotomy.

E. Adjacent Segment Decompensation

In the coronal plane, decompensation after surgical correction of deformity may occur due to (a) deformity progression in the mobile lumbar spine, (b) arthrodesis of the spine to the level of the sacrum, effectively limiting compensation in caudal segments, or (c) the exclusion of a structural curve from the segments chosen for arthrodesis. Fusion to the lower lumbar spine or the sacrum remains an area that lacks consensus among deformity surgeons (153). Eck et al. (154) demonstrated distal segment degeneration in 7 of 44 patients fused short of the sacrum and concluded that long fusion short of the sacrum in adult deformity is unreliable and does not have predictable long-term results. In

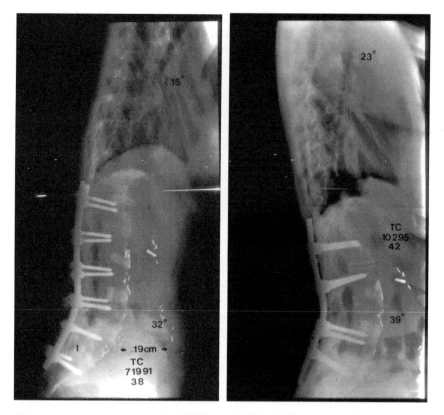

Case 4 Preoperative and postoperative lateral films of a 38 yo female with lumbar kyphotic decompensation after a multilevel circumferential arthrodesis of the spine done initially for the treatment of back pain. The patient's preoperative sagitttal balance was offset by 19cm from C7 to the posterior margin of the sacrum, and this improved to 2cm on post-operative standing films after a transpedicular wedge resection at L4.

contrast, Berven et al. (155) demonstrated improved function and reduced complications in patients fused to L4 or L5 compared with patients fused to the sacrum. The development of progressive lumbar deformity after selective thoracic fusion or fusion to the mobile lumbar spine is an important cause of postoperative degenerative changes, pain, and decompensation in the coronal plane (156–158). Cochran et al. (159) reported a high incidence of retrolisthesis, facet joint changes, and disk degeneration subjacent to the fused levels in patients fused below L3 with Harrington instrumentation (159). Accurate identification of structural and nonstructural deformity in the lumbar spine is important in deciding when the lumbar curve may spontaneously correct after a selective thoracic fusion and when the lumbar curve is likely to progress. Lenke et al. (160) demonstrated that in King II deformity, spontaneous correction of the lumbar curve was predictable after selective thoracic fusion using either an anterior or a posterior approach, with an anterior approach resulting in improved thoracic and lumbar curve correction. Differentiation of a King type II and type III deformity is essential in determining the risk of decompensation through progressive deformity in the lumbar mobile segments. Overall, the maintenance of mobile segments in the lumbar spine remains an important goal of deformity correction surgery in the child and in adults, and an accurate assessment of the integrity of the lumbosacral spine and of the mobility of the lumbar compensatory curve is important in choosing to end a fusion in the mobile lumbar spine.

The choice of fusion level in the upper end of a spinal deformity construct may also have a significant impact upon coronal decompensation. Recognition and inclusion of a structural upper thoracic curve is important in the preoperative planning of the cephalad extent of spinal arthrodesis for deformity. Lenke et al. (161) demonstrated that the failure to identify and include a structural upper thoracic curve may lead to shoulder asymmetry and postoperative coronal plane decompensation. The authors recommend extending a posterior fusion to the level of T2 when specific preoperative criteria are present, including a proximal thoracic curve measuring more than 30 degrees and correcting to more than 20 degrees on side-bending films, the presence of rotation or translation at the apex of the thoracic curve, and preoperative shoulder elevation on the convex side of the upper thoracic curve, or T1 tilt into the concavity of the upper thoracic curve. Subsequently, Kuklo et al. (162) demonstrated that spontaneous curve correction of the unfused upper thoracic curve occurs more reliably after anterior fusion of the main thoracic curve than after posterior fusion. The authors identified T1 tilt toward the concavity of the upper thoracic curve of > 5 degrees, shoulder asymmetry with elevation of the shoulder on the convex side of the upper thoracic curve, and bending correction to greater than 25 degrees as factors that may predict postoperative shoulder asymmetry and coronal decompensation after selective thoracic anterior spine fusion. Overall, careful radiographic assessment of the thoracic spine is useful in predicting postoperative decompensation in the upper thoracic region.

VII. SPECIAL CONSIDERATIONS IN THE ELDERLY

The elderly patient population is at significant risk for developing spinal deformity and complications related to the surgical management of deformity (163). Osteoporosis is an important comorbidity in the elderly population, and compromise of bone mineral density may lead to the development of spinal deformity. Sagittal plane deformity resulting from vertebral compression fractures is the most characteristic manifestation of osteoporosis of the spine (164). Back pain, height loss, and kyphotic deformity comprise the characteristic clinical presentation for vertebral compression fractures.

The impact of compression fractures and progressive kyphosis on quality of life and on mortality has been well-documented (165–169). The relationship between deformity in the coronal plane, rotatory subluxation, and spondylolisthesis and aging is not as direct as that for sagittal plane deformities. Healey and Lane (170) estimated an incidence of structural scoliosis in osteoporotic women of nearly 50%, with a predominance of lumbar and thoracolumbar curves (170). Curves were generally small, with only 10% measuring greater than 30 degrees. The authors also observed a high percentage of osteoporotic patients with rotatory subluxation and anterolisthesis. The presence of rotatory subluxation has been identified as a predictor of scoliosis morbidity and is a feature of unstable scoliosis and accelerated rate of deformity progression (171). Velis et al. identify osteoporosis as a distinct characteristic of patients with unstable scoliosis and not associated with stable scoliosis. Therefore, elderly patients are an important and substantial portion of the population presenting with symptomatic spinal deformity. Recognition of potential complications in this population is important for informed choice by the patient and the physician.

Age and age-related factors contribute significantly to the rate of complications in spine surgery. In the surgical management of degenerative conditions of the spine, Deyo et al. (172) identified age as an important predictor of complications after lumbar fusion surgery, with patients over 75 years old having an overall complication rate of 18%. Similarly, in evaluating the outcome of laminectomy for lumbar stenosis, Katz et al. (173) identified age and comorbidities as the most important predictor of outcome from surgery. In deformity surgery, elderly patients have less effective correction of deformity and increased complications compared with younger patients with spinal deformity. In an age-related assessment of outcome in spinal deformity surgery, Takahashi et al. (174) reported significantly less correction of deformity and inadequate restoration of lumbar lordosis in patients over 50 years of age. The overall complication rate was 29% and was unrelated to age. The authors identified factors that contribute to potential complications and surgical difficulty in elderly patients including curve rigidity, osteoporosis, and comorbidities. In a study of perioperative complications after anterior spine surgery for deformity, McDonnell et al. (175) reported that patients between 61 and 80 years old had a significantly higher rate of perioperative complications than younger cohorts, with pulmonary complications identified as the most common. Other medical complications that have been reported with increased incidence in the elderly include cardiac morbidity and pancreatitis in the postoperative period (176,177). Age and comorbidities were identified as independent predictors of hospital stay, operative time, and intraoperative blood loss in patients undergoing lumbar decompression with segmental instrumentation (178). Kostuik et al. (179) identified age and preoperative American Society of Anesthesiologists (ASA) score as important predictors of minor and major complications in adult spinal deformity surgery, reporting an overall complication rate of 57%, with major complcations in 27% of patients. The authors concluded that age is an important preoperative consideration for surgical planning and avoidance of complications. Elderly patients present with complex and rigid deformity, osteoporosis and other comorbidities, and significant pain and dysfunction. The surgical management of spinal deformity in this patient population may be complicated by technical difficulties intraoperatively and by perioperative complications. Sharing knowledge of complication rates and risks empowers the patient to participate in an informed choice regarding his or her care.

VIII. CONCLUSIONS

Spinal deformity surgery intrinsically introduces the risk of significant intraoperative and perioperative complications. Identification and recognition of potential complications is valuable for the surgeon in guiding decision making and operative planning. The choice of surgical approach, fusion levels, and operative versus nonoperative care may be influenced by knowledge of potential complications, and adverse outcomes may be avoided or prevented with appropriate anticipation. Knowledge of expected outcomes and risks of complication is also valuable for the patient. Deformity surgery is a discretionary procedure, and there is tremendous variability in the decision making regarding the management of deformity between physicians and patients. In order for the patient to make an informed choice regarding surgical care for spinal deformity, knowledge of both the natural history of deformity progression and the risks of surgery are essential.

REFERENCES

1. Transfeldt EE. Complications of treatment. In: Lonstein JE, Bradford DS, Winter RB, Ogilvie JW, eds. Moe's Textbook of Scoliosis and other Spinal Deformities. 3rd ed. Philadelphia: WB Saunders, 1996:451–481.

2. Micheli LJ, Hall JE. Complications in the management of adult spinal deformities. In: Epps CH Jr., ed. Complications in Orthopaedic Surgery. 2nd ed. Philadelphia: JB Lippincott, 1986:1039–1072.

3. Clapham LM, Buckley J. Outcome-directed clinical practice in lumbar spine surgery. Clin Perform Qual Health Care 1999; 7(4):167–171.

4. Wenger DR, Mubarak SJ, Leach J. Managing complications of posterior spinal instrumentation and fusion. Clin Orthop 1992; 284:25–33.

5. Bunch WH, Chapman RG. Patient preferences for surgery in scoliosis. J Bone Joint Surg (Am) 1985; 67:794–799.

6. Weinstein SL, Dolan LA, Spratt KF, Peterson KK, Spoonamore MJ, Ponseti IV. Health and function of patients with untreated idiopathic scoliosis: a 50-year natural history study. JAMA 2003; 289(5):559–567.

7. Nilsonne U, Lundgren KD. Long-term prognosis in idiopathic scoliosis. Acta Orthop Scand 1968; 29:456–458.

8. Kim YJ, Otsuka NY, Flynn JM, Hall JE, Emans JB, Hresko MT. Surgical treatment of congenital kyphosis. Spine 2001; 26(20):2251–2257.

9. Cusick JF, Jyklebust J, Syvoloski M, et al. Effects of vertebral column distraction in the monkey. J Neurosurg 1982; 57:651–659.

10. Naito M, Owen JH, Bridwell KH, Sugioka Y. Effects of distraction on physiologic integrity of the spinal cord, spinal cord blood flow, and clinical status. Spine 1992; 17:1154–1158.

11. Dolan EH, Transfeldt EE, Tater CH, et al. The effect of spinal distraction on regional spinal cord blood flow in cats. J Neurosurg 1980; 53:756–764.

12. Brodkey JS, Richards DE, Blasingame JP, Nulsen FE. Reversible spinal cord trauma in cats: additive effects of direct pressure and ischemia. J Neurosurg 1972; 37:591–593.

13. Bridwell KH, Kuklo TR, Lewis SJ, Sweet FA, Lenke LG, Baldus C. String test measurement to assess the effect of spinal deformity correction on spinal canal length. Spine 2001; 26(18):2013–2019.

14. MacEwen GD, Bunnell WP, Sriram K. Acute neurological complications in the treatment of scoliosis. J Bone Joint Surg 1975; 57A:404–411.

15. Winter RB. Neurologic safety in spinal deformity surgery. Spine 1997; 22:1527–1533.

16. Thompson GH, Wilbur RG, Shaffer JW, Scoles PR, Nash CL. Segmental spinal instrumentation in idiopathic scoliosis: a preliminary report. Spine 1985; 10:623–630.

17. Wilburg G, Thompson GH, Shaffer JW, Brown R, Nash CL. Postoperative neurological deficits in segmental spinal instrumentation. J Bone Joint Surg (Am) 1984; 66:1178–1187.

18. Zielke K, Pellen B. The neurological risk of Harrington procedures. Arch Orthop Unfall Chir 1975; 83:311–322.

19. Bridwell KH, Lenke LG, Baldus C, Blanke K. Major intraoperative neurologic deficits in pediatric and adult spinal deformity patients. Spine 1998; 23(3):324–331.

20. Winter RB. Neurologic safety in spinal deformity surgery. Spine 1997; 22:1527–1533.

21. Barr SJ, Schuette AM, Emans JB. Lumbar pedicle screws versus hooks. Results in double major curves in adolescent idiopathic scoliosis. Spine 1997; 22(12):1369–1379.

22. Hamill CL, Lenke LG, Bridwell KH, Chapman MP, Blanke K, Baldus C. The use of pedicle screw fixation to improve correction in the lumbar spine of patients with idiopathic scoliosis. Is it warranted? Spine 1996; 21(10):1241–1249.

23. Liljenqvist U, Lepsien U, Hackenberg L, Niemeyer T, Halm H. Comparative analysis of pedicle screw and hook instrumentation in posterior correction and fusion of idiopathic thoracic scoliosis. Eur Spine J 2002; 11(4):336–343.

24. Belmont PJ, Klemme WR, Dhawan A, DW Polly Jr. In vivo accuracy of thoracic pedicle screws. Spine 2001; 26:2340–2346.

25. Belmont PJ, Klemme WR, Robinson M, DW Polly Jr. Accuracy of thoracic pedicle screws in patients with and without coronal plane spinal deformities. Spine 2002; 27:1558–1566.

26. Suk SI, Kim WJ, Lee SM, Kim JH, Chung ER. Thoracic pedicle screw fixation in spinal deformities. Are they really safe. Spine 2001; 25(18):2049–2057.

27. Mooney JF, Bernstein R, Hennrikus WL, MacEwen GD. Neurologic risk and management in scoliosis surgery. J Ped Orthop 2002; 22:683–689.

28. Transfeldt EE. Complications of treatment. In: Lonstein JE, Bradford DS, Winter RB, Ogilvie JW, eds. Moe's Textbook of Scoliosis and other Spinal Deformities. 3rd ed. Philadelphia: WB Saunders, 1996:451–481.

29. Bradford DS, Heithoff KB, Cohen M. Intraspinal abnormalities and congenital spinal deformities: a radiographic and MRI study. J Pediatr Orthop 1991; 11:36–41.

30. McMaster MJ. Occult intraspinal anomalies and congenital scoliosis. J Bone Joint Surg 1988; 66:588–601.

31. Nordwall A, Wikkelso C. A late neurological complication of scoliosis surgery in connection with syringomyelia. Acta Orthop Scand 1979; 50:407–410.

32. Prahinski JR, Polly DW Jr, McHale KA, Ellenbogen RG. Occult intraspinal anomalies in congenital scoliosis. J Pediatr Orthop 2000; 20(1):59–63.

33. Zadeh HG, Sakka SA, Powell MP, Mehta MH. Absent superficial abdominal reflexes in children with scoliosis. An early indicator of syringomyelia. J Bone Joint Surg 1995; 77:762–767.

34. Suh SW, Sarwark JF, Vora A, Huang BK. Evaluating congenital spine deformities for intraspinal anomalies with magnetic resonance imaging. J Pediatr Orthop 2001; 21(4): 525–531.

35. Zadeh HG, Sakka SA, Powell MP, Mehta MH. Absent superficial abdominal reflexes in children with scoliosis. An early indicator of syringomyelia. J Bone Joint Surg 1995; 77:762–767.

36. Mejia EA, Hennrikus WL, Schwend RM, Emans JB. A prospective evaluation of idiopathic left thoracic scoliosis with magnetic resonance imaging. J Pediatr Orthop 1996; 16:354–358.

37. Schwend RM, Hennrikus WL, Hall JE, Emans JB. Childhood scoliosis: clinical indications for magnetic resonance imaging. J Bone Joint Surg 1995; 77:46–53.

38. Basu PS, Elsebaie H, Noordeen MH. Congenital spinal deformity: a comprehensive assessment at presentation. Spine 2002; 27(20):2255–2259.

39. Lonstein JE, Winter RB, Moe JH, Bradford DS, Chou SN, Pinto WC. Neurologic deficits secondary to spinal deformity A review of the literature and report of 43 cases. Spine 1980; 5(4):331–355.

40. Vogel LC, Lubicky JP. Neurologic and vascular complications of scoliosis surgery in patients with Ehlers-Danlos syndrome. Spine 1996; 21(21):2508–2514.

41. Kim YJ, Otsuka NY, Flynn JM, Hall JE, Emans JB, Hresko MT. Surgical treatment of congenital kyphosis. Spine 2001; 26(20):2251–2257.

42. Tribus CB. Transient paraparesis: a complication of the surgical management of Scheuermann's kyphosis secondary to thoracic stenosis. Spine 2001; 26:1086–1089.

43. Vauzelle C, Stagnara P, Jouviroux P. Functional monitoring of spinal activity during spinal surgery. Clin Orthop 1973; 93:173–178.

44. Brustowicz RM, Hall JE. In defense of the wake-up test. Anesth Analg 1988; 67(10):1019.

45. Seyal M, Mull B. Mechanisms of signal change during intraoperative somatosensory evoked potential monitoring of the spinal cord. J Clin Neurophysiol 2002; 19(5):409–415.

46. Nuwer MR, Dawson EG, Carlson LG, Kanim LEA, Sherman JE. Somatosensory evoked potential spinal cord monitoring reduces neurologic deficits after scoliosis surgery: results of a large multicenter survey. Electroencephalogr Clin Neurophysiol 1995; 96(1):6–11.

47. Dawson EG, Sherman JE, Kanim LE, Nuwer MR. Spinal cord monitoring. Results of the Scoliosis Research Society and the European Spinal Deformity Society survey. Spine 1991; 16(8 suppl):S361–S364.

48. Ginsburg HH, Shetter AG, Raudzens PA. Postoperative paraplegia with preserved intraoperative somatosensory evoked potentials. J Neurosurg 1985; 63:296–300.

49. Ben-David B, Haller G, Taylor P. Anterior spinal fusion complicated by paraplegia. A case report of a false-negative somatosensory-evoked potential. Spine 1987; 12:536–539.

50. Lesser RP, Raudzens P, Luders H, Nuwer MR, Goldie WD, Morris HH 3rd, Dinner DS, Klem G, Hahn JF, Shetter AG, Ginsburg HH, Gurd AR. Postoperative neurological deficits may occur despite unchanged intraoperative somatosensory evoked potentials. Ann Neurol 1986; 19(1):22–25.

51. Pelosi L, Jardine A, Webb JK. Neurological complications of anterior spinal surgery for kyphosis with normal somatosensory evoked potentials (SEPs). J Neurol Neurosurg Psychiatry 1999; 66(5):662–664.

52. Pelosi L, Lamb J, Grevitt M, Mehdian SMH, Webb JK, Blumhardt LD. Combined monitoring of motor and somatosensory evoked potentials in orthopaedic spinal surgery. Clin Neurophysiol 2002; 113:1082–1091.

53. Cotrel Y, Dubousset J, Guillaumat M. New universal instrumentation system in spinal surgery. Clin Orthop 1988; 227:10–23.

54. Winter RB. Neurologic safety in spinal deformity surgery. Spine 1997; 22:1527–1533.

55. Hall JE, Levine CR, Sudhir KG. Intraoperative awakening to monitor spinal cord function during Harrington distraction instrumentation and spine fusion: description of the procedure and report of three cases. J Bone Joint Surg 1978; AM 60:533–536.

56. Been HD, Kalkman CJ, Traast HS, Ongerboer de Visser BW. Neurologic injury after insertion of laminar hooks during Cotrel-Dubousset instrumentation. Spine 1994; 19(12):1402–1405.

57. Mooney JF, Bernstein R, Hennrikus WL, MacEwen GD. Neurologic risk and management in scoliosis surgery. J Ped Orthop 2002; 22:683–689.

58. Pelosi L, Lamb J, Grevitt M, Mehdian SMH, Webb JK, Blumhardt LD. Combined monitoring of motor and somatosensory evoked potentials in orthopaedic spinal surgery. Clin Neurophysiol 2002; 113:1082–1091.

59. Bridwell KH, Lenke LG, Baldus C, Blanke K. Major intraoperative neurologic deficits in pediatric and adult spinal deformity patients. Spine 1998; 23(3):324–331.

60. Kling TF Jr., Fergusson NV, Leach AB, Hensinger RN, Lane GA, Knight PR. The influence of induced hypotension and spine distraction on canine spinal cord blood flow. Spine 1985; 10(10):878–883.

61. Letts RM, Hollenberg C. Delayed paresis following spinal fusion with Harrington instrumentation. Clin Orthop 1977; 125:45–48.

62. Winter RB. Congenital kyphoscoliosis with paralysis following hemivertebra excision. Clin Orthop 1976; 119:116–125.

63. Ponte A. Postoperative paraplegia due to hypercorrection of scoliosis and drop in blood pressure. J Bone Joint Surg 1974; 56A:444.

64. Rittmeister M, Leyendecker K, Kurth A, Schmitt F. Cauda equina compression due to a laminar hook: a late complication of posterior instrumentation in scoliosis surgery. Eur Spine J 1999; 8:417–420.

65. Eismont FJ, Simeone FA. Bone overgrowth as a cause of late paraparesis after scoliosis fusion. J Bone Joint Surg 1981; 63:1016–1019.

66. Kornberg M, Herndon WA, Rechtine GR. Lumbar nerve root compression at the site of hook insertion: late complication of Harrington rod instrumentation for scoliosis. Spine 1985; 10:853–855.

67. Krodel A, Rehmet JC, Hamburger C. Spinal cord compression caused by a rod of a Harrington instrumentation device: a late complication in scoliosis surgery. Eur Spine J 1997; 6:208–210.

68. Dahlin LB, Danielsen N, Ehira T, Lundborg G, Rydevik B. Mechanical effects of compression of peripheral nerves. J Biomech Eng 1986; 108(2):120–122.

69. Geisler FH, Laich DT, Goldflies M, Shepard A. Anterior tibial compartment syndrome as a positioning complication of the prone-sitting position for lumbar surgery. Neurosurgery 1993; 33(6):1117.

70. Nambisan RN, Karakousis CP. Axillary compression syndrome with neurapraxia due to operative positioning. Surgery 1989; 105(3):449–454.

71. Warner MA, Warner ME, Martin JT. Ulnar neuropathy. Incidence, outcome, and risk factors in sedated or anesthetized patients. Anesthesiology 1994; 81(6):1332–1340.

72. Lee CT, Espley AJ. Perioperative ulnar neuropathy in orthopaedics: association with tilting the patient. Clin Orthop 2002; 396:106–111.

73. Hoshowsky VM. Surgical Positioning. Orthop Nurs 1998; 17(5):55–65.

74. Dillavou ED, Anderson LR, Bernert RA, Mularski RA, Hunter GC, Fiser SM, Rappaport WD. Lower extremity iatrogenic nerve injury due to compression during intraabdominal surgery. Am J Surg 1997; 173(6):504–508.

75. Mirovsky Y, Neuwirth M. Injuries to the lateral femoral cutaneous nerve during spine surgery. Spine 2000; 25(10):1266–1269.

76. Myers M, Hamilton SR, Bogosian AJ, Smith CH, Wagner TA. Visual loss as a complication of spine surgery. A review of 37 cases. Spine 1997; 22(12):1325–1329.

77. Stevens WR, Glazer PA, Kelley SD, Lietman TM, Bradford DS. Ophthalmic complications after spinal surgery. Spine 1997; 22(12):1319–1324.

78. McAfee PC. Complications of anterior approaches to the thoracolumbar spine. Emphasis on Kaneda instrumentation. Clin Orthop 1994; 306:110–119.

79. McAfee PC, Regan JR, Zdeblick T, Zuckerman J, Picetti GD, Heim S, Geis WP, Fedder IL. The incidence of complications in endoscopic anterior thoracolumbar spinal reconstructive surgery. A prospective multicenter study comprising the first 100 cases. Spine 1995; 20(14):1624–1632.

80. Baker JK, Reardon PR, Reardon MJ, Heggeness MH. Vascular injury in anterior lumbar surgery. Spine 1993; 18(15):2227–2230.

81. Rajaraman V, Vingan R, Roth P, Heary RF, Conklin L, Jacobs GB. Visceral and vascular complications resulting from anterior lumbar interbody fusion. J Neurosurg 1999; 91(1 suppl):60–64.

82. Bianchi C, Ballard JL, Abou-Zamzam AM, Teruya TH, Abu-Assal ML. Anterior retroperitoneal lumbosacral spine exposure: operative technique and results. Ann Vasc Surg 2003 Mar 6 (epub ahead of print).

83. Oskouian RJ Jr, Johnson JP. Vascular complications in anterior thoracolumbar spinal reconstruction. J Neurosurg 2002; 96(1 suppl):1–5.

84. Lieberman IH, Willsher PC, Litwin DE, Salo PT, Kraetschmer BG. Transperitoneal laparoscopic exposure for lumbar interbody fusion. Spine 2000; 25(4):509–515.

85. Regan JJ, Aronoff RJ, Ohnmeiss DD, Sengupta DK. Laparoscopic approach to L4-L5 for interbody fusion using BAK cages: experience in the first 58 cases. Spine 1999; 24(20):2171–2174.

86. Goodkin R, Laska LL. Vascular and visceral injuries associated with lumbar disc surgery: medicolegal implications. Surg Neurol 1998; 49(4):358–372.

87. Papadoulas S, Konstantinou D, Kourea HP, Kritikos N, Haftouras N, Tsolakis JA. Vascular injury complicating lumbar disc surgery. A systematic review. Eur J Vasc Endovasc Surg 2002; 24(3):189–195.

88. Raskas DS, Delamarter RB. Occlusion of the left iliac artery after retroperitoneal exposure of the spine. Clin Orthop 1997; (338):86–89.

89. Kulkarni SS, Lowery GL, Ross RE, Ravi Sankar K, Lykomitros V. Intimal injury and thrombosis of the iliac vessels is a significant problem in older patients with arteriosclerotic disease. Eur Spine J 2003; 12(1):48–54.

90. Choi JB, Han JO, Jeong JW. False aneurysm of the thoracic aorta associated with an aorto-chest wall fistula after spinal instrumentation. J Trauma 2001; 50(1):140–143.

91. Kassah F, Sucato D, Dempsey M. Thoracoscopic anterior spinal instrumentation and fusion for idiopathic scoliosis: a CT analysis of screw placement and completeness of discectomy. American Academy of Orthopaedic Surgeons, Poster #275, Dallas, TX, 2002.

92. Clements DH, Betz RR, Newton PO, Lenke LG, Lowe TG, Merola AA, Haher TR, Marks M. Incidence of vascular complications associated with anterior thoracic instrumentation for adolescent idiopathic scoliosis. Scoliosis Research Society, Poster #E10, Seattle, 2002.

93. Grossfeld S, Winter RB, Lonstein JE, Denis F, Leonard A, Johnson L. Complications of anterior spinal surgery in children. J Pediatr Orthop 1997; 17(1):89–95.

94. Weis JC, Betz RR, Clements DH 3rd, Balsara RK. Prevalence of perioperative complications after anterior spinal fusion for patients with idiopathic scoliosis. J Spinal Disord 1997; 10(5):371–375.

95. Shapiro G, Green DW, Fatica NS, Boachie-Adjei O. Medical complications in scoliosis surgery. Curr Opin in Ped 2001; 13:36–41.

96. Evarts C, Winter R, Hall J. Vascular compression of the duodenum with the treatment of scoliosis. J Bone Joint Surg 1971; 53A(3):431.

97. Crowther MAA, Webb FJ, Eyre-Brook IA. Superior mesenteric artery syndrome following surgery for scoliosis. Spine 2002; 27(2):E528–E533.

98. Wilkie DPD. Chronic duodenal ileus. Br Med J 1921; 2:262.

99. Dorph MH. The cast syndrome: review of the literature and report of a case. N Engl J Med 1950; 243:440–442.

100. Vitale MG, Higgs GB, Liebling MS, Roth N, Roye DP. Superior mesenteric artery syndrome after segmental instrumentation: A Biomechanical analysis. Am J Orthop 1999; 28(8): 461–467.

101. Flynn JC, Price CT. Sexual complications of anterior fusion of the lumbar spine. Spine 1984; 9(5):489–492.

102. Johnson RM, McGuire EJ. Urogenital complications of anterior approaches to the lumbar spine. Clin Orthop 1981; (154):114–118.

103. Escobar E, Transfeldt E, Garvey T, Ogilvie J, Graber J, Schultz L. Video-assisted versus open anterior lumbar spine fusion surgery. A comparison of four techniques and complications in 135 patients. Spine 2003; 28(7):729–732.

104. Hu R, Jaglal S, Axcell T, Anderson G. A population-based study of reoperations after back surgery. Spine 1997; 22(19):2265–2271.

105. Malter AD, McNeney B, Loeser JD, Deyo RA. 5-year reoperation rates after different types of lumbar spine surgery. Spine 1998; 22(7):814–820.

106. Cook S, Asher M, Lai SM, Shobe J. Reoperation after primary posterior instrumentation and fusion for idiopathic scoliosis. Spine 2000; 25(4):463–468.

107. Connolly PJ, Von Schroeder HP, Johnson GE, Kostuik JP. Adolescent idiopathic scoliosis: Long-term effect of instrumentation extending to the lumbar spine. J Bone Joint Surg [Am] 1995; 77:1210–1216.

108. Dickson JH, Mirkovic S, Noble PC, Nalty T, Erwin WD. Results of operative treatment of idiopathic scoliosis in adults. J Bone Joint Surg (Am) 1995; 77:513–523.

109. Harrington PR, Dickson JH. An eleven-year clinical investigation of Harrington instrumentation: a preliminary report on 578 cases. Clin Orthop 1973; 93:113–130.

110. Richards BS, Herring JA, Johnston CE, Birch JG, Roach JW. Treatment of adolescent idiopathic scoliosis using Texas Scottish Rite Hospital instrumentation. Spine 1994; 19:1598–1605.

111. Sponseller PD, Cohen MS, Nachemson AL, Hall JE, Wohl ME. Results of surgical treatment of adults with idiopathic scoliosis. J Bone Joint Surg Am 1987; 69(5):667–675.

112. Lonstein JE. Salvage and reconstructive surgery. In: Lonstein JE, Bradford DS, Winter RB, Ogilvie JW, eds. Moe's Textbook of Scoliosis and Other Spinal Deformities. 3rd ed Philadelphia: WB Saunders, 1995:387–398.

113. Steinmann JC, Herkowitz HN. Pseudarthrosis of the spine. Clin Orthop 1992; 284: 80–90.

114. Etminan M, Girardi FP, Khan SN, Cammisa FP Jr. Revision strategies for lumbar pseudarthrosis. Orthop Clin North Am 2002; 33(2):381–392.

115. Raiszadeh R, Heggeness M, Esses SI. Thoracolumbar pseudarthrosis. Am J Orthop 2000; 29(7):513–520.

116. Frymoyer JW, Metteri JD, Hanley EN, et al. Failed lumbar disc surgery requiring a second operation. Spine 1978; 3:7–11.

117. Stauffer RN, Coventry MB. Anterior interbody lumbar spine fusion. J Bone Joint Surg 1972; 54:756–768.

118. Larsen JM, Capen DA. Pseudarthrosis of the lumbar spine. J Am Acad Orthop Surg 1997; 5(3):153–162.

119. Heggeness MH, Esses SI. Classification of pseudarthrosis of the lumbar spine. Spine 1991; 16(8S):S449–S454.

120. Dawson EG, Clader TJ, Bassett LW. A comparison of different methods used to diagnose pseudarthrosis. J Bone Joint Surg 1986; 67(8):1153–1159.

121. Deckey JE, Court C, Bradford DS. Loss of sagittal plane correction after removal of spinal implants. Spine 2000; 25(19):2453–2460.

122. DePalma AF, Rothman RH. The nature of pseudarthrosis. Clin Orthop 1968; 59:113–118.

123. Dawson EG, Lotysch M 3rd, Urist MR. Intertransverse process lumbar arthrodesis with autogenous bone graft. Clin Orthop 1981; (154):90–96.

124. Kim DH, Albert TJ. Update on use of instrumentation in lumbar spine disorders. Best Pract Res Clin Rheumatol 2002; 16(1):123–140.

125. Cook S, Asher M, Lai SM, Shobe J. Reoperation after primary posterior instrumentation and fusion for idiopathic scoliosis. Spine 2000; 25(4):463–468.

126. McAfee PC, Lee GA, Fedder IL, Cunningham BW. Anterior BAK instrumentation and fusion: complete versus partial discectomy. Clin Orthop 2002; (394):55–63.

127. Berven S, Tay BK, Kleinstueck FS, Bradford DS. Clinical applications of bone graft substitutes in spine surgery: consideration of mineralized and demineralized preparations and growth factor supplementation. Eur Spine J 2001; 10(suppl 2):S169–S177.

128. Cleveland M, Bosworth DM, Thompson FR. Pseudarthrosis in the lumbosacral spine. J Bone Joint Surg 1948; 30:302–S312.

129. Boden SD, Sumner DR. Biologic factors affecting spine fusion and bone regeneration. Spine 1995; 20(24S):S102–S112.

130. Brown CW, Orme TJ, Richardson HD. The rate of pseudarthrosis (surgical nonunion) in patients who are smokers and patients who are nonsmokers: a comparison study. Spine 1986; 11:942–943.

131. Saer EH III, Winter RB, Lonstein JE. Long scoliosis fusion to the sacrum in adults with non-paralytic scoliosis: an improved method. Spine 1990; 15:650–653.

132. O'Brien JP, Dawson MH, Heard CW, Momberger G, Speck G, Weatherly CR. Simultaneous combined anterior and posterior fusion. A surgical solution for failed spinal surgery with a brief review of the first 150 patients. Clin Orthop 1986; (203):191–195.

133. Albert TJ, Pinto M, Denis F. Management of symptomatic lumbar pseudarthrosis with anteroposterior fusion. Spine 2000; 25:123–129.

134. Byrd JA III, Scoles PV, Winter RB, et al. Adult idiopathic scoliosis treated by anterior and posterior spinal fusion. J Bone Joint Surg Am 1987; 69:843–850.

135. Floman Y, Micheli LJ, Penny JN, et al. Combined anterior and posterior fusion in seventy-three spinally deformed patients: Indications, results and complications. Clin Orthop 1982; 164:110–122.

136. Winter RB. Combined Dwyer and Harrington instrumentation and fusion in the treatment of selected patients with painful adult idiopathic scoliosis. Spine 1978; 3:135–141.

137. Boachie-Adjei O, Dendrinos GK, Ogilvie JW, Bradford DS. Management of adult spinal deformity with combined anterior-posterior arthrodesis and Luque-Galveston instrumentation. J Spinal Disord 1991; 4(2):131–141.

138. Lapp MA, Bridwell KH, Lenke LG, Riew KD, Linville DA, Eck KR, Ungacta FF. Long-term complications in adult spinal deformity patients having combined surgery. A comparison of primary to revision patients. Spine 2001; 26(8):973–983.

139. Berven SH, Deviren V, Smith JA, Hu SS, Bradford DS. Management of fixed sagittal plane deformity: outcome of combined anterior and posterior surgery. Spine 2003; 28(15): 1710–1715.

140. Weis JC, Betz RR, Clements DH, Balsara RK. Prevalence of perioperative complications after anterior spinal fusion for patients with idiopathic scoliosis. J Spinal Disord 1997; 10(5):371–375.

141. Hu SS, Fontaine F, Kelly B, Bradford DS. Nutritional depletion in staged spinal reconstructive surgery. The effect of total parenteral nutrition. Spine 1998; 23(12):1401–1405.

142. Shufflebarger HL, Grimm JO, Bui V, Thomson JD. Anterior and posterior spinal fusion. Staged versus same-day surgery. Spine 1991; 16(8):930–933.

143. Ferguson RL, Hansen MM, Nicholas DA, Allen BL Jr. Same-day versus staged anterior-posterior spinal surgery in a neuromuscular scoliosis population: the evaluation of medical complications. J Pediatr Orthop 1996; 16(3):293–303.

144. Powell ET 4th, Krengel WF 3rd, King HA, Lagrone MO. Comparison of same-day sequential anterior and posterior spinal fusion with delayed two-stage anterior and posterior spinal fusion. Spine 1994; 19(11):1256–1259.

145. Hefti FL, McMaster MJ. The effect of the adolescent growth spurt on early posterior spinal fusion in infantile and juvenile idiopathic scoliosis. J Bone Joint Surg Br 1983; 65:247–254.

145a. Dubousset J, Herring JA, Shufflebarger H. The crankshaft phenomenon. J Pediatr Orthop 1989; 9(5):541–550.

146. Sanders JO, Herring JA, Browne RH. Posterior arthrodesis and instrumentation in the immature (Rissergrade-0) spine in idiopathic scoliosis. J Bone Joint Surg Am 1995; 77: 39–45.

147. Hamill CL, Bridwell KH, Lenke LG, Chapman MP, Baldus C, Blanke K. Posterior arthrodesis in the skeletally immature patient. Assessing the risk for crankshaft: is an open triradiate cartilage the answer? Spine 1997; 22(12):1343–1351.

148. Saunders JO, Little DG, Richards S. Prediction of the crankshaft phenomenon by peak height velocity. Spine 1997; 22(12):1352–1356.

149. Burton DC, Asher MA, Lai SM. Scoliosis correction maintenance in skeletally immature patients with idiopathic scoliosis. Is anterior fusion really necessary? Spine 2000; 25(1):61–68.

150. D'Andrea LP, Betz RR, Lenke LG, Harms J, Clements DH, Lowe TG. The effect of continued posterior spinal growth on sagittal contour in patients treated by anterior instrumentation for idiopathic scoliosis. Spine 2000; 25(7):813–818.

151. Doherty JH. Complications of fusion in lumbar scoliosis. J Bone Joint Surg 1973; 55A:438.

152. Farcy JP, Schwab F. Posterior osteotomies with pedicle subtraction for flatback and associated syndromes. Technique and results of prospective study. Bull Hosp Joint Dis 2000; 59(1):11–16.

153. Horton WC, Holt RT, Muldowny DS. Controversy: fusion of L5-S1 in adult scoliosis. Spine 1996; 21(21):2520–2522.

154. Eck KR, Bridwell KH, Ungacta FF, Riew D, Lapp MA, Lenke LG, Baldus C, Blanke K. Complications and results of long adult deformity fusions down to L4, L5, and the sacrum. Spine 2001; 26(9):E182–E192.

155. Berven S, Deviren V, Smith J, Hu S, Bradford D. Adult lumbar and thoraco-lumbar scoliosis: fusion to L4, L5, or sacrum. International Society for Surgery of the Lumbar Spine, Edinburgh, Scotland, 7/01.

156. Thompson JP, Transfeldt EE, Bradford DS, Ogilvie JW, Boachie-Adjei O. Decompensation after Cotrel-Dubousset instrumentation of idiopathic scoliosis. Spine 1990; 15:927–931.

157. Bridwell KH, McAllister JW, Betz RR, Huss G, Clancy M, Schoenecker PL. Coronal decompensation produced by Cotrel-Dubousset "derotation" maneuver for idiopathic right thoracic scoliosis. Spine 1991; 16:769–777.

158. Kalen V, Conklin M. The behavior of the unfused lumbar spine following selective thoracic fusion for idiopathic scoliosis. Spine 1990; 15:271–274.

159. Cochran T, Irstam L, Nachemson A. Long-term anatomic and functional changes in patients with adolescent idiopathic scoliosis treated by Harrington rod fusion. Spine 1983; 8(6): 576–584.

160. Lenke LG, Betz RR, Bridwell KH, Harms J, Clements DH, Lowe TG. Spontaneous lumbar curve coronal correction after selective anterior or posterior thoracic fusion in adolescent idiopathic scoliosis. Spine 1999; 24(16):1663–1672.

161. Lenke LG, Bridwell KH, O'Brien MF, Baldus C, Blanke K. Recognition and treatment of the proximal thoracic curve in adolescent idiopathic scoliosis treated with Cotrel-Dubousset instrumentation. Spine 1994; 19(14):1589–1597.

162. Kuklo TR, Lenke LG, Won DS, Graham EJ, Sweet FA, Betz RR, Bridwell KH, Blanke KM. Spontaneous proximal thoracic curve correction after isolated fusion of the main thoracic curve in adolescent idiopathic scoliosis. Spine 2001; 26(18):1966–1975.

163. Bradford DS. Adult scoliosis: current concepts of treatment. Clin Orthop 1988; 229:70–87.

164. Cortet B, Roches E, Logier R, Houvenagel E, Gaydier-Souquieres G, Puisieux F, Delcambre B. Evaluation of spinal curvatures after a recent osteoporotic vertebral fracture. J Bone Spine 2002; 69(2):201–208.

165. Matthis C, Weber U, O'Neill WO, Raspe H, and the European Vertebral Osteoporosis Study Group. Health impact associated with vertebral deformities: results from the European Vertebral Osteoporesis Study (EVOS). Osteoporosis Int 1998; 8:364–372.

166. Jinbayashi H, Aoyagi K, Ross PD, Ito M, Shindo H, Takemoto T. Prevalence of vertebral deformity and its association with physical impairment among Japanese women: The Hizen-Oshima Study. Osteoporosis Int 2002; 13:723–730.

167. Ettinger B, Black DM, Nevitt MC, Rundle AC, Cauley JA, Cummings SR, Genant HK. Contribution of vertebral deformities to chronic back pain and disability. The study of osteoporotic fractures research group. J Bone Miner Res 1992; 7(4):449–456.

168. Cooper C, Kinson EJ, Atkinson J, et al. Population based study of survival after osteoporotic fractures. Am J Epidemiol 1993; 137:1001–1005.

169. Gold JW. The clinical impact of vertebral fractures: quality of life in women with osteo-porosis. Bone 1996; 18(3S):185S–189S.

170. Healey JH, Lane JM. Structural scoliosis in osteoporotic women. Clin Orthop 1985; 195:216–223.

171. Velis KP, Healey JH, Schneider R. Osteoporosis in unstable adult scoliosis. Clin Orthop 1988; 237:132–141.

172. Deyo RA, Cherkin DC, Loeser JD, Bigos SJ, Ciol MA. Morbidity and mortality in association with operations on the lumbar spine. The influence of age, diagnosis, and procedure. J Bone Joint Surg Am 1992; 74(4):536–543.

173. Katz JN, Lipson SJ, Larson MG, McInnes JM, Fossel AH, Liang MH. The outcome of decompressive laminectomy for degenerative lumbar stenosis. J Bone Joint Surg Am 1991; 73(6):809–816.

174. Takahashi S, Delecrin J, Passuti N. Surgical treatment of idiopathic scoliosis in adults: an age-related analysis of outcome. Spine 2002; 27(16):1742–1748.

175. McDonnell MF, Glassman SD, Dimar JR 2nd, Puno RM, Johnson JR. Perioperative complications of anterior procedures on the spine. J Bone Joint Surg Am 1996; 78(6):839–847.

176. Shapiro G, Green DW, Fatica NS, Boachie-Adjei O. Medical complications in scoliosis surgery. Curr Opin in Ped 2001; 13:36–41.

177. Laplaza FJ, Widmann RF, Fealy S, Moustafellos E, Illueca M, Burke SW, Boachie-Adjei O. Pancreatitis after surgery in adolescent idiopathic scoliosis: incidence and risk factors. J Pediatr Orthop 2002; 22(1):80–83.

178. Zheng F, Cammisa FP Jr, Sandhu HS, Girardi FP, Khan SN. Factors predicting hospital stay, operative time, blood loss, and transfusion in patients undergoing revision posterior lumbar spine decompression, fusion, and segmental instrumentation. Spine 2002; 27(8):818–824.

179. Kostuik JP, Chang JY, Sieber AN, Cohen DB. Complications of spinal fusion in treatment of adult spinal deformity. Poster #308, American Academy of Orthopedic Surgeons, New Orleans, 2003.

31

Iatrogenic Fixed Sagittal Imbalance in the Treatment of Lumbar Degenerative Disease: Prevention and Management

Anthony S. Rinella
Loyola University, Maywood, Illinois, U.S.A.

Keith H. Bridwell
Barnes-Jewish Hospital and Washington University in St. Louis School of Medicine, St. Louis, Missouri, U.S.A.

"Fixed sagittal imbalance syndrome" is the term most commonly used to describe iatrogenic lumbar hypolordosis created by Harrington distraction instrumentation that contributes to global sagittal imbalance. Harrington instrumentation is effective in correcting coronal plane abnormalities, but often at the expense of sagittal balance. More specifically, fixed sagittal imbalance can be defined as a syndrome in which the patient is unable to stand erect without flexing the knees and extending the hips. This is usually due to segmental loss of lumbar lordosis that fails to balance normal or exaggerated thoracic kyphosis. As the weight of the upper torso and head move anteriorly relative to the sacrum, it becomes increasingly difficult to maintain neutral weight-bearing alignment. The patient may become symptomatic and try to offset his or her spinal imbalance by extending the hips and bending the knees. Patients often complain of tenderness in the lumbar spine due to fatigue of the spinal extensor muscles or from coexistent pseudar-throses. Whether the etiology is due to distraction instrumentation or other processes, global sagittal imbalance most commonly implies segmental loss of lumbar lordosis.

The normal ranges of sagittal curvatures in the spine vary considerably between individuals. Bernhardt and Bridwell (1) studied 102 adolescents noting wide ranges of thoracic kyphosis (9–53°, SD ± 10°) and lumbar lordosis (−14 to −69°, SD ± 12°). Lumbar lordosis increased segmentally with 67% of lordosis located between L4 and the sacrum. Jackson and McManus (2) provided similar measurements, further noting that the upper thoracolumbar junction (T10–T12) averaged 5.5° of kyphosis, while the lower thoracolumbar junction (T12–L2) averaged −3° of lordosis.

Further definitions of position and flexibility of the sagittal imbalance are important when considering treatment strategies. According to the Scoliosis Research Society definition, positive sagittal balance reflects the C7 plumb line lying anterior to the

L5-S1 disk on the standing, long-cassette lateral radiograph. Similarly, negative sagittal balance implies that the sagittal C7 plumb line is positioned posterior to this point. From a literature perspective, positive sagittal "imbalance" describes the sagittal C7 plumb line lying > 5 cm anterior to the sacrum (3). Standing radiographs must be studied carefully to determine whether alterations in sagittal balance are due to regional hyperkyphosis or hypolordosis or a fixed abnormality. A supine lateral radiograph or bolstered view will demonstrate whether the positive sagittal balance is reduced in the supine position (flexible sagittal balance) or the head remains elevated relative to the bed (fixed sagittal imbalance).

I. ETIOLOGY

As noted previously, Harrington distraction instrumentation is the most common iatrogenic cause of positive sagittal imbalance (4–6). This is a contemporary concern because many patients treated in the 1970s and 1980s are becoming symptomatic (3). Several other processes can lead to fixed sagittal imbalance. In the realm of scoliosis surgery, segmental lumbar hypolordosis may be caused by disk degeneration below a long fusion. Long hypolordotic fusions to L4 or L5 are at particular risk for imbalance. With time, the distal unfused levels degenerate and lose their ability to compensate for the lack of proper lordosis proximally (7). Sagittal decompensation has also been reported as the result of anterior compression instrumentation (Dwyer or Zielke) without the use of structural interbody grafts or settling of a long posterior lumbar fusion without structural grafting (8). The placement of structural grafts within the disk spaces, rod contouring, and dual rod constructs have limited this phenomenon. D'Andrea et al. (9) recently described a process analogous to the crankshaft phenomenon after anterior spinal instrumentation in the treatment of adolescent idiopathic scoliosis. They noted up to 15° of sagittal kyphosis resulting from continued growth of the posterior elements after anterior fusion.

Several processes unrelated to scoliosis may lead to fixed sagittal imbalance. Patients with ankylosing spondlylitis can present with lumbar hypolordosis or progressive thoracic or cervical kyphosis (10). These patients typically cannot compensate for their deformity due to rigidity in their thoracic and lumbar spine. Similarly, malalignments may be caused by thoracolumbar fracture(s) leading to posttraumatic kyphosis. Farcy and Schwab (11) described the kyphotic decompensation syndrome in which either lumbar fracture or previous lumbar or lumbosacral fusion leads to imbalance.

Fixed sagittal imbalance may be caused by a number of degenerative etiologies. Loss of lordosis can occur after multiple level lumbar fusions due to iatrogenic causes or increased anterior settling over time. Spondylolistheses may contribute to the deformity (Case 1). Several studies have noted the kyphosing and lordosing effects of various operating room tables. Stephens et al. (12) analyzed the lordosis of 10 asymptomatic volunteers in the standing position, prone on the Jackson table, and prone on the Andrews table with the hips flexed at various positions. They noted that the Andrews frame significantly reduced lumbar lordosis whether the hips were flexed to 60° or 90°. The knee-chest position can similarly create regional loss of lordosis. Tribus et al. (13) retrospectively reviewed the effect of the knee-chest position on 28 patients after segmental lumbar instrumented fusions. They noted decreased lordosis across the fused segments that lead to a transfer of lordosis proximally. In contrast, as demonstrated by Marsicano et al. (14) the Jackson OSI frame tends to maintain lumbar lordosis, but may decrease natural kyphosis in the thoracic spine and thoracolumbar junction.

2-Level Stenosis / 2-Level Spondylo / Segmental Kyphosis

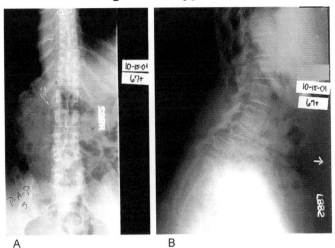

A   B

Segmental Kyphosis/Positive Sagittal Balance

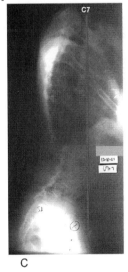

C

Case 1 Lumbar segmental kyphosis, spondylolisthesis, and spinal stenosis. (A,B,C). AP and lateral radiographs and long cassette lateral of a 67-year-old woman with kyphosis at L4-5 > L3-4 and subluxations at both levels. (D,E) Flexion-extension radiographs demonstrating that the L4-5 kyphosis does not completely reduce. (F,G) Axial MRI views at L3-4 and L4-5 shows spinal stenosis at both levels. (H,I) AP and lateral postoperative radiographs showing a posterior fusion from L3-S1/pelvis with decompressions at L3 to L5. (J,K) Long-cassette standing radiographs. This case demonstrates the importance of considering sagittal balance prior to a decompression procedure. If this patient had simply been treated with pedicle screws at L3, L4, and L5, her sagittal balance would not have been improved and in all likelihood would have been worse postoperatively than pre-operatively. Our options were either circumferential treatment (ALIF or PLIF) at those two segments (L3-L4 and L4-L5) or extending down to the sacrum and ilium, which is what was done to provide control of the L3, L4, and L5 segments with a stable distal anchor (the S1 and iliac screws).

Incomplete Reduction of the Kyphosis At L4-L5

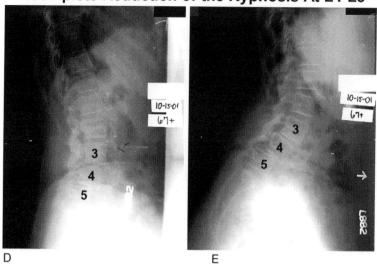

How to Balance the Patient?

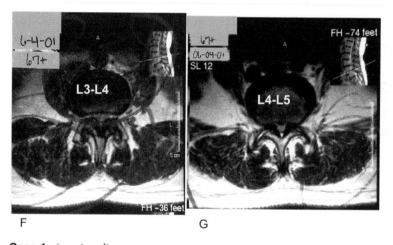

Case 1 (*continued*)

Lumbar segmental hypolordosis may be caused by distractive forces placed across an instrumented segment or disruption of the natural posterior tension band. The global effects of distractive instrumentation have been documented with Harrington instrumentation, but similar regional effects may occur with shorter constructs. The vertebrae may be distracted to offset foraminal narrowing, coronal deviations, or other regional losses in disk height. Similarly, disruption of the posterior ligamentous tension band and posterior musculature may contribute to loss of lordosis. These structures lie posterior to the rotational axis of the spine and thus contribute significantly to offsetting kyphotic forces. During any posterior procedure that exposes the posterior elements, the lumbodorsal fascia must be incised and the supraspinous or interspinous ligaments may be disrupted. This is especially true after multilevel laminectomies, particularly in patients with naturally hypolordotic lumbar spines or after prior posterior procedures. Furthermore,

Upright Postop

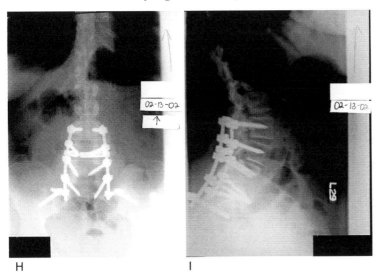

H   I

Status Post 2-Level Decompression and Fusion
Instrumentation L3 to the Sacrum and Pelvis

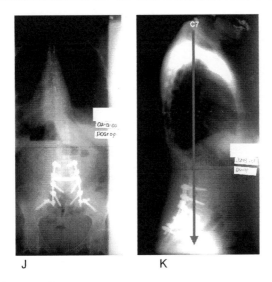

J   K

Case 1 (*continued*)

the ligaments above or below an intended fusion level may be compromised during exposure or decompression. Postlaminectomy kyphosis occurs more frequently than anticipated, even in expert hands.

Further degenerative etiologies may contribute to sagittal imbalance. Anterior settling is more likely with regional pathology, such as two-level degenerative spondylolisthesis or isthmic spondylolisthesis (Case 1). Settling of the disks can occur, especially if structural grafts or cages are not placed anteriorly after an anterior spinal fusion (see Cases 2 and 3). If an anterior structural graft or cage is present, it may lack

Degenerative Spondylolisthesis
(2-Level) Allowed To Heal In Kyphosis

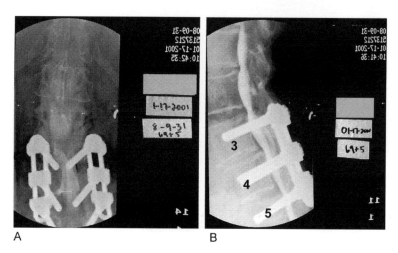

A   B

Solidly Fused Now, But With Fixed
Sagittal Imbalance

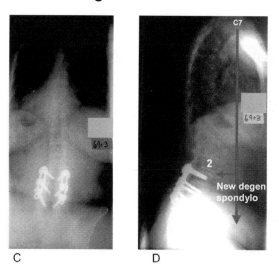

C   D

Case 2 Lumbar kyphosis after prior decompressions/short posterior fusion. (A,B) Preoperative AP and lateral radiographs demonstrating lumbar kyphosis after decompressions at L3-4 and L4-5 and a prior fusion of L5-S1. The decompressed segments settled into kyphosis and a spondylolisthesis developed at L2-3 with resultant positive sagittal balance. (C,D) Standing radiographs 10 months after a pedicle subtraction osteotomy at L4 with extension of her fusion and instrumentation to L2 (E,F). The fusion was extended to L2 because of the spondylolisthesis that developed above the previous fusion. Because she had a previous fusion at L5-S1, it was not necessary to do iliac screws. This case points out that a relatively minor loss of lordosis in the distal lumbar spine can easily cause a substantial sagittal imbalance. It also points out that it is not uncommon for screws to loosen at L5, which is what happened to this patient.

Fixed Sagittal Imbalance Treated With PSO At L4

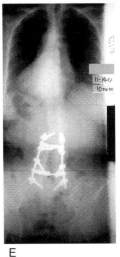 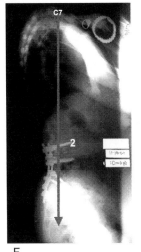

E   F

Case 2 (*continued*)

the proper height or lordosis or may not lie squarely against the endplates. The majority of lumbar lordosis occurs at the disk level, as opposed to the natural sagittal wedging of the thoracic vertebra that contributes to kyphosis (1). These phenomena occur most often in the distal lumbar spine, where 67% of lumbar lordosis naturally resides (1). Any degree of kyphosis in the distal lumbar spine may have significant global effects because of the length of the spinal lever arm.

Regional kyphosis also occurs after long fusions to the distal lumbar spine or sacrum, especially if there is loosening of the distal screws or pseudarthrosis. Edwards et al. (15) demonstrated that with long fusions to L5, there may be loosening of the distal screws and distal settling. The incidence of L5 screw loosening correlated with how "deep-seated" the L5 vertebra was relative to the proximal iliac crest. L5 seating was characterized by the distance from the midpoint of the L5 pedicles to the intercrestal line. A deep-seated L5 was defined by the L5 pedicles > 10 mm below the intercrestal line. Although a deep-seated L5 protected against subsequent L5-S1 disk degeneration, there was a higher rate of L5 screw loosening. With fusion to the sacrum, loosening of the sacral screws can occur with settling at L5-S1. This can be reduced by structural grafting anteriorly at L5-S1 and protecting the sacral screws with iliac screws (16) (see Table 1).

II. PATIENT ASSESSMENT

A thorough patient evaluation is important in assessing sagittal imbalance. Patients typically try to compensate for their loss of segmental lumbar lordosis with hyperlordosis through unfused lumbar, thoracic, or cervical motion segments; hip extension; and knee flexion in an effort to keep the head centered over the sacrum. Alteration in the normal weight-bearing line may contribute to overloading of the facets, disk degeneration, lumbar back pain, spondylolysis, or spondylolisthesis. Lagrone et al. (17) reported that almost all

Preop

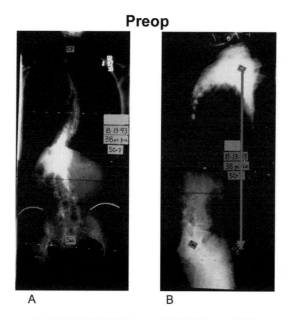

A   B

8+2 Years Postop

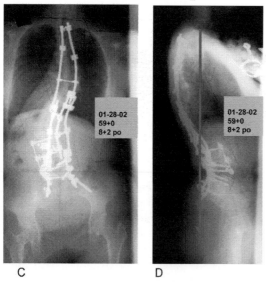

C   D

Case 3 (A,B) Standing AP and lateral radiographs of a patient with prior fusion from the upper thoracic spine to L3 without instrumentation. Radiographs demonstrate kyphosis with subsequent disk degeneration from L3-S1 leading to positive sagittal imbalance. (C,D) AP and lateral radiographs 8 years after extension of the fusion to the sacrum, several Smith-Petersen osteotomies at the thoracolumbar junction, and anterior structural grafting from L3-S1. (E,F) Clinical photos pre- and postop. This case illustrates the importance of anterior structural grafting when extending a fusion down to the sacrum. In addition, her sacral screws were protected with iliac screws.

Preop   ## Postop

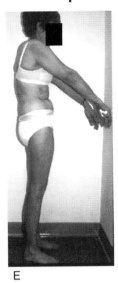

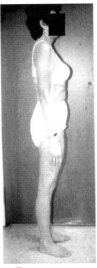

E   F

Case 3 (*continued*)

patients with sagittal imbalance (95%) were unable to stand erect, 89% had back pain that increased with prolonged activity, and 27% had to bend their knees to stay erect. Compensatory hip and knee positions can lead to gluteal and thigh pain and fatigue. The erector spinae muscles can become contracted in an effort to restore balance and eventually fatigue. Ultimately the patient may develop the inability to stand erect and true sagittal imbalance exists. The state of the patient's position in this progression can be noted by analyzing the patient's gait and standing postures.

The patient's age, past medical and surgical history, and medical comorbidities are important to consider. With age, osteoporosis becomes an increasing concern and may influence surgical indications. Dexa scans analyzing the hip (not spine) can be helpful in this regard. Older patients may develop degenerative loss of lumbar lordosis or increased thoracolumbar or thoracic kyphosis. It is important to remember that elderly patients may lack the physiological reserves to tolerate a posterior and/or anterior procedure, even if they are very active and appear healthy relative to their age. A thorough understanding of the patient's past surgical history is also important. Significant loss of lordosis is

Table 1 Steps to Prevent Fixed Sagittal Imbalance

Avoid distraction instrumentation posteriorly
Evaluate sagittal balance carefully in operating room
Maintain 2:1 ratio of lumbar:thoracic sagittal curvature
Place appropriate sagittal contour in lumbar rods
Protect facets and intraspinous/supraspinous ligaments above and below fusion
Place structural grafts or cages anteriorly with long fusions, especially in the distal segments
Protect L5 screws and S1 screws (protect L5 screws with anterior column support; protect S1 screws with both anterior column support and iliac screws)

unlikely after a single-level fusion, but may occur in fusions of two or more levels. Old operative reports are helpful if prior spinal surgery was performed, and any prior surgical complications should be elucidated. Medical comorbidities and smoking history are helpful in identifying high-risk patients.

As noted previously, physical exam can define the type and extent of sagittal imbalance. Patients should be examined while standing and walking. It is important to note differences in position when sitting versus lying supine or prone. In the supine position, the compensatory effects of hip extension and knee flexion are removed, and the rigidity of the kyphosis can be assessed. Similarly, the flexibility of the sagittal imbalance can be assessed in the prone position. This is also important when considering the patient's position on the operating table. Furthermore, any areas of spinal stenosis may become symptomatic in the hyperextended prone position, necessitating a thorough posterior decompression prior to any further maneuvers.

Various routine and special radiographs may help elucidate this complex degenerative process. Routine x-rays include standing long-cassette anteroposterior and lateral radiographs. The lateral radiographs should be taken with the hips and knees in full extension. Walkers or other external supports should not be used in order to truly assess the patient's global sagittal balance. The goal in each radiograph is to assess regional and global balance by examining the C7 plumb line intersection with the S1 superior endplate. In the sagittal plane, the C7 plumb line is measured from the posterior aspect of the S1 superior endplate [also known as the sagittal vertical axis (SVA)]. Any deviation more than 5 cm anterior to this point may be pathological and represent positive radiographic sagittal balance (3). An assessment of pelvic incidence helps define the relationship of the distal lumbar spine and sacrum to the pelvis and hips. The measurement is defined by the angle between the perpendicular to the sacral endplate at its midpoint and the line connecting this point to the midpoint of a line connecting the femoral heads (18,19). Long-cassette flexion-extension radiographs may help define regional and global flexibility of the spine. Supine hyperextension lateral radiographs are helpful in defining flexibility. Short-cassette radiographs may be useful in focusing evaluation on certain aspects of the spine. Similarly, a prone hyperextension lateral will help identify the patient's position on the operating table.

III. TREATMENT AND SURGICAL OPTIONS

Once sagittal imbalance has been thoroughly assessed, treatment options can be considered. In all cases typical modalities of conservative management should be offered. Anti-inflammatory medications, physical therapy, and aerobic exercise should be recommended if the patient can tolerate such treatments. Lifestyle modifications are often required. Bracing should only be considered with acute compression fractures or soft braces used for minor short-term myofascial pain exacerbations. Long-term bracing weakens the trunk muscles and is an ineffective long-term solution. If the positive sagittal balance is only mildly symptomatic and the imbalance is relatively minor, these modalities may obviate the need for surgery. Fluoroscopically guided transforaminal or epidural steroid injections may help relieve symptoms of neurological impingement and serve a diagnostic and therapeutic purpose. Often it is difficult to completely define the pain generators among multiple levels of relative stenosis. Sequential injections can help define the relative areas of impingement.

Table 2 Causes of Fixed Sagittal Imbalance

Ankylosing spondylitis
Congenital scoliosis (pre- and postfusion)
Iatrogenic
   Anterior instrumentation without structural graft/cage
   Distraction instrumentation posteriorly
   Long fusions to the distal lumbar spine or sacrum with
     settling of the distal segments into relative kyphosis
Multilevel laminectomies
Thoracolumbar trauma

Treatment of fixed sagittal imbalance requires rebalancing of the spine with one or several osteotomies (3). It is important to consider the type of sagittal imbalance that is present. Fixed sagittal imbalance can be divided into two major types: Type 1 (segmental) and Type 2 (global) (3) (see Table 2). Characteristics of a Type 1 sagittal imbalance deformity are segmental hypolordosis or kyphosis across fused lumbar segments in which the body of C7 remains centered over the lumbosacral disk. The disks below the fusion are typically hyperextended (≥ 5 mm taller anteriorly than posteriorly) to maintain sagittal balance and are without severe degeneration. The goal of surgery in these patients is to maintain normal sagittal balance with a more normal trapezoidal configuration of the disks below the fusion (anterior disk height ≤ 2 mm greater than the posterior disk height) as described by Bernhardt and Bridwell (1) and Wambolt and Spence (20). Type 2 sagittal imbalance deformity is defined as having the plumb line of C7 fall more than 5 cm anterior to the lumbosacral disk with either significant disk degeneration below the fusion or fusion to the sacrum. The goal of treatment is to improve sagittal balance by centering the C7 vertebra over or behind the lumbosacral disk. This is accomplished by restoring lumbar lordosis 10–30° greater than the thoracic kyphosis for the given patient (maintaining the normal 2:1 lumbar:thoracic sagittal curvature ratios).

Several spinal osteotomies have been described in the treatment of sagittal imbalance (11,15,21–34). Options include fracturing the spine after decompression with the patient awake (29), supplementing osteotomies with instrumentation (25,28,29,31,32), decancellating the posterior vertebral body with preservation of the pedicles (26), and combined anterior and posterior osteotomies (16). The two most common osteotomies at our institutions are the Smith-Petersen osteotomy and the pedicle subtraction osteotomy. In general, only closing wedge osteotomies should be performed. Using posterior–based osteotomies, approximately 1° of sagittal correction is usually achieved for every millimeter of bone resected (35). How much correction can be achieved at one level versus multiple levels depends on the patient's age, biology, and connective tissues (see Table 3 and Fig. 1).

Table 3 Treatments of Sagittal Imbalance

Smith-Petersen osteotomy (Fig. 1)
Pedicle subtraction osteotomy (Fig. 2)
Anterior/Posterior osteotomies
Vertebral resection

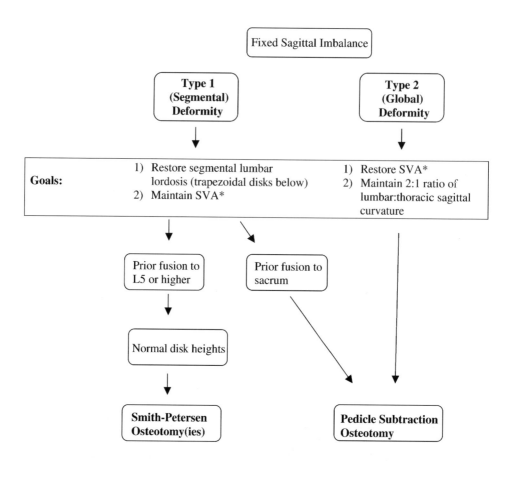

Figure 1   Treatment algorithm for fixed sagittal imbalance.

IV. SMITH-PETERSEN OSTEOTOMY

In 1945, Smith-Petersen described a V-shaped osteotomy of the posterior elements with exposure down to the dura (21) (see Fig. 2). During the bony resection, the nerve roots are completely decompressed and the fusion mass is beveled to allow room for the neural elements after closure of the osteotomy. The osteotomy hinges on the posterior disk and

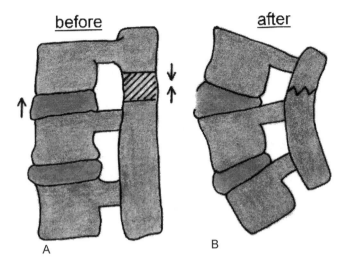

Figure 2 Smith-Petersen osteotomy. (A) The sagittal plane osteotomy: the cross-hatched area is the osteotomy site. (B) The resultant lordosis after the osteotomy is closed. (From Ref. 3.)

therefore depends on a mobile disk or an anterior osteotomy. The technical steps include the following (35):

1. Patient positioning—Denis (6) described extending the table after the osteotomy is performed. At our institutions, patients are placed on an open OSI table with two pads under the chest and four pads under the thighs in order to allow gravity to close the osteotomy site. If the patient is markedly kyphotic or very osteoporotic, hinging the operating table during exposure and the osteotomy followed by extending the table is advisable.
2. After exposure, thin down the fusion mass with a combination of osteotomies, lexelles, and curettes.
3. Thin the anterior cortex of the fusion mass as much as possible with a high-speed burr.
4. Enter the canal centrally (where the epidural space is largest) and make initial cuts in the bone with a small Kerrison rongeur between the cortex and ligamentum flavum. Note: In patients with ankylosing spondylitis, dural deficiencies may exist.
5. Extend the osteotomy laterally through the facets bilaterally. Note: Inspect the symmetry of the osteotomy sites prior to completing the lateral component because the osteotomy site tends to close down once the osteotomy is completed. Laminar spreaders are helpful in holding the osteotomy site open.
6. Resect the ligamentum flavum after the bony work is complete.

In general it is usually possible to close an osteotomy that is 10–15 mm in height without "releasing" the disk as long as the disk space measures at least 5 mm in height without bridging osteophytes (35). Larger osteotomies are possible with an anterior release of the disk. Osteotomies should be centered at the apex of the most kyphotic segments for maximum benefit. L3-4 is often an ideal level because its position is the natural apex of the lumbar spine and is above the bifurcation of the aorta (35,36). Levels with foraminal stenosis should be avoided because the osteotomy narrows the foramen at the osteotomy level. If a dural tear occurs, a patch graft should be applied with fibrin glue. Tightly closing the osteotomy reduces the likelihood of a cerebrospinal fluid (CSF) fistula.

V. PEDICLE SUBTRACTION OSTEOTOMY

The pedicle subtraction osteotomy or transpedicular wedge resection procedure has the advantage of obtaining three-column correction via a closing wedge osteotomy without lengthening the anterior column (7) (see Fig. 3). Correction occurs in the vertebral body as opposed to relying on disk extension and can obtain anterior and posterior bony fusion. The lack of lengthening of the anterior column maximizes healing potential while avoiding stretch on the major vessels and viscera anterior to the spine.

The Operative Procedure

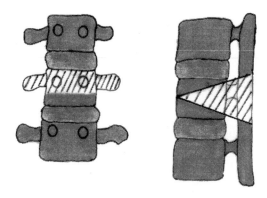

Resection of the Posterior Elements
Around the Pedicles and Then
Decancellation of the Pedicles and
Vertebral Body

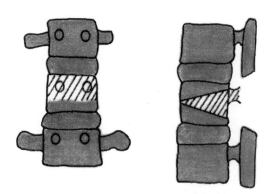

Figure 3 Pedicle subtraction osteotomy. The cross-hatched area represents the osteotomy location in the coronal and sagittal planes. (From Ref. 3.)

Green Sticking the Posterior Vertebral Cortex With a Woodson Elevator or Reverse Angled Curette

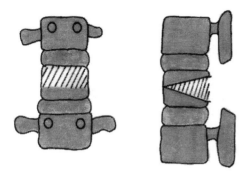

Resection of the Lateral Vertebral Cortex with Leksell Bilaterally

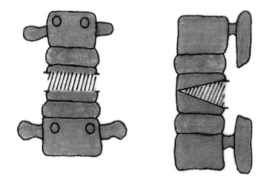

Closure of the Osteotomy by Compression/Cantilever/Extension of Chest/Lower Extremities

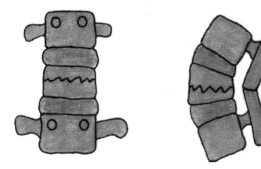

Figure 3 (*continued*)

The operative procedure consists of a posterior instrumented arthrodesis combined with a posterior-based closing wedge osteotomy. As with the Smith-Petersen osteotomy, 1 mm of bone resection generally leads to 1° of lordosis. The stepwise the procedure includes:

1. Establishing fixation points above and below the osteotomy site—usually at least four fixation points above and below (if pedicle screws are used; eight fixation points proximally if hooks are used). However, there are many exceptions to this rule, and it may, at times, be possible to get away with using fewer fixation points than this.

2. Decompress the epidural space and identify appropriate nerve roots. Widely decompress the epidural space centrally.

3. Remove bone surrounding the pedicles bilaterally (with exception of the vertebral body).

4. Through the pedicle, curette the pedicle and vertebral body by decancellating the posterior vertebral body. Carefully preserve the pedicle walls and vertebral cortex to protect the dura and epidural vessels.

5. Thin the posterior vertebral body from within using curved curettes.

6. Resect the pedicles with special attention to the exiting nerve roots below the pedicle.

7. Greenstick the posterior vertebral body with a Woodson elevator or reverse angled curette using an anterior directed force pushing the posterior bone into the vertebral body.

8. Place a Penfield elevator subperiostally along the lateral margin of the vertebral body, then resect the lateral vertebral cortex in a wedge-shaped fashion. Maintain the anterior cortex continuity to serve as a hinge to prevent translation.

9. Hyperextend the patient's hips and knees to close the osteotomy site. The operating room table can be hinged at the level of the osteotomy to assist with closing the osteotomy site.

In general, we try to perform the osteotomy at a level below the conus medullaris and in the site of previously fused segments. The more distal the osteotomy level, the more sagittal the correction that will be obtained. If a long fusion to the distal lumbar spine is required, arthrodesis is stopped at L5 only if the L5-S1 disk appears well preserved or is completely collapsed and stable. Otherwise, the arthrodesis is extended to S1 and is protected by iliac screws bilaterally (unless a fusion already exists at L5-S1). As reported by Kuklo et al. (37), we have had high fusion rates with high-grade spondylolisthesis and long fusions to the sacrum when iliac screws are used in addition to bicortical S1 screws. We commonly perform the osteotomy through a site of a previous laminectomy. The surgical goal is to restore the sagittal balance to normal (C7 sagittal plumb line falling within the L5-S1 disk or slightly behind it).

In terms of postoperative management, a substantial percentage of the older degenerative sagittal imbalance patients are often treated with a postoperative TLSO for several months postoperatively. Younger patients who have prior idiopathic scoliosis fusions subsequently extended down to the sacrum are not usually treated with a postoperative brace.

The decision of whether to perform the posterior procedure in one or two stages depends on the difficulty of removing existing instrumentation and establishing new fixation points, as well as how many "surprises" are anticipated. When these steps are especially difficult, the osteotomy, harvesting of bone graft, and completion of definitive instrumentation occurs 5–7 seven days after these initial steps are completed. Patients are typically placed on parenteral nutrition between stages.

Although the pedicle subtraction osteotomy achieves three-column correction, it does not obviate the need for an anterior procedure. The main circumstances requiring an anterior procedure are the presence of multiple pseudarthroses or when a long fusion is extended to the sacrum. In both cases, a thorough discectomy is performed with structural grafts or cages placed anteriorly. When a long fusion is extended by just two or three segments to the sacrum, a paramedian approach is quite useful. The role of bone morphogenic protein in this scenario is evolving.

Bridwell et al. (7) recently reported their results with 27 consecutive patients who underwent a pedicle subtraction osteotomy for fixed sagittal imbalance. The average increase in lordosis was 34°. One patient developed a pseudarthrosis through the osteotomy site in an area of a previous laminectomy and nonunion. Six patients developed thoracic pseudarthrosis, and 2 patients developed increased kyphosis at L5-S1 below the fusion resulting in some loss of sagittal correction. There was one neurological complication: urinary retention due to neural compression that improved after the osteotomy site was further decompressed centrally. After this occurrence, they emphasized the wide central decompression noted in the steps above. Loss of correction did not occur outside of the patients with pseudarthroses. There were significant improvements in overall Oswestry scores and pain scores.

VI. CONCLUSION

There are multiple surgical options for patients with fixed sagittal imbalance of various etiologies. In all cases the goal is to maintain neutral or negative sagittal balance with normal relationships between the thoracic and lumbar sagittal curvatures. In addition to the time-honored Smith-Petersen osteotomy, the pedicle subtraction osteotomy can be performed in patients with acceptable clinical and radiographic results and minimal loss of correction over time using modern instrumentation techniques.

REFERENCES

1. Bernhardt M, Bridwell KH. Segmental analysis of the sagittal plane alignment of the normal thoracic and lumbar spines and thoracolumbar junction. Spine 1989; 14:717.
2. Jackson RP, McManus AC. Radiographic analysis of sagittal plane alignment and balance in standing volunteers and patients with low back pain matched for age, sex, and size. Spine 1994; 19:1611.
3. Booth KC, Bridwell KH, Lenke LG, et al. Complications and predictive factors for successful treatment of flatback deformity (fixed sagittal imbalance). Spine 1999; 24:1712–1720.
4. Doherty JH. Complications of fusion in lumbar scoliosis: Proceedings of the Scoliosis Research Society. J Bone Joint Surg Am 1973; 55:438.
5. Bradford DS, Tribus CB. Current concepts and management of patients with mixed decompensated spinal deformity. Clin Orthop 1994; 306:64–72.
6. Denis F. The iatrogrenic loss of lumbar lordosis, The flat back and flat buttock syndromes. In: Farcy J-P, ed. Complex Spinal Deformities, Spine: State of the Art Reviews. Philadelphia: Hanley & Belkfus Inc., 1994; 659–680.
7. Bridwell KH, Lewis SH, Lenke LG, et al. Pedicle subtraction osteotomy for the treatment of fixed sagittal balance. J Bone Joint Surg Am 2003; 85(3):454–463.

8. DeWald RL. Revision surgery for spinal deformity. Adult Spinal Deformity. American Academy of Orthopaedic Surgeons, Instructional Course Lecture 105, San Francisco, CA, 1993.

9. D'Andrea LP, Betz RR, Lenke LG, et al. The effect of continued posterior spinal growth on sagittal contour in patients treated by anterior instrumentation for idiopathic scoliosis. Spine 2000, 25:813.

10. Bradford DS, Schumacher WL, Lonstein JE, Winter RB. Ankylosing spondylitis: experience and surgical management of 21 patients. Spine 1987; 2:238–243.

11. Farcy J-PC, Schwab FJ. Management of flatback and related kyphotic decompensation syndromes. Spine 1997; 22:2452–2457.

12. Stephens GC, Yoo JU, Wilbur G. Comparison of lumbar sagittal alignment produced by different operative positions. Spine 1996; 21:1802.

13. Tribus CB, Belanger TA, Zdeblick TA. The effect of operative position and short segment fusion on maintenance of sagittal alignment produced by different operative positions. Spine 1999; 24:58.

14. Marsicano JH, Lenke LG, Bridwell KH, et al. The lordotic effect of the OSI frame on operative adolescent idiopathic scoliosis patients. Spine 1998; 23:1341–1348.

15. Edwards CC, Bridwell KH, Patel A, et al. Thoracolumbar deformity arthrodesis to L5 in adult scoliotics: the fate of the L5-S1 disk: is it protected by a deep-seated L5? Presented at the Scoliosis Research Society 37th Annual Meeting, Seattle, WA, September 19–22, 2002.

16. Kostuik JP, Maurais GR, Richardson WJ, et al. Combined single stage anterior and posterior osteotomy for correction of iatrogenic lumbar kyphosis. Spine 1988; 13:257–266.

17. Lagrone MO, Bradford DS, Moe JH, et al. Treatment of symptomatic flatback after spinal fusion. J Bone Joint Surg 1988, 70-A:569.

18. Legaye J, Duval-Beaupere G, Hecquet J, Marty C. Pelvic incidence: a fundamental pelvic parameter for three-dimensional regulation of spinal sagittal curves. Euro Spine J 1998; 7:99–103.

19. Hanson DS, Bridwell KH, Rhee JM, Lenke LG. Correlation of pelvic incidence with low and high-grade isthmic spondylolisthesis. Spine 2002; 27(18):2026–2029.

20. Wambolt A, Spencer DL. A segmental analysis of the distribution of lumbar lordosis in the normal spine. Orthop Trans 1987; 11:92–93.

21. Smith-Petersen MH, Larson CB, Aufracn OE. Osteotomy of the spine for the correction of flexion deformity in rheumatoid arthritis. J Bone Joint Surg 1945; 27:1–11.

22. Emneus H. Wedge osteotomy of the spine in ankylosing spondylitis. Acta Orthop Scand 1968; 39:321–326.

23. Camargo FP, Cordiero EN, Napoli MM. Corrective osteotomy of the spine in ankylosing spondylitis. Experience with 66 cases. Clin Orthop 1986; 208:157–167.

24. Floman Y, Penny JN, Micheli LJ, et al. Osteotomy of the fusion mass in scoliosis. J Bone Joint Surg 1982; 64-A: 1307–1316.

25. Goel MK. Vertebral osteotomy for correction of fixed flexion deformity of the spine. J Bone Joint Surg 1968; 50-A:287–294.

26. Herbert JJ. Vertebral osteotomy for kyphosis, especially in Marie-Strumpell arthritis. J Bone Joint Surg 1959; 41-A:291–302.

27. Halm H, Metz-Stavenhagen P, Zielke K. Results of surgical correction of kyphotic deformities of the spine in ankylosing spondylitis on the basis of the Modified Arthritis Impact Measurement scales. Spine 1995; 20:1612–1619.

28. Hehne HJ, Zielke K, Bohm H. Polysegmental lumbar osteotomies and transpedicled fixation for correction of long-curved kyphotic deformities in ankylosing spondylitis. Report on 177 cases. Clin Orthop 1990; 258:49–55.

29. Jaffray D, Becker V, Eisenstein S. Closing wedge osteotomy with transpedicular fixation in ankylosing spondylitis. Clin Orthop 1992; 279:122–126.

30. LaChapelle EH. Osteotomy of the lumbar spine for correction of kyphosis in a case of ankylosing spondylarthritis. J Bone Joint Surg 1946; 28:851–858.

31. McMaster MJ. A technique for lumbar spinal osteotomy in ankylosing spondylitis. J Bone Joint Surg 1985; 67-B:204–210.
32. Simmons EH. Kyphotic deformity of the spine in ankylosing spondylitis. Clin Orthop 1977; 128:65–77.
33. Styblo K, Bossers GT, Slot GH. Osteotomy for kyphosis in ankylosing spondylitis. Acta Orthop Scand 1985; 56:294–297.
34. Weale AE, Marsh CH, Yeoman PM. Secure fixation of lumbar osteotomy. Surgical experience with 50 patients. Clin Orthop 1995; 321:216–222.
35. Bridwell KH. Osteotomies for fixed deformities in the thoracic and lumbar spine. In: Bridwell KH, DeWald RL, eds. The Textbook of Spinal Surgery. 2nd ed. Philadelphia: Lippincott-Raven, 1977:821–835.
36. Simmons EH. Relation of vascular complication to the level of lumbar extension osteotomy in ankylosing spondylitis. Paper 215, presented at the annual meeting of the American Academy of Orthopaedic Surgeons, New Orleans, LA, 1994.
37. Kuklo TR, Bridwell KH, Lewis SJ, et al. Minimum 2-year analysis of sacropelvic fixation and L5-S1 fusion using S1 and iliac screws. Spine 2001; 26:1976–1983.

32

Complications of Minimally Invasive Spinal Surgery—Part I: Cervical and Posterior Lumbar Spine

Larry T. Khoo and Anthony Virella
UCLA Medical Center, Los Angeles, California, U.S.A.

I. INTRODUCTION

With the advent of modern surgical technologies such as digital fluoroscopy, image guidance, high-resolution endoscopy, and surgical lasers, the use of minimally invasive techniques in the treatment of a variety of spinal pathologies has increased exponentially. These procedures offer both the real and potential advantages of decreased iatrogenic tissue trauma, smaller corridors of approach, reduced postoperative pain, truncated hospital stays, foreshortened recovery times, and a more rapid return to full function. To date, minimally invasive procedures are actively being applied in nearly all areas of the spinal column from the cervical (1,10,19,21,25) to the thoracic (23,38) to the lumbar region (4,5,8,11,12,17,22,24,26,28,29,31,32,35).

With minimalism, however, often comes a degree of increased technical difficulty as the corridors or approach and the degree of visualization becomes more narrowed. The learning curve necessary for mastering these techniques may be lengthy and cannot be easily circumvented. As endoscopic viewing by definition provides a nonlinear view of the pathology through the spatial separation of a two-dimensional video monitor, a certain amount of visual disorientation must be expected during the first dozen endoscopic-type cases. This is further compounded by the kinesthetic retardation caused by working through restrictive minimal access portals that are often under 2 cm in diameter. Most surgeons must modify their existing hand movements to accommodate for the restricted working space and learn to work with the hands closely together or with only one instrument at a time. These visual and spatial limitations thus magnify the risk of complication during minimally invasive spinal procedures. Inability to appreciate depth and accidental hand movements are often responsible for inadvertent durotomy, vessel laceration, and bony violation (7,10–12,19,22,26,35).

Although most minimally invasive procedures utilize instruments familiar to most spinal surgeons, they are much longer and more cumbersome to manuever than those typically used in equivalent open operations. In the case of thoracoscopic surgery,

513

for example, the chest wall, portals, and long instruments keep the surgeons hands far from the pathology. As a result, even simple tasks such as placing a screw over a K-wire can be become difficult and trying to the novice (23). Furthermore, simply lengthening or altering existing instruments and implants used for open procedures is often inadequate. In many cases, special "minimalist" modifications of the tools themselves creates even further unfamiliarity that can add to the learning curve. As such, many complications of minimally invasive spinal procedures can be attributed to accidental injury during placement or manipulation of the surgical tools during the procedure. This often occurs "blindly" as the instruments are being inserted away from the field of view or during percutaneous placement without adequate fluoroscopic or image-guided tracking of the instrument (1,11,24). Finally, technical considerations unique to some minimally invasive procedures such as insufflation during thoracoscopy and laparoscopy pose unique risks not encountered during standard open surgical techniques. A lack of a thorough understanding of the mechanics of insufflation are ultimately responsible for many of the commonly encountered complications during these "gas-dependent" procedures.

Lastly, operative disorientation is a major factor that leads to increased risk during minimally invasive spinal procedures. Whereas anatomical orientation is readily maintained in a wide extensile exposure, it is often difficult even for the seasoned surgeon to know where he is at all times while working through a small 1.5 cm field of view. For techniques such as that of percutaneous discectomy or vertebroplasty where the corridor of approach is under 5 mm in size, wide anatomical visualization is rendered nearly impossible. As such, the "minimalist" surgeon must have an even more initimate knowledge of the anatomy than his or her "traditional" surgical counterparts. Adjunctive visualization and guidance techniques such as endoscopy, fluoroscopy, intraoperative computed tomography (CT), electromyelogram (EMG), and vertebrograms become even more critical in order to avoid inadvertent injury to vital adjacent structures.

II. CERVICAL PROCEDURES

A. Posterior Cervical Procedures

The effectiveness of posterior cervical laminoforaminotomy (LF) for decompression of the lateral recess and neural foramen has been well documented in numerous publications over the last four decades (13,15,33). When compared to standard anterior cervical techniques, the posterior approach via a "keyhole"-type LF may provide better exposure for decompression of the exiting root and for removal of posterior or antero-lateral osteophytes (37,40). The posterior approach also avoids the additional risks of injury to the anterior structures of the neck, including the trachea, esophagus, thyroid, thymus, carotid arteries, jugular veins, vagus nerve, recurrent laryngeal nerve, superior laryngeal nerve, ansa cervicalis, and thoracic duct. Lastly, cervical laminoforaminotomy is an operation that treats the offending pathology without necessitating a fusion. The overall clinical popularity of laminoforaminotomy has also been tempered by technical limitations including a limited surgical view, difficulty in resecting osteophytes, limited visualization of the distal foramen, and often generous epidural venous plexi and associated bleeding (9,27). Furthermore, the muscle dissection often needed to obtain an adequate surgical exposure in the traditional procedure of open laminoforaminotomy has been associated with increased postoperative muscle spasm, neck pain, and recovery time.

Roh et al. described the use of the microendoscopic (MED) system for posterior cervical laminoforaminotomy in human cadaveric spines (40). In those microendoscopic foraminotomy (MEF) validation studies, the authors demonstrated that the average vertical and transverse diameters of the laminotomy defect were essentially identical for both the open and endoscopic groups. The average proportion of facet removal and length of nerve root decompression was actually greater in the MEF than the open decompressions. Since then, Adamson (1) and Khoo et al. (25) have described their surgical experience with MEF in over 125 patients. These procedures were performed in a series of patients in whom a cervical MEF was performed in either a prone or sitting position with the use of a muscle-dilating tubular retractor and endoscopic visualization. These authors separately reported decreased postoperative length of stays, decreased blood loss, and decreased postoperative narcotic pain requirements for the endoscopic patients (25) (Fig. 1).

In terms of the actual operative procedure, prior reports have cited a 2–9% incidence of operative complications, with durotomy and cerebrospinal fluid (CSF) leak being the most common for traditional open posterior cervical laminoforaminotomy (13,33,37,41). Operative blood loss data have ranged from 50–60 cc in Henderson's series (15) to 150–200 cc in earlier studies (41). As such, the MEF technique would seem to represent an improvement over open LF with an average blood loss of only 28.4 cc. Few data on the length of surgery are available from earlier published series. Complications such as incidental durotomy have been reported to have an 8% incidence encountered early on in the MEF learning curve (1,25). Adamson et al., reported two cases of minor durotomy repaired through simple tamponade with Gelfoam and only one superficial wound infection. In the series of Khoo et al., three durotomies (8%) were encountered in the treatment of 25 patients, all managed via tamponade and lumbar drainage only with no long-term sequelae or chronic CSF leakage (25). Since this report, the authors have gone on to perform the MEF procedure in over 200 patients with a 2–3% durotomy incidence. No cases of reported neural injury or paralysis have been reported to date for the procedure. Of note, the majority of incidental dural violations occurred early on in both series learning curves and has been reduced with experience in performing this technique over time. It is important to advise the patients preoperatively of this potential complication and to inform them that there are no adverse clinical consequences in the vast majority of appropriately managed cases (43). Sitting position has been employed in both the traditional and endoscopic versions of the foraminotomy. To date there have been few cases of symptomatic or relevant venous embolism during the procedure (1,15,25,30,41).

During many of these less invasive procedures, percutaneous K-wire or Steinmann pin placement is a common initial step followed by subsequent serial dilatation using a tubular retractor system such as the METRx tubes (Medtronic, Sofamor-Danek, Memphis, TN) (11,12) (Fig. 2). During this approach to the posterior cervical region, the fascia typically encountered is far thicker and tenacious than that found in the thoracodorsal fascia. As a result, excessive force is often needed to persuade the dilators through this dense layer. This can result in inadvertent "plunging" of the dilators if too much force is used. Although this complication has not been reported in the literature, it is often observed during the training of attending surgeons, residents, and fellows. As such, it is often recommended that the posterior cervical fascia be directly cut to avoid injury during serial dilation with the tubes. Direct visualization under lateral fluoroscopy is important to assess the depth of penetration of the K-wire or pin during initial placement. Furthermore, anteroposterior fluoroscopic imaging is also helpful to ensure safe docking on the facet complex. Medial migration can lead to durotomy or direct neural injury to the cord. Lateral migration can result in damage to the exiting nerve root or the

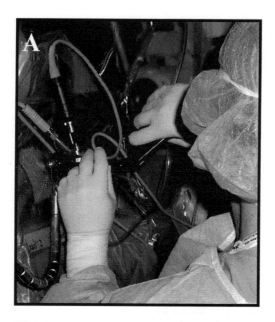

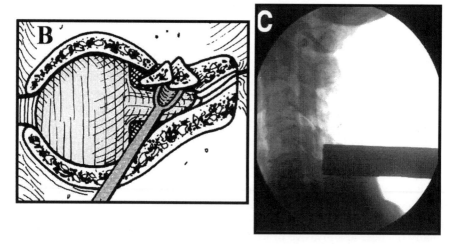

Figure 1 The microendoscopic foraminotomy is performed here with the patient in the prone position with the surgeon working through the access portal under fluoroscopic and endoscopic guidance (A). The medial aspect of the dura, nerve root axilla, and proximal nerve root are decompressed (B). Lateral intraoperative fluoroscopic confirmation of the position of the working cannula is needed to confirm proper placement at the targer level (C).

vertebral artery in the foramen transversarium. Similarly, caution is required to avoid such injury during passage of the sequential tubular dilators.

In addition to foraminotomy, endoscopic and percutaneous techniques have also been used in the posterior cervical spine for wider decompressions including laminectomy, laminoplasty, and percutaneous instrumentation. Experiences with these have been extremely preliminary, with only initial experiences being reported at recent national

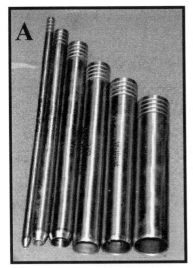

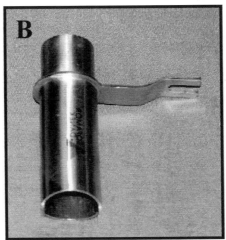

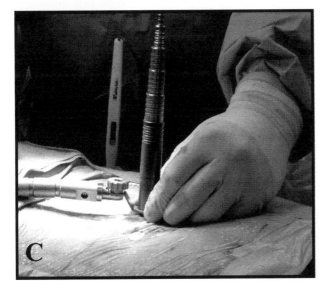

Figure 2 The METRx access system of tubular dilators (Medtronic Sofamor Danek, Memphis, TN) is comprised of sequential metallic tubes (A) and a final working channel that can be attached to a flexible snake-arm type bed-mounted arm (B). From smallest to largest, the tubes are progressively inserted to provide for less traumatic dilation of the musculature (C).

meetings and as technical notes in journals (36,44–46). In these reports, no significant untoward complications were noted or discussed. In all these papers, minimally invasive techniques are being pushed ahead to treat significant cervical pathology, including multilevel stenosis, fracture, deformity, and myelopathy. It is clear that as the spectrum of minimally invasive procedures grows in the posterior cervical spine, so too will the number of reported complications regarding neural injury, vascular injury, misplaced instrumentation, and failed arthrodesis.

B. Anterior Cervical Procedures

Endoscopic anterior cervical procedures have been only rarely reported in the literature due to the difficulty of percutaneously establishing a safe corridor of access. Whereas dorsal cervical approaches do not typically involve vital neurovascular and visceral structures, anterior cervical approaches carry the risk of potential injury to the carotid artery, jugular vein, esophagus, trachea, thyroid, and laryngeal nerves. In this manner, minimally invasive anterior approaches are no different from that of a standard anterior operation. The anterior cervical microforaminotomy and the endoscopic-assisted anterior cervical discectomy and fusion are the two most commonly utilized MIS procedures in the anterior cervical spine.

The anterior cervical microforaminotomy was first described in 1968 by Verbeist for the treatment of vertebral artery insufficiency (42). In essence, a slightly lateralized modification of the standard anterior approaches as described by Cloward, Smith, and Robinson has been advocated when using a minimally invasive method to approach the anterior cervical spine. Popularity of this approach for the treatment of spondylytic cervical radiculopathy has been limited due to concerns of vertebral artery injury and injury to the intervertebral disk complex (39). Most recently, this approach has been popularized in the literature by Jho and Johnson, who applied modern microsurgical techniques and instruments to the operation with great success (18–20).

During this procedure, the uncovertebral joint must often be drilled to fully expose the disk herniation, osteophyte, and nerve root compression. As such, the vertebral artery lies immediately adjacent and lateral to this position thereby placing it as risk (Fig. 3).

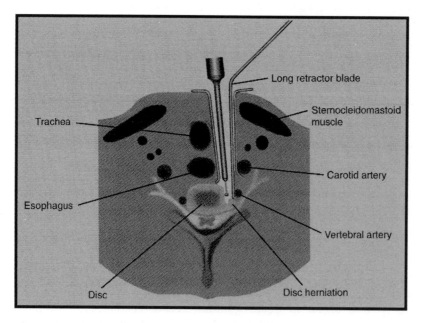

Figure 3 The paramedian corridor of approach seen during a microscopic anterior cervical foraminotomy requires the drilling of the uncovertebral joint to provide access to the lateral disk herniation or osteophyte. During this exposure, the vertebral artery typically lies immediately lateral to this corridor and should be protected through the use of a thin-bladed malleable retractor.

Jho, in his analysis of his experience, identified the three most common sites of vascular injury: at the level of C6-7, lateral to the uncinate process, and at the foramen transversarium (17). As the vertebral artery courses between the transverse process of C7 and the longus colli at the C6-7 level, it is particularly susceptible to injury as it is unshielded. To avoid this complication, Jho and Johnson have both recommended that the longus colli muscle be excised at the level of the C6 transverse process and then reflected as a stump caudally towards the C7 transverse process. In this fashion, the vertebral artery, which lies beneath the longus colli, is gradually exposed in a controlled fashion (18–20). The second most common site of injury, the uncinate process, is typically damaged due to drilling too deeply during the exposure of the lateral disk space. As such, it is prudent to leave a thin layer of cortical bone directly over the vertebral artery during the drilling process. This thin eggshell layer can then be gently removed with a microcurette while avoiding entry into the true transverse foramen (20). A cardinal sign of getting too close to the vertebral artery is brisk venous bleeding from the dense venous plexus that typically surrounds the artery in the transverse foramen. In general, injury to the vertebral artery during this approach can be very serious and extremely difficult to primarily repair due to the limited exposure afforded by the technique (6). Typically, aggressive tamponade with gel foam, bone wax, surgicel, or direct pressure should be undertaken for immediate control of the vessel. In some cases, direct exposure of the vessel by further drilling after tamponade can be attempted if feasible (2,14). To avoid this injury, a deep, thin, malleable retractor can be placed just medial to the vertebral artery during the procedure (20). Particular caution to avoid the perivertebral venous plexus by careful dissection around the uncovertebral joint can also facilitate less bleeding during the procedure.

Other structures at risk during anterior cervical microforaminotomy include the sympathetic chain and stellate ganglion. As these structures lie immediately anterior to the longus colli, they can be injured during section of the muscle as mentioned above or during overly aggressive retraction of the muscle strap. This can result in a Horner's syndrome. Careful attention to gradually retract the longus colli laterally and to limit cautery and section of the muscle can help to avoid these untoward complications.

As the anterior cervical microforaminotomy seeks to focally decompress the lateral nerve root without a fusion procedure, certain other unique complications have been encountered due to the technique itself. Incomplete decompression of the nerve root is often seen during the learning curve as the surgeon does not fully appreciate the three dimensional spatial relationship of the uncovertebral joint, lateral disk anulus, disk fragment, osteophyte, and nerve root. As such, the novice surgeon can often err either too medially or, more commonly, too lateral, thereby missing the actual pathological compressive point. Time spent in a cadaver lab setting to fully comprehend this regional anatomy as seen through a narrow corridor is the best way to circumvent this mistake. In addition, three-dimensional preoperative magnetic resonance imaging (MRI) and CT imaging can help to guide and focally direct the decompression as well. Poor patient selection can also result in poor outcomes and sequelae after anterior microforaminotomy. For patients with mechanical neck pain and advanced disk degeneration, removal of the uncovertebral joint may exacerbate the patients' symptoms due to removal of supporting tissue. Indeed, patients with asymptomatic contralateral foraminal narrowing have developed new postoperative contralateral radicular symptoms after anterior foraminotomy most likely due to the altered regional biomechanics and increased local hypermobility (20).

III. POSTERIOR LUMBAR PROCEDURES

In 1997 the Micro Endoscopic Discectomy (MED) system was introduced which allowed spinal surgeons to reliably decompress a symptomatic lumbar nerve root via an endoscopic, minimally invasive surgical (MIS) approach (11). Since January 1997, more than 6000 MED procedures have been performed in more than 500 institutions. This system offers many advantages over other MIS lumbar discectomy techniques described previously by reducing tissue trauma, allowing direct visualization of the nerve root and disk pathology, and allowing bony decompression. In addition, the system comes with long tapered instrumentation designed specifically for use in small working space. The approach used is anatomically familiar to spine surgeons, and excellent clinical results have been achieved on an outpatient surgical basis.

However, there were limitations to the initial MED system. The endoscope was not reusable, image quality was inconsistent, and the working space within the tubular retractor was limited. The next-generation system, called the METRx^{TM}, was developed to address these limitations. Compared to the MED system, the METRx system has additional advantages, including increased image quality, decreased endoscopic diameter, variable tubular retractor size, increased available working room within the tubular retractor, and decreased per-case cost. Unlike percutaneous approaches, the METRx system allows surgeons to address not only contained lumbar disk herniations, but also sequestered disk fragments and lateral recess stenosis. A prospective multicenter clinical study has shown the efficacy of this system in treating lumbar disk disease (3). The modularity of the METRx system also allows for the development of expanded application beyond lumbar nerve root decompression. To date, laminotomy, laminectomy, total discectomy, interbody fusion, schwannoma resection, and dural arteriovenousfistula ligation have all been performed through these tubes (24,26). With the advent of tubes designed for use with an operating microscope, the specific benefit of these techniques has become clear in that tubular dilatation of the dorsal musculoligamentous complex is associated with decreased pain and a more rapid return to function (16) (Fig. 2C).

The METRx system is very effective in performing microendoscopic lumbar discectomy on an ambulatory basis. However, there is a learning curve to using the system efficiently and safely. Since most surgeons use an operative microscope or loop magnification, looking up at a video monitor to perform microdiscectomy at first seems cumbersome. As the surgeon becomes more proficient, operative times decrease and overall satisfaction with this system increases. With the use of the METRx MD System of tubes, the operating microscope can be used in a standard fashion. In general, patients are very satisfied with the minimally invasive outcome.

The potential complications using the METRx system are not different from those encountered performing standard microdiscectomy. The most frequently stated risks are bleeding, neurological damage, damage to the surrounding soft tissue, and infection. In the early learning period there may be a slightly higher incidence of dural tears, but these can be avoided with careful attention to operative technique. Dural tears, if they occur, should be repaired primarily if possible; if not, then a small piece of DuraGen dural graft matrix (Integra NeuroSciences, Plainsboro, NJ) covered with fibrin glue can be applied. Early on in the learning curve, the initial steps of Steinmann pin docking can result in accidental dural violation. This avoidable injury can be prevented by using real-time lateral and anteroposterior fluoroscopy to ensure proper depth and targeting of the pin. Furthermore, avoidance of excessive force during passage of the dilators will prevent accidental "slippage" of the tubes deeper than desired. The potential for accidental cauda equina injury during overly aggressive placement of the METRx tubular dilators exists if caution is not exercised during their application.

Additional risks specific to the METRx system can include instrument malfunction, such as bending, fragmentation, loosening, and/or breakage (whole or partial). Since this is a delicate instrument, it is important not to force the endoscope into position on the tubular retractor. The locking lever that attaches the endoscope system to the tubular retractor must be fully released before rotating the endoscope into position on the tubular retractor. Also, to prevent inadvertently hitting the endoscope system during the procedure, the locking arm affixed to the operative table and METRx system and cables needs to be positioned out of the surgeon's way. High-energy radiation light emitted from the illuminating fiber at the distal end of the scope may give rise to temperatures exceeding 41°C within 8 mm in front of the scope. Therefore, do not leave the endoscope tip in direct contact with the patient's tissue or combustible materials, or burns may result.

The first 100 patients to undergo lumbar METRx MED were reported in 1997 (11). The versatility of this technique is seen in its ability to treat various lumbar disk pathology including far lateral disk herniations (11 patients), concomitant lateral recess stenosis (16 patients), and noncontained disk herniation (48 patients). Significant savings are reflected in reduced operative times with case proficiency (75 minutes last 30 cases), reduced hospital stays (mean 9.5 hours), and short return to work time (mean 20 days). Complications were few, including three (3%) patients with dural tears, all of which were repaired intra operatively and one patient with a delayed pseudomeningocele formation. Two patients had disk herniation recurrence. Using the modified Macnab criteria to grade patient outcome with a mean follow-up of 43 months (range 35–50 months), 85% had excellent, 11% good, 1% fair, and 3% poor outcome.

In a series of 87 patients treated via an operating microscope and tubular retractor, Hilton reported an overall 92% good outcome rate. There were two (2.2%) cases of dural tear and CSF leaks treated via fibrin glue, tight fascial closure, and bedrest with no long-term sequelae (16). He also observed that 10 patients complained of minor lumbar discomfort at the operative site, with some mild residual numbness at the incision. In the report of Perez-Cruet et al. (35) on 150 patients treated via the MED/METRx system, they observed eight total dural tears (5.3%), one delayed pseudomeningocele, one superficial wound infection, and four recurrent herniated disks. Aside from complications during initial tubular dilatation, complications of these procedures are essentially identical to those encountered during traditional open microdiscectomy and laminotomy. Comparing the rate of durotomy using a tubular retractor to that of a standard open operation, we found the rates of 2–5% to be quite comparable.

With more extensive procedures such as laminectomy for lumbar stenosis, it would be expected that the risk of durotomy and neural injury would increase given the more difficult nature of the pathology. Khoo and Fessler reported a prospective, non-randomized comparison of patients undergoing either open hemilaminotomy versus minimally invasive hemilaminotomy for the treatment of lumbar stenosis (24). The operative time for a single-level MEDL (microendoscopic dissection and hemilaminotomy) procedure ranged from 45 to 240 minutes, with an average of 109 minutes. This was only slightly longer than the 88-minute (range 60–198 min) mean operative time for the open control group and reflects the learning curve of the MEDL procedure. The opposite relationship was seen, however, in terms of the average operative blood loss per operated level: 68 cc (range 15–300cc) for the MEDL group and 193 cc (75–1000 cc) for the open group. No patients in the MEDL group required intraoperative or postoperative transfusions, whereas two control patients received 1 unit of packed red blood cells each. There were no cases of neural injury associated with either surgical group. For the MEDL group, there were 4 cases of dural violation and cerebrospinal fluid leak requiring 1–2 days of lumbar drainage. No long-term sequelae, delayed leaks, fluid collections, or pseudomeningoceles were seen. In the control group there were two cases of dural violation, with one case requiring an open repair of a chronic CSF collection. To date there have been no cases of iatrogenic or delayed spinal instability requiring fusion in the MEDL group, whereas three patients in the control group went on to have fusions. Palmer et al., in their experience with minimally invasive decompressive hemilaminotomy, observed similar results (34).

IV. SUMMARY

Minimally invasive spinal surgery represents an exciting evolution of traditional operative techniques. By achieving classical surgical objectives through less invasive corridors of access, patients can experience significantly reduced postoperative pain and disability, However, with such minimalism comes many technical challenges. These include constrained operative corridors, heightened anatomical disorientation, loss of three-dimensional visualization, a need for insufflation, a risk of inadvertent "blind" injury, and kinesthetic limitations of minimally invasive surgical tools. This myriad of operative factors leads to a significant relearning curve of common open surgical procedures for even the most experienced spinal surgeon. Inanimate labs, cadaver labs, animal labs, and performing surgery with an experienced thoracoscopic spine surgeon are highly recommended. Surgeons must develop skills of "tubeology"/"scopeology" (e.g., keeping the ports clean, keeping the scope clean, working away from the lens, keeping the scope stable, orienting the scope correctly), endoscopic navigation, and triangulation. In a sequential fashion, the training surgeon must overcome the various limitations of minimally invasive spinal procedures: safe placement of portals, narrow working corridors, restricted operative ergonomics, two-dimensional visualization, anatomical disorientation, unfamiliar surgical instruments, and specialized devices. Ultimately, a surgeon who wishes to become adept at minimally invasive spinal surgery must modify his or her existing surgical proficiencies as well as acquire a whole new operative skill set. Only through such a dedicated training process can the risk of complications during such "minimalist" procedures be avoided.

REFERENCES

1. Adamson TE. Microendoscopic posterior cervical laminoforaminotomy for unilateral radiculopathy: results of a new technique in 100 cases. J Neurosurg 2001; 95(suppl 1):51–57.
2. An HS, Simeone FA. Complications in cervical disk surgery. In: Balderston RA, An HS, eds. Complications in Spinal Surgery. Philadelphia: W.B. Saunders Co., 1991:41–59.
3. Brayda-Bruno M, Cinnella P. Posterior endoscopic discectomy (and other procedures). Eur Spine J. 2000; 9(suppl 1):S24–S29.
4. Chiras J. Percutaneous vertebral surgery: techniques and indications. J Neuroradiol 1997; 24:45–52.
5. Cortet B, Cotton A, Boutry R, Flipo RM, Duquesnoy B, Chastanet P, Delcambre B. Percutaneous vertebroplasty in the treatment of osteoporotic verterbral compression fractures: An open prospective study. J Rheumatol 1999; 26:2222–2228.

6. Cosgrove GR, Theron J. Vertebral arteriovenous fistula following anterior cervical spine surgery: report of two cases. J Neurosurg 1987; 66:297–299.
7. Cotton A, Dewatre F, Cortet B, Assaker R, Leblond D, DuquesnoyB, Chastanet P, Clarisse J. Percutaneous vertebroplasty for osteolytic metastases and myeloma: effects of the percentage of lesion filling and the leakage of methyl methacrylate at clinical follow-up. Radiology 1996; 200:525–530.
8. Ditsworth DA. Endoscopic transforaminal lumbar discectomy and reconfiguration: a postero-lateral approach into the spinal canal. Surg Neurol 1998; 49:588–598.
9. Ebersolf MJ, Raynor RB, Bovis GK, et al. Cervical laminotomy, laminectomy, laminoplasty, and foraminotomy. In: Benzel EC, ed. Spine Surgery: Techniques, Complication Avoidance and Management. Philadelphia: Churchill Livingstone, 1999; 251–253.
10. Fessler RG, Khoo LT. Minimally-invasive cervical microendoscopic foraminotomy: an initial clinical experience. Neurosurg 2002; 51(suppl 2):36–45.
11. Foley KT, Smith MM. Microendoscopic discectomy. Tech Neurosurg 1997; 3:301–307.
12. Foley KT, Gupta SK, Justis JR, Sherman MC. Percutaneous pedicle screw fixation of the lumbar spine. Neurosurg Focus 2001; 10:1–8.
13. Frykholm R. Cervical nerve root compression resulting from disk degeneration and root sleeve fibrosis. Acta Chir Scand 1951; 160:1–149.
14. Golfinos JG, Dickman CA, Zabramski JM, Sonntag VKH, Spetzler RF. Repair of vertebral artery injury during anterior cervical decompression. Spine 1994; 19: 2552–2556.
15. Henderson CM, Hennessy RG, Shuey HJ, Shackelford EG. Posterior-lateral foraminotomy as an exclusive operative technique for cervical radiculopathy: a review of 846 consecutively operated cases. Neurosurgery 1983; 13:504–521.
16. Hilton DL. Microdiscectomy with a minimally invasive tubular retractor. In: Perez-Cruet MJ, Fessler RG, eds. Outpatient Spinal Surgery. St. Louis: Quality Medical Publishing Inc., 2002: 159–170.
17. Jenson ML. Percutaneous polymethylmethacrylate vertebroplasty in the treatment of osteoporotic vertebral body compression fractures: technical aspects. AJNR Am J Neuroradiol 1997; 18:1897–1904.
18. Jho HD. Microsurgical anterior cervical foraminotomy for radiculopathy: a new approach to cervical disk herniation. J Neurosurg 1996; 84:155–160.
19. Jho HD. Decompression via microsurgical anterior foraminotomy for cervical spondylytic myelopathy: technical note. J Neurosurg 1997; 86:297–302.
20. Johnson JP, Filler AG, McBride DQ, Batzdorf U. Anterior cervical foraminotomy for unilateral radicular disease. Spine 2000; 25:905–909.
21. Johnson JP, Obasi C, Hahn MS, Glatleider P. Endoscopic thoracic sympathectomy. J Neurosurg 1999; 91:90–91.
22. Kambin P, Gellman H. Percutaneous lateral discectomy of the lumbar spine: a preliminary report. Clin Orthop 1983; 174:127–132.
23. Khoo LT, Beisse R, Potulski M. Thoracoscopic-assisted treatment of thoracic and lumbar fractures: a series of 371 consecutive cases. Neurosurg 2002; 51(suppl 2):105–117.
24. Khoo LT, Fessler RG. Microendoscopic decompressive laminotomy for the treatment of lumbar stenosis. Neurosurg 2002; 51(suppl 2):146–154.
25. Khoo LT, Laich DT, Perez-Cruet MJ, Fessler RG. Posterior cervical microendoscopic foraminotomy. In: Perez-Cruet MJ, Fessler RG, eds. Outpatient Spinal Surgery. St. Louis: Quality Medical Publishing Inc., 2002:71–93.
26. Khoo LT, Palmer S, Laich DT. Minimally invasive percutaneous posterior lumbar interbody fusion. Neurosurg 2002; 51(suppl 2):166–181.
27. Kubo Y, Waga S, Kojima T, et al. Microsurgical anatomy of the lower cervical spine and cord. Neurosurgery 1994; 34:895–902.
28. Liebschner MAK, Rosenberg WS, Keaveny TM. Effects of bone cement volume and distribution on vertebral stiffness after vertebroplasty. Spine 2000; 26:1547–1554.

29. Lew SM, Mehalic TF, Fagone KL. Transforaminal percutaneous endoscopic discectomy in the treatment of far-lateral and foraminal lumbar disk herniations. J Neurosurg 2001; 94(suppl 2):216–220.

30. Losasso TJ, Muzzi DA, Dietz NM, Cucchiara RF. Fifty percent nitrous oxide does not increase the risk of venous air embolism in neurosurgical patients operated upon in the sitting position. Anesthesiology 1992; 77:21–30.

31. Matthews HH. Transforaminal endoscopic microdiscectomy. Neurosurg Clin North Am 1996; 7:59–63.

32. Mayers HM, Brock M. Percutaneous endoscopic discectomy: surgical technique and preliminary results compared to microsurgical discectomy. J Neurosurg 1993; 78:216–225.

33. Murphey F, Simmons JCH, Brunson B. Cervical treatment of laterally ruptured cervical disks: review of 648 cases, 1939–1972. J Neurosurg 1973; 38:679–683.

34. Palmer S, Turner R, Palmer R. Bilateral decompression of lumbar spinal stenosis involving a unilateral approach with microscope and tubulat retractor system. J Neurosurg 2002; 97(2 suppl):L213–L217.

35. Perez-Cruet MJ, Foley KT, Isaacs RE, Rice-Wyllie L, Smith MM, Fessler RG. Micro-endoscopic lumbar discectomy: technical note. Neurosurgery 2002; 51(suppl 2):129–136.

36. Perez-Cruet MJ, Sandhu FA, Kelly K, Fessler RG. Minimally invasive multi-level decompressive cervical laminectomy. Presented at 19th Annual Meeting of the AANS/CNS Section on Disorders of the Spine and Peripheral Nerves, March 5, 2003.

37. Raynor R. Anterior or posterior approach to the cervical spine: an anatomical and radiographic evaluation and comparison. Neurosurgery 1983; 12:7–13.

38. Regan JJ, Guyer RD. Endoscopic techniques in spinal surgery. Clin Orthop 1997; 335:122–139.

39. Robinson R, Smith G. Anterolateral cervical disk removal and interbody fusion for cervical disk syndrome. Bull Johns Hopkins Hosp 1955; 96:223–224.

40. Roh SW, Kim DH, Cardoso AC, Fessler RG. Endoscopic foraminotomy using MED system in cadaveric specimens. Spine 2000; 25(2):260–264.

41. Scoville WB, Whitcomb BB. Lateral rupture of cervical intervertebral disks. Postgrad Med 1966; 39:174–180.

42. Verbeist H. A lateral approach to the cervical spine: technique and indications. J Neurosurg 1968; 28:191–203.

43. Wang JC, Bohlman HH, Riew KD. Dural tears secondary to operations on the lumbar spine: management and results after a two-year minimum follow-up of eighty-eight patients. J Bone Joint Surg Am 1998; 80A:1728–1732.

44. Wang MY, Green BA, Coscarella E, Baskaya MK, Levi AD, Guest JD. Minimally invasive cervical expansile laminoplasty: an initial cadaveric study. Neurosurgery 2003; 52(2):370–373.

45. Wang MY, Green BA, Oh BC, Levi AD, Gruen JP. Minimally invasive cervical expansile laminoplasty: cadaveric study and initial clinical results. Presented at 19th Annual Meeting of the AANS/CNS Section on Disorders of the Spine and Peripheral Nerves, March 5, 2003.

46. Wang MY, Prusmack CJ, Green BA, Gruen JP, Levi AD. Minimally invasive lateral mass screws in the treatment of cervical facet dislocations: technical note. Neurosurgery 2003; 52(2):444–448.

33

Complications of Minimally Invasive Spinal Surgery—Part II: Thoracoscopy

John J. Regan and Neel Anand
Cedar-Sinai Institute for Spinal Disorders, Los Angeles, California, U.S.A.

Larry T. Khoo and Anthony Virella
UCLA Medical Center, Los Angeles, California, U.S.A.

Michael A. Pahl and Alexander R. Vaccaro
Thomas Jefferson University and the Rothman Institute, Philadelphia, Pennsylvania, U.S.A.

I. INTRODUCTION

A variety of surgical techniques have traditionally been used to deal with thoracic spinal disorders and deformity They include laminectomy, pediculectomy, costotransversectomy, lateral extracavitary, transverse arthropediculectomy, transthoracic-transpleural thoracotomy, and thoracoscopy (12,19,21,28,29,35,49,55,56). Fessler and Sturgill, based on a review of the literature over the last 60 years, compared relative rates of morbidity and mortality in surgical approaches for thoracic discectomy. They noted that mortality dropped to nearly zero after development of anterior and posterolateral approaches and suggested that laminectomy does not provide adequate access for the safe removal of these lesions (21). Bohlman and Zdeblick reported excellent results in 16 of 19 patients undergoing an anterior approach for thoracic disk removal. They recommended the transthoracic over the costotransversectomy approach for anterior decompression of a herniated thoracic disk, as it greatly improved visualization of the anatomical structures (5). However, this technique involves the use of a thoracotomy with rib resection and wide bony resection of vertebral structures to reach the anterior spinal canal. These procedures, whether extrapleural or intrapleural, result in significant perioperative morbidity secondary to pain, difficult ventilation, shoulder girdle dysfunction, and wound-healing problems (20,41,58,59).

The first reported application of video-assisted thoracoscopic surgery (VATS) to problems of the thoracic spine was in 1993 (33). Comparisons between thoracoscopy and open thoracotomy have demonstrated improvement in postoperative pain, shoulder girdle function and morbidity, reduced blood loss, time required in an intensive care unit, and overall hospital stay when endoscopic techniques were employed (27,47).

Mangione et al. (36) compared thoracoscopy with thoracotomy in thoracic spinal surgery. A series of 29 patients undergoing thoracoscopy for a spinal disorder was matched regarding the etiology of spine disease and type of surgical procedure with 24 patients undergoing open thoracotomy. This matching procedure yielded two similar groups of 20 patients. The criteria used for evaluation were duration of the procedure, blood loss, intraoperative complications, duration of stay in postoperative intensive care, duration and yield of pleural drainage, time to return to the upright position, duration of use of WHO grade 3 analgesics (morphine derivatives), postoperative complications, and the length of hospitalization. The authors showed a significant difference in three parameters: the duration of the procedure (thoracotomy, 172 min; thoracoscopy, 246 min; $p < 0.006$), intraoperative bleeding (thoracotomy, 837 mL; thoracoscopy, 447 mL; $p < 0.0009$), and duration of use of WHO grade 3 analgesics (thoracotomy, 4.5 days; thoracoscopy, 2.3 days; $p = 0.011$). There was no difference in intra- or postoperative complication rates between the two methods. The authors concluded that their data confirms the usefulness of thoracoscopy, which is less traumatizing, less hemorrhagic, and causes no more complications than open thoracotomy. The longer operative duration was felt to be a minor drawback that should shorten with experience and the development of specific instrumentation modifications.

Newton et al. (42) compared early outcomes and cost of thoracoscopic and open thoracotomy approaches for anterior release and fusion in pediatric spinal deformity. They reported that percent curve correction was similar between the thoracoscopic and open methods: scoliosis 56% and 60%, respectively; kyphosis, 88% and 94%, respectively. The blood loss and complication rates were similar between the two groups; however, the chest tube output was greater in the thoracoscopic group. The length of hospital stay was not reduced, and the cost of the open procedure was 29% less than the thoracoscopic approach. They also noted that the minimally invasive thoracoscopic approach avoided cutting the chest/shoulder musculature, greatly decreasing the morbidity of anterior spinal surgery.

Cunningham et al. (12) did a comparative radiographic, biomechanical, and histological analysis in a sheep model of VATS versus open thoracotomy for anterior thoracic spinal fusion. They concluded that thoracic interbody spinal fusions performed by thoracoscopy demonstrated histological, biomechanical, and radiographic equivalence to those performed by a thoracotomy approach. However, in the endoscopy group they noted that intraoperative complications causing longer operative times, higher estimated blood loss, and increased animal morbidity indicated a substantial learning curve associated with the adoption of this surgical technique.

Anand and Regan (1) reported a comprehensive, large consecutive series of patients treated with VATS for symptomatic thoracic disk herniation. They presented a new classification system and long-term functional outcome of VATS for refractory symptomatic thoracic disk disease. Patients were grouped according to their initial presenting symptoms and classified into one of five grades (Table 1). The leg pain in Grade 3B patients is often described as a dull aching pain without any specific dermatomal pattern, suggesting cord rather than upper lumbar root compression. All patients with leg pain in Anand and Regan's (1) series were patients with thoracic disk herniations below T6-7.

Long-term patient satisfaction was best seen in myelopathic (Grade 4) patients, followed by patients with axial and leg pain (grade 3B), then by patients with axial and thoracic radicular pain (Grade 3A), followed by patients with pure axial pain (Grade 1) and lastly pure thoracic radicular pain (Grade 2). Significant improvement in Oswestry functional scores at long-term follow-up with objective clinical success (greater than 20% improvement in Oswestry Score) was most marked in Grade 4 patients, followed by Grade 3A, Grade 3B, and Grade 1. Anand and Regan felt that the clinical classification

Table 1 Clinical Grades of Thoracic Disk Disease

Grade	Presenting symptoms
Grade 1	Predominant thoracic central (axial) pain
Grade 2	Predominant thoracic radicular pain
Grade 3A	Significant axial and thoracic radicular pain
Grade 3B	Significant axial and lower leg pain with or without thoracic radicular pain
Grade 4	Myelopathy, but no significant motor weakness
Grade 5	Paretic/Paralytic (significant motor weakness)

system helped in differentiating various presentations of thoracic disk disease and their final outcome. They also stated that patients with no prior spinal surgery and patients with Oswestry Disability Scores greater than 50 also showed significant improvement in long-term functional scores with the percentage improvement in Oswestry Disability Scores correlating with patient satisfaction rather than absolute scores at follow-up.

The authors further concluded that patients with pure thoracic radicular symptoms should be cautioned about the possibility of developing axial pain in the future. Similarly, patients with pure axial pain should be cautioned about postoperative thoracic radicular pain. They had an overall acceptable long-term outcome with an 84% subjective satisfaction rate, with objective clinical success achieved in 70% of patients.

Lately, thoracoscopy has been popular as an approach to various disorders such as scoliosis, burst fractures, sympathectomy, thoracic corpectomy, and infections.

II. ANTERIOR THORACIC PROCEDURES

Thoracoscopic spine surgery carries with it potential complications similar to those seen with open procedures. The benefits of this minimally invasive option include decreased postoperative pain, decreased pulmonary complications, and decreased intercostal neuralgia and scapular dysfunction (15,16,23). Potential complications of this technology include problems with port placement and access, anesthesia, patient positioning, and accurate manipulation of lengthy unfamiliar instruments with potential injury to the thoracic vascular structures and/or lung parenchyma (Fig. 1). Specialized training, preferably in the form of a formal fellowship, should be sought by individuals wishing to master these techniques (38,39,61).

Several comorbid conditions increase the likelihood that conversion to an open procedure will be necessary. These include prior thoracic surgery with resultant lung scarring and severely distorted anatomy such as that seen in kyphoscoliosis. The surgeon must be prepared to perform an open thoracotomy, as obtaining optimum exposure is vital to a successful surgical procedure.

Anesthesia during minimally invasive thoracoscopic procedures also carries with it inherent risks. During thoracoscopic surgery these risks relate mainly to single lung ventilation. Patients with a smoking history and chronic obstructive pulmonary disease should have a thorough preoperative evaluation, which includes pulmonary function tests, arterial blood gas evaluation, and cardiac workup. In patients with severe spinal deformity, surgery is usually performed on the convex side, necessitating ventilation through the smaller lung on the concave side. In children, selective blocking of specific

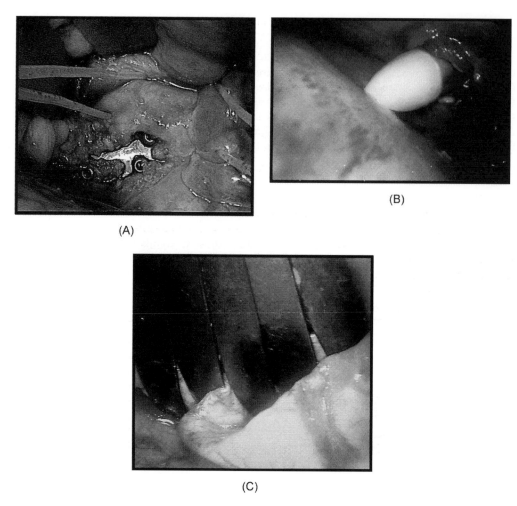

(A)

(B)

(C)

Figure 1 As in standard open thoracotomy, the structures of the chest and proximal abdomen are at risk for inadvertent injury. During thorascopic procedures, injury can often occur beyond the field of view or from accidental injury during retraction to the aorta (A), liver parenchyma (B), and lung parenchyma (C).

bronchi while ventilating adjacent bronchi can provide adequate space to perform the procedure while maximizing the amount of lung tissue being ventilated. Placement of the double lumen endotrachial tube can be fraught with complications. The tube may be malpositioned by being placed either too deep or too shallow with respect to the carina. The bronchial mucosa can also be injured via overinflation of the cuff. Underinflation of the cuff can lead to an air leak and further compromise the operative field (16).

Intraoperative arterial oxygen saturation under 90% should prompt an immediate pause in the surgical procedure. Fiberoscopy should then be utilized to confirm the position of the tube and to rule out migration of the tube during patient set-up and positioning. The resultant ventilation-perfusion mismatch that occurs with single-lung ventilation is more likely to occur in younger patients without structural pulmonary disease. Cardiovascular collapse can occur during insufflation to collapse the isolated lung.

Therefore, insufflation pressures should be kept below 15 mmHg in order to prevent mediastinal compression leading to cardiac tamponade and decreased cardiac output. Patients with central venous pressures (CVP) of < 5 mm Hg are especially prone to this complication. Therefore, albumin and normal saline are routinely used during surgery to maintain the CVP at 8–10 mmHg. Fatal CO_2 embolism may also occur with positive pressure ventilation.

Copious secretions may accumulate in the airways secondary to prolonged nonventilation of one lung. Therefore, aggressive pulmonary toilet should be performed in order to prevent atelectasis and pneumonia in the dependent lung. Furthermore, the use of intraoperative positive end-expiratory pressure on the ventilated lung and continuous positive airway pressure on the nonventilated lung can significantly reduce these complications (15).

Patients are usually placed in the lateral decubitis position. Therefore, adequate padding in the form of axillary rolls under the chest may help to minimize nerve damage and brachial plexus injuries. Overabduction of the arm should also be minimized. Other potential pressure points, such as the common peroneal nerve at the head of the fibula, should also be protected with padding to avoid iatrogenic postoperative neuropathies.

Complications can also occur during initial port placement. The initial port is the only port that is placed without direct vision. This can result in direct injury to the lung parenchyma and other vascular structures in the chest. Postoperative lung scarring from previous surgeries can result in adhesions connecting the lung to the chest wall, further increasing the likelihood of an injury. Therefore, a circumferential sweep with a gloved finger should be performed through the port site to release any adhesions before placement of the port. All subsequent ports should be placed under direct endoscopic vision to further minimize the increased risks of injury with the passage of additional ports.

Postoperative intercostal neuralgia can result from injury to the structures in the neurovascular bundle located on the inferior aspect of the rib. The use of rigid scopes can lead to an increase incidence of this phenomena. In the event of uncontrollable bleeding, a Foley catheter can be inserted into the port and the balloon can be inflated to tamponade the bleeding. If this fails to control the bleeding, one must be prepared to perform a formal thoracotomy to localize the source.

The use of endoscopic instruments can sometimes be traumatic to lung tissue and to the large vessels in the chest cavity, leading to postoperative air leaks and excessive intraoperative bleeding. A qualified thoracic surgeon should be consulted to repair excessive lung injury, which is outside the scope of practice for the neurosurgeon or orthopedic surgeon. The movement of endoscopic instruments within the chest cavity should be smooth and controlled in order to minimize the risks of injury to the neural and vascular elements of the pleural cavity. Fractured segments of endoscopic instruments can usually be retrieved endoscopically, but conversion to a formal thoracotomy is sometimes necessary to resolve this often frustrating complication. The tip of the endoscope can get quite hot secondary to the light source; therefore, great care should be taken when introducing the instrument, which should be placed with the tip up when outside the thoracic cavity. The risks of an intraoperative explosion also exists when using electrocautery and concentrated oxygen in a confined space. As mentioned previously, manipulation of the instruments should be done under direct vision, and caution should be used when introducing and removing these devices from the chest cavity. Infections are a ubiquitous complication of all surgery, including thoracoscopic spine surgery. Careful attention should be paid to the details of proper sterile surgical technique. The instruments need to be sterilized in a standardized fashion.

Thoracoscopic discectomy is a common surgical procedure (64). The management of a symptomatic disk herniation is usually conservative, but surgery should be reserved for patients who have failed conservative management and who have radiographic and clinically concomitant evidence of thoracic radiculopathy and/or myelopathy. Advances in instrumentation have facilitated the treatment of this condition (33,46,49,50).

The relative infrequency of symptomatic thoracic disk herniations and steep learning curves associated with thoracoscopy have limited its widespread use in the removal of a symptomatic disk herniation. Complication rates involving thoracoscopy vary per series. Most studies to date have concurred that thoracoscopic procedures have a lower incidence of costovertebral neuralgia, postoperative respiratory complications, and chest pain than traditional open procedures (16,51).

Thoracoscopic sympathectomy can result in a number of complications, some of which are related to injury of the sympathetic chain. These include compensatory hyperhidrosis syndrome (CHS), pneumothorax, vascular injury, intercostal neuralgia, and gustatory sweating. CHS results in increased sweating in nondenervated areas, including the back, abdomen, legs, and chest (26,54). The incidence of CHS after thoracic sympathectomy is somewhere between 40 and 73%. Rarely is this condition disabling, and most patients are satisfied with the resolution of their palmar hyperhidrosis.

Horner's syndrome can be prevented by sparing the rostral portion of the stellate ganglia. Intraoperative identification of the rostral stellate ganglion can be achieved by electrically stimulating the stellate ganglia while having an observer evaluate the pupil. Other complications tend to be more common with an open thoracotomy approach. Intercostal neuralgia can occur with injury to the neurovascular bundle on the inferior aspect of the rib. Pneumothorax is rare providing the visceral lung pleura is preserved during the procedure. The incidence of gustatory sweating is estimated to be 1–2% and is thought to result from aberrant synapses between sympathetic fibers and the vagus nerve (26). Major vascular injury is not common, but when it occurs it can be life threatening and requires immediate conversion to an open thoracotomy.

III. COMPLICATIONS RELATED TO THE APPROACH

Complications from a thoracoscopic approach to the spine are most often attributed to the learning curve of the surgeon; however, the entire operative team becomes exposed to the challenges of performing this procedure. As with any new technology, the surgeon and the operative team need to familiarize themselves with the new equipment and setup. There exists a learning curve for the anesthesiologists and nursing staff. Double-lumen endotracheal tube intubation is required with single-lung ventilation of the down lung during the procedure. A lateral decubitus approach is most commonly used. Prone thoracoscopy has been advocated for simultaneous anterior and posterior access to the thoracic spine. Supine thoracoscopy has also been advocated for thoracic sympathectomies.

Sucato et al. (57) reported a case of an 11-year-old patient with severe scoliosis who developed air in both chest cavities, mediastinum, peritoneum, retroperitoneum, and subcutaneous tissue after intubation with a double-lumen endotracheal tube. There also exists a learning curve for the anesthesiologist to become adept at obtaining single-lung ventilation and managing this throughout the operative procedure.

McAfee et al. (57) reported a complication in 16 out of 78 (20.5%) patients undergoing VATS. Six patients experienced intercostal neuralgia, 5 atelectasis, 2 excessive blood loss of more than 2500 cc, one patient was converted to an open thoracotomy, one patient had penetration of the hemidiaphragm from thoracoport in a patient with previous empyema, and one patient had transient hemiparesis related to spinal stenosis at a different vertebral level due to operative positioning. There were no cases of permanent iatrogenic neurological deficit and no cases of spinal wound infection in the above series.

Huang et al. (25) reported a series of 90 consecutive patients undergoing thoracoscopic spinal surgery, in which 30 complications were noted in 22 patients (24.4%). Two fatal complications occurred, resulting from massive blood transfusion in one case and postoperative pneumonia in another. Other nonfatal complications included four cases of transient intercostal neuralgia, three superficial wound infections, three cases of pharyngeal pain, two cases of lung atelectasis, two cases of persistent pneumothorax, two cases of subcutaneous emphysema, one inadvertent pericardial penetration due to adhesion, one chylothorax that resolved after conservative management, one vertebral screw malposition, and one graft dislodgement that needed late revision surgery. Three patients required ventilatory support for longer than 72 hours. Five patients with spinal metastases had an estimated intraoperative blood loss of more than 2000 mL. No injury to the internal organs or spinal cord was observed. There were four conversions to open procedures in two cases of severe pleural adhesions and two patients who tolerated one-lung ventilation poorly.

Anand and Regan reported on 21 patients (21%) who developed perioperative complications, all of which resolved uneventfully (1) (Table 2). No patient's neurological status worsened. There were no wound problems, dural tears, or postoperative infections. One patient with atelectasis also had a pneumothorax, while another with atelectasis had an ileus. One patient with severe intercostal neuralgia had decreased respiratory effort, developed pneumonia, and needed an epidural catheter for relief of pain. Four patients with intercostal neuralgia needed intercostal blocks to control the pain. All cases of postoperative intercostal neuralgia occurred early in the series. Avoidance of levering against the ribs as well as switching from a rigid to soft flexible plastic trocars has resulted in a decline in the incidence of postoperative intercostal neuralgia. None of the patients who underwent surgery with soft flexible trocars needed intercostal blocks to control postoperative pain. A total of five patients were reoperated on, four of whom

Table 2 Complications of Thoracoscopy

Perioperative complication	No. of patients
Pleuritic pain and pleural effusion	2
Pneumothorax	5
Atelectasis	6
Pneumonia	2
Intercostal neuralgia	6
Ileus	1
2500 cc blood loss	1
Converted to open	1

Source: Ref. 1.

had a secondary fusion procedure done for intractable axial pain at involved levels that were concordant on provocative discography. One patient, who had fusion with a BAK cage, developed a pseudarthrosis and was reoperated through a mini-thoracotomy. The cage was removed and autogenous rib was used to augment the fusion.

Dickman reported at the 2002 NASS annual meeting in Montreal his experience with the surgical treatment of large symptomatic thoracic disk herniations (14). Of the patients, 93% presented with myelopathy, 86% were found to have an ossified disk herniation, 43% of the disks had evidence of transdural erosion, and 36% of patients required fusion and instrumentation. Multiple surgeries were required to completely resect the disk in 64% of patients, and 43% experienced some degree of perioperative neurological deterioration. Selection of a thoracoscopic approach for a large thoracic herniation must take into account the above problems, and the prognosis and potential complications must be clearly discussed with the patient preoperatively.

IV. THORACOSCOPY FOR DEFORMITY

Huang et al. (25) compared the perioperative parameters and outcomes of VATS with open thoracotomy for anterior release and fusion in the treatment of pediatric spinal deformities. Blood loss, operative transfusion, and length of postoperative chest tube use were all decreased in the VATS patients compared with thoracotomy patients ($p \leq 0.05$). The average operating time for VATS was less than that for open thoracotomy but did not reach statistical significance. However, operating time was significantly shorter in the second 13 VATS patients compared with the first 13 VATS patients. No complications specifically related to the VATS approach were identified.

Early et al. (17) studied "small thoracoscopic children," defined as those weighing < 30 kg who had thoracoscopic spinal surgery, to "large thoracoscopic children" (> 30 kg, thoracoscopic surgery) and "small open children" (< 30 kg, open surgery). Preoperative, intraoperative, and postoperative parameters were analyzed. Small thoracoscopic children ($n = 33$) had greater estimated blood loss/kg body weight (13.6 vs. 6.2 mL/kg; $p = 0.003$), greater chest tube output (27.5 vs. 17.1 mL/kg; $p = 0.003$), and a longer intensive care unit stay (4.2 vs. 1.5 days; $p = 0.001$) than did large thoracoscopic children ($n = 48$). Conversion to an open thoracotomy occurred in one patient from each of the thoracoscopic groups. Small thoracoscopic children required more anesthesia preparation time (79.2 vs. 64.2 min; $p = 0.002$) than the small open children ($n = 25$). There was no significant difference in estimated blood loss, chest tube output, or intensive care unit stay between these two groups. Additionally, no significant difference was found between the three groups with regard to the number of disks excised, operative time, and total hospital stay. The authors concluded that anterior thoracoscopic surgery for spinal release and fusion can be performed as safely in "small" children as in "large" children; however, additional intraoperative challenges should be anticipated. Although the outcomes were similar in the small thoracoscopic children compared to the small open children, the authors stated that very small patients (< 20 kg) should remain a relative contraindication to thoracoscopic surgery, especially during a surgeon's learning curve.

Newton et al. (42) studied the pediatric spinal thoracoscopy learning curve and reported their first 65 consecutive cases. There was a slight decrease in the average operative time as the series progressed. The average number of disks excised was 6.5 ± 1.5 (range 3–10), and the number increased as the series progressed. The average operative time per disk was 29.3 ± 7.7 minutes in the first 30 patients compared with 22.3 ± 4.7 minutes in the next 35 patients ($p < 0.01$). The average blood loss during the thoracoscopic procedure was 301 ± 322 mL (range 25–2000 mL) and did not decrease as the series progressed. Initial postoperative scoliosis and kyphosis corrections were 59% $\pm$ 17% and 92% $\pm$ 12%, respectively. Complications occurred in six patients and were evenly distributed throughout the series.

Roush et al. (52) reported tension pneumothorax as a complication of VATS for anterior correction of idiopathic scoliosis in an adolescent female. This was a consequence of overadvancement of a Steinmann pin (guide wire). Symptoms were noted approximately 5 minutes after the overadvancement was corrected. These included a gradual increase in heart rate and a corresponding gradual decrease in oxygen saturation and systolic and diastolic blood pressure. After 35 minutes it was determined that the patient had sustained a tension pneumothorax of the left hemithorax. Urgent partial reinflation of the right lung and a tube thoracostomy of the left thoracic cavity was done. Vital signs quickly returned to stable levels, and the left lung easily reinflated with chest tube suction. The patient remained stable for the remainder of the surgery, and the postoperative course was uneventful.

REFERENCES

1. Anand N, Regan JJ. Video-assisted thoracoscopic surgery for thoracic disk disease—classification and outcome study of 100 consecutive cases with minimum 2-year follow-up. Spine 2002; 27(8):871–879.
2. Arce CA, Dohrmann GJ. Thoracic disk herniation Improved diagnosis with computed tomographic scanning and a review of the literature. Surg Neurol 1985; 23:356–361.
3. Awwad EE, Martin DS, Smith KR, Jr., et al. Asymptomatic versus symptomatic herniated thoracic disks: their frequency and characteristics as detected by computed tomography after myelography. Neurosurgery 1991; 28:180–186.
4. Balague F, Fankhauser H, Rosazza A, et al. Unusual presentation of thoracic disk herniation. Clin Rheumatol 1989; 8:269–273.
5. Bohlman HH, Zdeblick TA. Anterior excision of herniated thoracic disks. J Bone Joint Surg (Am) 1988; 70:1038–1047.
6. Boukobza M, Tebeka A, Sichez JP, et al. Thoracic disk herniation and spinal cord compression. MRI and gadolinium-enhancement. J Neuroradiol 1993; 20:272–279.
7. Broadhurst NA. The thoracic spine and its pain syndromes. Aust Fam Phys 1987; 16:738–739, 743, 745–746.
8. Brown CW, Deffer PA, Jr., Akmakjian J, et al. The natural history of thoracic disk herniation. Spine 1992; 17:S97–S102.
9. Bruckner FE, Allard SA, Moussa NA. Benign thoracic pain. J R Soc Med 1987; 80:286–289.
10. Bruckner FE, Greco A, Leung AW. 'Benign thoracic pain' syndrome: role of magnetic resonance imaging in the detection and localization of thoracic disk disease. J R Soc Med 1989; 82:81–83.
11. Carson J, Gumpert J, Jefferson A. Diagnosis and treatment of thoracic intervertebral disk protrusions. J Neurol Neurosurg Psychiatry 1971; 34:68–77.
12. Cunningham BW, Kotani Y, McNulty PS, Cappuccino A, Kanayama M, Fedder IL, McAfee PC. Video-assisted thoracoscopic surgery versus open thoracotomy for anterior thoracic spinal fusion. A comparative radiographic, biomechanical, and histologic analysis in a sheep model. Spine 1998; 23:1333–1340.
13. Delfini R, Di Lorenzo N, Ciappetta P, et al. Surgical treatment of thoracic disk herniation: a reappraisal of Larson's lateral extracavitary approach. Surg Neurol 1996; 45:517–523.

14. Dickman CA. Symposia: Controversies in Management of the Cervical Spine. North American Spine Society 17th Annual Meeting, Montreal, Quebec, Canada, Oct 29–Nov 2, 2002.

15. Dickman CA, Karahalio DG. Thorascopic spinal surgery. Clin Neurosurg 1996; 43: 392–422.

16. Dickman CA, Rosenthal D, Karahalios DG, Paramore CG, Mican CA, Apostolides PJ, Lorenz R, Sonntag VKH. Thoracic vertebrectomy and reconstruction using a microsurgical thorascopic approach. Neurosurgery 1996; 38:279–293.

17. Early SD, Newton PO, White KK, Wenger DR, Mubarak SJ. The feasibility of anterior thoracoscopic spine surgery in children under 30 kilograms. Spine 2002; 27:2368–2373.

18. Eleraky MA, Apostolides PJ, Dickman CA, et al. Herniated thoracic disks mimic cardiac disease: three case reports. Acta Neurochir 1998; 140:643–646.

19. el-Kalliny M, Tew JM, Jr., van Loveren H, et al. Surgical approaches to thoracic disk herniations. Acta Neurochir 1991; 111:22–32.

20. Faciszewski T, Winter RB, Lonstein JE, et al. The surgical and medical perioperative complications of anterior spinal fusion surgery in the thoracic and lumbar spine in adults. A review of 1223 procedures. Spine 1995; 20:1592–1599.

21. Fessler RG, Sturgill M. Review: complications of surgery for thoracic disk disease. Surg Neurol 1998; 49:609–618.

22. Fritsch EW, Heisel J, Rupp S. The failed back surgery syndrome: reasons, intraoperative findings, and long-term results: a report of 182 operative treatments. Spine 1996; 21:626–633.

23. Hannon JK, Faircloth WB, Lane DR, Ronderos JF, Snow LL, Weinstein LS, West JL III. Comparision of insuffflation vs. retractional technique for laparoscopic-assisted intervertebral fusion of the lumbar spine. Surg Endosc 2000; 14:300–304.

24. Horowitz MB, Moossy JJ, Julian T, et al. Thoracic discectomy using video assisted thoracoscopy. Spine 1994; 19:1082–1086.

25. Huang T, Hsu RW, Sum C, et al. Complications in thoracoscopic spinal surgery. A study of 90 consecutive patients. Surg Endosc 1999; 13:346–350.

26. Lai YT, Yang LH, Chio CC, Chen HH. Complications in patients with palmar hyperhidrosis treated with transthoracic endoscopic sympathectomy. Neurosurgery 1997; 41:110–113.

27. Landreneau RJ, Hazelrigg SR, Mack MJ, et al. Postoperative pain-related morbidity: video-assisted thoracic surgery versus thoracotomy. Ann Thorac Surg 1993; 56:1285–1289.

28. Larson SJ, Holst RA, Hemmy DC, et al. Lateral extracavitary approach to traumatic lesions of the thoracic and lumbar spine. J Neurosurg 1976; 45:628–637.

29. Le Roux PD, Haglund MM, Harris AB. Thoracic disk disease: experience with the transpedicular approach in twenty consecutive patients. Neurosurgery 1993; 33:58–66.

30. Lee YY, Huang TJ, Liu HP, et al. Thoracic disk herniation treated by video-assisted thoracoscopic surgery: case report. Chang Keng I Hsueh Tsa Chih 1998; 21:453–457.

31. Love JG, Schorn VG. Thoracic disk protrusions. Rheumatism 1967; 23:2–10.

32. Lyu RK, Chang HS, Tang LM, et al. Thoracic disk herniation mimicking acute lumbar disk disease. Spine 1999; 24:416–418.

33. Mack MJ, Regan JJ, Bobechko WP, et al. Application of thoracoscopy for diseases of the spine. Ann Thorac Surg 1993; 56:736–738.

34. Mack MJ, Regan JJ, McAfee PC, et al. Video-assisted thoracic surgery for the anterior approach to the thoracic spine. Ann Thorac Surg 1995; 59:1100–1106.

35. Maiman DJ, Larson SJ, Luck E, et al. Lateral extracavitary approach to the spine for thoracic disk herniation: report of 23 cases. Neurosurgery 1984; 14:178–182.

36. Mangione P, Vadier F, Senegas J. Thoracoscopy versus thoracotomy in spinal surgery: comparison of 2 paired series. Rev Chir Orthop [Fr] 1999; 85:574–580.

37. McAfee PC, Regan JR, Zdeblick T, et al. The incidence of complications in endoscopic anterior thoracolumbar spinal reconstructive surgery. A prospective multicenter study comprising the first 100 consecutive cases. Spine 1995; 20:1624–1632.

38. McKneally MF. Video-assisted thoracic surgery: standards and guidelines. Chest Surg Clin North Am 1993; 3:345–351.

39. McKneally MF, Lewis RJ, Anderson RJ, Fosburg RG, Gay WA Jr, Jones RH, Berringer MB. Statement of the AATS/STS joint committee on thoracoscopy and video-assisted thoracic surgery. J Thorac Cardiovasc.

40. Mulier S, Debois V. Thoracic disk herniations: transthoracic, lateral, or posterolateral approach? A review. Surg Neurol 1998; 49:599–608.

41. Naunheim KS, Barnett MG, Crandall DG, et al. Anterior exposure of the thoracic spine [see comments]. Ann Thorac Surg 1994; 57:1436–1439.

42. Newton PO, Cardelia JM, Farnsworth CL, et al. A biomechanical comparison of open and thoracoscopic anterior spinal release in a goat model. Spine 1998; 23:530–536.

43. North RB, Campbell JN, James CS, et al. Failed back surgery syndrome: 5-year follow-up in 102 patients undergoing repeated operation. Neurosurgery 1991; 28:685–691.

44. O'Leary PF, Camins MB, Polifroni NV, et al. Thoracic disk disease. Clinical manifestations and surgical treatment. Bull Hosp Joint Dis Orthop Inst 1984; 44:27–40.

45. Quast LM. Thoracic disk disease: diagnosis and surgical treatment. J Neurosci Nurs 1987; 19:198–204.

46. Regan JJ. Percutaneous endoscopic thoracic discectomy. Neurosurg Clin North Am 1996; 7:87–98.

47. Regan JJ, Ben-Yishay A, Mack MJ. Video-assisted thoracoscopic excision of herniated thoracic disk: description of technique and preliminary experience in the first 29 cases. J Spinal Disord 1998; 11:183–191.

48. Regan JJ, Guyer RD. Endoscopic techniques in spinal surgery. Clin Orthop 1997:122–139.

49. Regan JJ, Mack MJ, Picetti GD, 3rd. A technical report on video-assisted thoracoscopy in thoracic spinal surgery. Preliminary description. Spine 1995; 20:831–837.

50. Rosenthal D. Endoscopic approaches to the thoracic spine. Eur Spine J 2000; (suppl): S8–S16.

51. Rosenthal D, Dickman CA. Thorascoscopic microsurgical excision of a herniated thoracic disk. J Neurosurg 1988; 89:224–235.

52. Roush TF, Crawford AH, Berlin RE, Wolf RK. Tension pneumothorax as a complication of video-assisted thorascopic surgery for anterior correction of idiopathic scoliosis in an adolescent female. Spine 2001; 26:448–450.

53. Schellhas KP, Pollei SR, Dorwart RH. Thoracic discography. A safe and reliable technique [see comments]. Spine 1994; 19:2103–2109.

54. Shelley WB, Florence R. Compensatory hyperhidrosis after sympathectomy. N Engl J Med 1960; 263:1056–1058.

55. Stillerman CB, Chen TC, Couldwell WT, et al. Experience in the surgical management of 82 symptomatic herniated thoracic disks and review of the literature. J Neurosurg 1998; 88: 623–633.

56. Stillerman CB, Chen TC, Day JD, et al. The transfacet pedicle-sparing approach for thoracic disk removal: cadaveric morphometric analysis and preliminary clinical experience [see comments]. J Neurosurg 1995; 83:971–976.

57. Sucato DJ, Girgis M. Bilateral pneumothoraces, pneumomediastinum, pneumoperitoneum, pneumoretroperitoneum, and subcutaneous emphysema following intubation with a double-lumen endotracheal tube for thoracoscopic anterior spinal release and fusion in a patient with idiopathic scoliosis. Spinal Disord 2002; 15:133–138.

58. Sundaresan N, Shah J, Foley KM, et al. An anterior surgical approach to the upper thoracic vertebrae. J Neurosurg 1984; 61:686–690.

59. Turner PL, Webb JK. A surgical approach to the upper thoracic spine. J Bone Joint Surg [Br] 1987; 69:542–544.

60. Vanderburgh DF, Kelly WM. Radiographic assessment of discogenic disease of the spine. Neurosurg Clin North Am 1993; 4:13–33.

61. Visocchi M, Masferrer R, Sonntag VK, et al. Thoracoscopic approaches to the thoracic spine. Acta Neurochir 1998; 140:737–743.

62. Wall EJ, Bylski-Austrow DI, Shelton FS, et al. Endoscopic discectomy increases thoracic spine flexibility as effectively as open discectomy. A mechanical study in a porcine model. Spine 1998; 23:9–16.
63. Whitcomb DC, Martin SP, Schoen RE, et al. Chronic abdominal pain caused by thoracic disk herniation. Am J Gastroenterol 1995; 90:835–837.
64. Williams MP, Cherryman GR, Husband JE. Significance of thoracic disk herniation demonstrated by MR imaging. J Comput Assist Tomogr 1989; 13:211–214.
65. Wood KB, Garvey TA, Gundry C, et al. Magnetic resonance imaging of the thoracic spine. Evaluation of asymptomatic individuals. J Bone Joint Surg Am 1995; 77:1631–1638.
66. Wood KB, Schellhas KP, Garvey TA, et al. Thoracic discography in healthy individuals. A controlled prospective study of magnetic resonance imaging and discography in asymptomatic and symptomatic individuals. Spine 1999; 24:1548–1555.

34

Complications of Minimally Invasive Spinal Surgery—Part III: Laparoscopy

John J. Regan and Neel Anand
Cedar-Sinai Institute for Spinal Disorders, Los Angeles, California, U.S.A.

Larry T. Khoo and Anthony Virella
UCLA Medical Center, Los Angeles, California, U.S.A.

Michael A. Pahl and Alexander R. Vaccaro
Thomas Jefferson University and the Rothman Institute, Philadelphia, Pennsylvania, U.S.A.

There is considerable enthusiasm regarding minimally invasive surgical techniques. Laparoscopic surgical approaches have dramatically altered the field of general surgery. The advantages of transperitoneal laparoscopic surgery for the patient include smaller incisions with lessening postoperative pain, lack of postoperative ileus, and early hospital discharge. For the surgeon, there is improved visualization of the surgical anatomy and greater participation for the entire operating team, who can watch the monitor during the surgical procedure. Laparoscopic platform technology is merging with robotics and image guidance systems, which will likely lead to improved surgical accuracy and lower patient morbidity.

Spinal fusion has been used to treat various spinal disorders for most of the twentieth century. However, it was not until 1992, with the introduction of threaded spinal fusion cages, that the opportunity arose to combine the benefits of laparoscopy with the latest in fusion technology. A collaborative team consisting of a general and spine surgeon have become essential for success. In spite of these potential advantages, transperitoneal laparoscopic techniques have not gained wide acceptance. This relates to the technical challenges of this approach, which requires the expertise of a laparoscopic surgeon. Differences in clinical outcome have not been shown to be significant, leading most surgeons to adopt a mini-open retroperitoneal laparotomy as the preferred technique. Complications of laparoscopic approaches to the spine are divided into general complications of the endoscopic procedure and those specific to the spinal procedure (17,24).

I. INTRODUCTION

Transabdominal and retroperitoneal approaches for anterior lumbar interbody fusions are widely accepted, effective tools for the management of painful degenerative disk disease unresponsive to nonoperative measures. Recent advances in interbody fusion cage technology as well as recent FDA approval of bone morphogenic protein (BMP) have generated a great deal of interest in their application by laparoscopic and minimal access techniques (26). There are several potential advantages to a spinal fusion system that can be inserted using a laparoscopic or mini-open technique. This approach avoids posterior incisions with associated trauma to the paraspinal musculature. Epidural scarring, traction on nerve roots, and dural lacerations are avoided with the anterior approach. However, a team approach is essential to the success of this technology. The general and spinal surgeon must work together from the time of preoperative consultation, at surgery, and into early postoperative care to realize the full benefits of these surgical procedures and avoid the pitfalls of this surgical approach.

Appropriate patient selection is vital to success. The ideal candidate is a patient with discogenic pain related to isolated disk space collapse following a previous laminectomy. Stand-alone cages have better results at the L5-S1 level in patients with significant disk space collapse. Assessment of vascular anatomy on preoperative MRI scans and identification of anomalies or vascular disease is essential to avoid vascular injury. Monopolar cautery is avoided during surgery, and blunt dissection is used to avoid injury to the superior hypogastric plexus. The laparoscopic approach is best suited to the L5-S1 disk space, where the approach is between the iliac vessels. Fusion success is improved by excluding patients with osteoporosis. Achieving appropriate distraction with the cages and packing bone anterior to the cages or using BMP so that a sentinel fusion sign can be identified on plain x-rays is essential for a successful outcome.

II. INTERBODY FUSION CAGES

Interbody fusion cages offer the surgeon an alternative approach to fusion for discogenic pain syndromes. Arthrodesis is obtained by achieving immediate stability and long-term support with the ability to heal under compressive loads through and around the implant. Brantigan and Stefee developed a carbon fiber cage used with autogenous bone grafting. Bagby and Kuslich successfully introduced the first threaded titanium interbody cage (BAK, Spinetech, Inc., Minneapolis, MN) (1). A 91% clinical success and fusion rate has been reported with this cage. These results have recently been called into question as longer clinical outcome studies are available. Recent studies utilizing the LT cage (Medronics Sofamor Danek, Memphis, TN) with BMP have demonstrated a 95% fusion rate using cages as stand-alone devices for one level disease (4).

Obenchain reported the first laparoscopic anterior endoscopic lumbar discectomy (20). Mack et al. reported the application of thoracoscopy for disease of the spine in 1995 (12). Also in 1995, Mathews et al. (14), Zucherman et al. (31), and Regan et al. (23) reported the technique and preliminary results of laparoscopic lumbar fusion. Instruments have been designed to be placed laparoscopically for the purpose of disk space distraction, dcentering of the implant, and placement of two threaded titanium cylinders that engage both endplates of the disk space to be fused.

III. COMPLICATION AVOIDANCE DURING PATIENT SELECTION

Laparoscopic fusion techniques are indicated for use in patients with single-level symptomatic degenerative disk disease, internal disk disruption, and pseudarthrosis. Stable grade I spondylolisthesis and two-level degenerative disk disease may be considered if posterior instrumentation is also utilized. The ideal patient for laparoscopic fusion is one who has radiographic degenerative disk changes. These include disk space narrowing, endplate sclerosis, and osteophyte formation. This disease can be diagnosed in a patient with a strong history of mechanical back pain who has isolated changes at one level on radiographs and MRI scan. This diagnosis is best made in a young patient (45 years old) with normal disk intensity signal on magnetic resonance imaging (MRI) scan at adjacent disk levels. In older patients the diagnosis may be less clear because of the naturally occurring degenerative changes in the intervertebral disks.

In a patient with single-level disk disease and Modic changes confirmed on MRI, discography may not always be necessary (18). Patients with a strong mechanical back pain history who have conformed to a physical therapy program for 6 months without relief are good candidates for the procedure. Patients who have overlying psychological conditions and positive Waddell's signs and are habitual narcotics users are not candidates for fusion surgery.

Internal disk disruption patients are not ideal candidates for laparoscopic fusion. These patients have relatively normal plain radiographic examinations with decrease signal on MRI scan and concordant pain response and morphology on discography. These patients may be treated with laparoscopic techniques, but because of a tall disk height, it is more difficult to obtain the disk distraction required for stability. Anatomical fit is more difficult because larger cages are required.

Patients with extensive peritoneal adhesions from previous surgery or inflammatory or infectious diseases affecting the peritoneum should be excluded from the laparoscopic transperitoneal approach. Radiographs and MRI scans should also be examined for vascular calcifications, aneurysms, and anomalies, which may exclude the anterior approach altogether.

IV. COMPLICATIONS WITH THE SURGICAL TECHNIQUE

A. Anterior Lumbar Procedures

Anesthetic complications in laparoscopic surgery are usually related to insufflation of carbon dioxide (CO_2) (8) and patient positioning during these procedures. Increased intra-abdominal pressures created by the insufflation of CO_2 can impede the normal venous return from the lower extremities. Retention of CO_2 during the procedure can lead to hypercapnia, decreased diaphragmatic motion, and reduced lung compliance. Cardiac arrest may result from CO_2 emboli, which may result from the absorption of CO_2 at high pressures. Various arrhythmias including sinus bradycardia and ventricular fibrillation have been reported during laparoscopic insufflation. Postoperative pulmonary embolism can also occur from venous stasis in the lower extremities. The use of low-dose subcutaneous heparin and venous compression stockings can help reduce the incidence of this complication. The arms should be safely tucked away to the patient's side in order to prevent hyperextension injuries of the brachial plexus secondary to overextension and abduction of the arms.

CO_2 insufflation during laparoscopic spinal surgery can lead to several undesirable physiological effects, which include a rise in mean arterial pressure, a fall in cardiac output, and an increase in the systemic and pulmonary vascular resistance. Excessive insufflation can lead to hypoxemia by causing diaphragmatic pleural compression. Bowel injury can also occur, since CO_2 insufflation can force the bowel into the trocars. Visceral injury can also occur, resulting in pneumoperitoneum (10). The umbilicus should be elevated during the placement of the Veress needle for percutaneous insufflation. As with all thoracoscopic procedures, once the initial port is established, the remaining ports should be introduced under direct vision.

Other complications of the laparoscopic approach include ventral hernia, arterial thrombosis, and retrograde ejaculation (2,5,7,11,15,22,23). With laparoscopy, the surgeon regularly achieves access to the anterior lumbar spine at L5-S1 and L4-L5 (21,22). Injury to vessels in the retroperitoneal space can occur during the initial exposure. Care must be taken to dissect the common iliac arteries and veins to faciliatate placement of cages and dowels in the disk spaces (Fig. 1). Injury to the great vessels can occur during the initial exposure or placement of the instrumentation for the insertion of the bone grafts or cages.

The incidence of postoperative retrograde ejaculation is reported in 0.42–8% of cases after retroperitoneal lower interbody fusion (3,6,27). This is caused by injury to the superior hypogastric plexus that overlies the ventral portion of the lower lumbar segments. The majority of these patients will recover within 6–12 months, but 3–5% will be left with permanent disabilities. Several instruments, such as the harmonic scalpel, and techniques avoiding excessive electrocautery in this region have reduced the incidence of this complication. There is an increased incidence of retrograde ejaculation with laparoscopic insertion of interbody cages compared with the open procedure, making this approach less desirable in young males of childbearing age (19).

The incidence of complications with open anterior lumbar interbody fusion (ALIF) is similar to laparoscopic ALIF. The L4-L5 level can pose significant difficulties due to the overlying vascular anatomy. Zdeblick and David (30) noted a 20% versus 4% incidence of complications for laparoscopic versus open ALIF, respectively. This study ultimately

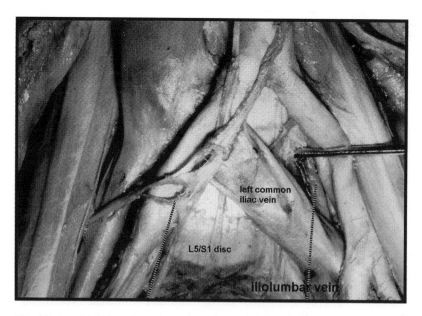

Figure 1 During laparoscopic anterior lumbar procedures, careful dissection to mobilize the adjacent vascular structures is critical to avoid inadvertent injury and to provide access to the underlying disk spaces. The aorta, vena cava, iliac veins, iliac arteries, and iliolumbar vein lie in close proximity to the L4-L5 and L5-S1 disk spaces.

concluded that there were no significant advantages to performing a laparoscopic ALIF at the L4-L5 level. Several other studies have described good results with laparoscopic ALIF at this level. Nonetheless, placement of two cages or bone grafts at this level can be technically demanding and should only be performed by individuals with ample experience in laparoscopic ALIF techniques.

B. L5-S1 Approach

A "four-stick" technique is used. A periumbilical Hasson trocar is used to place a 0 degree endoscope. This is followed by placement of two 5 mm trocars lateral to the inferior epigastric arteries, which run along the ventro-lateral border of the rectus abdominus muscle. This vessel can be injured during blind trocar insertion or inserting the trocar too close to the lateral border of the rectus abdominis, where the inferior epigastric artery can be seen internally as a pulsatile structure. If injury does occur, the artery must be tamponaded and ligated endoscopically. A 5 mm portal is placed in the suprapubic location after establishing the appropriate trajectory to the L5-S1 disk space by using lateral c-arm flouroscopy. The suprapubic trocar is placed above the bladder, which can be visualized endoscopically after it has been drained by a Foley catheter insertion. After insertion of the Hasson trocar and establishment of pneumoperitoneum, other trocar placements are made under direct vision. Percutaneous Veress needle technique is sometimes applied to achieve insufflation. Since this is a blind technique, bowel adhesions to the anterior abdominal wall may lead to bowel perforation. Therefore, this technique is avoided in the previously operated patient or those with a history of endometriosis or inflammatory bowel disorders or diverticulitis. The patient is positioned in 20–30 degrees of Trendelenburg, and graspers are placed in the 5 mm ports to facilitate packing the intestines into the superior portion of the abdomen. The location of the aortic bifurcation is identified, and the sigmoid colon mesentery is approached from the right side. The right ureter coursing over the right iliac artery must be identified prior to making this incision in the posterior peritoneum to avoid injury to it. Electrocautery is not used in making the incision to avoid injury to the superior hypogastric plexus. Blunt dissection using Kidner wands is then used to sweep the retroperitoneal tissue from right to left. This also avoids the possibility of dissecting through the hypogastric plexus. The sigmoid colon may travel close to the midline, requiring retraction. Preoperative laxative and a light dinner the day before surgery should result in colon evacuation, which will improve handling of the bowel.

After incising the peritoneum and mobilizing the sigmoid colon, the L5-S1 disk space is visualized along with the overlying middle sacral vessels. The median sacral vein and artery can be ligated with clips, or the harmonic scalpel may be used to coagulate the vessel. Sharp dissection and monopolar cautery are avoided to prevent injury to the hypogastric plexus. Kidner wands and endoscopic vascular retractors are used to retract the iliac vessels on either side. The vessels are mobilized until the sympathetic plexus can be seen on either side. This broad visualization of the disk space combined with a true AP lordotic fluoroscopic image of the L5-S1 disk space is essential in locating the true midline of the disk space. The midline is marked with a Steinman pin, and an AP and lateral x-ray is obtained. Once the center point is established, a trephine is used to enlarge the center hole. The appropriate-sized drill alignment guide determined from preoperative templating is used to create pilot holes on either side of midline. Failure to identify and work off the true midline can lead to asymmetrical cage placement with the result of encroachment on the neural foramen, resulting in leg pain or weakness and nerve root injury.

C. L4-L5 Approach

The L4-L5 disk space is visualized by making an incision in the posterior peritoneum to the right of the sigmoid mesocolon after visualizing the bifurcation of the aorta and vena cava. Preoperative MRI scans are evaluated to determine the location of the vascular bifurcation. The sigmoid colon is gently moved to the left of the midline and, if necessary, can be further retracted by placing a suture through the sigmoid mesocolon and bringing it to the anterior abdominal wall in the left lower quadrant. The L5-S1 disk space is identified and the dissection is carried in a cephalad direction between the bifurcation. It may be possible to approach the L4-5 disk from below the bifurcation, which can be determined at this time. Depending on the vascular anatomy, the L4-5 disk may be approached by retracting the left iliac artery and vein from left to right or going between the left iliac artery and vein.

1. Above the Bifurcation of the Vessels

This approach should be feasible in most patients, unless the bifurcation of the vessels is extremely high. The issue of autonomic nerve dysfunction is a concern with this approach. One critical step in successfully achieving visualization of the interspace is to identify and divide the ascending iliolumbar vein, which may be a single large vessel taking off obliquely from the left iliac vein or vena cava above or below the L4-L5 disk space or up to three or four small venous branches arising from the left iliac vein. The preferred method in dealing with the ascending iliolumbar vein is to apply a 5 mm clip to the vein and then to protect the iliac vein side with an Endoloop (Ethicon Endosurgery Inc., Cincinnati, OH). Loss of control of segmental vessels can often be recovered, but loss of control of the ascending lumbar vein often requires suture-ligature closure and may lead to conversion of the procedure to open surgery. The dissection is complete when the sympathetic plexus is seen on the patient's right side. In 1999 Regan et al. reported results of the laparoscopic approach to the L4-L5 level in 58 consecutive patients (22). This approach was used successfully in 50% of patients in this series.

2. Below the Bifurcation of the Vessels

This approach provides the easiest access to the L4-L5 disk space, but it involves significant dissection and possibly retraction in the area of the superior hypogastric plexus. All dissection is done with scissors, and no monopolar cautery is used at any time. The bifurcation is elevated, and retraction of the left and right iliac vessels is performed using a 5 mm vessel retractor. It is helpful to elevate the vessels off the surface of the vertebral body to facilitate drill tube insertion. In the Regan series reported above, they were able to approach the L4-L5 disk space by going under the bifurcation 33% of the time (21).

3. Between the Artery and Vein

This dissection is much easier than one would think and gives excellent exposure with minimal retraction on the iliac artery. A concern is when the disk procedure begins, as there are two vessels that can be injured instead of just one. Therefore, this approach requires more diligence than the other approaches. In cases of diseased arteries or difficult exposure, this approach is an option that minimizes traction on the left iliac artery. This approach was used 16% of the time in the series reported by Regan et al (21).

D. Lateral Endoscopic Fusion L1-L5

Retroperitoneal lumbar fusion and stabilization offers several advantages over conventional anterior transperitoneal laparoscopic approaches to the lumbar spine (16). Retroperitoneal approaches obviate the risk of small bowel obstruction. Additonally, there may be reduced risk of retrograde ejaculation compared to transperitoneal techniques. With the straight lateral position, it is easier to place an orthogonally directed fusion cage than anterior to posterior. There is minimal risk to nerve injury because the drilling and reaming is directed to the psoas on the opposite side as compared to conventional anterior surgery where the drilling is directed toward the spinal canal. There is minimal mobilization of the great vessels, especially at the L4-L5 disk space. The major difficulty in placing a lateral fusion cage is the psoas muscle.

The psoas muscle, which contains the lumbosacral nerve plexus, must be split at the lower lumbar levels to provide access for a laterally directed fusion cage. The genitofemoral and ilioinguinal nerves, which lie on the belly of the psoas muscle, must not be stretched during this procedure. Approaches through the psoas at L4-L5 carry an increased risk of injuring the descending nerve roots from L2 and L3, which may cross the disk space of L4-L5 within the psoas muscle and lie in the path of the direct lateral approach to the disk.

The surgical approach is facilitated with the patient in the straight lateral decubitus position on a radiolucent graphite table. A 1 cm incision is made at the anterior portion of the twelfth rib to approach the L1-L2 disk space. Below L2, a lateral fluoroscopic image is obtained, with a metal marker placed on the patient's back overlying the appropriate disk space. A dissecting trocar called an Optiview (Ethicon Endosurgery, Cincinnati, OH) is used with a 10 mm laparoscope to dissect through the three muscle layers to the retroperitoneal space. Insufflation of the retroperitoneal space is accomplished using a dissecting balloon or CO_2 insufflation. Additional trocars are placed after dissecting the peritoneum toward the midline. Once this space is created, our preference is to continue CO_2 insufflation during the entire case. Manual traction can also be utilized by increasing the size of the incision from 10 mm to 45 cm. The sympathetic ganglion is reflected in an anterior direction along with the ureter and great vessels. The anterior portion of the psoas will need to be split to facilitate lateral exposure of the disk space. If a single-level cage fusion is to be done, the segmental vessels can be protected.

V. RESULTS AND COMPLICATIONS

Patient stays following laparoscopic fusion have been dramatically shortened. In the Mahvi and Zdeblick series, mean hospital stay was 1.7 days, ranging from zero to 2 days in 20 consecutive patients (13). Nine of the last 18 patients were performed on an outpatient basis. Operative time averaged 125 minutes (range 70–160 min). Zdeblick prospectively compared the results of laparoscopic fusion (Group I) to posterolateral fusion with pedicle screws (Group II) and posterior interbody fusion with pedicle fixation (Group III) (28,29). Thirty-nine patients were randomized to these three groups in a prospective, randomized protocol for the treatment of L5-S1 degenerative disk disease. The hospital stay was 1.8 days for Group I, 5 days for Group II, and 5.1 days for Group III. The average return to work in the posterior fusion groups with pedicle fixation was 21 and 23 weeks, respectively, compared to 11 weeks for the laparoscopic group. Good to excellent clinical results were reported in 100% of the laparoscopic group compared to 73% for Group II and 91% for Group III.

Hisey et al. reported long-term survivability of threaded fusion devices implanted as stand-alone devices at one or two levels at one medical center by five surgeons (9). In a retrospective analysis of 190 patients with an average follow-up of 33 months (range 24–61 months) operated between 1994 and 1997, only 3 cases (1.6%) required posterior revision for pseudarthrosis and 3 cases (1.6%) cage removal for nerve impingement by cage or displaced disk material. A total of 3.2% of patients required revision surgery at the same level, and 6 patients (3.2%) had procedures at adjacent levels. There was no statistically significant difference in the revision rate of the laparoscopic group, which consisted of 80 patients (42%).

A prospective multimember study evaluating open and laparoscopic lumbar fusion in over 500 patients was reported by Regan et al. in 1999 (25). There were no major complications (i.e., great vessel damage, pulmonary embolism, implant migration, death) in the laparoscopic group, which consisted of 215 patients treated by 19 surgeons at 10 medical centers. Preliminary experience indicated a small conversion rate to open surgery resulting from preoperative scarring, bleeding, and poor visualization. Instruments and technique changed from the earliest experience, and no further conversions occurred. Intraoperative disk herniation from reaming and lateral cage placement with nerve irritation requiring posterior surgery was reported in 3.2% of the laparoscopic cases. Post-operative ileus rate was 4.7%, and incisional hernia did not occur in this group. Retrograde ejaculation occurred in 5.1% of laparoscopic cases, twice the rate of open cases. Almost all of these cases occurred early in the series as a result of monopolar cauterization. The discontinuation of monopolar cautery and use of blunt dissection after incising the peritonium to the right of the midline has almost eliminated this problem.

VI. CONCLUSION

Minimally invasive spine surgery has experienced significant gains in the past decade, primarily in anterior procedures such as thoracoscopy and laparoscopic surgery. Improvements in camera equipment, navigation systems, and robotics have enhanced this surgical approach. Ultimately, one must show improvements in the quality of the patient's life, with less pain, fewer complications, and a faster return to normal activity. Surgical training must keep up with the fast pace of technological advancements if these procedures are to have a broad appeal. At this time the surgical team approach has been successful, with a reduction in hospital time and a quicker return to work. Progress in spine surgery will come in small steps with the refinement of less invasive surgical technique, making the procedures both safer and more beneficial to our patients.

REFERENCES

1. Bagby G. Arthrodesis by the distraction-compression methods using a stainless steel implant. Orthopedics 1988; 11:931–934.
2. Baker JK, Reardon PR, Reardon MJ, Heggeness MH. Vascular injury in anterior lumbar surgery. Spine 1993; 18:2227–2230.
3. Belkoff SM, Mathis JM, Jasper LE, Deramond H. The biomechanics of vertebroplasty: the effect of cement volume on mechanical behavior. Spine 2001; 26:1537–1541.
4. Burkus JK, Dorchak JD, Sanders DL. Radiographic assessment of interbody fusion using recombinant human bone morphogenetic protein type 2. Spine 2003; 28:372–377.

5. Dewald CJ, Millikan KW, Hammerberg KW, Doolas A, Dewald RL. An open, minimally invasive approach to the lumbar spine. Am Surg 1999; 65:61–68.

6. Flynn JC, Price CT. Sexual complications of anterior fusion of the lumbar spine. Spine 1984; 9:489–492.

7. Hackenberg L, Liljenqvist U, Halm H, Winkelmann W. Occlusion of the left common iliac artery and consecutive thromboembolism of the left popliteal artery following anterior lumber interbody fusion. J Spinal Disord 2001; 14:365–368.

8. Hannon JK, Faircloth WB, Lane DR, Ronderos JF, Snow LL, Weinstein LS, West JL III. Comparision of insufflation vs. retractional technique for laparoscopic-assisted intervertebral fusion of the lumbar spine. Surg Endosc 2000; 14:300–304.

9. Hisey M, Regan J, Blumenthal S, Guyer R, Zigler J. Long term survivability of cages as stand alone devices. North American Spine Society Proceedings, October 1999, Chicago.

10. Jacobs M, Verdeja, Goldstein HS. Minimally invasive colon resection. Surg Laparosc Endosc 1991; 1:144–150.

11. Lieberman IH, Willsher PC, Litwin DE, Salo PT, Kraetschmer BG. Transperitoneal laparoscopic exposure for lumbar interbody fusion. Spine 2000; 5:509–514.

12. Mack MJ, Regan JJ, McAfee PC, Picetti G, Ben-Yishay A, Acuff TE. Video assisted thoracic surgery (VATS) for the anterior approach to the thoracic spine. Ann Thorac Surg 1995; 59:1100–1106.

13. Mahvi DM, Zdeblick TA. A prospective study of laparoscopic spinal fusion: technique and operative complications. Ann Surg 1996; 224:85–90.

14. Mathews HH, Evans MT, Molligan HJ, Long, BH. Laparoscopic discectomy with anterior lumbar interbody fusion. Spine 1995; 20(16):1791–1802.

15. Mayers HM. A new microsurgical technique for minimally invasive anterior lumbar interbody fusion. Spine 1997; 22:691–699.

16. McAfee PC, Regan JJ, Geiss P, Fedder I. Minimally invasive retroperitoneal approach to the spine. Spine 1998; 23(13):1476–1484.

17. McAfee PC, Regan JJ, Zdeblick T, Zuckerman J, Picetti GD 3rd, Heim S, Geis WP, Fedder IL. The incidence of complications in endoscopic anterior thoracolumbar spinal reconstructive surgery: a prospective multicenter study comprising the first 100 consecutive cases. Spine 1995; 20:1624–1632.

18. Modic MT, Steinberg PM, Ross JS, Masaryk TJ, Carter JR. Degenerative disk disease: assessment of changes in vertebral marrow. Radiology 1988; 166:193–199.

19. Mulholland RC. Cages: Outcome and complications. Eur Spine J 2000; (suppl):S110–S113.

20. Obenchain TG. Laparoscopic lumbar discectomy: a case report. J Laparoendosc Surg 1991; 1:145–149.

21. O'Dowd JK. Laparoscopic lumbar spine surgery. Eur Spine J 2000; 9(suppl):S3–S7.

22. Regan JJ, Aronoff, RJ, Ohmneiss DD, Sengtupa D. Laparoscopic approach to L4-L5 for interbody fusion using BAK cages: experience in the first 58 cases. Spine 1999; 24(20): 2171–2174.

23. Regan JJ, McAfee PC, Guyer RD, Aronoff RJ. Laparoscopic fusion of the lumbar spine in a multicenter series of the first 34 consecutive patients. Surg. Laparosc Endosc 1996; 6(6): 459–468.

24. Regan JJ, McAfee PC, Mack MJ. Atlas of Endoscopic Spine Surgery. St. Louis: Quality Medical Publishing, 1995.

25. Regan JJ, Yuan H, McAfee PC. Laparoscopic fusion of he lumbar spine. Minimally invasive spine surgery: a prospective multicenter cohort study evaluating perioperative complications in open and laparoscopic lumbar fusion using threaded fusion cages. Spine 1999; 24(20):402–411.

26. Regan JJ, Yuan H, McCullen, G. Minimally invasive approaches to the spine. Inkster Course Lecture 1997; 46:127–141.

27. Tiusanen H, Seitsalo S, Osterman K, Soini J. Retrograde ejaculation after anterior lumbar interbody fusion. Eur Spine J 1995; 4:339–342.
28. Zdeblick TA. A prospective randomized study of lumbar fusion: preliminary results. Spine 1993; 18(8):983–991.
29. Zdeblick TA. A prospective randomized study of the surgical treatment of L5-S1 degenerative disk disease. Presented at the Tenth Annual Meeting of the North American Spine Society, Washington, DC, October 20, 1995.
30. Zdeblick TA, David SM. A prospective comparison of surgical approach for anterior L4-L5 fusion: laparoscopic versus mini anterior lumbar interbody fusion. Spine 2000; 25:2682–2687.
31. Zucherman JF, Zdeblick TA, Bailey SA, Mahvi D, Hsu KY, Kohrs D. Instrumented laparoscopic spinal fusion: preliminary results. Spine 1995; 20:2029–2035.

35

Complications of Minimally Invasive Spinal Procedures and Surgery—Part IV: Percutaneous and Intradiscal Techniques

Anthony T. Yeung
Arizona Institute for Minimally Invasive Spine Care, Phoenix, Arizona, U.S.A.

Martin H. Savitz
*Royal College of Physicians and Surgeons (U.S.), American International University,
American Academy of Minimally Invasive Spinal Medicine and Surgery, and
Drexel University School of Medicine, Philadelphia, Pennsylvania, U.S.A.*

Larry T. Khoo and Anthony Virella
UCLA Medical Center, Los Angeles, California, U.S.A.

Michael A. Pahl and Alexander R. Vaccaro
Thomas Jefferson University and the Rothman Institute, Philadelphia, Pennsylvania, U.S.A.

I. INTRODUCTION

As the millennium dawns, it is interesting to note that the concept of operating on the spine through the least damaging route and by the most precise instrumentation originated in 1937. Pool (1) illuminated a simple cannula with a modified otoscope to perform myeloscopic examination of the dorsal nerve roots in cases of herniated nucleus pulposus, hypertrophied ligamentum flavum, adhesive arachnoiditis, benign neoplasm, and metastatic carcinoma. As early as 1939, Love (2) advanced the basic principles of microdiscectomy—interlaminar removal of disk material with a small incision and without resection of bone. Minimalism in neurosurgery became centered on microsurgical technique in 1955 when Malis (3) employed a binocular microscope to operate with bipolar coagulation. Percutaneous discectomy started with the work of Hijikata (4) and Kambin (5) in the early and mid-1970s. Ascher (6) in 1984 was the first to utilize a Nd:YAG laser to ablate the nucleus pulposus through an 18 gauge spinal needle.

One of the first truly minimally invasive techniques, chemonucleolysis by injection of chymopapain into the disk space, was the procedure of choice for young patients under 20 years of age with a contained herniation. Large double-blind series and numerous cohort studies validated the method introduced by Smith (7) in 1955. A few serious complications of anaphylaxis and transverse myelitis by at times poorly trained users caused most practitioners to shy away from the enzymatic denaturalization of the nucleus pulposus (8).

II. MINIMALLY INVASIVE APPROACH BY KEYHOLE INCISION

The minimally invasive approach to the spine by its nature is designed to limit the incidence of operative complications. Most surgeons equate minimalism with smaller incisions through traditional approaches where they are familiar with the anatomy. Keyhole incisions require no dissection of fascial or muscle planes. There is limited challenge to host defenses. Scheduling is most often a brief same-day procedure. Conscious sedation with local anesthetics avoids the sequelae of general anesthesia. Microinstrumentation produces little irritation or inflammation to local tissues. Blood loss is often insufficient to require transfusion. Constant irrigation with saline with standard minimally invasive techniques is designed to remove inflammatory detritus and debris. A single suture and Band Aid dressing are adequate for the majority of surgical wounds. Anesthetic requirements are frequently much lower than with open procedures. Mobilization, recovery, and return-to-work time periods have been truncated compared to open traditional procedures. Patient satisfaction averages over 90% in most reported series (9). The results at this time appear to be equivalent to open surgery with less morbidity in experienced hands. Why, then, has minimally invasive surgery become only slowly accepted?

The steep learning curve is the most daunting factor that prevents many surgeons from embracing minimally invasive spine surgery, especially foraminal endoscopic surgery, where surgical anatomy, approach, and anatomical relationships are different from the traditional approach. Most academic training centers do not offer relevant training, and interested surgeons have had to learn the technique after they became established and comfortable with traditional approaches. Early in the learning curve the success rate can be less than with traditional open approachs and the complication rate can increase due to unfamiliarity with endoscopic anatomy. The surgical success rate, however, soon increases if the surgeon conquers the learning curve. If a surgeon experiences his or her first complication or surgical failure in the early phase of this learning curve, there is a strong incentive for the surgeon to revert to old ways or perhaps to even argue against the techniques, especially if the surgeon concludes that, in his or her hands, the traditional approach is more efficacious. Minimally invasive surgery can also be discouraging to surgeons who are more comfortable with larger incisions and more generous exposure for visualization and exploration purposes. Once the learning curve is overcome, however, the advantages of minimally invasive spine surgery is very evident, and the accomplished and experienced minimally invasive surgeon soon learns to include minimally invasive techniques in his or surgical armamentarium.

III. THE POSTEROLATERAL (FORAMINAL) APPROACH

This approach was originally described by Kambin to access the lumbar spinal segment through the triangular zone between the traversing and exiting nerves (Fig. 1). The starting point for needle entry was estimated, but techniques for more accurately identifying the skin window have served to improve instrument placement. For more accurate instrument placement, standardization of the approach through topographic landmarks measured by intraoperative fluoroscopy created the concept of a skin window, anular window, and anatomical disk center (Fig. 2). Drawing lines on the patient's skin (Fig. 3) creates a reference line for adjusting the needle trajectory, decreasing the chance of inadvertent puncture of the exiting nerve by repeated needle passes to the anulus, especially at L5-S1, where the triangular zone is very small. The development of a two-hole obturator (Fig. 4) allows

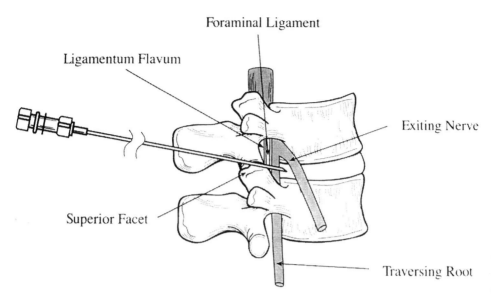

Figure 1 Kambin's triangular zone is the safe target zone for foraminal access to the disk and epidural space.

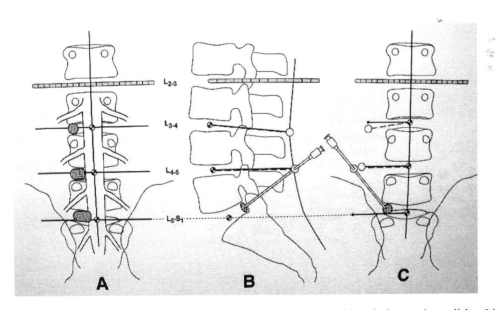

Figure 2 Fluoroscopic landmarks: (A) Spinous process centered in relation to the pedicles. Line drawn across each disk space to find trajectory parallel to each disk. (B) Line of inclination for each disk drawn in the lateral projection determines position of the skin window cephalad or caudal to the line in A. Distance from the disk center to the skin estimates the distance from the spinous process laterally. (C) Distance from the spinous process to the line of inclination determines the ideal position of the initial skin window.

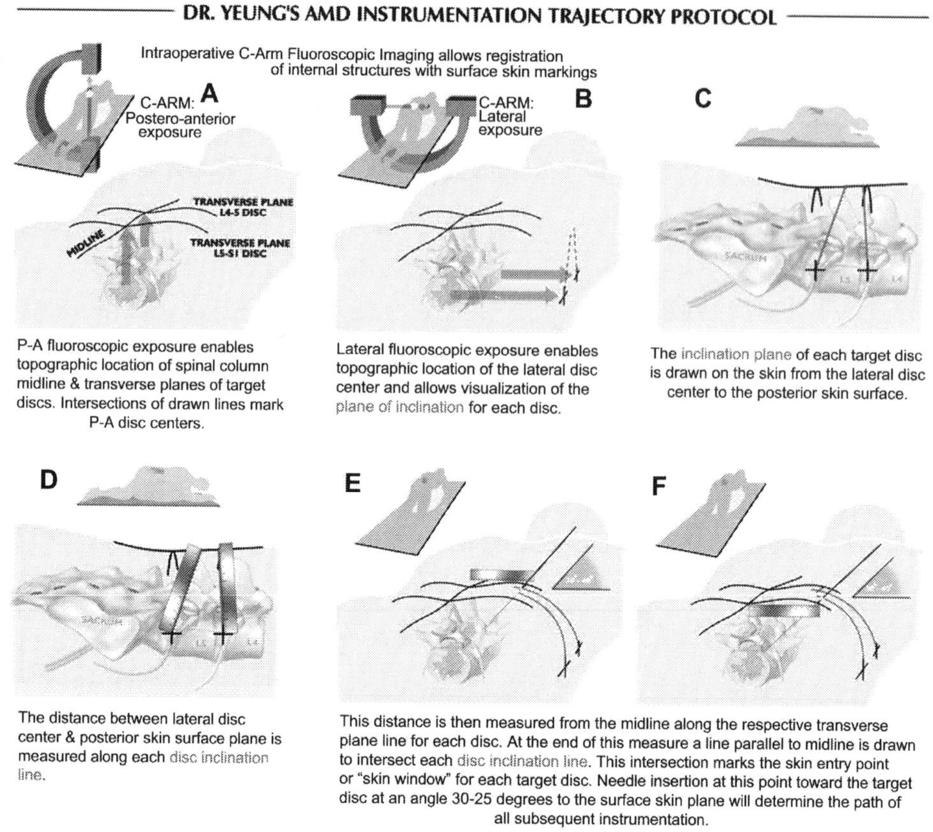

——————————— **DR. YEUNG'S AMD INSTRUMENTATION TRAJECTORY PROTOCOL** ———————————

Intraoperative C-Arm Fluoroscopic Imaging allows registration
of internal structures with surface skin markings

A C-ARM: Postero-anterior exposure

B C-ARM: Lateral exposure

C

TRANSVERSE PLANE L4-5 DISC
MIDLINE
TRANSVERSE PLANE L5-S1 DISC

P-A fluoroscopic exposure enables topographic location of spinal column midline & transverse planes of target discs. Intersections of drawn lines mark P-A disc centers.

Lateral fluoroscopic exposure enables topographic location of the lateral disc center and allows visualization of the plane of inclination for each disc.

The inclination plane of each target disc is drawn on the skin from the lateral disc center to the posterior skin surface.

D

E

F

The distance between lateral disc center & posterior skin surface plane is measured along each disc inclination line.

This distance is then measured from the midline along the respective transverse plane line for each disc. At the end of this measure a line parallel to midline is drawn to intersect each disc inclination line. This intersection marks the skin entry point or "skin window" for each target disc. Needle insertion at this point toward the target disc at an angle 30-25 degrees to the surface skin plane will determine the path of all subsequent instrumentation.

Figure 3 Protocol for determining cannula and instrument trajectory.

the surgeon to bluntly enter the foramen, using the side hole to anesthetize the instrument tract and anulus, pushing the exiting nerve aside if needed. Special cannulas with bevels and side openings (Fig. 5) allow the surgeon to protect vital structures and provide an opening to target specific pathology with various surgical instruments. Clear

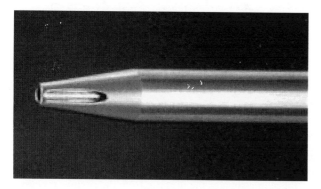

Figure 4 Two-hole obturator has side hole for needle palpation and for delivery of local anesthetic. Spinal probing identifies the pain generators in the foramen.

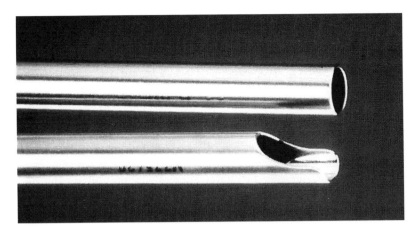

Figure 5 Slotted cannula exposes foraminal pathology and protects exiting nerve during endoscopic spine surgery.

visualization is imperative and is now possible with multichannel endoscopes (Fig. 6) utilizing pressure- and volume-controlled irrigation. A working channel in these endoscopes makes it possible to operate on pathology in the path of the cannula, and various radiofrequency tools and lasers also provide hemostasis and tissue modulation. Clear

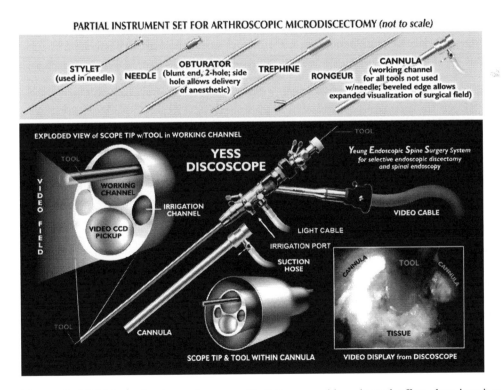

Figure 6 Multichannel spine endoscope with 2.8 mm working channel offers clear imaging in every case.

visualization of vital anatomy and proper cannula placement is the most important factor for avoiding complications in endoscopic surgery.

Complications can also be avoided by keeping the patient awake, and with minimal sedation. The patient will warn the surgeon if he or she feels any sensation of pain during the surgical procedure. Anomalous anatomy, i.e., conjoined nerves, furcal nerves, and autonomic nerves, have been documented endoscopically. With the advent of microsurgical techniques and 1 cm incisions, however, open surgical explorations are no longer the only operative option. A thorough review of all preoperative studies such as computed tomography (CT), magnetic resonance imaging (MRI), and the addition of chromodiscography provides a visual guide for endoscopic surgical exploration. The use of a vital dye for staining tissue through discography facilitates surgeon orientation during an endoscopic discectomy (10,11). Therapeutic measures like foraminal epidural steroids following a discogram and foraminal epiduralgram may also help the surgeon evaluate the foraminal approach and its efficacy in the surgical setting.

IV. MINIMALLY INVASIVE VERSUS TRADITIONAL SURGERY

Skepticism, disbelief, and hostility have continuously arisen over the concept of percutaneous endoscopic spinal surgery. Commenting on the multicenter report by Onik et al. (12) in 1990, Fager (13) predicted that all minimally invasive spinal techniques were doomed to the same oblivion as chemonucleolysis since he felt most patients who required surgery had sequestered or free fragments, and the most common finding at laminectomy was a large fragment ruptured through a small tear in the anulus. He felt that removal of the nucleus pulposus from within the disk space was impossible. In a letter to the editor (14) commenting on Savitz's (15) report on arthroscopic discectomy in 1994, he restated his opinion that intradiscal procedures lent nothing substantive to the treatment of lumbar spine disorders except for disk space infection and were certainly no better than "a non-surgical so-called aggressive conservative approach." In 1998, commenting on Ditsworth's (16) article on endoscopic transforaminal discectomy, Fager (17) reconsidered his initial skepticism and concluded that the superb technological approach and surgical technique advances effectively dispelled most of his previous criticism of minimally invasive procedures.

Endoscopically assisted microdiscectomy (18) and microendoscopic discectomy (19) were designed to introduce microsurgeons to endoscopic techniques. In the posterior lumbar endoscopic approach, the anatomy is familiar. The working space to access the spine is created by mechanical insertion of a special cannula that serves to retract muscle and provides access to the disk. The angle between the working channel and optics channel provides the triangulation necessary to keep the distal ends of the instruments constantly in view and allows bone removal with burrs and a micropunch. Even with an incision smaller than microdiscectomy with much less muscle dissection, in the early phases of the learning curve blood loss is often increased, and iatrogenic dural tears are not uncommon and often require open surgery for repair. Unfamiliarity with the anatomy through the endoscope may result in leaving behind retained disk fragments, which may result in continued lower extremity discomfort for the patient.

Fessler (20) most recently concluded that minimally invasive access spinal surgery allows decreases in operating time, blood loss, postoperative pain, medication use, hospital stays, and costs. Many percutaneous minimally invasive spinal surgery advocates propose very limited indications for fusion and attempt relief of discogenic pain by decompression of disk protrusions, strengthening of ligaments, soft tissue stabilization, and debridement of degenerating nucleus that produce phospholipase A_2, arachidonic acid, prostaglandins, leukotrienes, and other inflammatory agents (21). Other surgeons have limited the use of percutaneous minimally invasive spinal techniques solely for the relief of radicular pain through relief of foramenal stenosis or removal of symptomatic disk extrusions.

V.   NONVISUALIZED PERCUTANEOUS PROCEDURES

Nonendoscopic procedures are nonvisualized, with dependence on fluoroscopy for instrument localization and no intraoperative visualization of the pathoanatomy or actual disk removal. Chemonucleolysis (7) initially depended on unobserved enzymatic denaturalization of the nucleus pulposus. Craig (22) and Hijikata (4) performed a nucleotomy and an anatomical biopsy of the nucleus pulposus for contained disk protrusions with fluoroscopic monitoring. Ascher (6) introduced percutaneous laser discectomy through a large spinal needle or simple cannula to shrink the protruding disk material. Onik et al. (12) utilized an automated nucleotome to remove the nucleus pulposus from the center of the disk space. Intradiscal electrothermal treatment (23) and nucleoplasty by coblation (24) are relatively new nonendoscopic techniques for treating unremitting discogenic pain, but the clinical experience remains limited for both techniques, and lack of visual confirmation of patho-anatomy as well as insufficient scientific evidence has been gathered to evaluate efficacy.

VI.   POSTERIOR LUMBAR PROCEDURES

A.   Chymopapain

Chemonucleolysis via enzymatic digestion of the intervertebral nucleous pulposus has been used as an alternative to surgical treatment in lumbar disk herniations for nearly half a century. Discolysis with either chymopapain or collagenase is accomplished via cleavage of disk matrix proteoglycans with resultant shrinkage of the central nuclear volume and pressure. With this reduction in the nucleous pulposus, the indirect compression of the lumbar nerve roots by herniations is thereby felt to be reduced. As such, injection of patients with chymopapain has generally been limited to the same population of patients who would benefit from an open surgical excision of a proven herniated fragment. Despite FDA approval and over 40 years of overall successful findings from well-designed carefully controlled clinical trials, the indications, efficacy, and safety of chemonucleolysis continues to be hotly debated. As MacNab observed, "arguments regarding its efficacy changed chemonucleolysis into a cause rather than scientific grounds" (25).

Relative contraindications to the use of chymopapain include a history of previous laminectomy or chemonucleolysis, a rapidly progressing neurological deficit, evidence of cauda equina or conus compression syndrome, recurrent disk herniations at the same level, a spinal tumor, severe spinal stenosis, spondylolisthesis or severe deformity, multiple levels of disk herniations, sequestered disk fragments, cerebrospinal fluid leak or fistula, open or closed neural tube defects, severe allergies, diabetes, or pregnancy (23,26). A general rule of thumb is that chemonucleolysis should not be performed in a patient with a history of previous treatment (i.e., discectomy, laminectomy, or injection) at the same level (24). Chymopapain has the potential to induce hemorrhage if it enters the intrathecal compartment (subarachnoid space) , a phenomenon more frequent with revision procedures. As such, chemonucleolysis is not approved by FDA at previously operated levels. Allergic reactions to chymopapain and collagenase continue to be an issue of concern. Preoperative skin testing with ChymoFAST (Biowhitaker, Inc., Palo Alto, CA) or other similar systems is advocated as a screening tool to prevent the severe complication of anaphylaxis that can result from chymopapain exposure. Patients with any evidence of immunoglobulin E (IgE) antibody reaction to the enzyme should be excluded from treatment (27).

General anesthetic techniques increase the risk of complications as they can blunt systemic responses and mask anaphylactic reactions, thereby delaying proper treatment. Agents used during general anesthesia may also have an additive effect on histamine release (28). Furthermore, accidental nerve injury and improper needle placement can be avoided by having ready feedback from the awake patient. Inadvertent injection or penetration of a nerve root can occur in up to 7% of patients under general anesthesia. This unacceptably high complication rate falls precipitously when the patient is able to report any radicular numbness or pain radiating below the knee. Additionally, more fearsome complications such as transverse myelitis and systemic collapse due to anaphylaxis are also significantly more common in patients undergoing general anesthesia (29).

During needle insertion into the disk space, many clinicians will inject 1–3 cc of contrast media to perform a confirmatory discogram to ensure placement of the needle at the correct level. Anular tears and fistulas between the anulus and intrathecal space can often be visualized as well. Potential leakage of the enzyme into the epidural or subarachnoid space can occur in such cases. Others, however, have reported an increased incidence of complications with the use of concomitant contrast and enzyme injection. Experimental data from primate studies have suggested that there may be a synergistic harmful effect of chymopapain when combined with contrast material in the intrathecal space (29,30). Several of the more severe complications after chemonucleolysis have involved the use of simultaneous discograms as well (28). Once the needle is seated within the anulus of the desired disk level, approximately 1–3 mL of chymopapain-type enzyme is gently injected into the space until some resistance is encountered (Fig. 7). When no back-pressure is felt, up to 3 cc is typically infused. In cases where strong resistance is met or the patient complains of severe pain during injection, further forceful enzyme infusion is best deferred or abandoned. This cautious use of a slow, gradual injection may help prevent hydraulic extrusion of free disk fragments by reducing the fluid pressure and by allowing for feedback from the patient as an early warning sign of potential neural injury (28).

For most patients, the postprocedural course is typically short and uncomplicated, with the majority of patients being able to go home after 2–4 hours of observation. Of the possible immediate side effects, back pain and muscle spasm are the most common and limiting. Recent studies have suggested that lowering the dose of Chymodiactin to as little as 25% (1000 U) of the standard dosage (4000 U) can help to alleviate these uncomfortable sequelae. A prospective double-blind trial comparing the use of 2000 U versus 4000 U enzyme dosage did not, however, demonstrate any significant decrease in postinjection back pain (31). Injection of bupivacaine at the periphery of the disk anulus has also been described to reduce iatrogenic chemonucleolysis discomfort. A study utilizing such a technique found back pain in only 3.8% of 80 patients at 3 weeks after the procedure. Compared to the typical 30–40% reported incidence of pain in most series, this was felt to be a significant reduction (32).

As clinical experience with chemonucleolysis spans almost five decades, a large body of clinical retrospective and prospective data is available for review. Retrospective review of 7335 injected patients from 45 cohort studies in the period 1985–1993 found an average

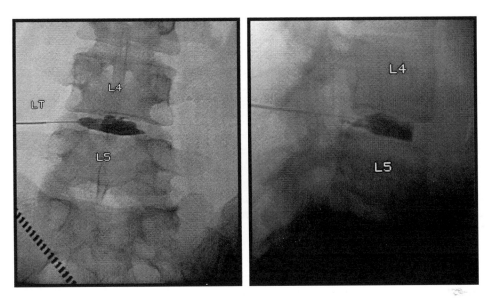

Figure 7 Prior to injection of the chymopapain enzyme, several clinicians have advocated the use of 1–3 cc of contrast media to ensure proper placement and to look for potential leakage of the enzyme into the peridural spaces. After injection, the location of the contrast dye is visualized under real-time AP and lateral fluoroscopy.

success rate of 76% (28). A subsequent meta-analysis of over 130,000 patients treated between 1975 and 1994 revealed an average success rate of 88% (33). Three large prospective randomized double-blind studies have been conducted comparing injection of chymopapain to placebo. From an open-label, double-blind, multicenter study of Chymodiactin conducted in 1498 patients, success rates ranging from 80 to 90% were reported. Patient selection in this series was especially strict regarding radicular symptoms, radiographic criteria, and patient demographics (34). The most definitive prospective clinical trial in the United States was conducted in 105 patients (35). At 6 weeks after injection, 75% of patients injected with the enzyme were significantly improved as compared to 45% of placebo patients ($p=0.003$). At 6 months the placebo success rate had fallen to 38% with no change in the injected group ($p > 0.001$). Placebo patients were then injected with chymopapain as well and achieved relief 91% of the time at one-year follow-up. Another double-blind study conducted in Australia found that 80% of patients injected with chymopapain still found their procedure efficacious at 10 years as compared to only 34% of patients injected with saline. Patients and physicians were both blinded to whether saline or enzyme was used during the course of the study (36). An overall efficacy rate of 50–80% for chemonucleolysis was agreed upon by several experienced authors who participated in a "diagnostic and therapeutic technology assessment" (DATTA) conducted by the American Medical Association (37).

As chymopapain use has been closely monitored by FDA for its safety and toxicity since 1982, outcomes from 135,000 patients are available from post-marketing surveillance (33). From these data, there were 7 fatalities from anaphylaxis, 24 infections, 32 hemorrhagic complications, 32 neurological complications, and 16 miscellaneous other problems. An overall mortality rate of 0.019% and complication rate of 0.090% were calculated. A subset analysis of 77,181 patients revealed 385 cases of some degree of reaction to chymopapain (0.5%). Most cases occurred within the first few years after chymodiactin's approval in 1982, with an allergy rate of only 0.2% seen in the last 5 years of the study. A decreased standard enzyme dosage, routine prescreening with the ChymoFAST test, avoidance of general anesthetics, and pretreatment with antihistamines are thought to account for this decreasing incidence.

For series with concomitant discography, up to 25% of chemonucleolysis procedures may result in some amount of enzyme leakage into the epidural space (37). However, numerous animal studies have consistently demonstrated that leakage of chymopapain and Chymodiactin into the epidural space at concentrations 100 times that used in humans has no harmful effects (30). Intrathecal injection, on the other hand, has been shown to be quite dangerous and can result in subarachnoid hemorrhage, paralysis, and other catastrophic consequences. All experienced authors have emphasized the need for correct needle placement with biplanar fluoroscopic confirmation to avoid such devastating complications. Widespread media publicity of such disastrous sequelae has greatly decreased the popularity of chemonucleolysis in the United States over the last decade (30,38).

An objective assessment of the available data, however, reveals a much lower incidence of serious sequelae. From FDA data, only 17 cases (21%) of the 80 hemorrhagic, neurological, and other serious miscellaneous events could be directly related to chymopapain or the manner in which it was administered. A serious complication rate of only 0.0125% is thus found among the 135,000 tracked cases. Similarly, another cohort of 80,000 patients treated with chemonucleolysis found only 46 cases of serious central nervous system complications for a rate of 1 in 2000 (0.05%) (39). Indeed, when compared to open surgical discectomy or laminectomy, chemonucleolysis has an objectively smaller procedural risk to the patient. A meta-analysis of 43,662 patients treated with chymopapain versus 2051 patients treated surgically revealed an overall complication rate of 3.7% and 26%, respectively (40). There were three surgically related deaths and no mortality from chemonucleolysis. When Nordby et al. compared the results of their extensive analysis with standard surgical outcome data, they found that surgery had a threefold higher mortality rate, a 15 times higher incidence of infection, and a 40 times higher rate of neurological or hemorrhagic sequelae (33). Although the efficacy of chemonucleolysis continues to be a point of controversy, it would seem that the procedure itself is relatively safe and carries little unwarranted risk to the patient.

B. Percutaneous Manual Lumbar Discectomy

As a result of the controversies surrounding chemonucleolysis, alternative mechanical means of decompressing the intervertebral disk space have been aggressively investigated and developed. Although varied in their exact technique, these procedures typically share two common goals. Like traditional open surgery, their first aim is to either directly or indirectly reduce the volume of a herniated disk fragment and to alleviate the patient's low back and radicular symptoms. Second, they seek to achieve this decompression through a minimally invasive percutaneous technique with little to no bony or soft tissue manipulation. Hijikata and colleagues reported the first successful use in 1975 of "percutaneous nucleotomy" to accomplish a partial decompression and removal of the nucleus pulposus via a small posterolateral skin incision (4). Typically, a working cannula ranging from 4 to 8 mm in diameter is passed from the skin down to the desired intervertebral level. Some combination of pituitary forceps, curettes, suction, and irrigation are then passed through this cannula to remove a variable quantity of intradiscal material. The technique involves a central decompression from within and typically does not utilize direct visualization to remove the herniated fragment. As such, most authors believe that the technique's success stems from an indirect decompression of the neural elements akin to that observed in chemonucleolysis.

From their initial experience in 100 patients, Hijikata et al. reported a 70% success rate with one case of infection and one case of vascular injury (4). Concurrently in the west, Kambin and Schaffer found a success rate of 85% in 100 patients treated via a similar percutaneous posterolateral approach (41). Hoppenfeld similarly reported an 86% success rate from the procedure and no significant complications at 10-year follow-up (42). Since these initial reports, numerous modifications of this procedure have been adopted worldwide (43,44).

From a theoretical standpoint, both chemonucleolysis and percutaneous discectomy techniques work on a similar hypothesis. APLD centrally decompresses the nucleus pulposus and thereby decreases the transmitted pressure through the anular tear into the herniated fragment. Although most of these techniques do not directly remove the herniations itself, it is thought that this indirect or secondary reduction in intradiscal pressure results in decreased pressure on the affected nerve root. It would follow that the clinical success rate of any percutaneous procedure would thereby be highly dependent on selecting patient's who have appropriate clinical pathology such as a protruding disk (45).

The large size of the surgical instruments and the working cannula used during the early studies were often associated with a significant risk of muscular trauma, nerve root injury, and major vessel damage. As such, Onik and his group developed an automated PLD technique utilizing a reciprocating suction cutting device for removal of disk material (45–47) (Fig. 8). This device was contained within an outer cannula of 2.8 mm diameter and utilized a guillotine-like blade that reciprocated across a side port enclosed in the blunt-tipped outer sheath at a rate of approximately 180 Hz. Much like chemonucleolysis, proper placement of the cannula and nucleotome was achieved via adequate anatomic

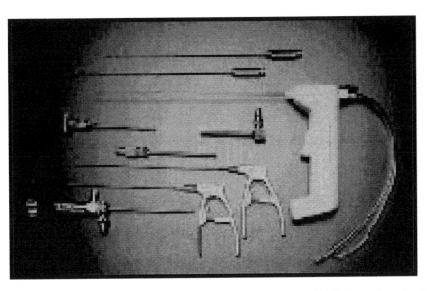

Figure 8 The automated posterior lumbar discectomy (APLD) tool and attachments were developed by Dr. Onik and his colleagues to perform an indirect decompression of the disk space through a minimally-invasive posterolateral approach through Kambin's triangle.

planning and biplanar fluoroscopic visualization. Due to its small size, the incidence of associated soft tissue injury was much smaller when compared with previous manual percutaneous techniques. As the outer cannula was passed first, the nucleotome itself did not encounter skin and was also associated with a lower infection rate. From their subsequent body of clinical experience in 200 consecutive patients, Onik et al. reported an overall success rate of 77.5% at a mean follow-up interval of 6 months (47). After a lag of many years, over 50,000 procedures were eventually performed in the United States. An extremely low morbidity rate of 0.2% was widely reported, with the most common complication being diskitis (48). From his review of 120,000 procedures performed worldwide, Onik could find no single case of death attributable to the procedure itself (49). Although controversy persists about the efficacy of and indications for the procedure, it is quite evident from the literature that APLD is one of the safest minimally invasive means of treating the intervertebral disk. From a review conducted of over 50 series comprising well over 5000 reported patients, there have been remarkably few complications, with no severe sequelae noted (49). Postprocedural back pain and muscle spasms were far less common (<10%) for APLD patients than chemonucleolysis patients and are typically very self-limited (50). When compared to the previous literature on manual percutaneous discectomy with the use of larger cannulas and pituitary type rongeurs, the incidence of soft tissue injury and hematoma is almost negligible for APLD (51). Compared to open discectomy, this rate is three to five times lower. Importantly, there is still no clear case of a mortality associated with APLD among the over 130,000 procedures performed worldwide (52). Most reported clinical failures have been due to retained free fragments or other factors. A re-herniation rate of 3–5% within the first 6 months has been demonstrated in several series of APLDs (53,54).

Despite these low complication rates, no discussion of APLD is complete without a brief mention of its controversial clinical results. Onik, the inventor of the modern nucleotome, conducted a prospective multi-institutional study of over 500 patients which carefully selected only patients with the "classic" criteria for disk herniations. With such stringent patient indications, the participating clinicians were able to achieve a 75% success rate at 6 months with the failures being attributed primarily to unrecognized free fragments. Interestingly only 15% of these failures required an open discectomy (55). Mayer, in a recent objective analysis of APLD outcome data, found significant errors and biases in many of the clinical series used to support APLD use. Applying the same criteria presently used for publication in the journal *Spine*, he found no report that met all selection criteria (48). Furthermore, he found an unacceptably high incidence of two- and three-level procedures, which were based primarily on multilevel discograms. From the few controlled, prospective trials available after screening the papers, the clinical success rates were quite varied. From a prospective, controlled multicenter trial of 327 patients, a clinical success rate of 75.2% was observed at 1 year. However, a smaller controlled, multi-institutional trial of 38 patients examined the actual pain and functional outcomes of patients after APLD and found that only 55% of those treated could return to work after one-year follow-up (56). Another prospective, randomized, multicenter trial comparing APLD and chemonucleolysis in 141 patients reported dismal 37% and 66% respective success rates at one-year follow-up (50). This study, however, has been appropriately criticized for its poor inclusion criteria, which allowed for many patients with disk herniations greater than 30–50% of the canal. From this global review of the APLD literature, Mayer (48) concluded, "there is no scientifically proven validity of automated percutaneous lumbar discectomy compared with standard surgical methods and chemonucleolysis. The majority of articles analyzed did not fulfill the selection criteria of *Spine*. Additional prospective, randomized and controlled studies are needed to define the eventual role of percutaneous lumbar discectomy on a scientific basis."

C. Percutaneous Laser Discectomy

With the advent and subsequent refinement of percutaneous discectomy techniques, it was simply a matter of time before alternative techniques of disk ablation were explored. In parallel with recent advances in technology, innovations in fiberoptics and miniaturization have brought laser technology into the realm of medical therapeutics. Laser energy is formed from focused light emitted from a lasing medium that has been excited by an external power supply. This energy must then be absorbed by biological tissue to have an effective surgical result. This effect is primarily one of ablation, necrosis, and cautery. The delivery of laser energy to the disk through a small percutaneous portal thus represents a logical union of the field of minimally invasive surgery and laser technology. Attractive aspects of percutaneous laser discectomy include (a) single-step insertion of a very small working cannula, as laser fibers are thin, (b) resultant easier access to the L5-S1 disk space, (c) more aggressive nucleotomy, as ablation can extend well beyond the reach of a standard manual nucleotome by increasing the power and pulse time of the laser, and (d) shortened treatment time.

Lasers are further defined by the characteristics of its emitted energy, which is monochromatic, coherent (i.e., nondivergent), and collimated within the same phase. Adjustments of these properties allow for alterations of the power level, pulse mode, and wavelength of each individual laser. Currently, lasers of the infrared, visible-light, and ultraviolet spectrum have been used clinically in surgical procedures. The first surgical use of a laser for disk removal was completed in 1984 when a CO_2 laser was used as an adjunct during standard open anterior cervical discectomy (57). Choy et al. reported the first clinical human use of a Nd:YAG ($1.32\,\mu m$ wavelength) for nonendoscopic percutaneous laser disk decompression and nucleotomy in 1986 (58). Since that time, numerous centers have adopted the use of laser energy for intradiscal ablation. As one of the newest means of nucleotomy, controlled prospective data is lacking. Most clinicians working with PLD agree that it is, in essence, a variation on the concept of manual and automated percutaneous discectomy techniques. Ultimately, all three techniques derive their benefit from achieving a volumetric decompression of the central nucleus pulposus without ever directly removing the disk herniation itself.

Although clinical experience with laser discectomy is not as extensive as other nucleotomy techniques, the concensus has been that the ideal PLD patient is one that meets all the "classic" radiographic and clinical criteria for a herniated disk (59). Some concerns have been raised, however, in cases with suspected severe scarring from either previous surgery, inflammation, or arachnoiditis. Whereas the nucleotomy of APLD is limited by the mechanical device and can be easily contained within the anulus by the operator, laser discectomy carries with it the potential for inadvertent local diffusion of the laser energy as well as distal thermal propagation. In cases where severe distortion of the normal anatomy has occurred, scarred neural and vascular structures may be much closer than anticipated. Laser discectomy may carry increased risk in such redo procedures due to the increased chance of inadvertent thermal transmission to these adherent vital structures (60).

From the available data, PLD may be as effective as other types of percutaneous nucleotomy. Choy and associates performed 333 percutaneous laser discectomies with a Nd:YAG laser and performed up to a one-year follow-up using MacNab's criteria

(61). In this prospective and uncontrolled study, they found that 261 patients (78.4%) had a fair to good response and 72 patients (21.6%) had a poor response to PLD. Eleven patients underwent a second laser discectomy, with 7 (64%) deriving subsequent benefit (62). They found a less than 1% overall complication rate, with diskitis being the most common of these (<0.2%).

Using the KTP/532 laser after its FDA approval, Yeung completed another prospective, uncontrolled study of 1000 patients undergoing PLD. The average dose was 1250 J of laser energy. Strict patient selection criteria were used to include only those with contained disk herniations on MRI or CT, no evidence of dye leak on discography, clinical findings consistent with sciatica, and a failure to respond to conservative therapy. Based on these indications, they reported good to excellent outcomes in 840 (84%) of their patients. Again they reported no mortality and a less than 1% incidence of significant complications (63).

Rhodes and colleagues utilized the Ho:YAG laser for percutaneous lumbar laser nucleotomy and delivered 1200 J of energy to 25 consecutive patients in a prospective but uncontrolled trial. Again utilizing quite stringent selection criteria and a Dallas Pain Questionnaire for follow-up assessment, they found that 20 patients (80%) reported significant improvement of their symptoms. Twenty-three (92%) had resolution of abnormal physical findings, and 21 (84%) were able to return to work (64). One of the largest studies of PLD patients was by Hellinger, who retrospectively analyzed more than 2535 patients treated between 1989 and 1993 (59). He found that 80% of lumbar patients and 86% of cervical patients reported some degree of symptomatic improvement. Additionally, thoracic cases seemed to do especially well. This subjective improvement rate lagged behind a reported 90% rate of improved physical findings. Whereas this series quoted a low rate of complications (<1%), like others in the published literature on PLD, this report is remarkable for the details of the few complications that were encountered. There was one case of diskitis requiring open debridement, one case of transient sympathectomy syndrome, one case of thermally induced paresis of the foot dorsiflexors, and one case of acute paraplegia after cervical laser discectomy. Although Hellinger reported an overall less than 1% complication rate, these sequelae serve as a reminder that laser discectomies are by no means risk-free.

D. Posterolateral Arthroscopic/Endoscopic Discectomy

Whereas chemonucleolysis, APLD, and laser discectomy were all classically nonvisualized means of indirect treatment of disk herniations, the advent of modern high-resolution arthroscopic and video-assisted endoscopic techniques made possible direct visualized removal of herniated disk fragments. In 1983, Forst and Hausmann reported the first insertion of a modified rigid arthroscope into the center of the intervertebral disk space for visualization purposes (65). Kambin would go on to apply this "discoscopic" view of a herniated disk fragment from within the disk in 1988 (66). As this group's experience with the technique grew, they applied these visualization techniques to percutaneous discectomy techniques to allow for direct visualization of resected herniated fragments from within the center of the disk space. Moving gradually outside of the disk itself, Kambin went on to describe and document a safe posterolateral triangular working zone known subsequently as "Kambin's triangle" (67). In 1996 Kambin would modify his approach to achieve an arthroscopic decompression of the neural foramen via mechanical decompression of the anulus and removal of an osteophyte (68). Simultaneously, Matthews described the first published report of a posterolateral arthroscopic approach to the lumbar neuroforamen in 1996 (69). Schreiber and coworkers went on to modify this technique in 1989 with the use of a biportal approach to allow for injection of indigo carmine to stain the abnormal nucleus pulposus, thereby allowing for direct, guided removal of the pathological fragment from the nerve root (44). Kambin et al. would utilize this endoscopic-assisted biportal transforaminal approach to excise both central and sequestered disk fragments in 59 cases with a satisfactory result rate in 88.2% of the patients (70). In 1997 Yeung would apply a rigid rod lens, multichannel, wide-angle endoscope designed specifically for spinal surgery. The beveled tubular shape of the access cannula allowed for same-field viewing of the epidural space, anular wall, and intradiscal space. The addition of working channels also allowed for multiple types of mechanical instruments, drills, and lasers to be applied (71) (Fig. 9). It is important to understand that

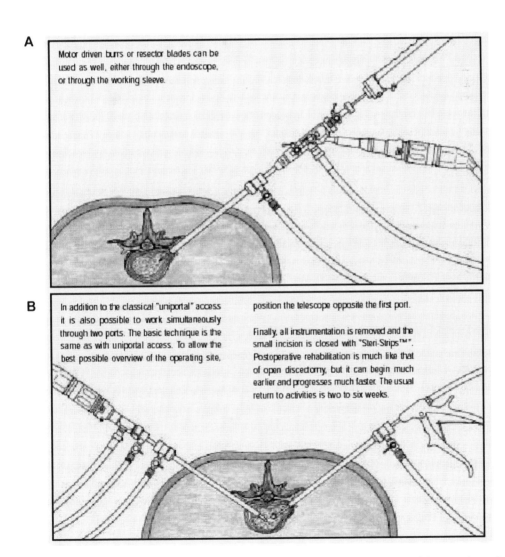

A

Motor driven burrs or resector blades can be used as well, either through the endoscope, or through the working sleeve.

B

In addition to the classical "uniportal" access it is also possible to work simultaneously through two ports. The basic technique is the same as with uniportal access. To allow the best possible overview of the operating site, position the telescope opposite the first port.

Finally, all instrumentation is removed and the small incision is closed with "Steri-Strips™". Postoperative rehabilitation is much like that of open discectomy, but it can begin much earlier and progresses much faster. The usual return to activities is two to six weeks.

Figure 9 Posterolateral endoscopic discectomy can be performed through either a uniportal (A) or biportal (B) technique. Various tools including motor drills, pituitary rongeurs, and suctions can be applied through the various portals.

the posterolateral approach utilized by these clinicians is essentially identical to that described for chymopapain and APLD. As such, the risks of the approach should be similar.

In their retrospective series of 307 patients treated via a posterolateral endoscopic technique, Yeung and Tsou reported an overall satisfactory outcome rate of 89.3%. Their combined major and minor complication rates were 3.5% (72). In contrast to the earlier reports of Kambin et al., Yeung and Tsou provided a clear documentation of their adverse outcomes and complications. In the 9.7% of patients who had poor outcomes requiring reoperations, they observed 1 durotomy, 2 cases of pyogenic disk space infection, 3 cases of congenital lumbar stenosis, 3 cases of persistent foraminal or lateral recess stenosis, 2 recurrent herniations, and 2 missed free disk fragments. Postoperatively, they reported dysesthetic leg pain for longer than 6 weeks in six patients and two patients who suffered thrombophlebitis or deep vein thrombosis. Of note, transient dysesthetic leg pain has been commonly described for the posterolateral transforaminal approach but typically resolves within a few days in the vast majority of cases (44,45,53,67–69,72–74). The exact nature and cause of this phenomenon has not been clearly elucidated. There were no cases of death or intraoperative vascular injuries.

In a review of the prior literature, Yeung et al. observed that the published complication rate for endoscopic excisions of disk herniations was quite low and not consistently reported (72,75). When compared with comparable standard microdiscectomy series and their complications rates, a 1–2% incidence of durotomy, diskitis, and reherniation appears appropriate (76). Hermantin et al. (7) in 1999 completed a prospective and randomized evaluation of surgical treatments for lumbar disk herniation with two surgical arms: standard microdiscectomy versus endoscopic discectomy. Their were 30 patients in each arm for a total of 60 patients. Rigid anatomical exclusionary criteria were used to ensure similar pathologies for both groups. Satisfactory outcomes were observed in 97% of the endoscopic group and 93% of the standard open group. No statistical difference with regards to outcome, recurrence, or complication rate was found (77). As such, it would appear that in the hands of surgeons skilled with the technique, posterolateral endoscopic directly visualized removal of disk fragments may be able to be accomplished with the same safety and efficacy as standard microdiscectomy.

E. Intradiscal Electrothermal Treatment

Unlike chemonucleolysis and percutaneous discectomies, for whom the ideal patient is one with a classical herniated disk protrusion, intradiscal electrothermal treatment (IDET) is typically indicated for treatment of the chronic discogenic back pain patient without frank herniation or "black-disk" disease. In the IDET technique, thermal energy is applied into the intervertebral disk space by means of either a coiled or linear radiofrequency catheter. Saal and Saal first reported the IDET procedure in 1998 in a preliminary series of 25 consecutive patients with chronic discogenic disk disease who had failed other conservative measures (78). Their thermal catheter protocol involved placement of a 17-gauge thin-wall needle placed into the center of the intervertebral disk space under biplanar fluoroscopic guidance. A steerable intradiscal catheter with a temperature controlled thermal resistive coil was then deployed through the needle and coiled within the disk space to rest along the inner posterior anulus under biplanar fluoroscopy (Fig. 10). The catheter was then heated to 90°C for 13 minutes and maintained at 90°C for 4 minutes to create anular temperatures of 60–65°C as observed in experimental studies. Cefazolin was then injected into the disk space with no anti-inflammatories or pain medications given. They observed pain relief as assessed by a visual analog score in

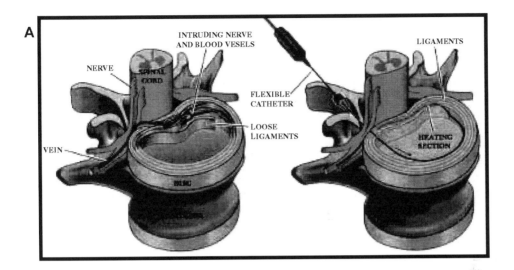

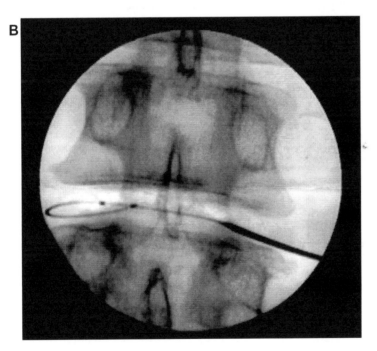

Figure 10 (A) The IDET catheter is threaded through a needle placed into the disk space via a standard discographic approach. The coil is deployed such that the catheter coils within the disk space with the thermal resistive coil resting along the annulus. (B) Placement and final confirmation of the catheter is done under fluoroscopic guidance.

80% of patients, with 72% reporting improvement in sitting tolerance and pain medication requirements (79).

In a cohort of 62 patients studied after 1-year follow-up, these same authors noted statistically significant improvements in 71% of the study patients by SF-36 criteria. They noted a mean decrease of 3 points on the VAS scores as well (80). In their study, the ideal IDET patient was one who had failed conservative measures, had a normal neurological examination, no tension signs, a negative systemic and metabolic work-up, no compressive lesion on MRI, and a positive provocative discogram with concordant pain. Exclusion criteria in their study were inflammatory arthritides, nonspinal conditions mimicking lumbar pain, confounding medical disorders, and prior spinal surgery at the symptomatic level. Thus, the IDET patient stands in stark contrast to the classical discectomy patient. These authors would go on to report 2-year data on 55 of the original cohort. The results were nearly identical to that observed in the original 1-year follow-up study with a 71% improvement on SF-36 and a 3.2 point decrease in the VAS (81). From a thorough review of all the Saals' literature, there were no reported operative or perioperative complications. The authors, however, admit that the sample size of their cohort was too small to predict the "true statistical significance rate of complications related to IDET in general use" (81).

Utilizing a simple literature review of some of the larger clinical series, a mixed cohort of 513 patients can be accrued (81–88). In this cohort, there were no reported immediate operative complications of the procedure. In their exhaustive review of the IDET procedure with regards to its safety, outcomes, and efficacy, Wetzel et al. concluded that even if IDET has no clinical efficacy, "there appears to be no undue risk in subjecting patients to a sham intradiscal lesion" as the reported complication rates of IDET have been negligible (88). Indeed, from a review of the literature, there is only one clear reported case of a complication after IDET with a patient developing acute cauda equina syndrome (89).

From a broader perspective, one must ask whether or not IDET causes untoward pathological changes within the disk space that could potentially lead to progressive degeneration, pain, or instability. From a clinical perspective, the data appear to be controversial. Whereas all studies suggest some degree of initial clinical benefit from the procedure, they do not agree on the sustainability of this improvement. In the Saal brothers' data, the improvements in SF-36 and VAS scores were maintained over the 2-year follow-up period (78–81). In the 60-patient cohort of Davis and Delamarter, they observed only a 37% good outcome rate at 1 year with 97% of patients still reporting significant back pain (82). In an independent non–industry-funded study of IDET, Karasek and Bogduk reported a success rate of as low as 23% and as high as 60% with confidence intervals of ± 16% depending on the stringency of outcome criteria employed (82). Heary, in a review of the topic, could not demonstrate any clear long-term efficacy of IDET over other noninvasive conservative measures (90).

To add further confusion to the topic, basic scientific evidence supporting the mechanism of IDET's action is also mixed. Whereas in a series of five cadavers, Lee et al. were able to demonstrate that there was a difference in segmental stiffness before and after IDET (91), the study of Kleinstueck et al. in five cadaveric specimens demonstrated that IDET-treated levels actually showed a consistent pattern of increased motion and decreased stiffness on biomechanical testing (92). To date, no cadaveric studies have been able to demonstrate an immediate posttreatment "stiffening" of the motion segment as suggested by Saal et al.(78). However, the application of thermal energy to affect structural changes via alterations in collagen has been described in other joint capsules. Hayashi et al. noted that laser energy applied to joint capsules resulted in shrinking of collagen fibers, thereby increasing capsular stiffness as the healing process ensued (93). As such, the effect of the IDET may not be seen in cadaveric studies, as this healing phase is not present. Indeed, clinical experience with the IDET procedure suggests that those patients who experience the most long-lasting relief from the procedure do so typically 4–6 weeks after treatment (88). In a light and electron microscopic study of cadaveric disks after IDET treatment, extensive collagen disorganization, decreased collage quantity, and fiber shrinkage were demonstrated (94). As such, IDET may indeed result in immediate changes in collagen that require a recovery period before providing improved biomechanical "stiffness" in the treated motion segment. A second mechanism by which IDET may work is that of nociceptive deafferentation of pain fibers. Kleinstueck et al. demonstrated perianular temperatures of 39–42°C (92). As cell death typically occurs at this temperature range, this mechanism of "burned" pain fibers would theoretically be supported. However, in the vast majority of clinically improved cases, patients do not experience immediate perioperative pain relief.

In summary, the IDET procedure appears to provide a clinical alternative in the treatment of a group of patients for whom there are few truly effective treatment regimens. Historically, patients with discogenic pain and "black-disk" disease on MRI have poor outcomes after either surgical or nonsurgical therapies. As such, IDET may provide a reasonable therapeutic option in these patients, as it appears to have a less than 1% clinical complication rate. Questions regarding the mechanism of action and the overall clinical efficacy of the IDET remain largely unanswered, however. As such, the benefit of IDET over placebo cannot be conclusively proven.

VII. THE EXPANSION OF ENDOSCOPICALLY MONITORED PROCEDURES

Kambin (5) and Hijikata et al. (4), in the early and mid-1970s, experimented with mechanical debulking of the nucleus for the management of contained disk herniation. Kambin (5) later evolved his technique to remove protruded and extruded disk herniations still contiguous with the disk. Yeung (95) in 1998 improved the instrumentation and optics of the spinal endoscope with a multichannel endoscope and specially configured cannulae that allowed for visualized surgical access to the spinal canal and foraminal zone, while the cannula also retracted and protected spinal nerves and dura. This technique allowed for true foraminal spine surgery through the foraminal approach with excellent visualization.

Knight et al. (96) developed visualized endoscopic laser foraminoplasty with a similar working channel endoscope utilizing a side-firing laser. As foraminal surgery evolved, foraminal enlargement included mechanical trephines, rasps, and various instruments that allowed the endoscopic surgeon to perform foraminal surgery by direct visualization. Other endoscopic surgeons embraced this operative portal for spondylolisthesis and stenosis in addition to disk excision. As the endoscopic technique evolved, however, so did the potential for complications (97). Dysesthesia, a neuropathic hypersensitive postoperative condition, is a potential complication experienced with endoscopic procedures in the foraminal zone. This complication is frequently underreported because it is almost always temporary. In a personal communication, Knight reports about a 29% incidence with foraminoplasty.

VIII. REPORTED AND UNREPORTED COMPLICATIONS

In a multicenter study (9) of over 26,000 cases combining percutaneous fluoroscopically techniques with endoscopic spine surgery, the overall complication rate of percutaneous endoscopic discectomy was less than 1%; dysesthesia, 0.45%; cerebrospinal fluid leak, 0.17%; diskitis, 0.25%; motor or sensory loss, 0.32%; disk recurrence, 0.79%. Postoperative dysesthesias were characterized by delay of onset, hypersensitivity, and allodynia.

Treatment consisted of anti-inflammatory agents, steroids, foraminal epidural blocks, sympathetic blocks, α-blockers, and neurontin titrated up to 3200 mg/day. Nine surgeons recorded all 48 cerebrospinal fluid leaks; none of the patients required surgical repair. Of the 61 cases of diskitis, only 11 were documented to be bacterial and septic. All patients recovered with appropriate antibiotic therapy. Not all of the 88 motor and sensory deficits were transient, but patient satisfaction ranged from 80 to 94%. Although the rate of second surgery was reported to be less than 1%, follow-up at many centers was only months, not years, and the real level of reoperation was very likely much higher. Disk recurrence rates reported by Hoogland (personal correspondence) and Yeung are approximately 4%. Other complications reported in the literature include cauda equina syndrome (98) and permanent foot drop (99–101).

Potential as well as rare complications not reported in the literature include severe complex regional pain syndrome, foot drop (even when laser or radiofrequency is not used), perforation of the bowel, penetration of the great vessels, spinal epidural hematoma, and mechanical injury of a nerve root. Some of these complications can also occur with open surgery and are not necessarily due to surgical mishap. The finding of nerve tissue in the surgical specimen does not automatically predict an injury to the traversing or exiting nerve crossing the disk space. The senior author (A.Y.) has personally removed a disk fragment adherent to the undersurface of a spinal nerve missed during posterior prior surgical discectomy. When the fragment was examined histologically, nerve filaments were found adherent to the discal fragment. Furcal nerve branches are also commonly seen branching from the exiting nerve and extending into the Psoas muscle

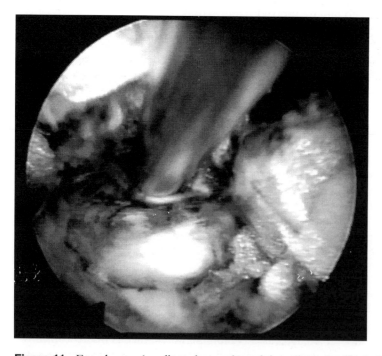

Figure 11 Furcal nerve (myelinated nerve branch in periannular fat) in Kambin's triangular zone. These 1–2 mm nerve branches can be found in the surgical specimen and are not part of the traversing or exiting nerve. The ability to clearly visualize pathology during endoscopic spine surgery is the best way to avoid complications inherent in any surgery.

or occasionally connecting with the traversing nerve. These furcal branches are usually only 1 or 2 mm in diameter and are myelinated (102,103) (Fig. 11). Surgical biopsy has confirmed that these furcal nerves are myelinated nerves. Removing these furcal branches may cause temporary neuropathic pain, but because they are not part of the main nerve trunk, there are usually no permanent functional residuals if treated with pain-management techniques.

IX. PREVENTION OF COMPLICATIONS

Most diskitis following endoscopic surgeries is sterile. Even with thorough tissue debridement for Gram stain and culture, these tissue samples, like the results following needle aspiration, are often negative for an illustrative organism. With repeat arthroscopic debridement, however, immediate relief of pain and rapid improvement in function often is seen. In order to prevent this potential complication, bacitracin and polymixin B may be added to all irrigating saline in bactericidal doses (103).

The delay in onset of neuropathic or sympathetic mediated pain suggests that the mechanism for postoperative dysesthesia, paresthesia, and anesthesia may be due to the close proximity of the dorsal root ganglion in the foraminal approach or from the furcal nerve branches that obstruct the foraminal access portal. Mechanical, electrothermal, and laser heat irritation of the dorsal root ganglion appear to be implicated most, but the symptoms of complex regional pain syndrome can occur from trauma distant to the apparent source of this neuropathic process. Neuromonitoring by EMG and SSEP are currently used to investigate the causes of nerve irritation in an attempt to lessen or prevent damage, but dysesthesia, a variant of complex regional pain syndrome, remains elusive and can occur even if there are no adverse events with neuromonitoring, and even if the patient experiences no pain during the operative procedure (104,105).

Complications of minimally invasive spine surgery can parallel those of traditional surgery. An increase in the complication rate during the initial learning curve can discourage surgeons who are more comfortable with traditional open procedures, but those surgeons who overcome the steep learning curve and master minimally invasive surgical techniques have added a new dimension to their surgical armamentarium.

REFERENCES

1. Pool JL. Myeloscopy: intraspinal endoscopy. Surgery 1942; 11:169–182.
2. Love JG. Removal of the protruded intervertebral discs without laminectomy. Proc Mayo Clin 1939; 14:800–806.
3. Malis JL. Technical contributions of Leonard I. Malis. Mt Sinai J Med 1997; 64:172–181.
4. Hijikata S, Yamagishi M, Nakayama T, et al. Percutaneous discectomy: a new treatment method for lumbar disk herniation. J Toden Hosp 1977; 5:5–13.
5. Kambin P. Arthroscopic microdiskectomy. Mt Sinai J Med 1991; 58:159–164.
6. Ascher PW. Application of the laser in neurosurgery. Lasers Surg Med 1984; 2:91–97.
7. Smith L. Enzyme dissolution of the nucleus pulposus in humans. JAMA 1964; 187:137–140.
8. Morrison PC, Felts M, Javid M. Overview of chemonucleolysis. In: Savitz MH, Chiu JC, Yeung AT, eds. The Practice of Minimally Invasive Spinal Technique. Richmond: AAMISMS Education, LLC, 2000:19–28.

9.   Chiu JC, Clifford TJ, Savitz MH, et al. Multicenter tudy of percutaneous endoscopic discectomy (lumbar, cervical, thoracic). J Minim Invasive Spinal Tech 2001; 1:33–37.

10. Yeung AT. The evolution of percutaneous spinal endoscopy and discectomy: state of the art. Mt Sinai J Med 2000; 67:327–332.

11. Rauschning W. Pathoanatomy of lumbar disk degeneration and stenosis. Acta Orthop Scand Suppl (Denmark) 1993; 251:3–12.

12. Onik G, Mooney V, Maroon JC. Automated percutaneous discectomy: a prospective multi-institutional study. Neurosurgery 1990; 26:228–232.

13. Fager CA. Comment on Onik G, Mooney, V, Maroon V, Maroon JC: Automated percutaneous discectomy: a prospective multi-institutional study. Neurosurgery 1990; 26:232.

14. Fager CA. Arthroscopic microdiscectomy (lett). J Neurosurg 1994; 81:639.

15. Savitz MH. Same-day microsurgical arthroscopic lateral-approach laser-assisted (SMALL) fluoroscopic discectomy. J Neurosurg 1994; 80:1039–1045.

16. Ditsworth DA. Endoscopic transforaminal lumbar discectomy and reconfiguration: a posterolateral approach into the spinal canal. Surg Neurol 1998; 49:588–597.

17. Fager CA. Comment on Ditsworth DA: Endoscopic transforaminal lumbar discectomy and reconfiguration: a posterolateral approach into the spinal canal. Surg Neurol 1998; 49:598.

18. Destandau J. A special device for endoscopic surgery of the lumbar spine. Neurol Res 1999; 21:39–42.

19. Perez-Cruet MJ, Foley KT, Isaacs RE, et al. Microendoscopic lumbar discectomy; technical note. Neurosurgery 2002; 51(5 suppl):129–136.

20. Fessler RG. Minimally invasive spine surgery. Neurosurgery 2002; 51(suppl 2):3–4.

21. Hadjipavlou AG, Simmons JW, Gaitanis IN. Etiopathogenisis of disk degeneration. In: Savitz MH, Chiu JC, Yeung AT, eds. The Practice of Minimally Invasive Spinal Technique. Richmond: AAMISMS Education, LLC, 2000:149–170.

22. Craig F. Vertebral body biopsy. J Bone Joint Surg 1956; 38:93–102.

23. Diaz JH, Connolly ES. Anesthetic management of chemonucleolysis with chymopapain. South Med J 1986; 79:1554–1561.

24. McCulloch JA. Chemonucleolysis: experience with 2000 cases. Clin Orthop 1980; 146:128–135.

25. MacNab I. Chemonucleolysis. Can J Surg 1971; 14:280.

26. Nachemson AL, Rydevik B. Chemonucleolysis for sciatica: a critical review. Acta Orthop Scand 1988; 59:56–62.

27. Grammer LC, Schafer M, Bernstein D, et al. Prevention of chymopapain anaphylaxis by screening chemonucleolysis candidates with cutaneous chymopapain testing. Clin Orthop 1988; 234:12–15.

28. Brown MD. Intradiscal Therapy: Chymopapain or Collagenase. Chicago: Yearbook Medical Publishers, 1983.

29. Agre K, Wilson RR, Brim M, McDermott DJ. Chymodiactin post-marketing surveillance. Spine 1984; 9:479–485.

30. Garvin P, Jennings RB, Smith L, Gessler RM. Chymopapain: a pharmacologic and toxicologic evaluation in experimental animals. Clin Orthop 1965; 41:204.

31. Benoist M, Bonneville JF, Lassale B, et al. [Foraminal and neuro-foraminal hernia. Mid-term results of percutaneous techniques nucleolysis-nucleotomyFrench]. Neurochirugie 1993; 39:110–115.

32. Abdel-Salam A, Eyres KS, Cleary J. A new paradiscal injection technique for the relief of back spasm after chemonucleolysis. Br J Rheumatology 1992; 31:491–493.

33. Nordby EJ, Wright PH, Schofield SR. Safety of chemonucleolysis: adverse effects reported in the USA 1982 to 1989. Clin Orthop 1993; 293:122–134.

34. Fraser RD. Chymopapain for the treatment of intervertebral disk herniations: The final report of a double-blind study. Spine 1984; 9:815–818.

35. Javid MJ. Efficacy of chymopapain chemonucleolysis: a long-term review of 105 patients. J Neurosurg 1985; 62:662–666.

36. Gogan WJ, Fraser RD. Chymopapain. A 10-year, double-blind study. Spine 1991; 17: 388–394.
37. Foley KT, Smith MM. Microendoscopic discectomy. Tech Neurosurg 1997; 3:301–307.
38. Smith L. Chemonucleolysis—personal history, trials, and tribulations. Clin Orthop 1993; 287:117–124.
39. Agre K. Serious neurological adverse events associated with administration of chymodiactin. In: Brown JE, ed. Chemonucleolysis. Thorofare, NJ: Slack Inc., 1985:203–215.
40. Bouillet R. Treatment of sciatica. A comparative survey of complications of surgical treatment and nucleolysis with chymopapain. Clin Orthop 1990; 251:144–152.
41. Kambin P, Schaffer JL. Percutaneous lumbar discectomy. Review of 100 patients and current practice. Clin Orthop 1989; 238:24–34.
42. Hoppenfeld S. Percutaneous removal of herniated lumbar discs. 50 cases with ten-year follow-up periods. Clin Orthop 1989; 238:92–97.
43. Friedman WA. Percutaneous discectomy: an alternative to chemonucleolysis? Neurosurgery 1983; 13:542–547.
44. Schreiber A, Suezawa MD, Leu H. Does percutaneous nucleotomy with discoscopy replace conventional discectomy? Eight years of experience and results in treatment of herniated lumbar disc. Clin Orthop 1989; 238:35.
45. Onik GM, Helms C. Nuances in percutaneous discectomy. Rad Clin North Am 1998; 36: 523–533.
46. Onik G, Helms CA, Ginsburg L, Hoaglund FT, Morris J. Percutaneous lumbar discectomy using a new aspiration probe. AJR 1985; 144:1137–1140.
47. Onik G, Maroon JC, Davis GW. Automated percutaneous discectomy at the L5-S1 level: use of a curved cannula. Clin Orthop 1988; 238:71–76.
48. Mayer HM. Spine update. Percutaneous lumbar disk surgery. Spine 1994; 23:2719–2723.
49. Onik GM. Automated percutaneous lumbar discectomy. In: White AH, Schofferman JA, eds. Spine Care. St. Louis: Mosby, 1995:1018–1027.
50. Regan JJ, McAfee PC, Guyer RD, Aronoff RJ. Laparoscopic fusion of the lumbar spine in a multicenter series of the first 34 consecutive patients. Surg Laparosc Endosc 1996; 6:459–468.
51. Onik G, Richardson D, Amaral J, et al. Percutaneous anterior discectomy under ultrasound guidance. Min Invas Neurosurg 1995; 38:90–95.
52. Gobin P. Percutaneous automated lumbar nucleotomy. J Radiol 1990; 71:401.
53. Luft C. Automated percutaneous lumbar discectomy (APLD)—method and 1-year follow-up. Eur Rad 1992; 2:292.
54. Phelip X, Troussier B, Chirossel JP. La nucleotomie percutanee automatisee dans le traitement des hernies discales lombaires. Presse Med 1992; 21(34):1604–1613.
55. Onik GM, Helms CA. Automated percutaneous lumbar discectomy. Am J Roentgenol 1991; 156:531–540.
56. Kahanovitz N, Viola K, Goldstein T, Dawson E. A multicenter analysis of percutaneous discectomy. Spine 1990; 15:713–715.
57. Gropper GR, Robertson JH, McClellan G. Comparative histologic and radiographic effects of CO_2 laser versus surgical anterior cervical discectomy in the dog. Neurosurgery 1984; 14:42–47.
58. Choy DSJ, Case RB, Ascher PW. Percutaneous laserablation of the lumbar disc. Ann Meet Orthop Res Soc 1987; 1:19.
59. Hellinger J. Technical aspects of the percutaneous cervical and lumbar laser-disc-decompression and -nucleotomy. Neuro Res 1999; 21:99–102.
60. Liebler WA. Percutaneous laser disk nucleotomy. Clin Orthop 1995; 310:58–66.
61. MacNab I. Negative disk exploration: an analysis of the causes of nerve root involvement in sixty-eight patients. J Bone Joint Surg 1971; 53A:891.
62. Choy DSJ, et al. Percutaneous laser decompression: a new therapeutic modality. Spine 1992; 17(8):949–956.

63. Yeung AT. Considerations for use of the KTP laser for disk decompression and ablation. Spine State Art Rev 1993; 7:67–70.

64. Rhodes A. Clinical use of the 2.1 micron holmium:YAG laser and percutaneous discectomy. Spine State Art Rev 1993; 7:49–54.

65. Forst R, Hausmann G. Nucleoscopy: a new examination technique. Arch Orthop Trauma Surg 1983; 101:219–221.

66. Kambin P. Percutaneous lumbar discectomy: current practice. Surg Rounds Orthop 1988; 2:31–35.

67. Kambin P. Posterolateral percutaneous lumbar discectomy and decompression. In: Kambin P, ed. Arthroscopic Microdiscectomy Minimal Intervention in Spinal Surgery. Baltimore: Williams & Wilkins, 1991:67–100.

68. Kambin P, Casey K, O'Brien E, et al. Transforaminal arthroscopic decompression of lateral recess stenosis. J Neurosurg 1996; 84:462–467.

69. Matthews HH. Transforaminal endoscopic microdiscectomy. Neurosurg Clin North Am 1996; 7:59–63.

70. Kambin P, O'Brien E, Zhou L, et al. Arthroscopic microdiscectomy and selective fragmentectomy. Clin Orthop 1998; 347:150–167.

71. Yeung AT. Spinal endoscopy with a multichannel, continuous irrigation discoscope with integrated inflow and outflow ports. Poster presentation. Fourth International Meeting on Advanced Spine Techniques, Bermuda, July 10–13, 1997.

72. Yeung AT, Tsou PM. Posterolateral endoscopic excision for lumbar disk herniation. Spine 2002; 27:722–731.

73. Hijikata S. Percutaneous nucleotomy: a new concept technique and 12 years' experience. Clin Orthop 1989; 238:9–23.

74. Kambin P, Gellman H. Percutaneous lateral discectomy of the lumbar spine: a preliminary report. Clin Orthop 1983; 174:127–132.

75. Boden SD, Herzog RJ, Rauschnig W, et al. Lumbar spine: the herniated disc. Instructional course number 249 presented at 67th Annual Meeting of the American Academy of Orthopaedic Surgeons, Orlando, FL, March 15–19, 2000.

76. Delamarter RB, McCulloch JA, Riew KD. Microsurgery for degenerative conditions of the lumbar spine. Instructional course number 381 presented at 67th Annual Meeting of the American Academy of Orthopaedic Surgeons Orlando, FL, March 15–19, 2000.

77. Hermantin FU, Peters T, Quartararo L. A prospective, randomized study comparing the results of open discectomy with those of video-assisted arthroscopic microdiscectomy. J Bone Joint Surg (Am) 1999; 81:958–965.

78. Saal JS, Saal JA. Management of chronic discogenic low back pain with a thermal intradiscal catheter. Spine 2000; 25:383–387.

79. Saal JA, Saal JS. Thermal characteristics of lumbar disc: evaluation of a novel approach to targeted intradiscal thermal therapy. Presented at the 13th Annual Meeting of the North American Spine Society, San Francisco, California, October 23–31, 1998.

80. Saal JA, Saal JS. Intradiscal electrothermal treatment for chronic discogenic low back pain: prospective outcome study with a minimum 1-year follow-up. Spine 2000; 25:2622–2627.

81. Saal JA, Saal JS. Intradiscal electrothermal treatment for chronic discogenic low back pain: prospective outcome study with a minimum 2-year follow-up. Spine 2002; 27(9):966–973.

82. Davis TT, Delamarter RB. The IDET procedure for chronic discogenic low back pain. Presented at North American Spine Society 16th Annual Meeting, Seattle, WA October 31-Nov 3,2001.

83. Karasek M, Bogduk N. Twelve-month follow-up of a controlled trial of intradiscal thermal anuloplasty for back pain due to internal disk disruption. Spine 2000; 25:2601–2607.

84. Endres SM, Fiedler GA, Larson KL. Effectiveness of intradiscal electrothermal therapy in increasing function and reducing chronic low back pain in selected patients. WMJ 2002; 101(1):31–34.

85. Spruit M, Jacobs WC. Pain and function after intradiscal electrothermal treatment (IDET) for symptomatic lumbar disk degeneration. Eur Spine J 2002; 11(6):589–593.

86. Thompson K, Eckel T. IDET Nationwide registry preliminary results 6-month follow-up data on 170. North American Spine Society, 15th Annual Meeting, New Orleans, LA, October 25–28, 2000.

87. Wetzel FT, Anderson GBJ, Peloza J, et al. Intradiscal electrothermal therapy (IDET) to treat discogenic low back pain: preliminary results of a multi-center prospective cohort study. North American Spine Society, 15th Annual Meeting, New Orleans, LA, October 25–28, 2000.

88. Wetzel FT, McNally TA, Phillips FM. Intradiscal electrothermal therapy used to manage chronic discogenic low back pain: new directions and interventions. Spine 2002; 27(22): 2621–2626.

89. Hsiu A, Isaac K, Katz J. Cauda equina syndrome from intradiscal electrothermal therapy. Neurology 2000; 55:320.

90. Heary RF. Intradiscal electrothermal annulopasty: the IDET procedure. J Spinal Disord 2001; 14(4):353–360.

91. Lee J, Lutz GE, Campbell D, Rodeo SA, Wright T. Stability of the lumbar spine after intradiscal electrothermal therapy. Arch Phys Med Rehabil 2001; 82(1):120–122.

92. Kleinstueck F, Diederich C, Nan W, et al. The IDET procedure: thermal distribution and biomechanical effects on human lumbar disk. North American Spine Society, 15th Annual Meeting. New Orleans, LA, October 25–28, 2000.

93. Hayashi K, Tabit G, Vailas AC. The effect of nonablative laser energy on joint capsular properties: An in-vitro histologic and biochemical study using a rabbit model. Am J Sports Med 1996; 24:640–646.

94. Shah RV, Lutz CE, Lee J, et al. Intradiscal electrothermal therapy: a preliminary histologic study. Arch Phys Med Rehab 2001; 82:1230–1237.

95. Yeung AT. Minimally invasive disk surgery with the Yeung Endoscopic Spine System (Y.E.S.S.). Surg Technol Int 1999; VIII:1–11.

96. Knight MTN, Goswami AKD, Patko J. Endoscopic laser foraminoplasty and aware state surgery; a treatment concept and outcome analysis. Arthroscopie 1999; 2:1–12.

97. Knight MTN, Goswami AKD. Endoscopic laser foraminoplasty. In: Savitz MH, Chiu JC, Yeung AT, eds. The Practice of Minimally Invasive Spinal Technique. Richmond: AAMISMS Education, LLC, 2000:337–338.

98. Epstein NE. Nerve root complications of percutaneous laser-assisted diskectomy performed at outside institutions: a technical note. J Spinal Disord 1994; 7:510–512.

99. Epstein NE. Laser-assisted diskectomy performed by an internist resulting in cauda equina syndrome. J Spinal Disord 1999; 12:77–79.

100. Gill K. New-onset sciatica after automated percutaneous discectomy. Spine 1994; 19:466–467.

101. Matsui H, Aoki M, Kanamori M. Lateral disk herniation following percutaneous lumbar discectomy: a case report. Int Orthop 1997; 21:169–171.

102. Yeung AT. Endoscopic spinal surgery: What future role? Musculoskel Med 2001; 18:518–528.

103. Yeung AT, Gore S. Evolving methodology in treating discogenic back pain by selective endoscopic discectomy (SED®) and thermal annuloplasty. J Min Invas Spinal Techn 2001; 1:8–15.

104. Savitz SI, Savitz MH, Goldstein HB. Topical irrigation within polymyxin and bacitracin for spinal surgery. Surg Neurol 1998; 50:208–212.

105. Zhu, P. Electrodiagnostic studies of radiculopathies + intraoperative monitoring. 3rd World Congress Minimally Invasive Spinal Surgery and Medicine, Phoenix, Az, Dec 8–11, 2002.

36

Complications of Spinal Injection Therapy and Discography

Mitchell K. Freedman and Zach Broyer
Thomas Jefferson University and the Rothman Institute, Philadelphia, Pennsylvania, U.S.A.

Ira Kornbluth
Thomas Jefferson University Hospital, Philadelphia, Pennsylvania, U.S.A.

I. INTRODUCTION

Spinal injection procedures are commonly performed for therapeutic and diagnostic purposes. Diagnosis of a spinal problem begins with the history and physical examination. Anatomical studies such as magnetic resonance imaging (MRI) and computed tomography (CT) scans should be viewed in the context of the clinical scenario. Abnormal findings may be seen in patients without any clinical complaints (1,2). Electrodiagnostic studies are a physiological tool used to identify lower motor neuron lesions. Sensitivity and specificity of EMG/NCV is not perfect (3).

Diagnostic injections provide a provocative tool to help to determine the pain generator in the spine. Injections are used to prognosticate potential for relief with surgical procedures (4). However, sensitivity and specificity have been questioned with spinal injection procedures as well (5). Therapeutic spinal injections can be a wonderful alternative to diminish pain, but they are not always successful.

Spinal injection as a therapeutic and diagnostic tool must thus be used in combination with other diagnostic and therapeutic strategies to maximize therapeutic outcomes. Diagnosis must not be made purely on the basis of the findings seen during an injection procedure. One must compare the results to the findings in the history and physical as well as the other diagnostic strategies. Provocative spinal injections should be ordered with a therapeutic goal in mind. Invasive procedures should not be performed for the sole reason of identification of the "pain generator." Treatment must also be approached with multiple possibilities under consideration. One must not approach the patient from the perspective of injection options alone. Consideration must be given to exercise strategies, medications, surgical options, etc.

In general, diagnostic and therapeutic injection procedures involve minimal morbidity or mortality. However, there is the potential to encounter severe complications; the cautious practitioner should be prepared for life-threatening events at all times. Physicians should be trained in advanced cardiac life support. Patients should have

573

their cardiovascular status monitored. Resuscitation equipment, including an automatic electrical defibrillator, laryngoscope and endotracheal tubes, oxygen, suction, and emergency drugs, should be available. Periodic mock codes should occur.

Complications may occur with any spinal injection such as epidurals, facet procedures (medial branch blocks, facet injections, and radiofrequency rhizotomy), sacroiliac procedures, and disk procedures (discography and IDET). The spinal care physician should be cognizant of the benefits as well as the diagnostic limitations of these minimally invasive spinal procedures. Strategies have been organized by many researchers and clinicians to limit complications and to treat problems when they do occur when performing spinal injections.

II. THE PHARMACOLOGY OF INJECTIONS

Multiple antiseptic agents are available to cleanse the skin. Commonly used agents include iodophors (Betadine), chlorhexidine (Hibiclens), hexachlorophene (Phisohex), and alcohol agents. Potential for local hypersensitivity reactions exists (6,7).

Local anesthetics consist of two chemical rings, one of which is hydrophilic and the other lipophilic. The two rings are linked by either an ester or an amide bond. The two major classes of anesthetics are defined by this bond (Table 1). Esters are hydrolyzed by the plasma enzyme cholinesterase. Metabolites include para-aminobenzoic acid (PABA), which carries a higher allergic potential. Amides are hydrolyzed by liver microsomal enzymes to inactive products and excreted by the kidney. Toxicity may be increased in patients with hepatic toxicity. In general, allergic reactions are rare but are more common in the esters than in the amides. Methylparaben is a bacteriostatic agent used as a preservative in local anesthetic solutions. It is structurally similar to PABA and may be a source of hypersensitivity reactions. Many manufacturers no longer use methylparaben. Cross-sensitivity among members of the ester group has been documented. Hypersensitivity to the amine group alone is rare but has been documented. There appears to be no cross-sensitivity between the esters and amides.

Adverse reactions to local anesthetics are generally caused by toxicity to the central nervous system or the cardiovascular system. Side effects may be dose related or secondary to inadvertent intravascular injections. The cardiovascular system is more resistant to side effects; seizures may occur at lower concentrations than doses required to produce cardiovascular collapse (Table 2).

Table 1 Local Anesthetics

Amides
   Lidocaine (xylocaine, lignocaine)
   Prilocaine(citanest, propitocaine)
   Mepivacaine (carbocaine)
   Buipivicaine (marcaine, sensorcaine)
   Etidocaine (duranest)
   Dibucaine
Esters
   Procaine (novocaine)
   2-Choloprocaine (nescaine)
   Tetracaine (pontocaine)
   Cocaine
   Benzocaine

Table 2   Acute Treatment of Seizures

Confirm diagnosis by observing seizure activity.
Oxygen by nasal cannula or mask; control head position and airway.
Monitor vital signs: BP, oxygen saturation and pulse. Establish ECG recording.
Obtain IV access and keep open with 0.9% saline.
Intubation if ventilatory assistance needed.
Diazepam 5 mg/min q 5 min up to 20 mg maximum.
If seizure persists, load with 20 mg/kg phenytoin no faster than 50 mg/kg in adults.
Must monitor ECG and BP.
9ll, neurological consult; check blood sugar; serum chemistries; hematology,
   toxicology, AED levels.

Central nervous system (CNS) toxicity is secondary to the concentration as well as the rate at which the anesthetic is presented to the central nervous system. Esters produce stimulant and euphoric symptoms, while amides produce sedation and amnesia. Common side effects include headache, lightheadedness, numbness in the distal extremities or around the mouth, metallic taste in mouth, tinnitus, anxiety, flushed or chilled sensation, blurred vision, and nausea. Slurred speech, obtundation, confusion, nystagmus, and muscle twitches can be observed. Seizures, coma, and respiratory arrest can occur.

Cardiovascular toxicity may be increased by hypoxia, acidosis, pregnancy, and hyperkalemia. Decreases in myocardial contractility, rates of electrical impulse conduction, and effects on smooth muscle contraction are dose dependent. CNS suppression may indirectly contribute to cardiac toxicity. Bupivicaine is more effective than lidocaine in blocking cardiac conduction. Peripheral vasodilatation, angina, bradycardia, arrhythmia, and cardiac arrest may occur (8–11).

Complications with glucocorticoids are common but vary greatly depending on the dose of a given agent, the frequency of injection, and the general medical condition of the patient. Caution must be taken when patients have concurrent liver or kidney disease. Labile diabetics can become hyperglycemic following exposure to steroids. Cardiac patients may be predisposed to congestive heart failure secondary to fluid retention. Adrenal cortical insufficiency may occur for 2–3 weeks following injections secondary to suppression of the hypothalamic pituitary axis. This may limit the body's ability to respond to stressful situations such as infection or surgery.

Local side effects of steroids from injections include skin and subcutaneous atrophy as well as changes in skin pigmentation. This can be limited if a separate needle is used to puncture the skin and if the injection needle is flushed with local anesthetic or saline.

Other systemic side effects to steroids include cushingoid symptoms resulting in a moon-face, hirsutism, buffalo hump, flushing, bruising, striae, and acne. Mobilization of calcium and phosphorus can result in osteoporosis and muscle wasting. Increased appetite can cause weight gain. Gastric upset may occur more commonly. Transient hypertension and edema may result from retention of salt and water. Menstrual irregularities, mood swings, and anxiety may occur (8,12–15).

III. ALLERGIC REACTIONS

Anaphylaxis is a type I hypersensitivity reaction caused by IgE-induced degranulation of tissue mast cells and basophils, which results in the release of potent mediators.

An anaphylactoid reaction is an event that mimics anaphylaxis, but is not due to an IgE antibody-antigen immune response. Symptoms generally occur within 20 minutes. However, a biphasic time course can occur. The late phase response can reappear within 3–12 hours and can be more profound than the first reaction.

Patients who suffer an anaphylactoid reaction to radiocontrast materials are at risk for a repeat reaction. The estimate of recurrence ranges from 16 to 44% with high-osmolality contrast agents. With the use of lower osmolar contrast agents and prophylaxis, the risk of repeat reaction is reduced to 1%. There is no link between allergy to shellfish and allergy to low-osmolar contrast agents. Overall frequency of adverse reactions is 5–8% with high-osmolality radiocontrast material (RCM); life-threatening reactions have a frequency of < 0.1%. Mortality is estimated to occur in one out of every 75,000 patients who receive high-osmolality RCM. The risk of anaphylactoid reactions with low-osmolality RCM is about 20% compared to conventional RCM.

Prophylaxis should be provided for patients with a previous reaction to radio-contrast agents if they must receive contrast for a given procedure. If a significant reaction has occurred in the past or if the patient has labile diabetes and contrast is not critical to the procedure, it may be wise not to utilize contrast. Prophylaxis should include prednisone 50 mg by mouth 13, 7, and 1 hour prior to the procedure. Diphenhydramine 50 mg IM should be given 1 hour prior to the procedure. Ranitidine 150 mg or cimetidine 300 mg orally is optional 3 hours before the procedure. Patients at high risk can also receive ephedrine 25 mg by mouth 1 hour before the procedure. This is contraindicated in the face of ischemic heart disease or angina (Table 3).

Classic features of anaphylactic reactions include laryngeal edema, bronchospasm, fainting and lightheadedness, and cardiovascular collapse. Patients may be flushed or pale, develop pruritus, itching of the palate or external auditory meatus, urticaria, conjunctivitis, nausea and vomiting, abdominal pain, and palpitations. The patient with a severe reaction must be monitored carefully; hospitalization may be wise since a biphasic reaction can occur. The patient should be recumbent with legs elevated. Oxygen at 8–10 L/min should be administered. If the patient demonstrates stridor, wheeze, or signs of shock, 0.3–0.5 ml of 1:1000 epinephrine solution should be administered IM into the thigh. This can be repeated every 15 minutes up to 2 doses.

Diphenhydramine 25–50 mg can be dispensed parenterally for urticaria. The airway should be maintained with an oropharyngeal airway device. Bronchospasm may require hydrocortisone, aminophyllin, or albuterol. Hypotension may require vasopressors. IV glucagon may be used for refractory hypotension (Table 4) (16–20).

Latex hypersensitivity is also a potential problem for healthcare workers as well as for patients. Children with spina bifida and genitourinary problems are at particular risk. Patients with spina bifida or a significant history of latex allergy should have procedures

Table 3 Prophylaxis for Anaphylaxis/Anaphylactoid Reaction to Radiocontrast Material

Prednisone 50 mg po 13, 7, and 1 h prior to administration of radiocontrast material (RCM)

Diphenhydramine 50 mg po or IM 1 h prior to RCM

Ephedrine 25 mg 1 h prior to RCM (omit with ischemic heart disease, angina, and cardiac arrhythmias and contraindications to sympathomimetics)

Optional use of H2 antagonist ranitidine 150 mg or cimetidine 300 mg po 3 h prior to RCM

Discontinue β-adrenergic blockers, ACE inhibitor, or ACE blocker if possible the morning of the injection

Table 4 Treatment of Anaphylaxis

Patient should be place in recumbent position with legs elevated
Monitor vital signs q 2–5 min
Administer oxygen 8–10 L/min
Maintain airway, intravenous access
Diphenhydramine 25–50 mg po, IM for urticaria
With stridor, wheeze, shock:
   Epinephrine: adults 0.2–0.5 cc of 1:1000 solution q 15 min into thigh IM
   up to total dose of 0.01 mL/kg
   Diphenhydramine 1–2 mg/kg (25–50 mg) IM or IV
Bronchospasm
   Albuterol 2 puffs q 15 min up to 3 doses
   Aminophyllin 5.6 mg/kg over 20 min
   Methylprednisolone 25 mg/kg q 6 hours
Hypotension
   IV fluids: 1 L isotonic NaCl q 20–30 min
   Epinephrine 1:10,000 solution at 1 mg/min initially then 2 mg/kg to maintain
   systolic >90 mmHg
   Glucagon 1 mg IV up to 5 mg/h if adrenergic agent complicates treatment

performed in a latex-controlled environment. No latex gloves or accessories with latex should contact the patient (21).

IV. ANTICOAGULANTS AND ANTIPLATELET AGENTS

Epidural injections resulting in bleeding and neurological complication is rare. It is clear that coumadin must be discontinued prior to spinal procedures. Current recommendations state that coumadin should be held for 5 days prior to injection procedures. A protime and INR should be checked on the morning of the procedure as well. Lovenox should be held for 2 days prior to a procedure (Table 5) (22).

Protocols for antiplatelet agents are less clear. Aspirin irreversibly inhibits platelet function for 7–10 days. Nonsteroidal anti-inflammatory drugs (NSAIDS) cause reversible competitive platelet inhibition; platelet function returns to normal in 1–3 days after withdrawal of the drug. Ticlopidine causes irreversible noncompetitive inhibition of platelet function. The effects on platelet function persist for 10–15 days after withdrawal of the drug. It has been suggested that a single antiplatelet agent does not need to be held; there are few case reports that link a single antiplatelet agent with epidural bleeding. Other sources suggest that aspirin and NSAIDS should be held for 7 days prior to a procedure (22,23).

Table 5 Coumadin Protocol

Establish if procedure is important and whether or not risk to patient is too great
   to stop the Coumadin
Hold Coumadin for 5 days prior to the day of the procedure
Check INR, PT on the morning of the procedure
Stop Lovenox 2 days prior to the day of the procedure

Table 6   Antiplatelet Agents

No definite contraindication to ongoing use of agent
If cautious or with cervical procedures, then stop:
    Aspirin 7–10 days prior to procedure
    Ticlopamide 7–10 days prior to procedure
    Ginkgo 36 hours prior to procedure
    Ginseng, garlic 7 days prior to procedure

Several herbal agents may increase the risk of bleeding in a surgical population. Ginkgo may alter platelet function by inhibiting platelet-activating factor. Preoperatively, it is held for 36 hours prior to surgery. Ginseng inhibits platelet aggregation and causes irreversible platelet inhibition for up to 7 days. Garlic inhibits platelet inhibition in a dose-dependent fashion; irreversible platelet fashion may occur for up to 7 days. Vitamin E inhibits platelet adhesiveness in vitro. However, in vivo there is no definite antiplatelet effect. Indeed, there is no definite evidence that any of these agents must be held prior to a spinal procedure (24–26) (Table 6).

V.   CONTRAINDICATIONS TO SPINAL INJECTIONS

Spinal injections are always elective procedures. If there is a question of safety, the procedure should not take place or it should be terminated. Absolute contraindications include coagulopathy or abnormal bleeding secondary to anticoagulation. Patients with local or systemic infection should not receive spinal injections. Abnormal anatomy secondary to congenital abnormalities or previous surgical procedures may prohibit certain types of spinal procedures. Patients with history of congestive heart failure may need to avoid steroid injections if they tend to retain fluid. Patients with labile diabetes mellitus should receive smaller doses of steroids or avoid exposure to steroids altogether.

VI.   FLUOROSCOPY

Fluoroscopy is routinely used to enable proper needle placement for spinal procedures. In general, it is a safe procedure. However, there are potential risks for both the operator and the patient. There are two classifications of potential biological effects of radiation. Stochastic effects include neoplasm and heritable effects in reproductive cells. Deterministic effects include cataracts and radiation burns.

Ionizing radiation can cause a neoplasm by inducing a change in a single cell. This can occur at any dose level but is more likely to happen with increasing dose levels. Doses in excess of 200 mGy can induce cancer. At this dose the risk is in the range of 0.2%–1.6%. In the first half of the twentieth century physicians who worked with radiography and fluoroscopy died of cancer at an increased rate relative to other physicians. While this is less of an issue now, there may still be a slight increased rate of multiple myeloma. It is also feasible that heritable changes in the genome of reproductive cells can affect the progeny of an individual. Risk is minimized by limiting dose and using gonadal shields.

Deterministic effects occur after a certain threshold is reached. Cell death occurs when the dose is high. Injuries to the hands of fluoroscopists are common. Radiation dermatitis results in fingernail changes, scaly and discolored skin, and diminished hair growth. Cumulative doses in excess of 10 Gy result in radiation dermatitis. The U.S. FDA has documented at least 40 cases of radiation induced burns to patients. Radiation-induced cataracts may also result from high doses of chronic exposure.

Exposure to personnel can be limited by the use of protective aprons, thyroid shields, sliding lead panels, and positioning of the patient and table as a shield. Lead gloves and glasses are available. Aprons should have shielding characteristics equal to 0.5 mm of lead. The x-ray tube should be at a maximal distance from the patient, and the image intensifier should be as close to the patient as possible. Personnel should be as far from the patient as possible. The dose rate decreases by the inverse of the inverse square of the relative increase in distance. Doubling the distance from the beam decreases exposure by four times. Beam-on time must be kept to a minimum. Pulsed fluoroscopy, collimation, and hold and store capabilities can all minimize exposure.

Radiation–monitoring devices should be worn on the collar. Doses of 100–400 mrem are high enough to consider extra shielding and to consider change in work habits. For doses in excess of 400 mrem, the practitioner must evaluate causes, work habits, and add shielding.

Pregnant women may wish to wear abdominal badges that can be monitored every 2 weeks to carefully monitor radiation exposure to the fetus. A wrap-around apron with 0.5 mm lead equivalent in front and 0.25 mm in back is recommended. Special 1 mm lead equivalent over the pelvis is available, or an extra 0.5 mm lap apron can be worn underneath the regular lead apron (8,10,27).

VII. GENERAL COMPLICATIONS

A. Infection

Minor infections resulting from spinal injections are not uncommon. The risk of infection is intimately related to sterile preparation. Severe infections that have been reported include meningitis (28,29) and epidural abscess (30–32). Diabetics are at higher infection risk and should be monitored closely for signs and symptoms of infection.

B. Bleeding

The epidural space is highly vascular and the risk of trauma to blood vessels is present. The risk of clinically significant bleeding is increased with cervical injections due to a smaller epidural space in the neck (33).

C. Dural Puncture

Even in the best hands, the dural membrane may be punctured during the performance of invasive injections. This is especially true with interlaminar epidural steroid injection (ESI). The posterior epidural space is 1.5–2 mm wide in the upper cervical spine and increases to 3–4 mm at the C7-T1 interspace. Derby suggests the use of extreme caution when doing cervical epidural injections above C7-T1. The posterior epidural space in the mid-lumbar region is 5–6 mm, and this narrows down to 2 mm at the S1 level (34).

In the event of a recognized dural puncture, the procedure should be aborted. Continuing the procedure at an adjacent level is not recommended as the injectate can flow in a caudal or cephalad direction through the dural defect (35). Fluoroscopy can identify

Table 7   Treatment of Dural Puncture Headaches

1.   Identify dural puncture
2.   If dural puncture is identified, inform patient of possible symptoms
3.   Prescribe analgesics as appropriate
4.   Encourage patient to ingest fluids, including caffeine, judiciously
5.   Advise relative bed rest
6.   If symptoms are prolonged and/or are debilitating, consider a blood patch

dural punctures. If the contrast is injected into the subdural space, a delayed, patchy, uneven blockade will occur (36). There is no fat, as in the epidural space, to prevent a more widespread blockade. Manifestations of an injection into the subarachnoid space are similar to those for an injection into the subdural space. Poor outcome from dural punctures and subsequent injection are rare but may include hypotension, cardiovascular arrest, spinal anesthesia, respiratory compromise, and death (10).

Arachnoiditis (37) as well as aseptic (38,39) and bacterial meningitis (28) have been attributed to the injection of steroids after a dural puncture. The polyethelene glycol component of methylprednisone may contribute to the development of arachnoiditis (8).

The most common symptom of dural puncture is delayed, persistent headache that is relieved by recumbence. Symptoms are due to leakage of Cerebrospinal fluid (CSF) through the dural defect, which causes a reduction in CSF pressure and downward traction on the pain-sensitive intracranial veins and meninges. Most dural puncture headaches resolve spontaneously. Patients should be prescribed analgesics, relative bed rest, and ample fluids as well as caffeine. There is not good evidence from randomized trials to suggest that routine bed rest after dural puncture is beneficial. Routine, prolonged bed rest should be avoided. Patients should be encouraged to mobilize as tolerated (40).

In cases of refractory headaches, an autologous blood patch may be necessary and highly effective (41). This involves the injection of approximately 20 cc of autologous blood into the extradural space around the dural puncture site. Blood coagulation factors are thought to help seal the dural defect (Table 7).

Not all headaches after ESI are due to dural puncture. In fact, an incidence of nondural puncture headache has been estimated at 2%. Possible mechanisms of non-dural puncture headaches after ESI include air injected into the epidural space and increased pressure from the injection (42).

D.   Paralysis

Neurological injury can occur from numerous mechanisms including direct penetrating trauma, compression from hematoma or abscess, injection following dural puncture, and intravenous injection. Seizures can be caused by intravenous injection of anesthetic agents. Nerve root injuries, tetraplegia, and paraplegia have all been reported as sequalae of interventional spine procedures.

E.   Syncope

Vasovagal reflex syncope is the most frequent cause of transient loss of consciousness (43). Syncope and vasovagal responses are not uncommon after interventional spine procedures

Table 8 Treatment of Syncope

1. Place patient in recumbent position, reverse Trendelenburg if needed
2. Identify the trigger (most commonly pain and/or volume depletion)
3. Assess ABC/vital signs
4. Secure the airway if necessary
5. Administer oxygen
6. Start IV (if not already placed), administer fluids
7. Cause specific interventions; use vasopressors as indicated

(36, 44–47). Before a procedure, patients should be queried about prior syncopal episodes. If patients have a history of syncope, proper precautions should be taken.

Premonitory symptoms such as nausea, diaphoresis, abdominal discomfort, and blurry vision frequently precede a syncopal event. These symptoms should be identified, and the patient should lie flat on the table, which will increase venous return to the heart (43) (Table 8).

F. Miscellaneous

Uncommon but reported complications include subdural hematoma (48), unilateral vitreous hemorrhage (49), retinal hemorrhage (50), persistent hiccups (51), pneumocephalus (52), complex regional pain syndrome (53,54), and dysphonia (55).

VIII. COMPLICATIONS AND LIMITATIONS OF VARIOUS EPIDURAL STEROID INJECTION TECHNIQUES

A. Complications of Caudal ESI

The risk of dural puncture is exceedingly rare as the needle is usually positioned below the thecal sac, which typically ends at the S2 vertebra. The thecal sac occasionally extends to the S4 vertebral level. Without fluoroscopy, incorrect needle placement has been estimated to occur 25–40% of the time (10).

In a large retrospective review, there were no major complications. Minor complications were noted after 15.6% of injections; the most common complication was insomnia the night of the injection (45).

B. Complications of Interlaminar ESI

The interlaminar approach should not be performed in patients whose anatomy prevents appreciation of this loss of resistance. For instance, patients should not undergo interlaminar ESI after laminectomy as their ligamentum flavum has been sacrificed. Fluoroscopy helps to assure proper placement. The needle is misplaced in 30% of cases without fluoroscopy (56).

Hodges reported two cases in which patients who were heavily sedated had new symptoms and MRI findings after cervical interlaminar ESI. In both cases, the needle was reintroduced at another level after a detected dural puncture. Patients should not be sedated to the point that they cannot communicate any undesirable symptoms. Derby also advised extreme caution with cervical interlaminar ESI above C7-T1 due to the narrowness of epidural space (35).

In a large retrospective study of cervical interlaminar ESI, the overall incidence of complications was 16.8%. The most common complication was increased neck pain. Only one dural puncture resulted from 345 injections (47).

C. Complications of Transforaminal ESI

Fluoroscopy is mandatory for proper needle placement and to decrease the chance of intravascular injection. Arteries travel with nerve roots in the neural foramen and can easily be injected inadvertently despite proper needle placement. The risk of significant morbidity from transforaminal ESI is higher in the cervical spine as the vertebral arteries run in close proximity to the target site for injection (Fig. 1). The steroid particulate matter can obstruct flow in the vertebral artery or flow upstream and lodge in the basilar artery. Tetraplegia has been reported from intra-arterial injection during cervical transforaminal ESI (57). In this case, the injection caused an anterior cord syndrome.

Paraplegia has been postulated from intra-arterial placement during lumbar transforaminal ESI. A recent case series reports that three patients developed paraplegia after lumbosacral nerve root blocks below the L2 vertebra. The authors suggest that the injectant was taken up by an abnormally low artery of Adamkiewicz (58).

Furman et al. showed that 11% of transforaminal ESI were intravascular and that aspiration was not a sensitive means to detect whether the injection was intravascular (59). Under fluoroscopy, the contrast should outline the nerve root and persist. If the dye is intravascular, it will dissipate rapidly.

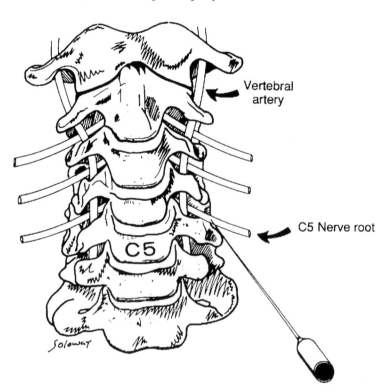

Figure 1 Anatomy of the cervical spine. Note the proximity of the vertebral artery to the target site for transforaminal injections. (From Ref. 56a. Adapted with permission from Lippincott, Williams, and Wilkins.)

In a retrospective study, 9.6% of patients had minor complications. The most common complication was a transient, nonpositional headache (46).

D. Limitations of ESI

Placebo response may be as much as 50%. There is a larger placebo response with more invasive procedures. Explanations for placebo response include positive relationship with the clinician, patient and clinician expectation of a positive outcome, endogenous endorphin release during a procedure, and reduction of stress and anxiety by the procedure (60).

In a study by North et al., patients with diagnoses of facet syndrome and radiculopathy underwent a series of diagnostic blocks in random order using equivalent doses (3 cc) of bupivicaine. Patients received significant, temporary relief from lumbosacral nerve root blocks, medial branch blocks, and sciatic nerve blocks. This study suggests that false-positive responses are quite common and that specificity of diagnostic blocks is low (5).

IX. ZYGAPOPHYSEAL JOINT INJECTIONS

A. Complications

Major complications from zygapophyseal joint injections are uncommon. In a study that included 42 zygapophyseal joint injections and 43 medial branch blocks, the only adverse effects reported were transient worsening of pain, headache, nausea, and paresthesias (61). Meningitis has been reported after lumbar zygapophyseal joint injection (62,63).

B. Limitations

Recent studies estimate that 15–40% of chronic low back pain is attributable to the zygapophyseal joints (64,65). However, diagnosis is difficult as response to injection is not clearly correlated with any aspect of the history or physical exam (66). Pain eminating from the zygapophyseal joint has been noted to radiate in overlapping regions. If the decision has been made to inject the zygapophyseal joints, it is often not clear which zygapophyseal joints to inject. This is especially true in the lumbar spine (67–70).

The gold standard for diagnosing zygapophyseal joint pain is through injections. The literature supports use of a double block paradigm to definitively establish the zygapophyseal joint as the pain generator. A double block paradigm entails the use of two anesthetic agents of two different durations on two different occasions to anesthetize the medial branches of the dorsal rami. For a positive response to the double block paradigm, there must be a positive response to both anesthetic agents, and the response must persist for the appropriate duration. In fact, a false-positive rate of 38% was found when a single block was used to diagnose zygapophyseal joint pain (66). Typically, a volume of 0.5 cc is used to perform median branch blocks. Larger volumes could theoretically spread to local structures and cause a false-positive response (71). Leakage from the facet capsule can occur if volumes in excess of 1 cc are used (68).

Common reasons for false-negative results include misplaced needles, inadequate injection volume, and injections performed at the incorrect zygapophyseal joint. Two dorsal rami innervate each zygapophyseal joint, and each must be adequately blocked to prevent a false-negative result.

X. RADIOFREQUENCY NERVE ABLATION

Radiofrequency is an effective means of treating zygapophyseal joint pain by ablating the medial branch of the dorsal ramus, which innervates the zygapophyseal joint (72,73). Dysesthetic pain is an untoward sequalae of radiofrequency nerve ablation (74).

The medial branch of the dorsal ramus also supplies the multifidi. One concern about ablation was that the multifidi would be weakened and unwanted weakness would result. Thus far, no significant multifidi weakeness has been attributed to radiofrequency nerve ablation (73).

If patients do not achieve significant relief from the procedure, an EMG of the multifidi can help to evaluate whether the desired denervation occurred. A false-negative result may be a consequence of technical failure if the patient reports no relief and there is no evidence of multifidi denervation (75).

XI. SACROILIAC JOINT INJECTIONS

No aspects of the history or physical exam firmly establish a diagnosis of sacroiliac joint pain (76–78). As in the zygapophyseal joint, injections are the gold standard for diagnosis. A double block paradigm using different duration anesthetics on separate occasions also helps to limit false-positive findings (77).

In one study, the mean total joint volume was determined to be 1.08 cc in symptomatic patients and 1.6 cc in asymptomatic volunteers (79). Escape of injectate may occur, and the injectate can communication with neural structures in the region. Communication to the lumbosacral plexus, the L5 spinal nerve, and the dorsal sacral foramina has been demonstrated (80). If excess volume is used, specificity may be poor.

Major complications from sacroiliac joint injections are uncommon. Complications from sacroiliac joint injections include bleeding, infection, adverse drug reactions, and nerve damage from inadvertent needle placement.

XII. COMPLICATIONS AND LIMITATIONS OF DISCOGRAPHY

A. Complications of Discography

The most notable complication of discography is diskitis. With the initiation of a two-needle technique, the incidence of bacterial diskitis has decreased. Rates of diskitis vary in the literature. Fraser et al. showed that the single-needle technique for lumbar discography had a 2.7% rate of diskitis, while the double-needle technique had only a 0.7% rate of diskitis (81). The rate of lumbar diskitis described by Guyer et al. (82) was 0.10% per patient or 0.05% lumbar diskitis per disk. In the cervical spine the rate of diskitis may be higher due to the fact that only the single needle technique is used. The rate of diskitis post–cervical discography has been described from 1.38 to 2.48% per patient and 0.37 to 1.49% per disk (82–84).

Diskitiswas thought to be a chemical process. The early literature assumed that diskitis was chemically induced because of an inability to culture bacteria from the disks. Agre et al. reviewed 29,075 patients with chymopapain injections; only 9 of the 22 cases of diskitis had positive bacterial culture (85). Fraser et al. (81) refuted the chemical explanation. In their study sheep disks were injected with *Staphylococcus epidermidis*. No matter how much bacteria was injected, there was no difference in the diskitis reaction.

Table 9 Diagnosis of Diskitis

1. Marked increase in back or neck pain
2. Increased ESR by 3 weeks (peak)
3. X-ray
   a. Loss of disk height
   b. Endplate irregularity
4. MRI evidence
   a. Abnormal signal intensity in vertebra and disk
   b. Decreased signal intensity on T1
   c. Increased signal intensity on T2
   d. Indistinct vertebral endplate
5. Bone scan with increased uptake — not accurate until 3 weeks after injection

Cultures of the disks at 6 weeks did not yield bacteria, perhaps explaining the lack of positive cultures in previous studies. Pathology specimens revealed nuclear protrusion into the endplates, with a resultant increase in vascularity and bacterial death by possible lymphoid infiltration (81).

After discography, diskitis should be suspected in patients with increased neck or back pain. The average time to increased neck or back pain is 17 days. The erythrocyte sedimentation rate may show elevation on average at 20 days. Bone scan is generally negative before 18 days. The bone scan will show evidence of increased uptake by an average of 33 days. MRI findings have not been noted before 35 days postdiscography. Diskitis typically appears on MRI as decreased signal intensity of the vertebra and disk on T1 images and increased signal intensity on T2 images with indistinct vertebral endplates (86). Disk space narrowing or endplate changes appeared on x-ray after at least 14 day (82). Cervical discography patients had earlier positive findings. Disk biopsies demonstrated S. epidermidis. Erythrocyte sedimentation rate does not normalize until 8–11 weeks in the lumbar patients and 6–7 weeks in the cervical patients (82) (Table 9).

Several other serious complications after discography have been described. Abscess has been reported in the lumbar spine (83) and in the cervical spine (87). A case of a hematoma in the right carotid sheath post-cervical discography has been described. This was thought to be caused by a puncture of the right internal jugular vein (88). There is also a case of occipital neuralgia in a patient with intermittent headaches after a motor vehicle accident. This was noted 2 days after the discogram and may be an incidental finding (88).

Quadraparesis secondary to subdural empyema has been reported one week postdiscography. Initial treatment with antibiotics was ineffective. Surgery was required

Table 10 Prevention of Diskitis

1. Clean aseptic room
2. Prepare skin over a wide area
3. Avoid contamination of radiographic equipment
4. Double needle technique
5. Avoid handling needle tip
7. IV antibiotics 30 minutes prior to injection or mixed with contrast:
   Cephalosporin
   Vancomycin or Cleocin are options in patient with penicillin allergy

Table 11   Treatment of Diskitis

1.   Aspiration of disk space for culture
2.   IV antibiotics for 4 weeks in cases of osteomyelitis
3.   Oral antibiotics afterwards for 2–4 weeks
4.   Follow ESR to assess effectiveness of treatment

because of lack of neurological improvement. Laminectomy and antibiotics resulted in some improvement, but spastic quadraparesis has persisted (84).

Increased fever and increased neck pain with subsequent quadriplegia without resolution of symptoms post-surgical decompression has been described. (89) There is also a case of acute quadriplegia within seconds of discography. At surgery, this patient was found to have multiple sequestered fragments of disk in the epidural space (90).

Diskitis without osteomyelitis is a self-limiting phenomenon; antibiotic treatment is of questionable efficacy. Osti et al. showed that cefazolin started one week after injection of bacteria into sheep disks had no effect on the outcome of diskitis. The addition of intravenous cefazolin 30 minutes prior to discography or intradiscal cefazolin during discography prevented diskitis. None of the sheep disks that received the aforementioned antibiotic prophylaxis developed diskitis (91). Patients who are allergic to penicillin may use vancomycin or cleocin for prophylaxis (Table 10). In certain cases biopsy may be warranted. This is to be followed by the appropriate antibiotics. Without osteomyelitis, the course of diskitis is self-limited because of bacterial destruction by the immune system (92) (Table 11).

B.   False-positive Results in Discography

False-positive results can be seen in specific populations. Patients can also develop new low back pain after discography. Patients with emotional issues or unrelated chronic pain problems may continue to have back pain for months after the procedure (93). Young patients and those without underlying psychological or chronic pain histories have been shown to have a low false-positive rate of pain reproduction under discography (94–96). On the other hand, patients with psychological or confounding socioeconomic issues have been shown to have a higher rate of positive responses (95). Older patients have a greater degree of disk degeneration. This has been shown to correlate with a higher rate of pain provocation in asymptomatic patients. However, the pain is usually of a dissimilar nature (97).

Patients with pain from another source may cause a false-positive discogram. Discography resulted in exact or similar pain in 85% of patients who had iliac bone graft pain. This calls into question whether patients can differentiate between pain of spinal and nonspinal origin in the pelvic region (98).

In symptomatic patients, concordant pain has been associated with annular pathology (97). It has been shown that patients with high-intensity zones on MRI have a higher percentage of painful disks during discography (99). However, the rate of high-intensity zone-injected disks that yielded pain in symptomatic and asymptomatic patients was equal. Location concordancy must be used to determine the disk causing the patient's pain (99).

Cervical discography is less selective than lumbar discography. The cervical disk may not be the most common source of pain. The zygapophyseal joints are significant pain generators as well (68,69). Only one half of patients with positive discograms have a single pain generator. The rest will have pain not only from the disk but from the zygapophyseal joint as well. Bogduk and Aprill proposed the need to block the zygapophyseal joints as well. They feel that a normal disk with a positive zygapophyseal joint segment may induce false-positive pain due to the mediation of impulses from branches of the same segmental nerves. Cervical discography loses its value in the patient with positive results due to both an abnormal disk and injured zygapophyseal joints. The yield for improvement of pain with surgery would be low (100).

Cervical discography in patients with cervical spondylotic myelopathy, radiculopathy, and amyotrophy is not specific. Fifty percent of pain-free patients demonstrated a positive discogram (101).

XIII. COMPLICATIONS OF PERCUTANEOUS DISK PROCEDURES

There are few percutaneous procedures for disk pathology. Intradiscal electrothermal therapy (IDET), is used to treat internal disk disruption and degenerative disk disease by running a thermal resistive coil into the nucleus of the disk and navigating it adjacent to the posterior anulus. The anulus is then heated. Improvement in pain has been substantiated (102). Coblation is performed using bipolar radiofrequency to cause thermal heating and coagulation with resultant back pain relief (103).

Very few of the studies about IDET or coblation mention any significant complications. Anecdotal stories about IDET include reports of bacterial diskitis, nerve root injury, and catheter breakage. Incidence of complications is not yet known (104). There has been one case of cauda equina reported post-IDET due to improper catheter placement within the spinal canal (105). Coblation may result in new numbness, tingling, and back pain (106).

REFERENCES

1. Boden SD, Davis DO, Dina TS, Patronas NJ, Wiesel SW. Abnormal magnetic-resonance scans of the lumbar spine in asymptomatic subjects. J Bone Joint Surg 1990; 72A:403–408.
2. Paajanen H, Erkintalo M, Kuusela T, Dahlstrom S, Kormano M. Magnetic resonance study of disk degeneration in young low-back pain patients. Spine 1989; 14:982–985.
3. American Association of Electrodiagnostic Medicine. Practice parameter for needle electromyographic evaluation of patients with suspected cervical radiculopathy: summary statement. Muscle Nerve 1999; S209–S211.
4. Derby R, Kline G, Saal JA, Reynolds J, Goldwaite N, White AH, Hsu K, Zucherman J. Response to steroid and duration of radicular pain as predictors of surgical outcome. Spine 1992; 17:S176–S183.
5. North RB, Kidd DH, Zahurak M, Piantadosi S. Specificity of diagnostic nerve blocks: a prospective, randomized study of sciatica due to lumbosacral spine disease. Pain 1996; 65:77–85.
6. Masterson BJ. Skin preparation. Clin Obstet Gynecol 1988; 31:736–743.
7. Sebben JE. Surgical antiseptics. J Am Acad Dermatol 1983; 9:759–765.
8. Lennard TA. Fundamentals of procedural care. In: Lennard TA, ed. Physiatric Procedures in Clinical Practice. Philadelphia: Hanley and Belfus, 1995:1–13.
9. Williams MJ. Local anesthetics. In: Raj PJ, ed. Pain Medicine: A Comprehensive Review. St Louis: Mosby, 1996:162–175.
10. Windsor RE, Pinzon EG, Gore HC. Complications of common selective spinal injections: prevention and management. Am J Orthop 2000; 29(10):759–770.

11. Willmore JL. Epilepsy emergencies: the first seizure and status epilepticus. Neurology 1998; 51:534–538.

12. Bogduk N. Information on steroids. ISIS 10th Annual Scientific Meeting, September 2002: 20–29.

13. Gottlieb NL, Riskin WG. Complications of local corticosteriod injections. JAMA 1980; 243:1547–1548.

14. Claman HN. Glucocorticosteriods I: anti-inflammation mechanisms. Hosp Pract 1983: 123–134.

15. Black DM, Filak AT. Hyperglycemia with non-insulin dependent diabetes following intraarticular steroid injection. J Fam Pract 1989; 28:462–463.

16. Lieberman PL, Seigle RL. Reactions to radiocontrast material. Clin Rev Allergy Immunol 1999; 17(4):469–496.

17. Winbery SL, Lieberman PL. Histamine and antihistamines in anaphylaxis. Clin Allergy Immunol 2002; 17:287–317.

18. Gompels LL, Bethune C, Johnston SL, Gompels MM. Proposed use of adrenaline in anaphylaxis and related conditions: a study of senior house officers starting accident and emergency posts. Postgrad Med J 2002; 78:416–418.

19. Rusznak C, Peebles RS. Anaphylaxis and anaphylactoid reactions. Postgrad Med 2002; 11:101–114.

20. Joint Task Force on Practice Parameters, American Academy of Allergy, Asthma and Immunology, American College of Allergy, Asthma and Immunology and the Joint Council of Allergy, Asthma and Immunology. J Allergy Clin Immunol 1998; 101:S465–S528.

21. Yunginger JW. Latex allergy in the workplace: an overview of where we are. Ann Allergy Asthma Immunol 1999; 83:630–663.

22. Andrews CL. Imaging methods for procedures, medication/radiation safety. ISIS 9th annual scientific meeting, Boston, September 2001: 1–4.

23. Urmey WF, Rowlingson J. Do antiplatelet agents contribute to the development of perioperative spinal hematoma? Reg Anesth Pain Med 1998; 23(6 suppl 2):S146–S151.

24. Huijgens PC, Vandenberg CA, Imandt LM. Vitamin E and platelet aggregation. Acta Haemat 1981; 65:217–218.

25. Stampfer MJ, Jakubowski JA, Faigel D. Vitamin E supplementation effect on human platelet function, arachidonic acid metabolism and plasma prostacyclin levels. Am J Clin Nutr 1988; 47:700–706.

26. Ang-Lee MK, Moss J, Yuan CS. Herbal medicines and perioperative care. JAMA 2001; 286:208–216.

27. Wagner LK, Archer BR. Minimizing Risks from Fluoroscopic X-Rays: Bioffects, Instrumentation and Examination. 2nd. The Woodlands, TX: Partners in Radiation Management, 1998.

28. Dougherty JH, Fraser RA. Complications following spinal injection procedures: reports of two cases. J Neurosurg 1978; 48:1023–1025.

29. Gutkencht DR. Chemical meningitis following injections of epidural steroids. Am J Med 1987; 82(3):570.

30. Goucke CR, Gradziotti P. Extradural abscess following local anesthetic and steroid injection for chronic low back pain. Br J Anesth 1990; 65(3):427–429.

31. Chan ST, Leung S. Spinal epidural abscess following steroid injection for sciatica. Spine 1984; 78(1):106–108.

32. Mamourian AC, Dickman CA, Drayer BP, Sonntag VK. Spinal epidural abscess: three cases following spinal epidural injection demonstrated with magnetic resonance imaging. Anesthesiology 1993; 78(1):204–207.

33. Williams KN, Jackowski A, Evans PJD. Epidural hematoma requiring surgical decompression following repeated cervical epidural steroid injections for chronic pain. Pain 1990; 42:197–199.

34. Woodward JL, Herring SA, Windsor RE. Epidural procedures in spine pain management. In: Lennard TA, ed. Pain Procedures in Clinical Practice. Philadelphia: Hanley and Belfus, 2000:341–376.

35. Derby R. Point of view: cervical epidural steroid injection with intrinsic spinal cord damage: two case reports. Spine 1998; 23(19):2141–2142.

36. Lehmann LJ, Pallares VS. Subdural injection of a local anesthetic with steroids: complications of epidural anesthesia. South Med J 1995; 88(4):467–469.

37. Bernat JL, Dadowsky Ch, Vincent FM. Sclerosing spinal pachymeningitis. J Neurol Neurosurg Psychiatry 1976; 39:1124–1128.

38. Plumb VJ, Dismukes WE. Chemical meningitis related to intrathecal corticosteroid therapy. South Med J 1977; 70:1241.

39. Morris JT, Konkol KA, Longfield RN. Chemical meningitis following methylprednisone injection. Infect Med 1994; 11:439–440.

40. Sudlow C, Warlow C. Epidural blood patching for preventing and treating post-dural puncture headache. Cochrane Database of Systematic Reviews (2) 2002.

41. Vercauteren MP, Hoffmann VH, Mertens E, Sermeus L, Adriaensen HA. Seven-year review of requests for epidural blood patches for headache after dural puncture: referral patterns and the effectiveness of blood patches. Anesthesiology 1999; 16(5):298–303.

42. Abram SE, O'Connor TC. Complications associated with epidural steroid injections. Regional Anesth 1996; 21(2):149–162.

43. Krediet CT, VanDijk N, Linzer M, VanLieshout JJ, Wieling W. Management of vasovagal syncope. Circulation 2002; 106(13):1684–1689.

44. Spaccarelli KC. Lumbar and caudal epidural steroid injections. Mayo Clin Proc 1996; 71: 168–178.

45. Botwin KP, Gruber RD, Bouchlas CG, Torres-Ramos FM, Hanna A, Rittenberg J, Thomas SA. Complications of fluoroscopically guided caudal epidural injections. Am J Phys Med Rehabil 2001; 80(6):416–424.

46. Botwin KP, Gruber RD, Bouchlas CG, Torres-Ramos FM, Freeman TL, Slaten WK. Complications of fluoroscopically guided transforaminal lumbar epidural injections. Arch Phys Med Rehabil 2000; 81:1045–1050.

47. Botwin, Thomas, Gruber, Torres, Bouchlas, Rittenberg. Complications of fluoroscopically guided cervical interlaminar epidural injections. ISIS 10th Annual Meeting, Austin, Texas, September 6–8, 2002.

48. Reitman CA, Watters W. Subdural hematoma after cervical epidural steroid injection. Spine 2002; 27(6):E174–E176.

49. Gibran S, Mizra K, Kinsella F. Unilateral vitreous hemorrhage secondary to caudal epidural steroid injection: a variant of Terson's syndrome. Br J Ophthalmol 2002; 86(3):353–354.

50. Kushner RH, Olson JC. Retinal hemorrhage as a consequence of epidural steroid injection. Arch Ophthalmol 1996; 113(3):309–313.

51. Slipman CW, Shin CH, Patel RK, Braverman DL, Lenrow DA, Ellen MI, Nematbakhsh MA. Persistent hiccups associated with thoracic epidural injection. Am J Phys Med Rehabil 2001; 80(8):618–621.

52. Mateo E, Lopez-Alarcon MD, Moliner S, Calabuig E, Vivo M, DeAndres J, Grau F. Epidural and subarachnoid pneumocephalus after epidural technique. Eur J Anesthesiol 1997; 86(6):413–417.

53. Siegfried RN. Development of complex regional pain syndrome after a cervical epidural steroid injection. Anesthesiology 1997; 86(6):1394–1396.

54. Hodges SC, Castelberg BA, Miller T, Ward R, Thornburg C. Cervical epidural steroid injection with intrinsic spinal cord damage: two case reports. Spine 2002; 23(19): 2137–2142.

55. Slipman CW, Chow DW, Lenrow DA, Blaugrund JE, Chou LH. Dysphonia associated with epidural steroid injection: a case report. Arch Phys Med Rehabil 2002; 83(9):1309–1310.

56. Renfrew DL, Moore TE, Kathol MH, el-Khoury GY, Lemke JH, Walker CW. Correct placement of epidural steroid injections: fluoroscopic guidance and contrast administration. Am J Neuroradiol 1991; 12(5):1003–1007.

56a. Macnab I, McCulloch J, Neck Ache and Shoulder Pain Baltimore, MD: Williams and Wilkins: 1994; 39.

57. Brouwers PJ, Kottink EJ, Simon MA, Prevo RL. A cervical anterior spinal artery syndrome after diagnostic blockade of the right C6 nerve root. Pain 2001; 91:397–399.

58. Houten JK, Errico, TJ. Paraplegia after lumbosacral nerve root block: report of three cases. Spine J 2002; 2:70–75.

59. Furman MB, O'Brien EM, Zgleszewski TM. Incidence of intravascular penetration in transforaminal lumbosacral epidural steroid injections. Spine 2000; 25(20):2628–2632.

60. Turner J, Deyo RA, Loesser J, Van Korff M, Fordyce WE. The importance of placebo effects in pain treatment and research. JAMA 1994; 271(20):1609–1614.

61. Marks RC, Houston T, Thulbourne T. Facet joint injection and facet nerve block: a randomized comparison in 86 patients with chronic low back pain. Pain 1992; 49:325–328.

62. Berrian T. Chemical meningism after lumbar facet joint block. Anesthesia 1992; 47:905–906.

63. Thomson SJ, Lomax DM, Collet BJ. Chemical meningism after lumbar facet joint nerve block with local anesthetic and steroid. Anesthesia 1993; 46:563–564.

64. Schwarzer AC, Wang SC, Bogduk N. Prevalence and clinical features of lumbar zygoapophyseal joint pain: a study in an Australian population with chronic low back pain. Ann Rheumatol Dis 1995; 54:100–106.

65. Schwarzer AC, Aprill CN, Fortin. The relative contribution of the disk and zygoapophyseal joint in chronic low back pain. Spine 1994; 19:801–806.

66. Schwarzer AC, Aprill CN, Derby R. Clinical features of patients with pain stemming from the zygoapophyseal joints. Is the lumbar facet syndrome a clinical entity? Spine 1994; 19:1132–1137.

67. Fukui S, Ohseto K, Shiotani M, Ohno K, Karasawa Hidetake, Naganuma Y. Distribution of referred pain from the lumbar zygoapophyseal joints and dorsal rami. Clin J Pain 1997; 13:303–307.

68. Dwyer A, Aprill C, Bogduk N. Cervical zygoapophyseal joint pain patterns I: a study in normal volunteers. Spine 1990; 6:453–457.

69. Dwyer A, Aprill C, Bogduk N. Cervical zygoapophyseal joint pain patterns II: a clinical evaluation. Spine 1990; 6:458–461.

70. Fukui S, Ohseto K, Shiotani M, Ohno K, Karasawa Hidetake, Naganuma Y, Yuda Y. Referral pain distribution of the cervical zygoapophyseal joints and cervical dorsal rami. Pain 1996; 68:79–83.

71. Barnsley L, Bogduk N. Medial branch blocks are specific for the diagnosis of cervical zygoapophyseal joint pain. Reg Anesth 1993; 18:343–350.

72. Lord SM, Barnsley L, Wallis BJ, McDonald GJ, Bogduk N. Percutaneous radiofrequency neurotomy for chronic cervical zygoapophyseal joint pain. N Eng J Med 1996; 335(23):1721–1726.

73. Dreyfuss P, Halbrook B, Pauza K, Joshi A, McLarty J, Bogduk N. Efficacy and validity of radiofrequency neurotomy for chronic lumbar zygapophysial joint pain. Spine 2000; 25(10):1270–1277.

74. Lord S, Barnsley L, Bogduk N. Percutaneous radiofrequency neurotomy in the treatment of cervical zygoapophyseal joint pain: a caution. Neurosurgery 1995; 36:732–739.

75. Dreyfus P, Rogers CJ. Radiofrequency neurotomy of the zygoapophyseal and sacroiliac joints. In: Lennard TA, ed. Pain Procedures in Clinical Practice. Philadelphia: Hanley and Belfus, 2000:395–420.

76. Fortin JD, Falco FJ. The Fortin finger test: an indicator of sacroiliac pain. Am J Orthop 1997; 26(7):477–480.

77. Maigne, J, Aivaliklis A, Pfefer F. Results of sacroiliac joint double block and value of sacro-iliac pain provocation tests in 54 patients with low back pain. Spine 1996; 21(16):1889–1892.

78. Dreyfuss P, Michaelsen M, Pauza K. The value of history and physical examination in diagnosing sacroiliac joint pain. Spine 1996; 21:2594–2602.

79. Fortin JD, Tolchin RB. Sacroiliac provocation and arthrography. Arch of Phys Med Rehabil 1993; 74:125–129.

80. Fortin JD, Washington WJ, Falco FJ. Three pathways between the sacroiliac joint and neural structures exist. Am J Neuroradiol 1999; 20(8):1429–1434.

81. Fraser RD, Osti OL, Vernon-Roberts. Diskitisafter discography. J Bone Joint Surg 1987; 69B:26–35.

82. Guyer RD, Collier R, Stith WJ, Ohnmeiss DD, Hochschuler SH, Rashbaum RF, Regan JJ. Diskitisafter discography. Spine 1988; 13(12):1352–1354.

83. Guyer RD, Ohnmeiss DD, Marson SL, Shelokow AP. Complications of cervical discography: findings in a large series. J Spinal Disord 1997; 10(2):95–101.

84. Lownie SP, Ferguson DD. Spinal subdural empyema complicating cervical discography. Spine 1989; 14(12):1415–1417.

85. Agre K, Wilson RR, Brim M, McDermott DJ. Chymodiactin postmarketing surveillance: demographic and adverse experience data in 29,075 patients. Spine 1984; 9:479–485.

86. Berquist TH. Musculoskeletal Imaging Companion. Philadelphia: Lippincott Williams and Wilkins, 2002.

87. Grubb SA, Kelly CK. Cervical discography: clinical implications from 12 years of experience. Spine 2000; 25:1382–1389.

88. Guyer R. Complications of cervical discography: findings in a large series. J Spinal Disord 1997; 10(2):95–101.

89. Connor PM, Darden BV. Cervcial discography complications and clinical efficacy. Spine 1993; 18(14):2035–2038.

90. Laun A, Lorenz R, Agnoli AL. Complications of cervical discography. J Neurosurg Sci 1981; 25:17–20.

91. Osti OL, Fraser RD, Vernon-Roberts B. Diskitisafter discography the role of prophylactic antibiotics. J Spinal Disord 1990; 72-B:271–274.

92. Fraser RD, Osti OL, Vernon-Roberts B. Iatrogenic diskitis: the role of intravenous antibiotics in prevention and treatment and experimental study. Spine 1989; 14(9):1025–1032.

93. Carragee EJ, Yung C, Tanner CM, Hayward C, Rossi M, Hagle C. Can discography cause long-term back symptoms in previously asymptoms in previously asymptomatic subjects? Spine 2000; 25(14):1803–1808.

94. Simmons JW, Aprill CN, Dwyer AP, Brodsky AE. A reassessment of Holt's data on: "the question of lumbar discography." Clin Orthop 1988; 237:120–124.

95. Carragee EJ, Tanner CM, Khurana S, Hayward C, Welsh J, Date E, Truong T, Rossi M, Hagle C. The rates of false-positive lumbar discography in select patients without low back symptoms. Spine 2000; 25(11):1373–1381.

96. Walsh T, Weinstein J, Spratt K, Lehmann TR, Aprill C, Sayre H. Lumbar discography in normal subjects: a controlled prospective study. J Bone Joint Surg 1990; 72A:1081–1088.

97. Vanharanta H, Sachs BL, Ohnmeiss DD, Aprill C, Spivey M, Guyer RD, Rashbaum RF, Hochschuler SH, Terry A, Selby D, Stith WJ, Mooney V. Pain provocation and disk deterioration by age. A CT/discogranhy study in a low back pain population. Spine 1989; 12:420–423.

98. Carragee EJ, Tanner CM, Yang B, Brito JL, Truong T. False-positive findings on lumbar discography. Reliability of subjective concordance assessment during provocative disk injection. Spine 1999; 24(23):2542–2547.

99. Aprill C, Bogduk N. High-intensity zone: a diagnostic sign of painful lumbar disk on magnetic resonance imaging. Br J Radiol 1992; 65:361–369.

100. Bogduk N, Aprill C. On the nature of neck pain, discography and cervical zygapophysial joint blocks. Pain 1993; 54:213–217.

101. Shinomiya K, Nakao K, Shindoh S, Mochida K, Furuya K. Evaluation of cervical discography in pain origin and provocation. J Spinal Disord 1993; 6(5):422–426.
102. Saal JA, Saal JS. Intradiscal electrothermal treatment for chronic discogenic low back pain. A prospective outcome study with minimum 1-year follow-up. Spine 2000; 25(20):2622–2627.
103. O'Neill C. Percutaneous discectomy using nucleoplasty. ISIS 10th Annual Meeting, Austin, Texas, September 6–8, 2002.
104. Heary Robert F. Intradiscal electrothermal annuloplasty: the IDET procedure. Journal of Spinal Disorders 2001; 14(4):353–360.
105. Hsia AW, Isaac K, Katz JS. Cauda equina syndrome from intradiscal electrothermal therapy. Neurology 2000; 55:320.
106. Nirschl M, Slipman CW, Isaac Z, Gilchrest R, Bhat A. Preliminary data: side effects and complications of lumbar nucleoplasty. ISIS 10th Annual Meeting, Austin, Texas, September 6–8, 2002.

37

Complications of Vertebroplasty and Kyphoplasty

Frank M. Phillips
Rush University Medical Center, Chicago, Illinois, U.S.A.

I. INTRODUCTION

A. Vertebral Compression Fractures

Pathologic vertebral compression fractures (VCFs) can result from a variety of disorders that cause osseous compromise, including osteoporosis, multiple myeloma, and metastatic tumors. Osteoporosis is a systemic disease characterized by decreased bone mass and microarchitectural deterioration. The resulting decrease in mechanical strength often manifests as fragility fractures. The number of people affected is quite large, and the National Osteoporosis Foundation estimates that over 100 million people worldwide, and nearly 44 million people in the United States, are at risk for developing fragility fractures secondary to osteoporosis. In the United States, an estimated 700,000 pathological, osteoporotic vertebral compression fractures occur each year (1).

Multiple myeloma is the second most prevalent blood cancer (after non-Hodgkin's lymphoma) and accounts for approximately 1% of all cancers. VCFs frequently occur in multiple myeloma patients as a result of the destruction of normal bone by the plasma cell tumor(s). In addition, bone loss is accelerated in multiple myeloma by the malignant plasma cells stimulation of bone-resorbing osteoclast activity (2,3). Up to 80% of breast, prostate, and lung cancer patients will have bone metastases, primarily to the spine, ribs, and pelvis (4,5). Like multiple myeloma, metastases from breast and lung cancer tend to be osteolytic, while metastases from prostate cancer tend to be osteoblastic (5). The fracture risk is higher for vertebrae harboring osteolytic tumors compared to those with osteoblastic tumors, but both types of tumors increase vertebral fracture risk.

Pathological vertebral fractures are leading causes of morbidity and disability in patients with osteoporosis, multiple myeloma, or bone metastases, (2,6,7). Pain associated with acute VCFs can be incapacitating. Although acute symptoms may subside over a period of weeks to months, severe pain may become chronic in a number of patients (7). Chronic pain may result from incomplete vertebral healing often associated with progressive bony collapse, with altered spine kinematics as a consequence of spinal deformity or with the development of a true pseudoarthrosis at the involved vertebra. In myeloma and metastatic disease, pain also may be caused by nerve stimulation in the endosteum and by increased intraosseous pressure from perilesional edema and tumor enlargement. Chronic pain associated with VCFs often leads to impaired quality of life and depression (7,8).

Regardless of the levels of pain related to the VCF, any resulting spinal deformity can adversely affect physical function (7,9), pulmonary function (10,11), gastrointestinal function (7), mental health (7,8), quality of life (7,8), and survival (12,13). Kyphotic deformity in the osteopenic spine may also create a biomechanical environment that promotes additional fractures (14,15).

B. Treatment

The symptoms of acute VCFs are routinely treated medically with some combination of analgesic medication, bed rest, or orthotics. Unfortunately, these treatments can have deleterious side effects. This patient population often tolerates anti-inflammatory and narcotic medications poorly, in part because these drugs may predispose to confusion, increased risk of fall, and gastrointestinal side effects. Extended bed rest promotes an overall physiological deconditioning and a further acceleration of bone loss. Bracing is also not well tolerated by older patients and may restrict diaphragmatic excursion. Surgical intervention is usually avoided except in rare cases in which the fracture is associated with neurological compromise or advanced spinal instability. Spinal surgery in this patient population is fraught with complications related not only to advanced patient age and comorbidities but also to difficulties in securing fixation in osteopenic bone.

Orthopedic fracture care emphasizes restoration of anatomy, correction of deformity, and preservation of function. These treatment goals have not been applied to a majority of patients with pathological VCFs. Vertebroplasty and kyphoplasty offer minimally invasive treatments that immediately stabilize the fracture, treat the fracture-related pain, and possibly improve the kyphotic deformity. As discussed below, both procedures address the pain associated with VCFs in part by stabilizing the fractured vertebra with bone cement. In addition, by using an inflatable bone tamp to raise vertebral endplates before cement placement, kyphoplasty has the potential to correct spinal sagittal malalignment.

II. VERTEBROPLASTY

A. Indications and Contraindications

Suggested indications for vertebroplasty include stabilization of painful osteoporotic and osteolytic vertebral fractures due to osteoporosis, metastases, multiple myeloma, hemangioma, and Kummell's disease. Contraindications and precautions include fractures that result in neurological compromise, result from high-energy injury, possess significant burst components, involve the posterior vertebral body wall, have a geometry that restricts vertebral body access, and have poor intraoperative radiographic visualization. Also, younger patients, patients with localized spine infections, with sepsis, with bleeding disorders, on anticoagulation therapy, or with cardiopulmonary compromise that precludes safely performing the procedure should not be treated by vertebroplasty.

B. Technique

In 1987 Galibert first described percutaneous vertebroplasty, which is a method for augmenting a vertebral body with bone cement (16). This procedure may be performed in a radiology suite or operating room and is typically performed under local anesthesia.

The patient is positioned prone with the spine extended by chest and pelvic bolsters. Typically, an 11- to 13-gauge needle is advanced towards the center of the vertebral body using a transpedicular or extrapedicular approach and fluoroscopic guidance. If needed, biopsy needles can be used to obtain samples before cement injection (17,18). The bone cement most commonly used is polymethylmethacrylate (PMMA)(e.g., Simplex P; Howmedica Osteonics, Allendale, NJ). PMMA is mixed with barium for opacification. While some physicians treat patients with intravenous antibiotics, some physicians add antibiotics to the cement mixture itself, especially when operating on immunocompromised patients (17,19–20) When the mixture attains the consistency of toothpaste, the cement is transferred to syringes. Between 2 and 10 mL of partially cured cement is injected into the vertebral body under live, multidirectional fluoroscopy. Cement injection is stopped if extravasation is detected. Ideally the vertebral body is completely filled with cement, but pain relief has been reported when the anterior two thirds of the vertebra contains cement (21). Using a cement injector tool has been shown to increase epidural cement leakage, while the position of the needle tip in the vertebral body does not predict leakage (22). The patient is not moved from the prone position until the leftover cement has solidified. Most patients rest supine under observation for at least 4 hours before discharge.

C. Results

Overall, vertebroplasty is a technically demanding procedure with a low rate of major complications reported (21,23). As summarized in Table 1, vertebroplasty has proven effective in reducing pain in 60–100% of patients from retrospective or consecutive cohort studies. Pain relief often occurs within 72 hours after surgery and is usually stable through follow-up visits that ranged from 6 months to 10 years (17,20,24–28). As a result of the decrease in pain, patient mobility was also reported to improve in many of these studies.

The mechanism of pain relief after vertebroplasty is not clear. Pain relief is not proportional to the percentage of lesion filling with cement (21,29), but one potential explanation may be a mechanical immobilization of the fracture and the support of the cortex by the cement (30). Another theory suggests that the heat produced during PMMA polymerization may cause deafferentation of the fractured vertebra.

Vertebroplasty is limited in that it does not address spinal deformity. In addition, bone cement is forced directly into cancellous bone, necessitating the use of high-pressure injection of relatively low-viscosity cement (17,21,23), which increases the risk for cement leaks and related complications (see below). In spite of the limitations, vertebroplasty has been shown to be an effective and relatively inexpensive technique for decreasing pain associated with osteoporotic VCFs.

III. KYPHOPLASTY

A. Indications and Contraindications

The indications and contraindications for kyphoplasty are similar to those for vertebroplasty. Currently, indications for kyphoplasty include painful or progressive osteoporotic and osteolytic vertebral compression fractures. The ideal timing of the kyphoplasty procedure is uncertain. In patients with acute VCFs and relatively minor degrees of vertebral collapse, many spine care providers will attempt a 6-week trial of conservative care during which serial radiographs are obtained. If there is progressive collapse of the vertebral body, kyphoplasty is recommended. Also, if the pain attributed

Table 1 Published Results from Percutaneous Vertebroplasty Studies

Study (Ref.)	Patients (fractured vertebrae)	Underlying disease	Successful pain reduction (successes/total)	Extravasation rate (leaks/total fractures)	Complication	Types of complication
Kaemmerlen et al., 1989 (75)	20 (33)	Metastases	80% (16/20)		2	Signs of cord compression
Gangi et al., 1994 (76)	5 (5)	Hemangiomas,			None	
	1 (1)	Metastasis				
	4 (8)	Osteoporosis				
	10 (14)	Total	100%	None		
Weill et al., 1996 (77)	37 (52)	Metastases	73%	38% (20/52)	5	3 transient radiculopathy (cement leakage, surgery required for 1) 2 transient difficulty swallowing (cement leakage)
Cotten et al., 1996 (29)	29 (30)	Metastases	97% (28/29)	77% (23/30)	3	2 nerve root compression (cement leak; decompression surgery required) 1 transient femoral neuropathy (cement leak)
Cortet et al., 1997 (26)	8 (10)	Multiple myeloma	100%	60% (6/10)		Severe nerve root pain (cement leakage into neural foramen)
	29 (30)	Metastases				
	8 (10)	Multiple myeloma				
Jensen et al., 1997 (17)	37 (40)	Total	97% (36/37)	73% (29/40)	2	2 nondisplaced rib fractures;
	29 (47)	Osteoporosis	90% (26/29)	23% (11/47) (ncc)	4	2 PMMA pulmonary embolisms (ncc)
Deramond et al., 1998 (55)	80 (n/r)	Osteoporosis	>90%	n/r	1	Intercostal neuralgia

Reference	n (levels)	Pathology	Success	Complication rate	Complications	Description
Cortet et al., 1999 (27)	16 (20)	Osteoporosis	88%	65% (13/20) (ncc)	None	
Cyteval et al., 1999 (24)	20 (23)	Osteoporosis	75% (15/20)	35% (8/23)	2	Painful cement leakage into the psoas muscle or foramina
Martin et al., 1999(78)	11	Osteoporosis	78% (7/9)			Radicular pain associated with cement leak; deep thrombosis of leg; broncho-aspiration pneumonia associated with general anesthesia
	7	Hemangioma	80% (4/5)			
	19	Metastases	72% (13/18)			
	2	Multiple myeloma	100% (1/1)			
	1	Bone lymphoma	100% (1/1)	n/r		
	40 (67)	Total	~80%			
Padovanni et al., 1999 (79)	1	Langerhans' cell vertebral histiocytosis		1	<6%/level 1	Fatal pulmonary embolization
Barr et al., 2000 (52)	8 (13)	Cancer	50% (4/8)	13% (1/8)		
	1 (1)	Hemangioma	0%	n/r		
	38 (70)	Osteoporosis	95% (36/38)	n/r		Dermatome radicular neuritis; nonbacterial urethritis
	47 (84)	Total	87% (40/46)			
Grados et al., 2000 (80)	25 (34)	Osteoporosis	~96% (24)	~21% (7) (ncc)	2 5	Transitory: 2 nerve root pain, 2 fever, 1 exacerbation of pain
Heini et al., 2000 (81)	17 (45)	Osteoporosis	76% (13/17)	20% (8/45) (ncc)	n/r	
Maynard et al., 2000 (38)	27 (35)	Osteoporosis	93%	n/r	n/r	
O'Brien et al., 2000 (82)	6 (6)	n/r	67% (4/6)	33% (2/6) (ncc)	None	

(Continued)

Table 1 (*Continued*)

Study (Ref.)	Patients (fractured vertebrae)	Underlying disease	Successful pain reduction (successes/total)	Extravasation rate (leaks/total fractures)	Complication	Types of complication
Amar et al., 2001 (44)	93	Osteoporosis				Cement leaks: 3 pulmonary embolisms (2 asymptomatic); 2 radicular pain and 1 quadriceps weakness; 1 persistent pain (possibly associated with cement leak); Other: Dual tear; fever secondary to atelectasis; transient intro-operative hypotension; death from respiratory failure after reversal of general anesthesia/extubation (preexisting pneumonia before surgery)
	4	Metastases or multiple myeloma				
Kaufmann et al., 2001 (83)	97 (258)	Total	98% (79/81)	n/r	11	
	75 (122)	Osteoporosis	n/r	n/r	n/r	
Minart et al., 2001 (18)	(37)	Osteoporosis				
	(14)	Metastasis				
	(3)	Myeloma				
	(2)	Amyloidosis				
	46 (57)	Total	n/r	n/r	None	
Chen et al., 2002 (48)	1				1	Fatal pulmonary embolism
Gaughen et al., 2002 (57)	48 (84)	Osteoporosis	95% (40/42)	61% (50/82) (ncc)	1	Cerebrospinal fluid leak during venography

Jang et al., 2002 (47)	27	Metastasis			3	Pulmonary embolism: 2 patients had transient dyspnea and discomfort, 1 patient was asymptomatic
Kim et al., 2002 (84)	49 (75)	n/r	90%	n/r	n/r	
Lee et al., 2002 (85)	1	Osteoporosis			1	Paraplegia
McGraw et al., 2002 (58)	61 (96)	n/r	n/r	~23%	n/r	
McGraw et al., 2002 (25)	100 (154)		93%		2	Sternal fracture; transient radiculopathy
Peh et al., 2002 (28)	37 (48)	Osteoporosis	47% complete 50% partial	44% (21/48) (ncc)	None	
Ryu et al., 2002 (22)	159 (347)	Osteoporosis	87% (89/102)	27% (92/347)	No neurological injuries	
Tsou et al., 2002 (86)	16 (17)	Osteoporosis	100%	12% (2/17)	None	
Vasconcelos et al., 2002 (59)	(171)	Osteoporosis			(None related to cement leaks)	Transient: arterial hypotension during cement injection (no leak); temporary cutaneous hypoesthesia at puncture site; radiculopathy
	(27)	Metastases				
	(4)	Multiple myeloma				
	(2)	Hemangioma				
	(1)	Osteogenesis imperfecta				
	137 (205)	Total	n/r	27% (55/205) (ncc)	3	
Zoarski et al., 2002 (87)	30 (54)	Osteoporosis	~97% (29/30)	~2% (1/54) (ncc)	None	

n/r = not reported; ncc=no clinical consequences.

to the VCF is incapacitating or does not respond to a period of conservative care, kyphoplasty is recommended. With advanced kyphosis at the time of presentation after a VCF, many physicians will consider immediate kyphoplasty to improve sagittal alignment. Thoracolumbar junction fractures, fractures due to steroid-induced osteoporosis, and fractures occurring in vertebrae with extremely low bone mineral density are predisposed to progressive collapse and deformity so that earlier kyphoplasty may be warranted.

The contraindications include systemic pathologies such as sepsis, prolonged bleeding times, or cardiopulmonary conditions, which would preclude the safe completion of the procedure. Other relative contraindications include nonosteolytic infiltrative tumor spinal metastases, vertebral bodies with deficient posterior cortices, or patients presenting with neurological signs or symptoms. In certain burst or vertebra plana fracture configurations, kyphoplasty may be technically difficult, and the feasibility of the procedure should be assessed on the merits of the case. The author does not advocate performing kyphoplasty (or vertebroplasty) on more than three vertebral levels during one procedure because of potential deleterious cardiopulmonary effects related to cement and/or fat embolization to the lungs.

B. Technique

In the early 1990s, vertebroplasty was modified by the addition of a step to elevate the compressed vertebral body endplates before deposition of bone cement. This technique became known as kyphoplasty. Although this procedure may be performed in a radiology suite or operating room using local, spinal, or general anesthesia, most kyphoplasty procedures are performed in an operating room with general anesthesia. The patient is positioned prone on a Jackson table with the spine extended by chest and pelvic bolsters. Care should be taken to ensure that all bony prominences are well padded. Simultaneous biplane fluoroscopy is used throughout the procedure. An 11-gauge Jamshidi needle is placed percutaneously into the posterior vertebral body through either a bilateral, transpedicular or bilateral, extrapedicular approach. The biopsy needles are exchanged over a guide wire for a working cannula. KyphX® Inflatable Bone Tamps (IBTs) (Kyphon, Inc., Sunnyvale, CA) are placed bilaterally into the vertebral body through working cannulas. The IBTs are inflated using visual (fluoroscopic) and manometric parameters. Inflation continues until vertebral body height is restored, the IBT contacts a vertebral body cortical wall, the IBT reaches 220 psi, or the maximal balloon volume is reached. After the IBTs are withdrawn, a stylet and bone filler cannula are used to place partially cured PMMA cement mixed with additional barium into the cavity within the fractured vertebral body. The cement volume approximates the volume of the cavity created by the IBT. The patient is not moved from the prone position until the leftover cement has solidified.

C. Results

Because kyphoplasty is a newer technique, fewer studies have been reported compared to vertebroplasty. Nonetheless, kyphoplasty, like vertebroplasty, is a technically demanding procedure with a low rate of major complications (21,23). As summarized in Table 2, kyphoplasty has proven effective in reducing pain in a majority of patients from retrospective or consecutive cohort studies. In a large series of kyphoplasty procedures, a 0.2% per fracture complication rate was reported (23).

Of importance, kyphoplasty has the potential to improve spinal deformity by elevating the vertebral endplates before fixation. Initial reports indicate that vertebral

Table 2 Published Results from Balloon Kyphoplasty Studies

Study (Ref.)	Patients (fractured vertebrae)	Underlying disease	Successful pain reduction (successes/total)	Extravasation rate (leaks/total fractures)	Complications	Types of complication
Wong et al., 2000 (21)	85 (143)	n/r	94% (80/85)	n/r	2 (These patients were also included in Garfin 2001)	Anterior cord syndrome (loss of segmental blood supply); transient fever/hypoxia, but no breathing difficulties (inadvertent administration of highly runny cement)
Garfin et al., 2001 (23)	340 (603)	n/r	90%	n/r	4	See above Epidural hematoma (due to heparin bolus administered 8 hours postoperatively); partial motor loss due to instrument placement and cement leak (significant recovery after additional surgery) Perioperative pulmonary edema and myocardial infarction (secondary to intraoperative fluid overload); rib fracture (2 patients)
Lieberman et al., 2001 (32)	24	Osteoporosis				
	6	Multiple myeloma				
	30 (70)		100%	8.6% (6/70)(ncc)	3	
Dudeney et al., 2002 (62)	18 (55)	Multiple myeloma	(significant improvements in SF-36 scores)	4% (2/55)(ncc)	None	
Theodorou et al., 2002 (33)	15 (24)	Osteoporosis	100%	n/r	None	
Phillips' 2002 (34)	29 (61)	Osteoporosis	92% (33/36 procedures)	9.8% (6/61)	3	Postoperative myocardial infarction; urinary retention; postoperative atrial fibrillation and exacerbation of congestive heart failure

n/r = not reported; ncc = no clinical consequences.

height could be restored partially or completely in the majority of fractures. In an ex vivo study, Belkoff and colleagues showed a 97% reversal of deformity with kyphoplasty compared with a 30% reversal with vertebroplasty (31). Lieberman and colleagues reported vertebral height restoration in 70% of 70 fractured vertebra treated with kyphoplasty. In those patients in whom the vertebral fractures were reduced by kyphoplasty, vertebral height was increased by a mean of 46.8 % (32). Wong and coauthors and Garfin and coauthors similarly noted increased vertebral body height after kyphoplasty (21,23).

Although these data confirm the ability of the IBT to elevate the vertebral body endplates, the ultimate value of the reduction maneuver is its effect on spinal sagittal alignment. These data have just begun to be reported. Theodorou and colleagues studied 15 patients (24) with osteoporotic VCFs. They reported a mean midline vertebral height restoration of 65.7% and a mean improvement in kyphosis of $62.4 \pm 16.7\%$, but did not indicate in how many of the 15 patients fracture reduction occurred. No data on the radiographic techniques used for measuring sagittal alignment were provided (33). Phillips and colleagues reported the effects of kyphoplasty on sagittal alignment using a radiographic technique previously validated for measurement of posttraumatic kyphosis. In the authors' early experience with kyphoplasty, local sagittal alignment was improved by a mean of 8.8° for all fractures and 14.2° in those fractures considered reducible (i.e., that experienced at least 5° of correction) (34). This degree of improvement in local sagittal alignment reported with kyphoplasty is similar to that reported for open reduction and internal fixation of traumatic burst fractures. Esses and colleagues reported 9.3° (anterior instrumentation) and 11.3° (posterior instrumentation) improvements in local kyphotic angle with open reduction and internal fixation of burst fractures (35).

IV. COMPLICATIONS

A. Errors in Patient Selection

Poor clinical outcomes may be predicted for vertebroplasty and kyphoplasty unless careful attention is given to patient screening and work-up. Treating old, healed VCFs is unlikely to affect the patient's symptoms. The VCF must be confirmed as the likely pain generator if either vertebroplasty or kyphoplasty is being considered. This will usually require a combination of clinical findings suggestive of fracture pain and confirmatory imaging studies. VCF pain often increases with weight-bearing activities and eases with recumbency. On history, the presence of abrupt onset of pain aggravated by activity and change of position and localized to the area of the radiographically documented fracture suggests that the fracture is responsible for the patient's symptoms.

The existence of multiple fractures may complicate the diagnosis, so the results from a physical exam and standard radiographs should be confirmed with bone scans or magnetic resonance (MR) images (36–38). On bone scan analyses, recently fractured vertebrae will show increased uptake of ^{99m}TC compared to nonfractured vertebrae. CT plus bone scans may be used when MR images cannot be obtained. Sagittal T1-weighted MR sequences can distinguish acute or nonhealed fractures from healed fractures. Edema associated with acute VCFs produces low signal intensity, whereas more chronic fractures tend to produce signals similar to those of nonfractured vertebrae. Sagittal short-tau inversion recovery (STIR; heavily T2-weighted) MR sequences are the most sensitive way to distinguish marrow fat from marrow edema. In STIR-MR images, edema in acute fractures produces a high-intensity signal (19,37). MR images have the additional advantage of assisting in the detection of potential infection or tumor involvement.

Malignant causes of VCF are usually associated with ill-defined margins, enhancement, pedicle involvement, and paravertebral soft tissue masses (39).

The pain related to the VCF must be differentiated from chronic back pain related to underlying conditions such as spinal arthritis. In addition, patients with multiple, old spinal fractures and kyphotic deformity may have chronic back pain related to the stretching of the posterior soft tissues and to paraspinal muscle fatigue secondary to the kyphotic posture. In contrast to acute fracture pain, the back pain of kyphosis typically worsens as the patient remains erect for periods of time and may not be exacerbated by changes in position. In this situation, back pain will not be improved by performing vertebroplasty or kyphoplasty unless the deformity is addressed. Patients with underlying painful spinal disorders and a recent painful VCF should be counseled preoperatively as to what degree of symptom relief might be achieved with vertebroplasty or kyphoplasty.

B. Vertebral Body Access Complications

Most vertebroplasty and kyphoplasty procedures are performed by accessing the vertebral body through a transpedicular approach. In the upper thoracic spine, the transpedicular route may not allow for adequate medial placement of the instruments, which may limit optimal IBT inflation. An alternative that may allow for better medialization of the tools is the extrapedicular approach. With either of these approaches, care must be taken to avoid injuring surrounding tissues while accessing the vertebral body. If the medial pedicle wall is breached, one risks injuring the neural elements of the spinal canal. Accessing the vertebral body caudal to the pedicle with an extravertebral approach may also place the segmental vessels and nerve roots at risk. In addition, perforation of the vertebral body cortex with instrumentation may result in vascular injury or injury to structures in the thoracic or retroperitoneal spaces. Multiple attempts at cannulating the vertebral body should be avoided because of the increased risk of cement leaks through these additional tracts.

Access to the vertebral body is dependent on excellent visualization of the bony landmarks using radiographic imaging techniques (Fig. 1). Typically, biplanar fluoroscopy is used for these procedures. With the transpedicular approach, the instrument should dock on the facet joint overlying the lateral aspect of the pedicle on the AP fluoroscopic image. With the extrapedicular approach, the instrument is docked at the junction of the transverse process, rib head, and superior lateral pedicle wall. The tip of the instrument will appear outside of the lateral pedicle wall on the AP image. With both approaches, as the instrument is advanced, the tip should remain lateral to the medial pedicle wall on the AP image until it has reached the posterior aspect of the vertebral body on the lateral image (Figs. 2, 3). This will ensure that the instrument is outside of the spinal canal. Once the vertebral body is entered, the tip of the instrument may be medialized as is appropriate. Proper needle placement is a key factor in reducing the complication rate with vertebroplasty and kyphoplasty.

C. Cement Leaks

1. Cement

Although acrylic cement has been used for the fixation of metal and plastic joint replacements and also for the fixation of pathological fractures (40–42), it has not been approved by FDA for use in the spine to treat vertebral compression fractures. Also, the cement used in vertebroplasty and kyphoplasty is often modified. First, more opacification

"True" AP Image

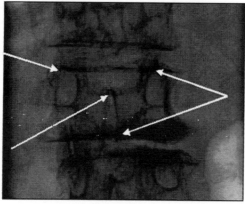

Pedicles in upper half of vertebral body

Spinous process equidistant between pedicles

Endplates parallel

"True" Lateral Image

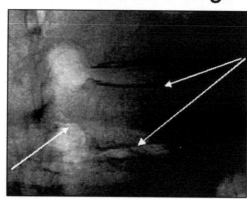

Endplates parallel

Pedicles superimposed

Figure 1 Optimal anteroposterior (AP) and lateral radiographic views. On the AP view, the endplates are parallel, the pedicles should be in the upper half of the vertebral body, and the spinous process should be centered between the symmetrically shaped pedicle "rings." The lateral image should be aligned so that the endplates are parallel and the pedicles are superimposed.

powder (usually barium sulfate, but often tantalum, tungsten or some combination) is added to the cement mixture. Second, the monomer-to-powder ratio recommended by manufacturers is often modified to create a thicker consistency (17,20,21,43).

Potential problems with PMMA include the exothermic reaction during the curing process when the temperature may reach 100°C, causing thermal damage to adjacent structures. Thermal damage may become problematic if extravertebral cement extravasation occurs. Cardiopulmonary toxicity of the unreacted cement monomer and the lack of biointegration of the cement are also concerns with the use of PMMA. Occasional cases of symptomatic and lethal PMMA pulmonary embolism with vertebroplasty have been reported (44–48). A recent study investigated the cardiopulmonary effects of cement injection during vertebroplasty in sheep. Immediately after cement injection, there was a fall in heart rate and arterial pressure with a second fall in arterial pressure occurring after

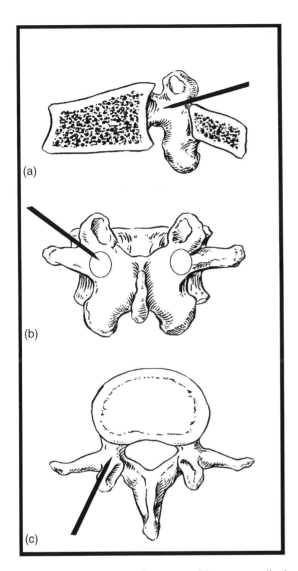

Figure 2 Instrument placement with a transpedicular approach (Views: (a) sagittal; (b) coronal; (c) axial). The instrument tip is half way across the pedicle ring on the coronal view (b) and half way down the pedicle on the sagittal view, (a) which should ensure that the medial pedicle wall is not breached as the instrument is advanced (c).

a mean of 18 seconds post–cement injection associated with fat emboli passing through the heart and being trapped in the lungs (49).

The ideal biomaterial for vertebral augmentation would have handling characteristics that allowed easy injection, no toxicity, a gradual transition from a viscous to a solid state with low exothermic temperatures, and adequate compressive strength to stabilize the fractured vertebral body. An osteoconductive, biodegradable material that is replaced by host bone (e.g., carbonated apatite cement or calcium phophate cement) may be advantageous, but the ability of osteoporotic bone to remodel and replace a biodegradable material with bone of adequate quality is uncertain and must be studied before such

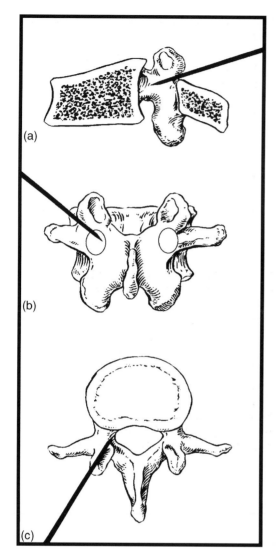

Figure 3 "Too-medial" instrument placement with a transpedicular approach (Views: (a) sagittal; (b) coronal; (c) axial). The instrument tip is at the medial pedicle wall on the coronal view (b) and only halfway down the pedicle on the sagittal view. (a) As the instrument is advanced, the medial pedicle wall will be breached (c).

materials are considered for clinical use. Several biomaterials, including carbonated apatite (50), bioactive cement (51), and calcium phosphate (52,53), were shown to provide significant improvement in compressive strength and load to failure of vertebral bodies. A more extensive understanding of the toxicity profiles and long-term stability of these materials is essential.

2. Vertebroplasty

As mentioned above, vertebroplasty has a higher risk of extravertebral cement extravasation during injection than kyphoplasty. During vertebroplasty, the high-pressure injection of low-viscosity cement directly into cancellous bone makes it difficult to control cement flow in the vertebral body, which creates an unpredictable risk of cement extravasation outside of the vertebral body (16). Extravertebral cement extravasation commonly occurs during vertebroplasty, with leak rates of up to 65% reported (Table 1) (27). A higher rate of extravasation has been noted in patients with metastases or hemangiomas compared to patients with osteoporosis (20,21). Studies in sheep models indicate that low-viscosity cement does not penetrate bone as well even under sustained pressurization. Instead, the low-viscosity cement tends to take the path of least resistance into the venous system (54).

Most of the complications associated with vertebroplasty are due to extra-vertebral cement leaks. Desite the high rate of cement leaks, reports indicate a 1–3% complication rate for patients with osteoporosis, 2–5% for patients with hemangiomas, and 10% for patients with metastatic disease. Of note, the higher rate of complications seen in patients with metastatic disease is likely due to the generally increased deterioration of vertebral bodies and poor overall health compared to other patient populations (55).

While most cement leaks are clinically silent, the complications associated with extravertebral cement can be devastating. The sites at risk with cement leaks include the paravertebral soft tissues, spinal canal, neural foramina, adjacent disks, and veins. The reported complications related to cement leak during vertebroplasty procedures include radiculopathies, pulmonary emboli, paraplegia, and spinal cord compromise (see also Table 1) (20,21,56).

The risks of cement leaks can be reduced with thorough technical training and high-quality imaging systems. Careful needle positioning is required, and the internal cortex of the pedicle must not be disrupted during the surgical approach (55). Intraosseous venography has also been used to detect potential sites of cement leakage and to ensure that the cement injector tool tip is not in contact with a major venous outlet. The different viscosity of the dye from cement, the potential allergic reactions and the potential for residual dye to obscure the view of cement during injection should be considered (57–59). Proponents of vertebroplasty have suggested that vertebroplasty may be safely performed without venography (57,59).

3. Kyphoplasty

In contrast to vertebroplasty, the reported rate of cement extravasation is less than 10% for kyphoplasty procedures (Table 2). With kyphoplasty, the creation of an intra-vertebral cavity surrounded by compacted bone allows for the placement of higher viscosity cement under lower pressure compared to the injection conditions needed for vertebroplasty. The author's recent intraosseous venography study showed significantly less vascular and transcortical extravasation of injected contrast with kyphoplasty than with vertebroplasty (60).

Kyphoplasty procedures have been associated with isolated cases of epidural bleeding, transient spinal cord injury, and transient acute respiratory distress (see also Table 2) (20,21). These complications occurred in the first 50 kyphoplasty procedures performed and were largely related to surgeon errors. For example, a patient with epidural bleeding had been anticoagulated in the immediate peri-kyphoplasty period; this practice has since been discontinued. The failure to add additional barium to the PMMA resulted in a spinal cord injury from cement extravasation into the spinal canal that was not detected during cement placement. The case of transient respiratory distress was thought to be related to pulmonary embolism from the use of runny cement. As experience with kyphoplasty has been gained, it has become apparent that the intra-vertebral cavity created by the IBT allows for placement of more viscous, partially cured cement. In a report on the initial multicenter experience with kyphoplasty to treat 2194 vertebral fractures in 1439 patients between 1998 and 2000, the serious adverse event rate was 0.2% per fracture (61). More recent studies of kyphoplasty have reported no neurological events (32–34,62).

D. Reduction Failure

The deleterious effects of spinal kyphosis on physical function and mental, respiratory, and gastrointestinal health are well established (7–13). As mentioned above, vertebroplasty tends to freeze the fracture in its deformed shape. Although occasional cases of postural fracture reduction have been reported, this is an infrequent phenomenon. Kyphoplasty attempts to reduce the fracture and associated deformity in a reliable and predictable fashion. Several groups have suggested that younger fractures (less than 10–12 weeks) have a better likelihood of reduction (20,21,34). To date, most kyphoplasty procedures have been performed later than 6 weeks from the time of fracture. If reduction of the deformity is a goal of treatment, it does seem reasonable that those patients presenting with an acute VCF and significant kyphosis might be best managed by earlier intervention in an attempt to maximize improvement in spinal sagittal alignment. This may be particularly important at the thoracolumbar junction, where a tendency for the development of significant kyphosis has been observed.

Some degree of fracture reduction has been achieved in more than 60% of treated fractures. Factors that seem to limit reduction achieved with kyphoplasty include partial healing of bone, suboptimal placement of the IBT, and collapse of vertebral endplates after IBT removal, prior to cement placement. In cases where healed bone limits IBT expansion and fracture reduction, high IBT pressures at low balloon volumes and distorted IBT inflation shapes will be observed. To improve reduction of partially healed bone, the author has developed a technique combining kyphoplasty with percutaneous osteotomy. Regarding instrument positioning, if the IBT is placed too far laterally in the vertebral body, balloon contact with the lateral vertebral body cortex early during inflation will limit the surgeon's ability to continue inflation and optimize vertebral endplate elevation. This may be salvaged by the use of directional balloon tamps that will preferentially inflate in a medial direction (under investigation); however, this situation is best prevented by creating a medial channel for IBT placement. In cases where loss of endplate reduction occurs with balloon deflation, it may be possible to maintain reduction with unilateral bone tamp inflation elevating the endplate while placing cement on the opposite side.

V. CEMENT AUGMENTATION OF SPINAL HARDWARE

As larger reconstructive spine surgeries are performed on older patients, the ability of the osteoporotic spine to support spinal implants must be considered. Posterior instrumentation failure has been shown to correlate with low bone mineral density (BMD) (63–65). In the osteoporotic spine, the implant/bone interface is the weakest part of the instrumentation construct. The majority of instrumentation failures involve screw loosening and pullout, which may lead to failure of fusion and the development of recurrent or de novo deformity.

At the time of pedicle screw insertion, the surgeon may recognize poor purchase in osteoporotic bone by the low insertion torque required to advance the screw. Screw pull-out has been correlated with low insertion torque and low BMD (66–68). If poor screw purchase is recognized intraoperatively, the surgeon should attempt to salvage the situation rather than rely on inadequate fixation to achieve the goals of instrumentation. One technique for improving stability at the bonescrew interface involves the injection of bone cement into the pedicle prior to screw placement. A two- to threefold increase in screw pullout forces has been demonstrated with the use of PMMA bone cement injected into the vertebral body through a cannulated pedicle (64,69). Other cements such as hydroxyapatite cement, calcium phosphate, and carbonated apatite have also been shown to enhance the screwbone interface and increase pedicle screw pullout strength (71–72). Cement augmentation of screws has been used in patients with osteoporosis and metastatic spinal tumors undergoing spinal instrumentation with acceptable clinical results and low rates of instrumentation failure (41,73,74).

Of note, PMMA is not bioabsorbable and could complicate revision surgery or hardware removal. Also, Moore and colleagues reported that the failure modes seen with PMMA and calcium phosphate cement differed in pullout tests (71). With PMMA augmentation, pedicle fracture occurred at or near the junction with the vertebral body in 83% (25 of 30) of the samples. In contrast, failure of calcium phosphate augmentation occurred at the cementscrew interface in 80% (24 of 30) of the samples. Another possible risk of cement augmentation of spinal hardware includes cement extravasation during injection, with potential damage from cement leakage into the spinal canal or neural foramina.

The vertebra adjacent to an instrumented fusion is also a concern in the osteoporotic spine. The osteoporotic adjacent vertebra is subject to large forces, and fractures of the adjacent vertebra are being seen with increasing frequency as longer, more rigid fusions are being performed in elderly patients. Prophylactic augmentation of the adjacent vertebra with cement at the time of instrumented fusion has been discussed, but current reports of success are only anecdotal. Further study is required to more precisely identify the role of prophylactic cement augmentation in this situation.

VI. CONCLUSIONS

To date, no controlled clinical trials have been reported for either vertebroplasty or kyphoplasty. The potential benefit to patients suffering from vertebral compression fractures warrants the continued study of the long-term effects of using bone cement in the spine. While vertebroplasty and kyphoplasty are effective in reducing the chronic pain associated with VCFs, kyphoplasty is the only treatment that attempts to reduce the fracture and correct spinal deformity. The use of bone cement in reconstructive spine surgery also offers the potential for prophylactic treatment to prevent or reduce the rate of fracture in "at-risk" vertebrae.

REFERENCES

1. Riggs BL, Melton LJ, 3rd. The worldwide problem of osteoporosis: insights afforded by epidemiology. Bone 1995; 17:505S–511S.
2. Barrick MC, Mitchell SA. Multiple myeloma. AJN 2001; 101(suppl):6–12.

3. Anderson KC, Kyle RA, Dalton WS, Landowski T, Shain K, Jove R, Hazlehurst L, Berenson J. Multiple myeloma: new insights and therapeutic approaches. Hematology (Am Soc Hematol Educ Program) 2000:147–165..

4. Janjan N. Bone metastases: approaches to management. Semin Oncol 2001; 28:28–34.

5. Mundy GR. Metastasis to bone: causes, consequences and therapeutic opportunities. Nat Rev Cancer 2002; 2:584–593.

6. Schachar NS. An update on the nonoperative treatment of patients with metastatic bone disease. Clin Orthop 2001:75–81.

7. Silverman SL. The clinical consequences of vertebral compression fracture. Bone 1992; 13(Suppl 2):S27–S31.

8. Gold DT. The clinical impact of vertebral fractures: quality of life in women with osteoporosis. Bone 1996; 18:185S–189S.

9. Lyles KW, Gold DT, Shipp KM, Pieper CF, Martinez S, Mulhausen PL. Association of osteoporotic vertebral compression fractures with impaired functional status. Am J Med 1993; 94:595–601.

10. Schlaich C, Minne HW, Bruckner T, Wagner G, Gebest HJ, Grunze M, Ziegler R, Leidig-Bruckner G. Reduced pulmonary function in patients with spinal osteoporotic fractures. Osteoporos Int 1998; 8:261–267.

11. Leech JA, Dulberg C, Kellie S, Pattee L, Gay J. Relationship of lung function to severity of osteoporosis in women. Am Rev Respir Dis 1990; 141:68–71.

12. Kado DM, Browner WS, Palermo L, Nevitt MC, Genant HK, Cummings SR. Vertebral fractures and mortality in older women: a prospective study. Arch Intern Med 1999; 159:1215–1220.

13. Cooper C, Atkinson EJ, Jacobsen SJ, O'Fallon WM, Melton LJ, 3rd. Population-based study of survival after osteoporotic fractures. Am J Epidemiol 1993; 137:1001–1005.

14. Belmont PJ, Jr., Polly DW, Jr., Cunningham BW, Klemme WR. The effects of hook pattern and kyphotic angulation on mechanical strength and apical rod strain in a long-segment posterior construct using a synthetic model. Spine 2001; 26:627–635..

15. White AA, 3rd, Panjabi MM, Thomas CL. The clinical biomechanics of kyphotic deformities. Clin Orthop 1977:8-17.

16. Galibert P, Deramond H, Rosat P, Le Gars D. Preliminary note on the treatment of vertebral angioma by percutaneous acrylic vertebroplasty. Neurochirurgie 1987; 33:166–168.

17. Jensen ME, Evans AJ, Mathis JM, Kallmes DF, Cloft HJ, Dion JE. Percutaneous polymethyl-methacrylate vertebroplasty in the treatment of osteoporotic vertebral body compression fractures: technical aspects. AJNR Am J Neuroradiol 1997; 18:1897–1904.

18. Minart D, Vallee JN, Cormier E, Chiras J. Percutaneous coaxial transpedicular biopsy of vertebral body lesions during vertebroplasty. Neuroradiology 2001; 43:409–412.

19. Mathis JM, Barr JD, Belkoff SM, Barr MS, Jensen ME, Deramond H. Percutaneous vertebroplasty: a developing standard of care for vertebral compression fractures. AJNR Am J Neuroradiol 2001; 22:373–381.

20. Watts NB, Harris ST, Genant HK. Treatment of painful osteoporotic vertebral fractures with percutaneous vertebroplasty or kyphoplasty. Osteoporos Int 2001; 12:429–437.

21. Wong WH, Reiley MA, Garfin SR. Vertebroplasty/kyphoplasty. J Women's Imaging 2000; 2:117–124.

22. Ryu KS, Park CK, Kim MC, Kang JK. Dose-dependent epidural leakage of polymethyl-methacrylate after percutaneous vertebroplasty in patients with osteoporotic vertebral compression fractures. J Neurosurg 2002; 96:56–61.

23. Garfin SR, Yuan HA, Reiley MA. New technologies in spine: kyphoplasty and vertebro-plasty for the treatment of painful osteoporotic compression fractures. Spine 2001; 26:1511–1515.

24. Cyteval C, Sarrabere MP, Roux JO, Thomas E, Jorgensen C, Blotman F, Sany J, Taourel P. Acute osteoporotic vertebral collapse: open study on percutaneous injection of acrylic surgical cement in 20 patients. AJR Am J Roentgenol 1999; 173:1685–1690.

25. McGraw JK, Lippert JA, Minkus KD, Rami PM, Davis TM, Budzik RF. Prospective evaluation of pain relief in 100 patients undergoing percutaneous vertebroplasty: results and follow-up. J Vasc Interv Radiol 2002; 13:883–886.

26. Cortet B, Cotten A, Boutry N, Dewatre F, Flipo RM, Duquesnoy B, Chastanet P, Delcambre B. Percutaneous vertebroplasty in patients with osteolytic metastases or multiple myeloma. Rev Rheum Engl Ed 1997; 64:177–183.

27. Cortet B, Cotten A, Boutry N, Flipo RM, Duquesnoy B, Chastanet P, Delcambre B. Percutaneous vertebroplasty in the treatment of osteoporotic vertebral compression fractures: an open prospective study. J Rheumatol 1999; 26:2222–2228.

28. Peh WC, Gilula LA, Peck DD. Percutaneous vertebroplasty for severe osteoporotic vertebral body compression fractures. Radiology 2002; 223:121–126.

29. Cotten A, Dewatre F, Cortet B, Assaker R, Leblond D, Duquesnoy B, Chastanet P, Clarisse J. Percutaneous vertebroplasty for osteolytic metastases and myeloma: effects of the percentage of lesion filling and the leakage of methyl methacrylate at clinical follow-up. Radiology 1996; 200:525–530.

30. Belkoff SM, Maroney M, Fenton DC, Mathis JM. An in vitro biomechanical evaluation of bone cements used in percutaneous vertebroplasty. Bone 1999; 25:23S–26S.

31. Belkoff SM, Mathis JM, Fenton DC, Scribner RM, Reiley ME, Talmadge K. An ex vivo biomechanical evaluation of an inflatable bone tamp used in the treatment of compression fracture. Spine 2001; 26:151–156.

32. Lieberman IH, Dudeney S, Reinhardt MK, Bell G. Initial outcome and efficacy of "kyphoplasty" in the treatment of painful osteoporotic vertebral compression fractures. Spine 2001; 26:1631–1638.

33. Theodorou DJ, Theodorou SJ, Duncan TD, Garfin SR, Wong WH. Percutaneous balloon kyphoplasty for the correction of spinal deformity in painful vertebral body compression fractures. Clin Imag 2002; 26:1–5.

34. Phillips FM, Ho E, Campbell-Hupp M, Kerr E, Wetzel FT, Gupta P. Balloon kyphoplasty for the treatment of painful spinal deformity resulting from osteoporotic vertebral compression fractures. Spine J 2002; 2:121S.

35. Esses SI, Botsford DJ, Kostuik JP. Evaluation of surgical treatment for burst fractures. Spine 1990; 15:667–673.

36. Gaughen JR, Jr., Jensen ME, Schweickert PA, Kaufmann TJ, Marx WF, Kallmes DF. Lack of preoperative spinous process tenderness does not affect clinical success of percutaneous vertebroplasty. J Vasc Interv Radiol 2002; 13:1135–1138.

37. Do HM. Magnetic resonance imaging in the evaluation of patients for percutaneous vertebroplasty. Top Magn Reson Imaging 2000; 11:235–244.

38. Maynard AS, Jensen ME, Schweickert PA, Marx WF, Short JG, Kallmes DF. Value of bone scan imaging in predicting pain relief from percutaneous vertebroplasty in osteoporotic vertebral fractures. AJNR Am J Neuroradiol 2000; 21:1807–1812.

39. Shih TT, Huang KM, Li YW. Solitary vertebral collapse: distinction between benign and malignant causes using MR patterns. J Magn Reson Imaging 1999; 9:635–642.

40. Bauer TW, Schils J. The pathology of total joint arthroplasty. I. Mechanisms of implant fixation. Skel Radiol 1999; 28:423–432.

41. Jang JS, Lee SH, Rhee CH. Polymethylmethacrylate-augmented screw fixation for stabilization in metastatic spinal tumors. Technical note. J Neurosurg 2002; 96:131–134.

42. Wada T, Kaya M, Nagoya S, Kawaguchi S, Isu K, Yamashita T, Yamawaki S, Ishii S. Complications associated with bone cementing for the treatment of giant cell tumors of bone. J Orthop Sci 2002; 7:194–198.

43. Belkoff SM, Sanders JC, Jasper LE. The effect of the monomer-to-powder ratio on the material properties of acrylic bone cement. J Biomed Mater Res 2002; 63:396–399.

44. Amar AP, Larsen DW, Esnaashari N, Albuquerque FC, Lavine SD, Teitelbaum GP. Percutaneous transpedicular polymethylmethacrylate vertebroplasty for the treatment of spinal compression fractures. Neurosurgery 2001; 49:1105–1115.

45. Levine SA, Perin LA, Hayes D, Hayes WS. An evidence-based evaluation of percutaneous vertebroplasty. Manag Care 2000; 63:56–60.

46. Perrin C, Jullien V, Padovani B, Blaive B. Percutaneous vertebroplasty complicated by pulmonary embolus of acrylic cement. Rev Mal Respir 1999; 16:215–217.

47. Jang JS, Lee SH, Jung SK. Pulmonary embolism of polymethylmethacrylate after percutaneous vertebroplasty: a report of three cases. Spine 2002; 27:E416–E418.

48. Chen HL, Wong CS, Ho ST, Chang FL, Hsu CH, Wu CT. A lethal pulmonary embolism during percutaneous vertebroplasty. Anesth Analg 2002; 95:1060–1062.

49. Aebli N, Krebs J, Davis G, Walton M, Williams MJ, Theis JC. Fat embolism and acute hypotension during vertebroplasty: an experimental study in sheep. Spine 2002; 27:460–466.

50. Schildhauer TA, Bennet AP, Wright TM, et al. Intravertebral body reconstruction with injectable in situ setting carbonated apatite: biomechanical evaluation of a minimally invasive technique. J Orthop Res 1999; 17:67–72.

51. Belkoff SM, Mathis JM, Erbe EM, Fenton DC. Biomechanical evaluation of a new bone cement for use in vertebroplasty. Spine 2000; 25:1061–1064.

52. Barr JD, Barr MS, Lemley TJ, McCann RM. Percutaneous vertebroplasty for pain relief and spinal stabilization. Spine 2000; 25:923–928.

53. Lim TH, Brebach GT, Renner SM, Kim WJ, Kim JG, Lee RE, Andersson GB, An HS. Biomechanical evaluation of an injectable calcium phosphate cement for vertebroplasty. Spine 2002; 27:1297–1302.

54. Breusch S, Heisel C, Muller J, Borchers T, Mau H. Influence of cement viscosity on cement interdigitation and venous fat content under in vivo conditions: a bilateral study of 13 sheep. Acta Orthop Scand 2002; 73:409–415.

55. Deramond H, Depriester C, Galibert P, Le Gars D. Percutaneous vertebroplasty with polymethylmethacrylate. Technique, indications, and results. Radiol Clin North Am 1998; 36:533–546.

56. Hardouin P, Grados F, Cotten A, Cortet B. Should percutaneous vertebroplasty be used to treat osteoporotic fractures? An update. Joint Bone Spine 2001; 68:216–221.

57. Gaughen JR, Jr., Jensen ME, Schweickert PA, Kaufmann TJ, Marx WF, Kallmes DF. Relevance of antecedent venography in percutaneous vertebroplasty for the treatment of osteoporotic compression fractures. AJNR Am J Neuroradiol 2002; 23:594–600.

58. McGraw JK, Heatwole EV, Strnad BT, Silber JS, Patzilk SB, Boorstein JM. Predictive value of intraosseous venography before percutaneous vertebroplasty. J Vasc Interv Radiol 2002; 13:149–153.

59. Vasconcelos C, Gailloud P, Beauchamp NJ, Heck DV, Murphy KJ. Is percutaneous verte-broplasty without pretreatment venography safe? Evaluation of 205 consecutives procedures. AJNR Am J Neuroradiol 2002; 23:913–917.

60. Phillips FM, Todd Wetzel F, Lieberman I, Campbell-Hupp M. An in vivo comparison of the potential for extravertebral cement leak after vertebroplasty and kyphoplasty. Spine 2002; 27:2173–2178.

61. Garfin S, Lin G, Lieberman I, Phillips FM, Truumees E, Yuan H, Lane JM, Ledlie JT, Rhyne A, James S, Logan S, Wong W, Vives M. Retrospective analysis of the outcomes of balloon kyphoplasty to treat vertebral body compression fracture (VCF) refractory to medical management. Eur Spine J 2001; 10(suppl 1):S7.

62. Dudeney S, Lieberman IH, Reinhardt MK, Hussein M. Kyphoplasty in the treatment of osteolytic vertebral compression fractures as a result of multiple myeloma. J Clin Oncol 2002; 20:2382–2387.

63. Coe JD, Warden KE, Herzig MA, McAfee PC. Influence of bone mineral density on the fixation of thoracolumbar implants. A comparative study of transpedicular screws, laminar hooks, and spinous process wires. Spine 1990; 15:902–907.

64. Soshi S, Shiba R, Kondo H, Murota K. An experimental study on transpedicular screw fixation in relation to osteoporosis of the lumbar spine. Spine 1991; 16:1335–1341.

65. Yamagata M, Kitahara H, Minami S, Takahashi K, Isobe K, Moriya H, Tamaki T. Mechanical stability of the pedicle screw fixation systems for the lumbar spine. Spine 1992; 17:S51–S54.

66. Lu WW, Zhu Q, Holmes AD, Luk KD, Zhong S, Leong JC. Loosening of sacral screw fixation under in vitro fatigue loading. J Orthop Res 2000; 18:808–814.

67. Okuyama K, Sato K, Abe E, Inaba H, Shimada Y, Murai H. Stability of transpedicle screwing for the osteoporotic spine. An in vitro study of the mechanical stability. Spine 1993; 18: 2240–2245.

68. Zdeblick TA, Kunz DN, Cooke ME, McCabe R. Pedicle screw pullout strength. Correlation with insertional torque. Spine 1993; 18:1673–1676.

69. Zindrick MR, Wiltse LL, Widell EH, Thomas JC, Holland WR, Field BT, Spencer CW. A biomechanical study of intrapeduncular screw fixation in the lumbosacral spine. Clin Orthop 1986:99–112.

70. Yerby SA, Toh E, McLain RF. Revision of failed pedicle screws using hydroxyapatite cement. A biomechanical analysis. Spine 1998; 23:1657–1661.

71. Moore DC, Maitra RS, Farjo LA, Graziano GP, Goldstein SA. Restoration of pedicle screw fixation with an in situ setting calcium phosphate cement. Spine 1997; 22:1696–1705.

72. Lotz JC, Hu SS, Chiu DF, Yu M, Colliou O, Poser RD. Carbonated apatite cement augmentation of pedicle screw fixation in the lumbar spine. Spine 1997; 22:2716–2723.

73. Noorda RJ, Wuisman PI, Fidler MW, Lips PT, Winters HA. Severe progressive osteoporotic spine deformity with cardiopulmonary impairment in a young patient. A case report. Spine 1999; 24:489–492.

74. Wuisman PI, Van Dijk M, Staal H, Van Royen BJ. Augmentation of (pedicle) screws with calcium apatite cement in patients with severe progressive osteoporotic spinal deformities: an innovative technique. Eur Spine J 2000; 9:528–533.

75. Kaemmerlen P, Thiesse P, Bouvard H, Biron P, Mornex F, Jonas P. Percutaneous vertebroplasty in the treatment of metastases. Technic and results. J Radiol 1989; 70:557–562.

76. Gangi A, Kastler BA, Dietemann JL. Percutaneous vertebroplasty guided by a combination of CT and fluoroscopy. AJNR Am J Neuroradiol 1994; 15:83–86.

77. Weill A, Chiras J, Simon JM, Rose M, Sola-Martinez T, Enkaoua E. Spinal metastases: indications for and results of percutaneous injection of acrylic surgical cement. Radiology 1996; 199:241–247.

78. Martin JB, Jean B, Sugiu K, San Millan Ruiz D, Piotin M, Murphy K, Rufenacht B, Muster M, Rufenacht DA. Vertebroplasty: clinical experience and follow-up results. Bone 1999; 25:11S-15S.

79. Padovani B, Kasriel O, Brunner P, Peretti-Viton P. Pulmonary embolism caused by acrylic cement: a rare complication of percutaneous vertebroplasty. AJNR Am J Neuroradiol 1999; 20:375–377.

80. Grados F, Depriester C, Cayrolle G, Hardy N, Deramond H, Fardellone P. Long-term observations of vertebral osteoporotic fractures treated by percutaneous vertebroplasty. Rheumatology 2000; 39:1410–1414.

81. Heini PF, Walchli B, Berlemann U. Percutaneous transpedicular vertebroplasty with PMMA: operative technique and early results. A prospective study for the treatment of osteoporotic compression fractures.. Eur Spine J 2000; 9:445–450.

82. O'Brien JP, Sims JT, Evans AJ. Vertebroplasty in patients with severe vertebral compression fractures: a technical report. AJNR Am J Neuroradiol 2000; 21:1555–1558.

83. Kaufmann TJ, Jensen ME, Schweickert PA, Marx WF, Kallmes DF. Age of fracture and clinical outcomes of percutaneous vertebroplasty. AJNR Am J Neuroradiol 2001; 22: 1860–1863.

84. Kim AK, Jensen ME, Dion JE, Schweickert PA, Kaufmann TJ, Kallmes DF. Unilateral transpedicular percutaneous vertebroplasty: initial experience. Radiology 2002; 222:737–741.

85. Lee BJ, Lee SR, Yoo TY. Paraplegia as a complication of percutaneous vertebroplasty with polymethylmethacrylate: a case report. Spine 2002; 27:E419–E422.

86. Tsou IY, Goh PY, Peh WC, Goh LA, Chee TS. Percutaneous vertebroplasty in the management of osteoporotic vertebral compression fractures: initial experience. Ann Acad Med Singapore 2002; 31:15–20.
87. Zoarski GH, Snow P, Olan WJ, Stallmeyer MJ, Dick BW, Hebel JR, De Deyne M. Percutaneous vertebroplasty for osteoporotic compression fractures: quantitative prospective evaluation of long-term outcomes. J Vasc Interv Radiol 2002; 13:139–148.

38

Pitfalls of Image-Guided Spinal Navigation

Iain H. Kalfas
Cleveland Clinic Foundation, Cleveland, Ohio, U.S.A.

I. INTRODUCTION

Image-guided spinal navigation is a computer-based surgical technology that was developed to improve intraoperative orientation to unexposed anatomy during complex spinal procedures (1,2). It evolved from the principles of stereotaxy, which have been used by neurosurgeons for several decades to help localize intracranial lesions. Stereotaxy is defined as the localization of a specific point in space using three-dimensional coordinates. The application of stereotaxy to intracranial surgery initially involved the use of an external frame attached to the patient's head. However, the evolution of computer-based technologies has eliminated the need for this frame and has allowed for the expansion of stereotactic technology into other surgical fields, in particular, spinal surgery.

The management of complex spinal disorders has been greatly influenced by the increased acceptance and use of spinal instrumentation devices as well as the development of more complex operative exposures. Many of these techniques place a greater demand on the spinal surgeon by requiring a precise orientation to that part of the spinal anatomy that is not exposed in the surgical field. In particular, the various fixation techniques that require placing bone screws into the pedicles of the thoracic, lumbar, and sacral spine, into the lateral masses of the cervical spine and across joint spaces in the upper cervical spine require "visualization" of often unexposed spinal anatomy. Although conventional intraoperative imaging techniques such as fluoroscopy have proven useful, they are limited in that they provide only two-dimensional imaging of a complex three-dimensional structure. Consequently, the surgeon is required to extrapolate the third dimension based on an interpretation of the images and a knowledge of the pertinent anatomy. This so-called "dead reckoning" of the anatomy can result in varying degrees of inaccuracy when placing screws into the unexposed spinal column.

Several studies have shown the unreliability of routine radiography in assessing pedicle screw placement in the lumbosacral spine. The rate of penetration of the pedicle cortex by an inserted screw ranges from 21 to 31% in these studies (3–5). The disadvantage of these conventional radiographic techniques in orienting the spinal surgeon to the unexposed spinal anatomy is that they display, at most, only two planar images. While the lateral view can be relatively easy to assess, the anteroposterior (AP) or oblique view can be difficult to interpret. For most screw fixation procedures, it is the position of the screw in the axial plane that is most important. This plane best demonstrates the position of the screw relative to the neural canal. Conventional intraoperative imaging cannot provide this view. To assess the potential advantage of axial imaging for screw placement, Steinmann et al. used an image-based technique for pedicle screw placement that combined computed tomography (CT) axial images of cadaver spine specimens with fluoroscopy. This study demonstrated an improvement in pedicle screw insertion accuracy with an error rate of only 5.5% (6).

Image-guided spinal navigation minimizes much of the "guesswork" associated with complex spinal surgery. It allows for the intraoperative manipulation of multiplanar CT images that can be oriented to any selected point in the surgical field. Although it is not an intraoperative imaging device, it provides the spinal surgeon with superior image data compared to conventional intraoperative imaging technology (i.e., fluoroscopy). It improves the speed, accuracy, and precision of complex spinal surgery while, in most cases, eliminating the need for cumbersome intraoperative fluoroscopy.

Despite its advantages, however, image-guided spinal navigation is not foolproof. If used inappropriately or incorrectly it can provide inaccurate information that can lead to added time of the surgery or intraoperative judgment errors based on the surgeon relying too heavily on the incorrect data. This chapter will focus on the errors and pitfalls of using image-guided technology in the spine.

II. PRINCIPLES OF IMAGE-GUIDED SPINAL NAVIGATION

The use of an image-guide navigational system for localizing intracranial lesions has been previously described (7,8). Image-guided navigation establishes a spatial relationship between preoperative CT image data and its corresponding intraoperative anatomy. Both the CT image data and the anatomy can be viewed as a three-dimensional coordinate system, with each point in that system having a specific x, y, and z Cartesian coordinate. Using defined mathematical algorithms, a specific point in the image data set can be "matched" to its corresponding point in the surgical field. This process is called registration and represents the critical step of image-guided navigation. A minimum of three points needs to be matched, or registered, to allow for accurate navigation.

A variety of navigational systems have evolved over the past decade. The common components of most of these systems include an image-processing computer workstation interfaced with a two-camera optical localizer (Fig. 1). When positioned during surgery, the optical localizer emits infrared light towards the operative field. A hand-held navigational probe mounted with a fixed array of passive reflective spheres serves as the link between the surgeon and the computer workstation (Fig. 2). Alternatively, passive reflectors may be attached to standard surgical instruments. The spacing and positioning of the passive reflectors on each navigational probe or customized trackable surgical instrument is known by the computer workstation. The infrared light that is transmitted towards the operative field is reflected back to the optical localizer by the passive reflectors. This information is then relayed to the computer workstation, which can then calculate the precise location of the instrument tip in the surgical field as well as the location of the anatomical point on which the instrument tip is resting.

The initial application of navigational principles to spinal surgery was not intuitive. Early navigational technology applied to intracranial surgery used an external frame mounted to the patient's head to provide a point of reference to link preoperative image data to intracranial anatomy. This was not practical for spinal surgery. The current generation of intracranial navigational technology uses reference markers or fiducials that

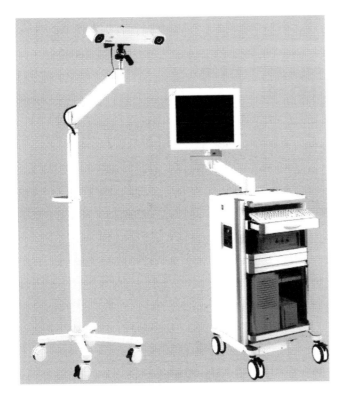

Figure 1 Image-guided navigational workstation with infrared camera localizer system.

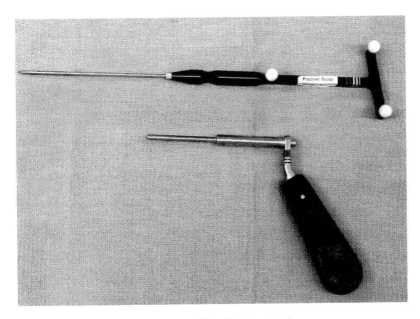

Figure 2 Navigation probe and drill guide for spinal surgery.

are glued to the patient's scalp prior to imaging. However, the use of these surface-mounted fiducials for spinal navigation is not practical because of accuracy issues related to a greater degree of skin movement over the spinal column (9,10). This is less of a problem with intracranial applications because of the relatively fixed position of the overlying scalp to the attached fiducials.

The application of navigational technology to spinal surgery involves using the rigid spinal anatomy itself as a frame of reference. Bone landmarks on the exposed surface of the spinal column provide the points of reference necessary for image-guidance navigation. Specifically, any anatomic landmark that can be identified intraoperatively as well as in the preoperative image data set can be used as a reference point. The tip of a spinous or transverse process, a facet joint, or a prominent osteophyte can serve as a potential reference point (Fig. 3). Since each vertebra is a fixed, rigid body, the spatial relationship of the selected registration points to the vertebral anatomy at a single spinal level is not affected by changes in body position. Two different registration techniques can be used for spinal navigation; paired point registration and surface matching. Paired point registration involves selecting a series of corresponding points in a CT or magnetic resonance imaging (MRI) data set and in the exposed spinal anatomy. The registration process is performed immediately after surgical exposure and prior to any planned decompressive procedure. This allows for the use of the spinous processes as registration points.

A specific registration point in the CT image data set is selected by highlighting it with the computer cursor. The tip of the probe is then placed on the corresponding point in the surgical field, and the reflective spheres on the probe handle are aimed towards the camera. Infrared light from the camera is reflected back, allowing the spatial position of the probe's tip to be identified. This initial step of the registration process effectively "links" the point selected in the image data with the point selected in the surgical field.

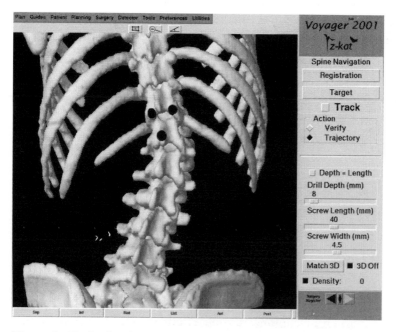

Figure 3 Navigational workstation screen demonstrating a paired point registration plan. Three discrete bony landmarks are selected at a single vertebral level. In this case the tips of the two transverse processes and the spinous process have been selected at the level to be instrumented (T12).

When a minimum of three such points are registered, the probe can be placed on any other point in the surgical field and the corresponding point in the image data set will be identified on the computer workstation.

Alternatively, a second registration technique, surface matching, can be used. This technique involves arbitrarily selecting multiple nondiscrete points only on the exposed and debrided surface of the spine in the surgical field. This technique does not require the selection of points in the image set, although several points in both the image data set and in the surgical field are frequently required to improve the accuracy of surface mapping. The positional information of these points is transferred to the workstation, and a topographic map of the selected anatomy is created and "matched" to the patient's image set (11).

Typically, paired point registration can be done more quickly than surface mapping. The average time needed for paired point registration is 10–15 seconds. The time needed for surface mapping is much longer, with difficult cases requiring as much as 10–15 minutes. With the need to perform several registration processes during each surgery, this time difference can significantly affect the length of the navigational procedure and the surgery itself (12).

The purpose of the registration process is to establish a precise spatial relationship between the image space of the data with the physical space of the patient's corresponding surgical anatomy. If the patient is moved after registration, this spatial relationship is distorted, making the navigational information inaccurate. This problem can be minimized by the optional use of a spinal tracking device, which consists of a separate set of passive reflectors mounted on an instrument that can be attached to the exposed spinal anatomy (Fig. 4). The position of the reference frame can be tracked by the camera system. Movement of the frame alerts the navigational system to any inadvertent movement of the spine. The system can then make correctional steps to keep the registration process accurate and eliminate the need to repeat the registration process. The disadvantage of using a tracking device is the added time needed for its attachment to the spine, the need to maintain a line of sight between it and the camera, and the inconvenience of having to perform the procedure with the device placed in the surgical field. It is particularly cumbersome when image-guided navigation is used during cervical procedures. Alternatively, image-guided spinal navigation can be performed without a tracking device (1,12). This involves acknowledging the effect of patient movement on the accuracy of image-guided navigation and maintaining reasonably stable patient position during the relatively short amount of time needed (10–20 s) for the selection of each appropriate screw trajectory. Patient movement can potentially occur with respiration, from the surgical team leaning on the table or from a change of table position. Movement associated with patient respiration is negligible and does not require any tracking even in the thoracic spine. Although movement associated with leaning on the table or repositioning the table or the patient will affect registration accuracy, it can be easily avoided during the short navigational procedure. If inadvertent patient movement does occur, the registration process can be repeated. Repeating the registration process is easiest when using the shorter paired point technique as opposed to the more time-consuming surface mapping technique.

When the registration process has been completed, the probe can be positioned on any surface point in the surgical field and three separate reformatted CT images centered on the corresponding point in the image data set are immediately presented on the workstation monitor. Each reformatted image is referenced to the long axis of the probe. If the probe is placed on the spinal anatomy directly perpendicular to its long axis, the

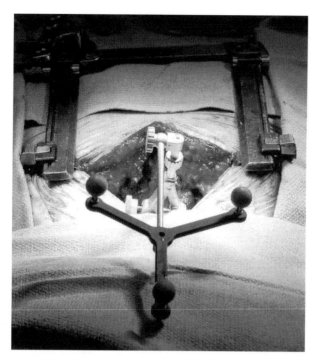

Figure 4 Reference frame attached to a spinous process in the surgical field. The reference frame monitors inadvertent movement of the spinal anatomy that may affect navigational accuracy.

three images will be in the sagittal, coronal, and axial planes. A trajectory line representing the orientation of the long axis of the probe will overlay the sagittal and axial planes. A cursor representing a cross section through the selected trajectory will overlay the coronal plane. The insertional "depth" of the trajectory can be adjusted to correspond to selected screw lengths. As the depth is adjusted, the specific coronal plane will also adjust accordingly with the position of the cursor demonstrating the final position of the tip of a screw placed at that depth along the selected trajectory. As the probe is moved to another point in the surgical field, the reformatted images as well as the position of the cursor and trajectory line will also change. The planar orientation of the three reformatted images will also change as the probe's angle relative to the spinal axis changes. When the probe's orientation is not perpendicular to the long axis of the spine, the images displayed will be in oblique or orthogonal planes. Regardless of the probe's orientation, the navigational workstation will provide the surgeon with a greater degree of anatomical information than can be provided by any intraoperative imaging technique.

The application of image-guided navigation to spinal surgery is directed by the complexity of the procedure and, specifically, by the need to "visualize" the unexposed spinal anatomy. Image-guided navigation can be used with or without standard intra-operative imaging techniques (i.e., fluoroscopy). In either case, image-guided navigation provides the surgeon with an improved orientation to the pertinent spinal anatomy, which subsequently facilitates the accuracy and effectiveness of the procedure. It is currently used for pedicle fixation of the thoracic and lumbosacral regions (Fig. 5), C1-2 screw fixation (Fig. 6), transoral surgery (Fig. 7), anterior cervical, thoracic, and thoracolumbar surgery, and for the removal of spinal tumors (1,12–16).

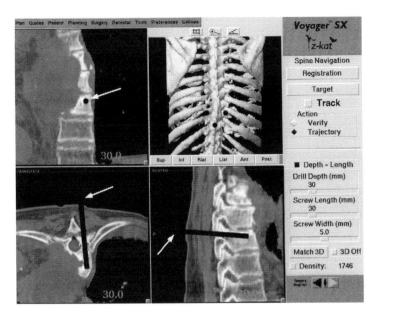

Figure 5 Workstation screen demonstrating navigation for a T9 pedicle screw in a patient with a mycotic aneurysm of the aorta (Screw trajectory and tip location highlighted by arrows).

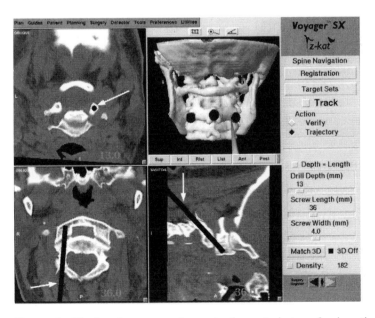

Figure 6 Workstation screen demonstrating a trajectory for insertion of a C1-2 transarticular screw. The lower right screen shows the trajectory in the sagittal plane. The lower left screen represents an orthogonal plane lying between the axial and coronal planes. It conveys the medial-lateral trajectory. The upper left screen represents a plane that is perpendicular to the two other images. It demonstrates the location of the screw tip inserted along the selected trajectory at the indicated depth (screw trajectory and tip location highlighted by arrows).

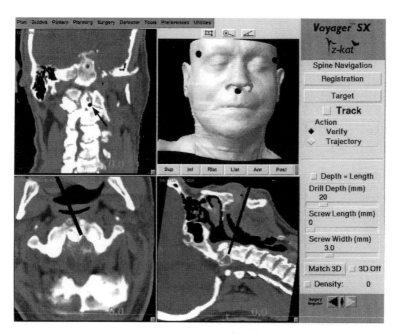

Figure 7 Workstation screen demonstrating navigational information during transoral decompression (Probe tip location and trajectory highlighted by arrows).

III. PITFALLS AND ERRORS

While image-guided spinal navigation has proven to be a versatile and effective tool for facilitating complex surgical procedures, it can be prone to several potential problems prior to and during its use. In general, these pitfalls and errors are related to issues of accuracy, technique, and overall ease of use of the technology during surgery. A thorough understanding of these potential problems is required to assure the efficient and effective use of image-guided navigation for spinal surgery.

A. Accuracy

When using image-guided technology for spinal surgery it is important to understand the difference between the ideal accuracy of a computer-based system and the realistic accuracy demands of spinal surgery. While absolute accuracy is desirable, it is not necessary in the majority of spinal procedures. A more realistic approach to spinal navigational accuracy is termed "clinically relevant accuracy." This concept implies that for each spinal procedure, a certain level of accuracy is needed, and that once it is achieved, making efforts to acquire more is unnecessary. Placing a 6 mm diameter pedicle screw through a lumbar pedicle that may be 15 mm in diameter does not require submillimetric accuracy. While placement of a transarticular screw at the C1-2 level may require more accuracy than a lumbar pedicle screw placement, it still does not require submillimetric accuracy. It only requires a level of accuracy that is greater than the standard of fluoroscopic guidance and to a degree that safely positions the screw thorough the desired trajectory. Attempts to achieve anything more than clinically relevant does nothing more than contribute to the complexity of the technology, making it more time-consuming and difficult to use.

The accuracy of image-guided navigation in the spine depends on several factors. The inherent quality of the image data is a critical factor. The initial process in assuring that the image data are of sufficient quality is the compatibility testing that occurs when a system is installed. This typically requires an evaluation of the imaging scanners that will provide the data to the image-guided system. A precise interface between the CT scanner and the image-guided system needs to be established so that the images can be properly read.

Computed tomography scan limitations allow for image slice thickness of no less than 1 mm. Therefore, the smallest error and the greatest degree of accuracy that can be achieved when using image-guidance is 1 mm. Submillimetric accuracy with image-guided technology does not exist. Typically, scans with 1 or 2 mm slice thickness are recommended for the use of image-guidance in the spine.

The quality of the image data can also be affected by patient movement during image acquisition. This may result in blurred or fragmented images that are not adequate for use. Typically, these images appear on the workstation screen as one segment of the image clearly disconnected from the remaining image. However, with advances in spiral CT imaging, current scanners are capable of acquiring large amounts of image data in a very short period of time, limiting the problem of poor image quality secondary to patient movement.

As the quality of image-guided technology has improved, the problems of inaccuracy related to system or image factors has declined. The inherent accuracy and precision of this technology has been demonstrated (17). The majority of accuracy problems associated with current image-guided spinal navigational technology is directly related to surgeon error and a failure to use correct registration and navigational techniques.

B. Technique

A number of image-guided systems are currently available for use during spinal surgery. Each system has its own specific technique of operation that must be adhered to in order to achieve accurate and reliable information. The surgeon and operating room staff typically receive an instructional course on the correct technique when the system is installed.

The initial step in using the acquired images for intraoperative navigation is the proper transfer of the data to the workstation. This is done using a network link between the workstation and the CT scanner or transferring the data via optical disk. Failure to follow the appropriate protocol for transferring image data can result in significant errors that may prevent the use of the system for that particular surgery.

The most important technical step in the use of image-guided technology is the registration process. Failure on the part of the surgeon to adequately perform the specific registration technique will guarantee inaccurate navigational data that, unless recognized as flawed, may result in misplaced spinal fixation screws or other intraoperative judgment errors. An incorrect registration technique also contributes significantly to the added time that many image-guided systems bring to spinal surgery.

Each individual image-guided system has its own registration technique requirements using a paired point method, a surface matching method, or a combination of both. If the paired point method is used, the surgeon selects three to five anatomical points in the image data set at each level to be instrumented. The points selected should not lie on the same plane or the same line, and they should not be close together. They should be points that can be easily identified in the surgical field (i.e., tip of a spinous or transverse process), and they should ideally be peripheral to the intended target(s) (i.e., vertebral pedicles). Following selection of the registration points in the image data set, the corresponding points in the surgical field need to be correctly identified and registered. If the surgeon selects the proper anatomical structure but does so at the wrong level or on the wrong side, a significant registration error will result. Therefore, it is important that the surgeon know the spinal anatomy and be able to transfer his or her interpretation of the spinal image data to the surgical field. This is no different than the demands of spinal surgery without the use of image-guided technology.

If the surface matching registration method is used, the surgeon must adequately debride the surface of the spinal anatomy to be registered. Failure to adequately expose the bone surface for registration of 15–30 separate points can result in a significant registration error. Furthermore, most surface matching methods require that the system be oriented in some way to facilitate the registration process. This usually involves adding some element of the paired point technique to the surface matching method to improve registration accuracy. The previously mentioned potential errors of the paired point method apply to this combined technique.

When the registration process is completed, each system will provide the surgeon with a measurement of registration error typically expressed in millimeters. It is important to recognize that this error is not a linear error but rather a volumetric error. It represents the difference in the volume of space contained between the registration points selected in the image data set and the corresponding volume in the surgical field. It is, at best, a relative indicator of registration accuracy. A more absolute indicator of accuracy is obtained by placing the navigation probe on a landmark in the surgical field (i.e., spinous process) and confirming that the workstation screen is localizing the same point. If there is a discrepancy between the surgical field and the workstation screen, the registration process needs to be repeated (Fig. 8).

Another potential pitfall related to the registration process is the use of registration at one spinal segment to navigate at a distant spinal segment. While this non-segmental registration method may occasionally provide acceptable data when used at an immediately adjacent level, it is not recommended for use at levels that are not adjacent. The potential change in position of the spinal segments from their preoperative scanned position to the intraoperative position introduces the potential for significant navigational error if segmental registration is not used.

Following a satisfactory registration, the surgeon needs to use the correct navigational technique for the particular system employed. Typically this involves place-ment of the navigation probe through a drill guide and onto the selected pedicle entry point. The surgeon assesses the anatomical landmarks in the surgical field and selects the appropriate trajectory prior to looking at the workstation screen. When the surgeon feels that the appropriate entry point and trajectory have been selected, the workstation screen is checked to assess the selection. This is an important principle in the use of image-guidance for spinal surgery. The navigational images created need to be correlated with the surgeon's own knowledge of the surgical anatomy and the appropriate screw trajectories through that anatomy. Image-guided navigation is not a replacement for the surgeon knowing the pertinent spinal anatomy and surgical technique. It merely serves to help confirm a surgeon's estimation of the nonexposed anatomy by providing image information that typically exceeds that of intraoperative fluoroscopy.

Depending on which system is used, a spinal tracking system may or may not be required. If it is used, the tracking device should be placed in the surgical field as close to the spinal segment undergoing registration and navigation. Care must be

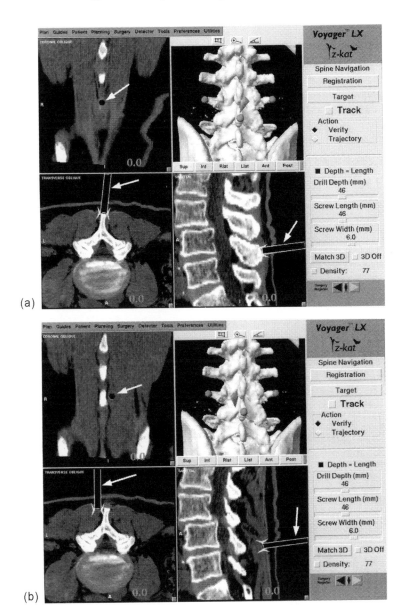

Figure 8 (a) Navigational workstation screen demonstrating satisfactory verification of registration accuracy. While the navigational probe is positioned on the L4 spinous process in the surgical field, the workstation screen should show the cursor and trajectory line in a correlative position in the CT image set. (b) Navigational workstation screen demonstrating an unsatisfactory verification of registration accuracy. If the navigational probe is positioned on the L4 spinous process in the surgical field but the workstation screen shows the cursor and trajectory line is a noncorrelative position (i.e., not on the L4 spinous process), accurate registration has not been achieved, and the registration process needs to be repeated before proceeding with navigation.

taken to assure that the localizer camera can visualize both the probe as well as the tracking device. The tracking device must also be firmly attached to the spinal anatomy. Any movement of the device will result in incorrect information being provided by the system.

As mentioned previously, the use of a tracking device is not an absolute requirement. Systems are available that allow the surgeon the option of using or not using a tracking device. If no tracking device is used, the surgeon needs to recognize the need to maintain the patient reasonably still during the registration and navigational process. This approach is best done with a system that utilizes a short registration time. This allows for an easy and rapid reregistration if any inadvertent movement of the patient occurs following the initial registration process.

Correct navigational technique is also best achieved when performed immediately following registration at that particular segment. Registering multiple spinal segments prior to navigation does not reduce the time of navigation and may result in significant navigational errors.

C. Ease of Use

The problems and pitfalls mentioned above contribute to the overall difficulty in using image-guided technology for spinal surgery. Some current image-guided systems are far more difficult to use than others, contributing to unacceptable added operative time. However, as image-guided technology and its clinical usage have evolved, the ease of use of many of the available systems has significantly improved. This ease-of-use factor can significantly reduce the amount of time needed to apply the technology to spinal procedures.

The ease of use of a particular image-guided navigational system is directly related to the technique requirements. Systems that require the use of surface matching registration and the use of a tracking device require more time and are therefore more difficult to use than systems that employ paired point registration and make the tracking device optional. The ease of use of a particular system also relates to the surgeon understanding the capabilities and limitations of image-guided technology in general as well as the technique requirements for the specific system being used. Ultimately, image-guided technology should be made easy enough to use so that it does not interfere with the standard surgical routine. Any system that adds time to the procedure needs to be modified.

III. FLUOROSCOPIC NAVIGATION

Fluoroscopic navigation is the combination of standard fluoroscopy with image-guided navigational technology. It was developed to counter the user difficulties of some earlier image-guided systems that typically took much longer to use than standard fluoroscopy. The presumed advantage of fluoroscopic navigation is that a preoperative CT image is not required and the navigational image can be updated at any point during the surgical procedure. The advantage over conventional fluoroscopic techniques is that the amount of fluoroscopic time is reduced.

With the patient in position prior to surgery, an anteroposterior and lateral fluoroscopic view of the pertinent spinal anatomy is obtained. This is done with a customized reference frame attached to the C-arm or to the patient. This frame serves to superimpose a specific grid on the two images obtained. The navigational workstation can then take the two images and relate the spatial position of the imaged anatomy to a navigational probe. A navigational trajectory line and cursor can then be superimposed on the lateral and anteroposterior images, respectively. As the probe is moved over the exposed spinal anatomy during surgery, the trajectory line and cursor will adjust their position on the stationary fluoroscopic images (18).

The disadvantage of fluoroscopic navigation is that it is still only fluoroscopy. The same difficulties experienced with standard fluoroscopy are present with fluoroscopic navigation. Specifically, only an anteroposterior and lateral images are provided. The critical plane for most spinal screw fixation procedures is the axial plane, which is the only plane that can definitively demonstrate violation of the spinal canal by a medially displaced screw. Only CT-based image-guided navigation can demonstrate this view, although current developments with standard fluoroscopy will eventually allow for axial reconstructions. Furthermore, any region of the spinal column that is difficult to image with standard fluoroscopy (i.e., upper thoracic) will be difficult to image with fluoroscopic navigation.

The early goals of image-guided spinal navigation were to improve the surgeon's orientation to the intraoperative spinal anatomy in a time- and cost-efficient manner and to ultimately replace fluoroscopy. Many of these earlier CT-based image-guided systems were difficult to use and time-consuming. This led to the application of fluoroscopy to image-guided technology. However, several years of clinical experience have helped modify and improve CT-based navigational technology, making these systems easier to use than earlier systems. This improved ease of use coupled with the ability to obtain axial imaging as well as its superior accuracy, image manipulation, and orientation capabilities provides image-guided technology with a clear advantage over any fluoroscopic-based technology.

IV. CONCLUSION

Image-guided navigational technology has been successfully applied to spinal surgery. By linking digitized image data to spinal surface anatomy, image-guided spinal navigation facilitates the surgeon's orientation to unexposed spinal structures, improving the precision and accuracy of the surgery. It is typically used to optimize the placement of spinal fixation screws and to monitor the extent of complex decompressive procedures. It can also be used as a preoperative planning tool.

While image-guided spinal navigation is a versatile and effective technology, it is not a replacement for the surgeon having thorough knowledge of the pertinent spinal anatomy as well as correct surgical techniques. It merely serves as an additional source of information used by the surgeon to make selected intraoperative decisions. In this way it is similar to more conventional intraoperative imaging techniques (i.e., fluoroscopy) except that it provides a much greater degree of information to the surgeon.

The use of image-guided technology is highly dependent on the surgeon understanding its capabilities and limitations. Several potential pitfalls can occur prior to and during its use for spinal surgery. Unless recognized, these pitfalls can result in significant errors in navigational accuracy and can make the use of image-guidance difficult and time-consuming. However, by recognizing their potential and using correct registration and navigational techniques, these pitfalls can all be avoided.

REFERENCES

1. Kalfas IH, Kormos DW, Murphy MA, McKenzie RL, Barnett GH, Bell GR, Steiner CP, Trimble MB, Weisenberger JP. Application of frameless stereotaxy to pedicle screw fixation of the spine. J Neurosurg 1995; 83:641–647.

2. Murphy MA, McKenzie RL, Kormos DW, Kalfas IH. Frameless stereotaxis for the insertion of lumbar pedicle screws: a technical note. J Clin Neurosci 1994; 1(4):257–260.

3. George DC, Krag MH, Johnson CC, Van Hal ME, Haugh LD, Grobler LJ. Hole preparation technique for transpedicle screws: effect on pull-out strength from human cadaveric vertebrae. Spine 1991; 16:181–184.

4. Gertzbein SD, Robbins SE. Accuracy of pedicle screw placement in vivo. Spine 1990; 15:11–14.

5. Weinstein JN, Spratt KF, Spengler D, Brick C, Reid S. Spinal pedicle fixation: reliability and validity of roentgenogram-based assessment and surgical factors on successful screw placement. Spine 1988; 13:1012–1018.

6. Steinmann JC, Herkowitz HO, El-Kommos H, Wesolowski DP. Spinal pedicle fixation: confirmation of an image-based technique for screw placement. Spine 1993; 18:1856–1861.

7. Barnett GH, Kormos DW, Steiner CP, Weisenberger J. Use of a frameless, armless stereotactic wand for brain tumor localization with two-dimensional and three-dimensional neuroimaging. Neurosurgery 1993; 33:674–678.

8. Barnett GH, Kormos DW, Steiner CP, Weisenberger J. Intraoperative localization using an armless, frameless stereotactic wand. Technical note. J Neurosurg 1993; 78:510–514.

9. Brodwater BK, Roberts DW, Nakajima T, Friets EM, Strohbehn JW. Extracranial application of the frameless stereotactic operating microscope: experience with lumbar spine. Neurosurgery 1993; 32:209–213.

10. Bryant JT, Reid JG, Smith BL, Stevenson JM. A method for determining vertebral body positions in the sagittal plane using skin markers. Spine 1989; 14:258–265.

11. Pellizzari CA, Levin DN, Chen GTY, Chen CT. Image registration based on anatomic surface matching. In: Maciunas RJ, ed. Interactive Image-Guided Neurosurgery. Park Ridge, IL: AANS Publications, 1993:47–62.

12. Kalfas IH. Image-guided spinal navigation. Clin Neurosurg 1999; 46:70–88.

13. Kalfas IH. Spinal Surgery. In: Barnett GH, Roberts DW and Maciunas RJ, eds. Image-Guided Neurosurgery: Clinical Applications of Surgical Navigation. St. Louis: Quality Medical Publishing, 1998:117–134.

14. Kalfas IH. Image-guided spinal navigation: application to spinal metastasis. In: Maciunas RJ, ed. Advanced Techniques in Central Nervous System Metastasis. Lebanon, NH: AANS Publications, 1998:245–254.

15. Kalfas IH. Frameless stereotaxy assisted spinal surgery. In: Renganchary SS, ed. Neurosurgery Operative Color Atlas. Lebanon, NH: AANS Publications, 2000:123–134.

16. Welch WC, Subach BR, Pollack IF, Jacobs GB. Frameless stereotactic guidance for surgery of the upper cervical spine. Neurosurgery 1997; 40(5):958–964.

17. Kitchen ND, Lemieux L, Thomas DG. Accuracy in frame-based and frameless stereotaxy. Sterotact Functional Neurosurg 1993; 61:195–206.

18. Foley KT, Simon DA, Rampersaud YR. Virtual fluoroscopy: computer-assisted fluoroscopic navigation. Spine 2001; 26(4):347–351.

39

Complications Related to the Surgical Management of Achondroplasia

Michael C. Ain, B. M. Cascio, R. G. Geocadin, and Daniele Rigamonti
Johns Hopkins Hospital, Baltimore, Maryland, U.S.A.

I. INTRODUCTION

Achondroplasia is an autosomal dominant disorder that affects the endochondral growth of bone. It is caused by a point mutation in fibroblast growth factor receptor 3 located on chromosome 4p16.3. Over 80% of the cases result from new mutations in a child born to normal parents. The defective endochondral growth of bone results in rhizomelic dwarfism that has characteristic macrocephaly and hypoplasia of the midface. The disorder is also associated with a delay in achieving milestones such as balanced sitting and walking, which plays a role in the development of the unique achondroplastic spinal deformities.

II. PATHOANATOMY

The complications encountered in surgery on the achondroplastic spine include those encountered with the nonachondroplastic spine with some unique additions. The complications shared with all spine surgery, such as dural tears and neural injury, are more common in the achondroplast. The reason for the increased risk of typical spinal surgery complications as well as for the additional, unique operative complications is secondary to the characteristic pathoanatomy of the achondroplastic spine.

The defect in endochondral growth of the achondroplastic spine produces a shortened, stenotic spinal column with characteristic abnormal features originally described by Donath and Vogl in 1925 (1). These features include abnormalities in the vertebral bodies, intervertebral disks, pedicles, ligaments, facets, and the overall curvature of the spinal column.

The vertebral bodies grow in height by endochondral bone formation at the superior and inferior epiphyseal plate just as in the long bone (2). Thus, the disease causes a shortened vertebral body that is enlarged and mushroomed at the superior and inferior aspects and also concave on its posterior border (3–5). The formation of the neural arch is also affected, and as a result the spinal canal is abnormally small while the neural elements are normal sized. Specifically, the pathoanatomical changes include thickened, short pedicles and thickened lamina (4). The spinal canal is also trefoil shaped due to the facet hypertrophy that usually occurs with age. The resulting size of the spinal canal is reduced by one third to one half (5). This size mismatch is at the root of the nerve compression syndromes that plague the achondroplastic spine. The size mismatch is most significant at the L2-L3 level, explaining the increased incidence of cauda equina syndrome in achondroplasts (6,7).

The intervertebral disks of the achondroplastic spine are hyperplastic (8). The disks, in addition, have the tendency to bulge, further impinging upon the already stenotic spinal canal, lateral gutter, and intervertebral foramen. The problem is further complicated by the frequent presence of a hypertrophic ligamentum flavum (9).

There is also a characteristic sagittal deformity of the achondroplastic spine. The cause is attributed to the increase in stress placed on the achondroplastic spine by the associated macrocephaly. This increased stress, compounded with the flat, relatively unsupportive thoracic cage, generalized hypotonia, and the interaction of the globus abdomen, diaphragm, and abdominal muscles, manifests itself as a hypokyphosis of the upper thoracic spine, a hyperkyphosis of the lower thoracic and upper lumbar spine, and a lordosis of the lumbosacral junction (10). The kyphosis of the thoracic and lumbar spine usually correct upon the achondroplastic child beginning to ambulate. However, some kyphoses persist and even progress (11). The lumbosacral junction lordosis is attributed to the horizontal orientation of the sacrum, caused by the characteristic flexion contracture of the hips.

The dura is notoriously thin and fragile in the achondroplastic spine. One of the larger series of achondroplastic spine surgery demonstrated a greater than 50% dural tear rate (12) There is lack of the normal amount of epidural fat in achondroplasts, resulting in even less protection for the neural elements (13).

The aging achondroplastic spine manifests the same changes as the nonachondroplastic spine, including facet hypertrophy, disk degeneration and narrowing, and osteophyte formation.

III. PRESENTATION

The two main pathological mechanisms that affect the achondroplastic spine are persistent thoracolumbar kyphosis and lumbar or cervical stenosis (14). Between the ages of 5 and 15, the most common spine pathology is persistence of the thoracolumbar kyphosis (14). The achondroplast begins to suffer neural complications from spinal stenosis as early as infancy, but usually symptoms begin by 30 years of age (14–16). There are four main presentations of neurological dysfunction: (a) Progressive, insidious; (b) Intermittent claudication; (c) nerve compression causing radiculopathy; and; (d) acute paraplegia (7). The first two are more prevalent.

IV. IMAGING

The typical imaging modalities are used in evaluation of the achondroplastic spine with one major exception. Lumbar puncture for myelography is difficult and many times impossible to perform, but is also dangerous in the stenotic achondroplastic spine because removing even a small amount of spinal fluid from the lumbar canal can remove the only cushion preventing the direct compression of neural elements. High cervical puncture is recommended instead (17). The myelogram produced possesses distinctive features with

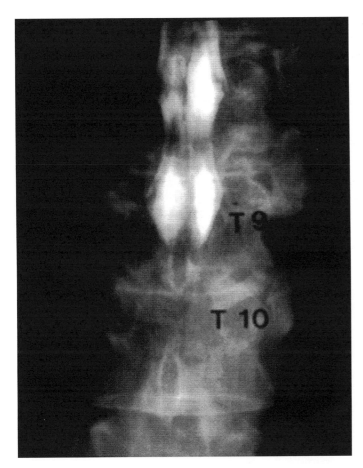

Figure 1 This distinctive myelogram of the stenotic achondroplastic spine demonstrates alternating levels of stenosis and filling defects, representing areas corresponding to disk protrusion, with areas of pooling, representing areas posterior to the concave vertebral bodies. This myelogram also demonstrates a complete block of dye at the T9 vertebral level.

alternating levels of stenosis and filling defects, representing areas corresponding to disk protrusion, with areas of pooling, representing areas posterior to the concave vertebral bodies (Fig. 1).

V. SURGICAL INDICATIONS AND PROCEDURES

There are few absolute indications and accepted surgical procedures for achondroplastic spine surgery due to the lack of any large clinical studies.

For stenosis, surgery is performed for objective nerve deficits, progressive symptoms, and urinary retention. A decompression without fusion is usually performed. A common cause of failure is the insufficient release of compressed neural tissue. The medial aspect of the facets must be addressed to enlarge the lateral recess, and a wide laminectomy must be performed to decompress the stenotic spinal canal. The literature is not clear as to how many levels to decompress, but it is certain that hypertrophic scar tissue invading the already stenotic neighboring regions is the cause for many revisions. One author suggests lower thoracic spine to sacrum decompression for thoracolumbar level compression (17). Early intervention is also recommended because while early intervention is associated with better outcomes, delayed intervention is associated with permanent dysfunction (17). Fusion is added to decompressions when a kyphosis is present, when $> 50\%$ of the facets are removed bilaterally, or when patients have not reached skeletal maturity, even with a normal sagittal profile.

For kyphotic deformity, surgery is performed for symptoms as well as structural deformity. Patients less than 5 years of age with a kyphosis greater than 50° and who have failed conservative treatment are treated with anterior discectomy and strut grafting with instrumentation and a posterior fusion. If there is anterior impingement or apical wedging, the patient is treated with anterior corpectomy and strut graft fusion with instrumentation and posterior fusion. Patients greater than 5 years old with a kyphosis that corrects to less than 50° and with adequately sized pedicles are treated with posterior fusion with pedicle screws (Fig. 2). Patients who do not correct to less than 50° are treated with an anterior

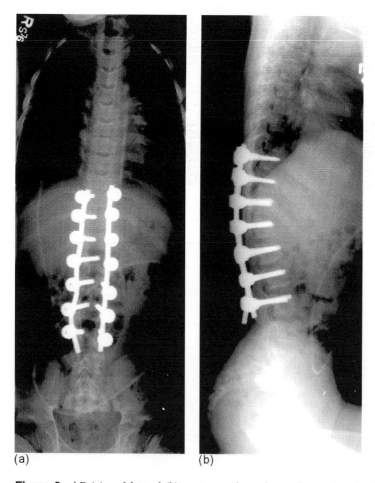

(a)   (b)

Figure 2 AP (a) and lateral (b) postoperative spine radiographs of a 6-year-old boy who underwent multiple level lumbar laminectomy for stenosis and prophylactic posterior fusion to prevent progression of a thoracolumbar kyphosis that did not correct to less than 50° preoperatively.

and posterior fusion. The goal for correction is established by a lateral hyperextension view over a bolster. This view is obtained during the preoperative workup, approximately one week before surgery. The patient is able to report at that time if any neurological changes occur with hyperextension.

VI. RESULTS

A review of cases of achondroplastic spinal surgery elucidates some trends (6–25). Mild or modest neurological deficits that are present for less than 3 years tend to do better than those that are more chronic. Severe preoperative deficits, including paraplegia and sphincter dysfunction, do not benefit greatly from surgery unless treated acutely (24). Good long term results are associated with older age at the time of onset of symptoms, acute onset of symptoms and signs, prompt wide thoracolumbosacral decompression, complete neurologic functional recovery within one week of surgery, and no presence of cervical stenosis (12).

VII. COMPLICATIONS

A. General

The hyperlordosis of the lumbosacral junction essentially forces the surgeon to work in a narrow, deep hole. This fact, combined with the stenotic spinal canal, places both the dura and spinal elements at increased risk. Electrocautery is used as little as possible in order to preserve the facet capsules and prevent deinnervation and resultant atrophy of the paraspinal muscles (17).

The following significant complications were noted to have occurred in a review of reported cases of adult achondroplastic spine patients (12,17–19):

Postoperative anemia
Hypertension
Failure of relief of symptoms
Pseudarthrosis
Vertebral artery ischemia
Bacterial meningitis
Hypotension/hypovolemia
Laryngeal edema
Ileus
Death
Urinary tract infection
Paraplegia/quadriplegia
Recurrence or worsening of symptoms
Vertebral column instability
Cerebral infarction
Dural tear
Congestive heart failure
Urinary retention
Epidural hematoma

B. Positioning

The characteristic abnormalities of the achondroplastic skeleton make intraoperative positioning a source of potential complications. The stenotic foramen magnum and cervical spine and macrocephaly demand increased vigilance during the preoperative positioning of the head and neck. Specifically, hyperextension should be carefully avoided. The achondroplastic elbow does not possess normal extension or supination, the shoulder lacks normal abduction, and the hip possesses a flexion contracture between 15 and 20°. These structural abnormalities have to be considered during positioning. A Jackson table is used to maximally decompress the abdomen to facilitate venous drainage. Increased venous pressure due to the stenotic Jugular foramen has been thought to have contributed to at least one case of intracranial hemorrhage (26). Somatosensory-evoked potentials (SSEPs) and motor-evoked potentials (MEPs) must be monitored during surgery.

C. Respiratory

The achondroplastic patient is at a substantially increased risk of respiratory problems due to an abnormally flat and relatively weakened thoracic cage and upper airway obstruction due to midface hypoplasia. In the perioperative period, the achondroplastic tendency for sleep apnea due to the stenosis of the foramen magnum must be met with continuous monitoring and even airway assist devices if necessary. One reported death after revision spine surgery occurred due to a cardiac arrest secondary to acute respitory insufficiency after a 24-hour delay in extubation (20). The prone position of patients during surgery leads to dependent edema in the face and the upper airway. If significant soft tissue swelling, especially in the facial area is noted, delay in extubation should be considered because of increased chances of airway compomise due to upper airway edema.

D. Instrumentation

No instrumentation such as lamina wires or hooks should be placed in the spinal canal. Placement of such devices has proved to be a great risk for developing iatrogenic neurological deficits due to the stenotic spinal canal (14). Pedicle screws are used when pedicles are large enough to accept them. Pedicle screws have replaced casting.

E. Dural Tears

The dura associated with the achondroplastic spine is notoriously thin and fragile and is easily torn. Working on the dura in the narrow, deep hyperlordotic region of the achondroplastic spine is complicated by the fact that there is a lack of epidural fat to cushion the dura from instruments and the dura is often adherent to the thickened ligamentum flavum (13). Dural tears were reported to occur in over half of the cases in one study (12). The surgeon is advised to use Kerrison punches with extreme caution when decompressing the spinal canal due to the intimate relationship of the neural elements and dura with the ligamentum flavum and neural arch. Preferably, a high-speed bur is used to create an eggshell thin layer of bone, which is then carefully picked away.

When a tear occurs, it is not uncommon for part of the cauda equina to extrude into the operative field due to the increased pressure in the spinal canal. Often, many of the nerve roots escape the dural sac and fill the operative wound. Neural elements should be gently repositioned into the dural sac. Then the tear should be primarily repaired and sealed with fibrin glue. A Valsalva test should be performed intraoperatively to confirm the satisfactory level of the repair. If there is no leak at 40 mmHg, the patient is kept with head flat for 2 days and then head elevation is allowed as tolerated.

F. Infection

Two main types of infection are most commonly associated with surgery on the achondro-plastic spine. The first is urinary tract infections associated with urinary retention. In many instances, the patient has urinary retention preoperatively. When urinary retention is chronic, it is unlikely that decompression will reverse neural damage. The second type of infection is wound infection. Decompression of the hyperlordotic segment of the achondroplast spine produces a deep dead space that may cause a pseudomeningocoele, hematoma, or seroma formation. To close this potential dead space, the paraspinal muscles are overlapped to create an additional protective layer. One case series found that wound infections occurred in 4 of 22 cases and urinary tract infections occurred in 8 of 22 cases (14). Another case series found that bacterial infection occurred in 34% of 50 spine

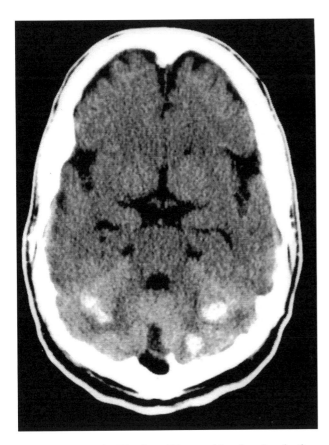

Figure 3 Head CT of a 37-year-old achondroplastic male who sustained an intracerebral hemorrhage status post–spine surgery. It is thought that the complication was partially attributable to the jugular foramen stenosis found in achondroplasts, which increases central venous pressure. This occurrence underlines the importance of decompressing the abdomen by allowing it to hang freely during surgery.

patients, about half of which were urinary tract infections (19). Other types of infection found in achondroplastic spine surgery include those expected of any major spine surgery, namely, bacterial meningitis and pneumonia.

G. Epidural Hematoma/Intracranial Hemorrhage

One instance of epidural hematoma has been reported in the literature. The specific instance was attributed to a relative overdose of subcutaneous heparin therapy 24 hours postoperatively (6). There is one reported episode of an intracranial hemorrhage after a revision (Fig. 3) (26). This was attributed to elevated venous pressure secondary to congenital jugular foramen stenosis exacerbated by prolonged recumbency. This intracranial hemorrhage underlines the importance of decompressing the abdomen by appropriate positioning during surgery.

H. Instability

One author noted a pseudarthrosis in a series of 5 cases (4). No other instances of pseudarthroses were found. A review of achondroplastic spine revisions found that revision surgery caused destabilization requiring fusion in 4 of 8 patients (20).

I. Reoperation/Failure

Insufficient initial laminectomy is the primary reason for failed surgery (17). Pyeritz et al. reported that 10 of 22 patients required additional laminectomies (12). Another study of 20 spines demonstrated improvement in 14 postoperatively, no change in 5, and worsening of symptoms/signs in 1 (18). Another study of 35 patients demonstrated 25 with complete recovery and 2 with no benefit (6). The achondroplastic spine is unforgiving to a conservative decompression because postoperative scar formation has no extradural space in which to form and therefore displaces neural structures in an already stenotic spinal canal adjacent to the initial decompression. Several authors have recommended that an extensive decompression be performed at the initial operation (12,17,23). Three general guidelines include decompressing three levels cephalad to the myelographic block, decompressing caudal to the second sacral level, and decompressing lateral to the facet joints (12).

Revision surgery in achondroplasts, as in nonachondroplasts, increases the risk of nerve injury, instability, and dural tears. The benefits to the patient, however, outweigh the potential complications. Specific improvements seen in one study of achondroplastic spine revisions include improvements in strength, claudication, pain, bladder dysfunction, and bowel disturbance (20). Restenosis can be quite disabling for achondroplasts, and repeated operation can successfully lessen pain and neurological symptoms in most of these patients (20).

REFERENCES

1. Donath J, Vogel A. Untersuchungen über den chondrodystrophischen Zwergwuchs. Wiener Arch Inn Med 1925; 10:1–44.
2. Bick EM, Copel JW. Longitudinal growth of the human vertebra. JBJS 1950; 32-A(4):803–814.
3. Alexander E. Significance of the small lumbar spinal canal: cauda equina compression syndromes due to spondylosis. Part 5. Achondroplasia. J Neurosurg 1969; 31:513–519.

4. Duvoisin RC, Yahr MD. Compressive spinal cord and root syndromes in achondroplastic dwarfs. Neurology 1962; 12:202–207.
5. Lutter LD, Lonstein JE, Winter RB, Langer LO. Anatomy of the achondroplastic lumbar canal. 1977; 126:139–142.
6. Thomeer RT, van Dijk JM. Surgical treatment of lumbar stenosis in achondroplasia. J Neurosurg (Spine 3) 2002; 96:292–297.
7. Lutter LD, Langer LO. Neurological symptoms in achondroplastic dwarfs—surgical treatment. JBJS 1977; 59-A:87–92.
8. Morgan DF, Young RF. Spinal neurological complications of achondroplasia. J Neurosurg 1980; 52:463–472.
9. Uematsu S, Wang H, Kopits SE, Hurko O. Total craniospinal decompression in achondroplastic stenosis. J Neurosurg 1994; 35(2):250–258.
10. Kopits SE. Thoracolumbar kyphosis and lumbosacral hyperlordosis in achondroplastic children. In: Nicoletti B, Kopits SE, Ascani E, McKusick VA, eds. Human Achondroplasia: A Multidisciplinary Approach. New York: Plenum, 1986:241–255.
11. Lonstein JE. Treatment of kyphosis and lumbar stenosis in achondroplasia. In: Nicoletti B, Kopits SE, Ascani E, McKusick VA, eds. Human Achondroplasia: A Multidisciplinary Approach. New York: Plenum, 1986:283–292.
12. Pyeritz RE, Sack GH, Udvarhelyi GB. Thoracolumbosacral laminectomy in achondroplasia: long-term results in 22 patients. Am J Med Gen 1987; 28:433–444.
13. Hancock DO, Philips DG. Spinal compression in achondroplasia. Paraplegia 1965; 3:23–33.
14. Tolo VT. Spinal deformity in short-stature syndromes. In: Bridwell KH, DeWald RL, eds. The Textbook of Spinal Surgery. 2nd ed. Philadelphia: Lippincott-Raven, 1996:399–405.
15. Hahn YS, Engelhard HH, Naidich T, McLone DG. Paraplegia resulting from thoracolumbar stenosis in a seven-month-old achondroplastic dwarf. Pediatr Neurosci 1989; 15:39–43.
16. Kahanovitz N, Rimoin DL, Sillence DO. The clinical spectrum of limbar spine disease in achondroplasia. Spine 1982; 7(2):137–140.
17. Hurko O, Uematsu S. Surgical considerations in skeletal dysplasias. Neurosurg Q 1993; 3(3):192–217.
18. Streeten E, Uematsu S, Hurko O, Kopits S, Murphy E, Pyeritz R. Extended laminectomy for spinal stenosis in achondroplasia. In: Nicoletti B, Kopits SE, Ascani E, McKusick VA, eds. Human Achondroplasia: A Multidisciplinary Approach. New York: Plenum, 1986:261–273.
19. Geocadin R, Johnson C, Conway JA, Bendebba M, Lower J, Mirski MA, Ain M, Rigamonti D. Spinal surgery in achondroplastic patients: a 5 year post-operative and intensive care experience at The Johns Hopkins Hospital 1995–2000. 31st Congress of the Society of Critical Care Medicine, San Diego, CA, January 2000.
20. Ain, MC, Elmaci I, Hurko O, Clatterbuck RE, Lee RR, Rigamonti D. Reoperation for spinal restenosis in achondroplasia. J Spinal Disord 2000; 13(2):168–173.
21. Dubousset J, Masson JC. Spinal disorders: kyphosis and lumbar stenosis. In: Nicoletti B, Kopits SE, Ascani E, McKusick VA, eds. Human Achondroplasia: A Multidisciplinary Approach. New York: Plenum, 1986:299–303.
22. Epstein JA, Malis LI. Compression of spinal cord and cauda equina in achondroplastic dwarfs. Neurology 1955; 5:875–881.
23. Fortuna A, Ferrante L, Acqui M, Santoro A, Mastronardi. Narrowing of thoraco-lumbar spinal canal in achondroplasia. J Neuro Sciences 1989; 33(2):185–196.
24. Nelson MA. Kyphosis and lumbar stenosis in achondroplasia. In: Nicoletti B, Kopits SE, Ascani E, McKusick VA, eds. Human Achondroplasia: A Multidisciplinary Approach. New York: Plenum, 1986:305–311.
25. O'Donnell HD, Uematsu S, Hurko O, Kopits S, Wang H. Craniospinal stenosis in achondroplasia: a 10-year surgical experience with 64 cases (abstr.). J Neurosurg 1992; 76:378–379.
26. Elmaci I, Ain MC, Wright MJ, Lee RR, Sheppard JM, Rigamonti D, Hurko O. J Neurosurg Anesthesiol 2000; 12(3):217–220.

40

Complications Related to the Surgical Management of Patients with Skeletal Dysplasias and Connective Tissue Diseases

Paul D. Sponseller
Johns Hopkins University, Baltimore, Maryland, U.S.A.

In addition to complications of spine surgery in achondroplasia (Chapter 39), many other skeletal dysplasias and connective tissue disorders may cause spinal problems. This chapter will first cover other skeletal dysplasias, followed by connective tissue disorders such as Marfan syndrome and Ehlers-Danlos syndrome. In each section we will summarize the unique features and challenges of each condition, followed by a discussion of intraoperative complications, postoperative surgical complications, and postoperative medical complications.

I. SKELETAL DYSPLASIAS

A. Mucopolysaccharidoses

The mucopolysaccharidoses are a group of heritable disorders caused by deficiency of lysosomal enzymes required for degradation of acid mucopolysaccharides (also termed glycosaminoglycans). Deficiency of the specific hydrolase results in partial degradation of the molecules and lysosomal storage of the residual fragment. This leads to intralysosomal accumulations of the glycosaminoglycans, progressive physical (and sometimes mental) deterioration, and, in severe forms, death. Some of the more common disorders falling in this category include Morquio's, Hunter-Hurler, and Maroteaux-Lamy syndromes. Common spinal problems associated with these conditions include odontoid hypoplasia with atlantoaxial instability, thoracolumbar kyphosis and/or instability, and spinal stenosis. Extradural soft-tissue thickening has occasionally been reported (1).

1. Intraoperative Complications

Anesthetic management of these patients is difficult. It is advisable to know the stability of the cervical spine no matter which part of the spine is being operated upon. Vigorous hyperextension of the neck may cause cord compromise. Fiberoptic intubation is considered the safest way to handle these patients and prevent complications. Complications may arise from turning the patient with an unstable neck. Spinal cord monitoring should be used before and during patient positioning. Loss of fixation has been reported in both the cervical and thoracolumbar portions of the spine due to the small size of the vertebrae and frequent osteoporosis. In the cervical spine, Koop et al. have described an effective technique of immobilization of the spine if internal fixation proves problematic (2). Halo-vest immobilization is used until fusion is solid.

2. Postoperative Surgical Complications

Surgical treatment does not guarantee that there will be no further spinal problems. Some patients after fusion have developed a deformity at the region of the kyphosis fusion due to continued anterior growth (3). Large kyphoses should be fused anteriorly and posteriorly. Some patients have been noted to have kyphosis at another location; the entire thoracolumbar spine should be carefully examined prior to the initial surgery.

3. Postoperative Medical Complications

Airway obstruction continues to be a concern after surgery. Death from obstruction has occurred after extubation, so observation should be carried out in an intensive care setting until stable respiratory status is assured. Even in the nonacute setting, ventilation should be assessed during sleep since sleep apnea is also more frequent in these patients. Patients with Morquio syndrome often have cardiac problems, such as valvular thickening and insufficiency, as well as conduction defects.

B. Diastrophic Dysplasia

Diastrophic dysplasia is caused by a disorder in proteoglycan sulfation. Thus, cartilage at all locations develops abnormal properties. Patients develop short stature, joint contractures, severe foot deformities, and a characteristic "hitchhiker thumb." The most characteristic cervical spine deformity is kyphosis with spina bifida occulta, seen in 5–10% of patients (4,5). This sometimes improves with time (6,7). Spinal deformity becomes severe in the minority: approximately 20% develop a curve exceeding 50 degrees. The usual thoracolumbar spinal deformity is a double-major scoliosis with junctional kyphosis between the two curves. The curves tend to be very stiff, most likely due to premature degenerative changes in the facets and disks (8). This results in small amounts of correction with surgery. The pedicles tend to be short, leading to relative spinal stenosis (8).

1. Intraoperative Complications

Intraoperative neurological deficit has been reported. It may be due to the focal kyphosis, spinal stenosis, and canal intrusion with hooks. For this reason, pedicle screws are preferable when they can be used.

2. Postoperative Complications

Prolonged mechanical ventilation may be needed because of preexisting restrictive lung disease. Patients should be counseled about this possibility. Failure of fixation is seen more commonly than in many other disorders, most likely because of decreased size and strength of laminae and pedicles, as well as curve rigidity. Use of halo traction for large curves without focal remaining kyphosis may decrease the stress on the fixation. Pseudarthrosis is seen in over 10% of these patients (9), and this is one of the reasons for recommendation of anterior and posterior fusion in diastrophic dysplasia.

C. Spondyloepiphyseal Dysplasia

Due to a disorder of type II collagen, this disorder is more severe in the congenita form. Atlantoaxial instability occurs in nearly half of these children, and this level should be fused if there is clinical or radiographic evidence of cord compression (10). Scoliosis is also common in the thoracolumbar spine.

Intraoperative problems may include inability to obtain or maintain reduction of the atlantoaxial translation, in which case decompression is needed. Another problem may be the finding of a bifid arch of the atlas, in which fusion to the occiput may be indicated if adequate bone surface is not available for fusion. Preoperative imaging with computed tomography (CT) or magnetic resonance imaging (MRI) is recommended to look for this.

Postoperative problems may include either nonunion or extension of the fusion.

D. Larsen Syndrome

Larsen syndrome is characterized by multiple joint dislocations (hips, knees, and elbows), combined with unusual facial features and foot deformities as well as an accessory calcaneal apophysis. The genetic etiology is still unknown. The spinal deformity of Larsen syndrome is cervical spina bifida with resultant kyphosis having an apex at the fourth or fifth cervical vertebrae. The frequency of this is unknown, but appears to involve a minority of patients. Unlike diastrophic dysplasia, this kyphosis does not improve with time. Early posterior fusion in infancy or early childhood is indicated as soon as the deformity is identified. Also, thoracolumbar scoliosis, kyphosis, or spondylolisthesis may occur and occasionally require surgery (11).

1. Intraoperative Complications

During these often difficult intubations, the anesthesiologist should try to avoid further flexion of the cervical spine in order to prevent compression from the anterior side. Ideally, spinal cord monitoring should be performed during positioning as well as surgery. Dissection posteriorly should be performed carefully in order to avoid cord damage at the levels with open laminae. Localization of levels should be precise in order to avoid extension to levels above or below the desired fusion. Anteriorly, if corpectomy is indicated, it should begin at the upper and lower end of the gibbus where the cord is least compressed, so that a perspective can be obtained. If portions of the cartilage components of the vertebral bodies are left in place, they can later enlarge and lead to recurrent deformity.

2. Postoperative Complications

Patients need to be immobilized until the fusion is solid. Quadriparesis has been reported postoperatively from a fall in patients whose deformity has not been able to be completely reduced. Postoperative progression is possible after a posterior fusion if the kyphosis is greater than about 50 degrees, although the indications for an anterior arthrodesis have not been clearly defined (12). If an anterior fusion is performed, the excision of anterior growth cartilage should be as complete as possible, or continued anterior growth may occur and cause progressive myelopathy (Fig. 1). On the other extreme, early posterior fusion for smaller curves may lead to progressive lordosis with growth, and this may contribute to

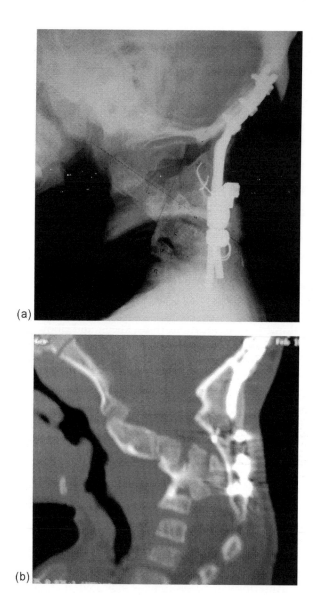

(a)

(b)

Figure 1 (a) Six-year-old with Larsen syndrome and worsening myelopathy kyphosis despite anterior and posterior spinal fusion. (b) CT scan confirms persistent open growth plates of apical vertebral bodies, causing increased deformity.

myelopathy from posterior compression (13). If this scenario develops, an anterior epiphyseodesis of the involved levels may be indicated in addition to posterior decompression.

II. OTHER CONNECTIVE TISSUE DISORDERS

A. Marfan Syndrome

Marfan syndrome (MFS) is a connective tissue disorder caused by mutations in the gene encoding fibrillin-1. Diagnosis of MFS is made clinically according to the Ghent criteria, which rely on multiple organ system involvement, most notably skeletal, ocular, and cardiovascular manifestations. In this classification system there are major and minor criteria; diagnosis requires at least two major findings and one minor. The major criteria are dilation or dissection of the ascending aortic arch, subluxation of the lens of the eye, dural ectasia of the spine, and a genetically proven fibrillin mutation.

Spinal deformities are also relatively common in MFS. Sponseller et al. radiographically screened MFS patients and found scoliosis greater than 10 degrees in 63% and an unusual sagittal plane in over half of patients (14). Marfan patients typically present to the spinal surgeon with one of four problems: scoliosis, kyphosis, spondylolisthesis, or complex revision deformity, usually involving both scoliosis and kyphosis. The scoliosis often presents at a young age, before adolescence, and the risk of infantile scoliosis is higher.

1. Unique Features

There are special challenges in treating spinal deformities in the setting of MFS. Bracing for scoliosis in MFS is successful in only 17% of patients (15). This contrasts with 45–75% success rates reported for selected patients braced for idiopathic scoliosis. It is successful even less often in infantile Marfan curves. About 12% of Marfan individuals eventually develop scoliosis of a degree that requires surgical intervention.

The unique sagittal profile of the Marfan spine—deformity onset at a younger age, and higher operative risks due to aortic dilatation, risk of dissection, anticoagulation for prosthetic cardiac valves, and risk of pulmonary complications—should be taken into account. Altered lumbosacral anatomy in MFS, commonly including thinned posterior elements and dural ectasia, make instrumentation more difficult (16) (Fig. 2). Bone mineral density, often decreased in MFS, may also weaken fixation stability. Finally, connective tissue changes may adversely affect wound healing and ligamentous stability.

Clinical research has shown that patients with MFS have increased blood loss and rates of infection, instrumentation failure, pseudarthrosis, and coronal and sagittal decompensation. We recommend obtaining preoperative MRI on all Marfan patients undergoing deformity surgery in order to look for dural ectasia (Fig. 3) (17). We also recommend preoperative lumbar CT in order to assess the lumbar pedicles and laminae and to assess the sacrum for erosions that may affect fixation.

2. Intraoperative Complications

Blood loss is generally greater in Marfan syndrome than in the general spinal deformity population, although there is considerable variability. Some Marfan patients do not have any greater bleeding than normal, but many others do. It is somewhat hard to sort out how much of this is due to the increasing complexity of their deformities, but it is the author's impression that some of these patients do seem to have decreases in their tissue and vascular clotting ability. Preoperative bleeding tests do not seem able to predict this. This is compounded by the fact that the anesthesiologist may have a harder time maintaining usual degrees of hypotension due to preexisting medical management. Nevertheless, it is worthwhile to have extra blood available in the blood bank and to use the cell saver. The amount of bleeding may also affect the decision as to whether to perform circumferential fusion in one stage or two.

Cerebrospinal leak is often a risk in Marfan syndrome. In one series (18), the incidence was 12%. This increased incidence is caused by the bulging of the dura and as well as its fragility. The bulging is greatest distally below L3. Often the enlarged dural

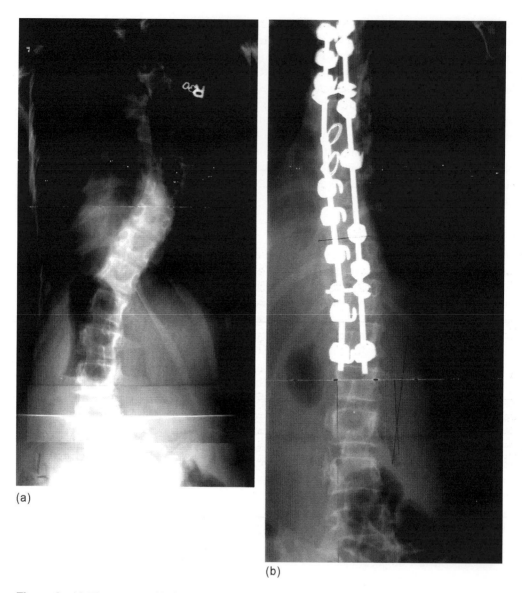

(a)

(b)

Figure 2   (a) Eleven-year-old girl with Marfan syndrome and 66 degree scoliosis. Sagittal plane is nearly straight without junctional kyphosis. (b) Anterior and posterior fusion of major curve to stable L1 vertebra produced satisfactory balance on AP, and lateral radiographs. Within 18 months, the curve had added on in both the coronal (c) and sagittal. (d) Planes. (e,f) Extension of the fusion down to L4 then became necessary.

sleeve will displace epidural fat and present directly under the ligamentum flavum. The prominence can be decreased somewhat by placing the patient in relative Trendelenburg during the deep dissection and instrumentation of the lower lumbar spine. Once visualized, it is evident that the dura is extremely thinned, presenting not the usual bluish-grey opalescence but rather a clear translucence. Dissection inside the canal should be kept to a minimum. If a leak occurs, it is often difficult to suture due to the extreme fragility

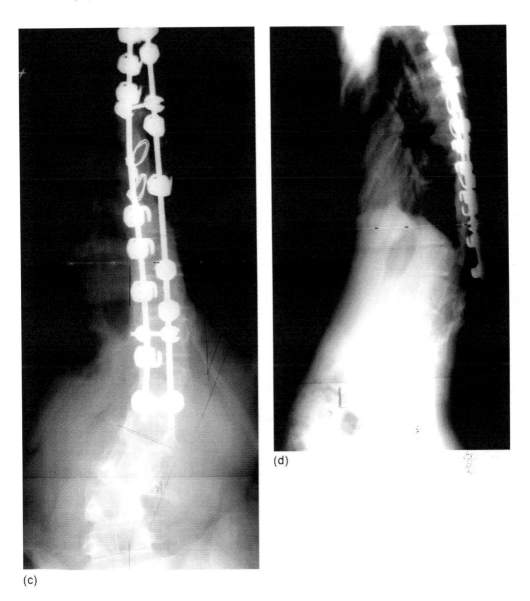

(d)

(c)

Figure 2 (*continued*).

of the dura and can sometimes be handled by increasing the Trendelenburg and using fibrin glue and an occlusive tissue patch in the exposed spinal "window." Postoperatively an increased period of recumbency should be ordered. A proximal cerebrospinal fluid (CSF) drain can be employed in difficult cases.

Obtaining adequate fixation can be difficult intraoperatively. The very thinned pedicles may preclude adequate use of pedicle screws, even in the lower lumbar spine. Sponseller et al. found that pedicle widths were below 5 mm in the majority of pedicles at or above L3, and in 10% even at L5 (16). The lumbar laminae are also somewhat thinner than average. The sacrum may be extremely scalloped, precluding medially directed S1 screws. All of these changes are largely attributed to dural ectasia, although

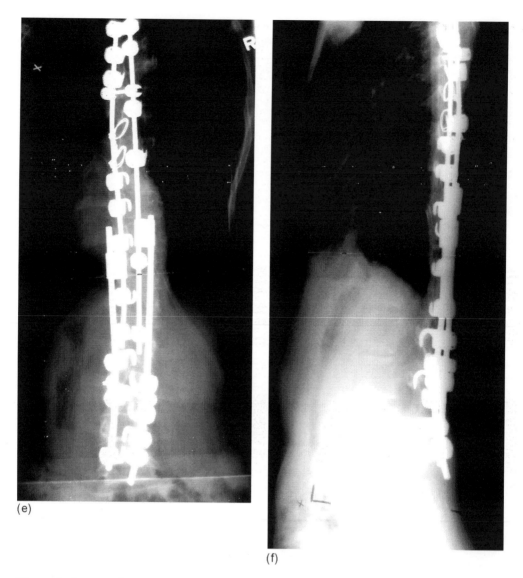

(e)

(f)

Figure 2 (*continued*).

some component of them may be due to the "Marfan morphology." Suggestions for dealing with this problem include the following: a) carefully assess and target the pedicles with fluoroscopy or other imaging systems, staying lateral rather than medial; b) plan multiple points of fixation in cases where critical pedicles do not have adequate size or strength; c) extend the instrumentation distally if needed; d) in the sacropelvis, consider iliac fixation whenever the sacrum seems severely eroded. This is especially relevant in spondylolisthesis surgery.

3. Postoperative Surgical Complications

Deep wound infection occurred in about 12% of patients. Although there was no comparison population of non-MFS patients with the same deformity mix, it seems that the risk

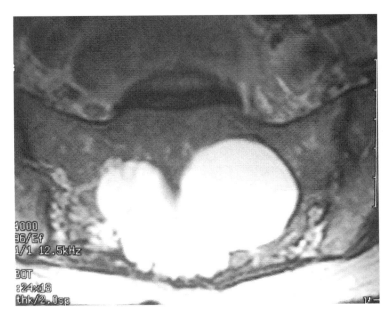

Figure 3 Dural ectasia causing sacral erosions. This may impair fixation and lead to cerebrospinal fluid leak.

of infection is higher in MFS, possibly due to the increased blood loss and surgical time. It may also be an intrinsic factor of the syndrome. Close surveillance and prompt treatment are indicated using standard methods. Postoperative failure of fixation is not uncommon. This was often seen in infantile Marfan syndrome patients treated with the older style of "growing rods" (19). Newer styles of rods, with segmental fixation, seem to have better results. An additional factor causing loss of fixation is the altered sagittal plane anatomy. Instrumentation that controls the coronal plane may end on a level of kyphosis and therefore become dislodged. These factors should be taken into account during preoperative surgical planning.

Curve decompensation or "adding on" is a frequent complicating factor in Marfan syndrome. This was seen in almost one quarter of the patients (18). It is attributable to several factors. First, patients often develop deformities at a young age and growth and crankshaft may play a role. Second, the ligamentous characteristics of the syndrome seem to allow progression of secondary curves and fractional curves, which would not progress in idiopathic deformity. Many clinicians are now recommending that in MFS the surgeon should not attempt extreme degrees of correction and to avoid the concepts of "fuse short" or "save levels" as is more and more often being done in idiopathic scoliosis. Applying idiopathic decision-making rules to Marfan syndrome, the surgeon may often end up reoperating for residual deformity. Pseudarthrosis has also been reported in MFS with increased frequency.

4. Postoperative Medical Problems

Patients with Marfan syndrome often take longer to recover their strength and endurance than do idiopathic patients. They also need to be watched more carefully to avoid cardiovascular stress. If the patient was on a betablocker preoperatively, remember to restart it postoperatively. Tachycardia and elevations of blood pressure should be kept to a minimum in order to avoid further aortic dilatation. It is often advisable to have Marfan patients conjointly followed by an internist, pediatrician, or cardiologist. Valvular incompetence and cardiac failure has been reported in the postoperative period, although fortunately it is not very common. Pneumothorax may occur spontaneously in patients with MFS and hemothorax may develop as well. Superior mesenteric artery syndrome has been reported in MFS and should be considered because these patients often have significant kyphosis that is being corrected and are asthenic to begin with.

5. Conclusions

Marfan patients should be evaluated preoperatively for aortic root dilatation and valvular insufficiency. The anesthesia team should be notified in advance so that they may plan for appropriate staffing and cardiac monitoring.

Pre-operative MRI of the entire spine should be used to evaluate for dural ectasia. CT of any region of the spine where pedicle screws are to be used is indicated to assess the adequacy of pedicles. DEXA to detect osteopenia is useful in some patients.

To prevent curve decompensation, preoperative bending radiographs can help to plan fixation and correction. We recommend avoiding short or selective fusion and limiting correction to 50–60%. Consideration must also be paid to the sagittal profile, which can have an especially caudal transition between kyphosis and lordosis. Fusion should extend to neutral and stable vertebrae in both planes.

The possibility of larger blood loss should be anticipated with Marfan patients. Procedures can be staged to avoid cardiovascular compromise from larger cumulative losses. Anticoagulation for prosthetic valves should be noted and managed appropriately.

Every attempt should be made to limit soft-tissue dissection and increase the number of points of solid fixation in the Marfan spine to minimize wound and hardware complications as well as curve decompensation.

B. Ehlers-Danlos Syndrome

Ehlers-Danlos syndrome (EDS) is caused by a deficiency in collagen in most cases. The most recent classification system is the Berlin nosology, according to which there are nine types of Ehlers-Danlos syndrome. Scoliosis is most common in types I (classic) and VI (ocular-scoliotic). However, spinal deformity does not appear to be as common as it is in Marfan syndrome. Beighton and Horan reviewed 100 patients with EDS and found severe scoliosis in only 6 (20). Spondylolisthesis is also slightly more common in this condition (21). Atlantoaxial instability has been reported in type IV EDS but does not often cause impairment or require intervention (22).

1. Intraoperative Complications

These primarily involve bleeding. McMaster reported five patients with spinal deformity in EDS treated by posterior spinal fusion (23). There is an increased incidence of vascular fragility in this condition, leading to bleeding from small muscular and periosteal vessels during posterior spine fusion. This is usually possible to control using standard methods. Adequate blood replacement, as well as the cell saver, should be available. Use of a drain is advised. McMaster reported wound hematoma in two of five patients (23). Anterior spine fusion should be approached with more caution, especially in type I EDS. The retroperitoneal vessels, especially the veins, are friable and at risk for tear during dissection.

They may be very difficult to repair and may require vascular consultation or ligation. Vogel and Lubicky reported a patient who experienced avulsion of two segmental arteries from the aorta despite careful handling (24). This required repair with a pericardial patch (24). Anterior approaches should only be carried out when deemed essential, and the posterior approach should be used whenever it can effectively be done. During posterior exposure, the presence of thin, possibly ectatic, dura increases the risk of CSF leak, and the surgeon should be aware of this.

Neurological deficits during spinal deformity correction may be more common in EDS. Two patients were reported with paraplegia and one with a partial but permanent neurological injury. The frequency of this complication cannot be assessed because the total number of patients seen during this period was not listed. However, it is likely to be greater than in the general population. Several factors are hypothesized to account for the neurological deficits. The ligamentous laxity may allow for greater distraction or more focal distraction than in non-EDS patients. Vascular fragility may be an additive factor, compromising perfusion to a cord during distraction. In addition, the large focal deformities sometimes seen in this syndrome are undoubtedly risk factors. The presence of focal kyphosis is known to pose an increased neurological risk (Fig. 4). It is recommended that patients with EDS undergo preoperative MRI to look for dural ectasia or focal cord distortion (24). Motor and sensory monitoring of the spinal cord should be done, if possible.

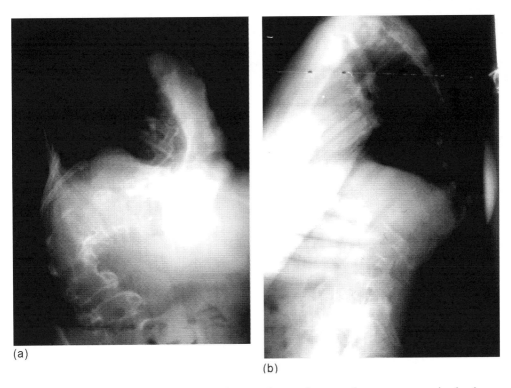

(a)

(b)

Figure 4 Thirteen-year-old male with Ehlers-Danlos syndrome and severe, progressive kyphoscoliosis (a,b). Anterior and posterior fusion was performed, but was complicated by disintegration of the iliac vein, requiring ligation. The patient tolerated this with development of collateral circulation. Note development of postoperative proximal junctional kyphosis (c,d) due to ligamentous laxity.

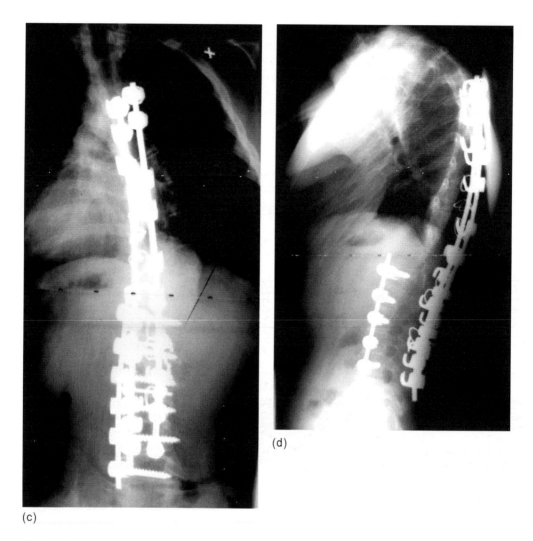

(d)

(c)

Figure 4 (*continued*).

2. Postoperative Complications

In the consecutive series of McMaster, there were no permanent complications (23). Post-operative wound hematomas were seen in 40%, and wound dehiscence was common. These responded to secondary closure. Wound infection and pseudarthrosis were not seen.

C. Stickler Syndrome

Stickler syndrome (hereditary arthro-ophthalmopathy) is an autosomal dominant disorder of collagen types II or XI. It is characterized by ocular abnormalities (retinal degeneration or myopia), craniofacial abnormalities (cleft palate, retrognathia), hearing loss, hip and/or spine abnormalities (25,26). It is about as common as Marfan syndrome. Common spinal abnormalities include vertebral endplate irregularity, disk degeneration, and kyphosis. Severe scoliosis is uncommon. Back pain is almost universal in adults with the syndrome.

The occurrence of Scheuermann-like spinal endplate changes along with epiphyseal changes in the hips should make the surgeon suspect this syndrome.

Data on complications of spine surgery are scarce. However, mitral valve prolapse and retinal detachment are also common in this syndrome. Patients should be screened preoperatively for any cardiac or ophthalmologic problems that may require management. The anesthesiologist may experience difficulty in airway management due to a small jaw or midface hypoplasia.

D. Osteogenesis Imperfecta

Osteogenesis imperfecta (OI) is due to a defect in type I collagen. It is one of the more common genetic disorders presenting to the spine surgeon. Numerous different mutations have been identified, which in part explains the spectrum of severity and manifestations seen in this disorder. In general, problems are more common in nonambulatory patients than in ambulatory ones, and bone quality decreases progressively from patients who have straight diaphyses and normal vertebral contours to those with biconcave vertebrae, to thinning of the diaphyses, to absence of a definite diaphyseal cortex (27). Common spinal problems include basilar invagination, scoliosis, and kyphosis (28). Bracing is not very effective in controlling curves except perhaps in ambulatory patients (27). In patients with lower bone density, it has been reported to cause rib cage distortion (29). Spinal surgery may be effective in slowing declining pulmonary function if due to scoliosis (Fig. 5). It also appears to stabilize or partially reverse neurological deficits due to basilar invagination.

Preoperative assessment should be extensive in order to prevent complications. Patients undergoing spine surgery at any level should have lateral radiographs of the cervical spine in order to rule out basilar invagination if they have not had these in the past. Questions about pulmonary function, such as exercise tolerance and history of pneumonia, should be used to assess need for postoperative ventilatory support. Pulmonary function tests may help quantify this. If there is adequate time (more than 6 months) before surgery, bisphosphonate treatment should be considered in order to prevent failure of fixation. Halo-gravity traction may be helpful in providing gradual correction and decreasing the forces on the instrumentation (30).

1. Intraoperative Complications

Anesthetic preparation is often extensive and time-consuming. Fiberoptic intubation is sometimes called for. Dissection is often difficult since usually the ribs protrude posteriorly on both sides of the spine and render access to these narrow spinal elements difficult. Bleeding tends to be greater than in non-syndromic cases (27). In some cases this may be a factor limiting the performance of same-day anterior and posterior fusion. It is variable, for some patients do not bleed excessively. Fixation problems are the biggest source of intraoperative complications. Segmental fixation, with a hook, wire, or screw at as many levels as possible, can help minimize the risk. Intraoperative traction can help to evenly distribute the corrective forces. The rods used should be malleable so that they have as much "give" as the bone. Large, rigid rods are more likely to cut out of the bone. The surgeon should use discretion in applying corrective forces to the spine. A modest amount of correction that is tolerated by the bone is better than a dramatic degree which then causes implant cut-out. Care should be especially used in correction of kyphosis. This correction involves posterior column shortening, which depends significantly upon the support of the instrumentation. In osteoporotic bone, this will fail sooner or later.

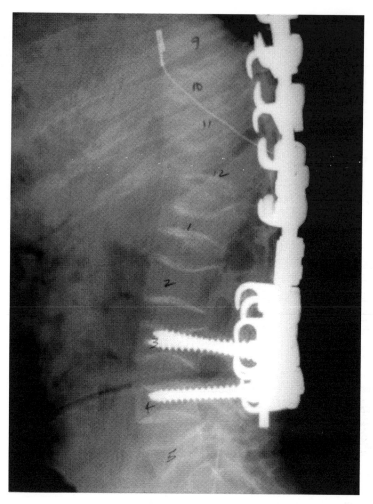

Figure 5   Scoliosis in an 18-year-old with osteogenesis imperfecta was treated surgically. The distal three pairs of hooks cut out within 6 weeks, requiring revision with pedicle screws reinforced with methylmethacrylate.

If the surgeon finds himself or herself "levering" the rod down to meet the spine, that same force will eventually cause a dorsal rod displacement. The use of methylmethacrylate has been advocated both anteriorly and posteriorly when needed to augment fixation (31). Anteriorly, the surgeon may use it to supplement the vertebral body before a through-and-through hole is prepared. Posteriorly, it is useful for pedicle screws but not as practical for hooks.

Anteriorly, if instrumentation is used, structural anterior column support in the disk spaces can minimize the force on the instrumentation. Another intraoperative factor for the patient with osteogenesis imperfecta is that the dura is often thinner than in normal patients. Cerebrospinal leaks may occur. Awareness of this when dissecting around the ligamentum flavum may help minimize problems.

Occasionally there are patients with osteogenesis imperfecta whose spines cannot support any instrumentation. The goal of experienced preoperative selection is to counsel these patients against surgery. However, if such a situation occurs, the use of non-resorbable suture-tapes to act as sublaminar wires along with a thin rod may occasionally salvage some situations. If this is not successful, bone graft with autograft and long allograft struts may permit a fusion to occur after immobilization in a cast.

2. Postoperative Complications

The patient with OI cannot be allowed activity "ad lib" as has become the custom for many idiopathic patients. The surgeon should make this assessment based upon the quality of the fixation. Postoperative bracing for 3–6 months may be needed. Loss of correction is the norm, but will likely stabilize as long as the fixation is maintained. Dislodgement of fixation at the ends of the construct should be repaired if possible by using alternate means of anchorage (i.e., using pedicle screws, methylmethacrylate, or extending the fusion (31). Prolonged pain is common but usually abates as the fusion matures.

REFERENCES

1. Herman MJ, Pizzutillo PD. Cervical spine disorders in children. Orthop Clin North Am 1999; 30(3):457–466, ix.
2. Koop SE, Winter RB, Lonstein JE. The surgical treatment of instability of the upper part of the cervical spine in children and adolescents. J Bone Joint Surg Am 1984; 66(3):403–411.
3. Tandon V, Williamson JB, Cowie RA, Wraith JE. Spinal problems in mucopolysaccharidosis I (Hurler syndrome). J Bone Joint Surg Br 1996; 78(6):938–944.
4. Remes V, Tervahartiala P, Poussa M, Peltonen J. Cervical spine in diastrophic dysplasia: an MRI analysis. J Pediatr Orthop 2000; 20(1):48–53.
5. Remes VM, Marttinen EJ, Poussa MS, Helenius IJ, Peltonen JI. Cervical spine in patients with diastrophic dysplasia—radiographic findings in 122 patients. Pediatr Radiol 2002; 32(9):621–628.
6. Forese LL, Berdon WE, Harcke HT, et al. Severe mid-cervical kyphosis with cord compression in Larsen's syndrome and diastrophic dysplasia: unrelated syndromes with similar radiologic findings and neurosurgical implications. Pediatr Radiol 1995; 25(2):136–139.
7. Herring JA. The spinal disorders in diastrophic dwarfism. J Bone Joint Surg Am 1978; 60(2):177–182.
8. Remes V, Tervahartiala P, Poussa M, Peltonen J. Thoracic and lumbar spine in diastrophic dysplasia: a clinical and magnetic resonance imaging analysis. Spine 2001; 26(2):187–195.
9. Matsuyama Y, Winter RB, Lonstein JE. The spine in diastrophic dysplasia. The surgical arthrodesis of thoracic and lumbar deformities in 21 patients. Spine 1999; 24(22):2325–2331.
10. Kornblum M, Stanitski DF. Spinal manifestations of skeletal dysplasias. Orthop Clin North Am. 1999; 30(3):501–520, x.
11. Bowen JR, Ortega K, Ray S, MacEwen GD. Spinal deformities in Larsen's syndrome. Clin Orthop 1985:(197) 159–163.
12. Johnston CE, 2nd, Birch JG, Daniels JL. Cervical kyphosis in patients who have Larsen syndrome. J Bone Joint Surg Am 1996; 78(4):538–545.
13. Johnston CE, 2nd, Schoenecker PL. Cervical kyphosis in patients who have Larsen syndrome. J Bone Joint Surg Am 1997; 79(10):1590–1591.
14. Sponseller PD, Hobbs W, Riley LH, 3rd, Pyeritz RE. The thoracolumbar spine in Marfan syndrome. J Bone Joint Surg Am 1995; 77(6):867–876.
15. Sponseller PD, Bhimani M, Solacoff D, Dormans JP. Results of brace treatment of scoliosis in Marfan syndrome. Spine 2000; 25(18):2350–2354.

16. Sponseller PD, Ahn NU, Ahn UM, et al. Osseous anatomy of the lumbosacral spine in Marfan syndrome. Spin 2000; 25(21):2797–2802.

17. Ahn NU, Sponseller PD, Ahn UM, et al. Dural ectasia in the Marfan syndrome: MR and CT findings and criteria. Genet Med 2000; 2(3):173–179.

18. Lipton GE, Guille JT, Kumar SJ. Surgical treatment of scoliosis in Marfan syndrome: guidelines for a successful outcome. J Pediatr Orthop 2002; 22(3):302–307.

19. Sponseller PD, Sethi N, Cameron DE, Pyeritz RE. Infantile scoliosis in Marfan syndrome. Spine 1997; 22(5):509–516.

20. Beighton P, Horan F. Orthopaedic aspects of the Ehlers-Danlos syndrome. J Bone Joint Surg Br 1969; 51(3):444–453.

21. Stanitski DF, Nadjarian R, Stanitski CL, Bawle E, Tsipouras P. Orthopaedic manifestations of Ehlers-Danlos syndrome. Clin Orthop 2000; (376):213–221.

22. Halko GJ, Cobb R, Abeles M. Patients with type IV Ehlers-Danlos syndrome may be predisposed to atlantoaxial subluxation. J Rheumatol 1995; 22(11):2152–2155.

23. McMaster MJ. Spinal deformity in Ehlers-Danlos syndrome. Five patients treated by spinal fusion. J Bone Joint Surg Br 1994; 76(5):773–777.

24. Vogel LC, Lubicky JP. Neurologic and vascular complications of scoliosis surgery in patients with Ehlers-Danlos syndrome. A case report. Spine 1996; 21(21):2508–2514.

25. Rose PS, Ahn NU, Levy HP, et al. Thoracolumbar spinal abnormalities in Stickler syndrome. Spine 2001; 26(4):403–409.

26. Letts M, Kabir A, Davidson D. The spinal manifestations of Stickler's syndrome. Spine 1999; 24(12):1260–1264.

27. Hanscom DA WR, Lutter L, LOnstein JE, Bloom BA, Bradford DS. Osteogenesis imperfecta. Radiographic classification, natural history, and treatment of spinal deformities. J Bone Joint Surg 1992; 74-A(4):598–616.

28. Nakamura M, Yone K, Yamaura I, et al. Treatment of craniocervical spine lesion with osteogenesis imperfecta: a case report. Spine. 2002; 27(8):E224–E227.

29. Cristofaro RL, Hoek KJ, Bonnett CA, Brown JC. Operative treatment of spine deformity in osteogenesis imperfecta. Clin Orthop 1979; (139):40–48.

30. Janus GJ, Finidori G, Engelbert RH, Pouliquen M, Pruijs JE. Operative treatment of severe scoliosis in osteogenesis imperfecta: results of 20 patients after halo traction and posterior spondylodesis with instrumentation. Eur Spine J 2000; 9(6):486–491.

31. Benson DR, Newman DC. The spine and surgical treatment in osteogenesis imperfecta. Clin Orthop 1981; (159):147–153.

41

Complications Related to the Surgical Management of Patients with Cerebral Palsy

Peter G. Gabos
Jefferson Medical College, Philadelphia, Pennsylvania and Alfred I. duPont Hospital for Children, Wilmington, Delaware, U.S.A.

Spinal surgery in the child with cerebral palsy is a challenging undertaking. The procedures are technically demanding and require a total awareness of the complications that can occur during and after the surgery to avoid a poor outcome. The patients are frequently medically fragile, often with extensive previous medical and surgical histories. Family and social histories become important, and the surgeon needs to take into account possible postoperative care requirements and the environment to which the patient may be returned after surgery. A multidisciplinary approach is helpful to assure optimization of medical and social parameters prior to surgery, typically involving pediatricians, pulmonologists, gastroenterologists, physical therapists, and social workers when necessary.

This chapter is as much about *avoiding* complications as it is about managing them when they arise. Preoperative considerations and intraoperative and early and late postoperative complications are described in detail, with an emphasis on steps that can be taken to help preclude an untoward event, followed by suggested management considerations should such an event occur. Ultimately, the orthopedic surgeon must recognize whether or not the necessary resources are in place to allow for the safe management of spinal deformity in the child with cerebral palsy. The responsibility that comes with performing a spinal fusion in this patient population extends well past the mere technical exercise.

I. PREOPERATIVE CONSIDERATIONS

A. Nutritional Status

In children with cerebral palsy, significant scoliosis tends to occur in those children with more severe neurological involvement. These patients may have accompanying medical conditions such as malnutrition, gastrointestinal disorders, swallowing and feeding problems, frequent pneumonia, and seizure disorders that put them at higher risk for postoperative complications. Several studies have looked at the impact of nutrition on complication rates, suggesting optimization of these parameters prior to surgery (1–3). Jevsevar and Karlin (2) found that patients with a preoperative serum albumin of less than

35 g/L and a total blood-lymphocyte count of less than 1.5 g/L had a significantly higher rate of infection, a longer period of endotracheal intubation after surgery, and a longer period of hospitalization. Similarly, Mandelbaum and colleagues (3) found a higher rate of postoperative urinary tract infection in their patients using similar laboratory criteria for malnutrition. In a review of 107 patients with cerebral palsy who had undergone a posterior spinal fusion using unit rod instrumentation at the Alfred I. duPont Institute, Lipton and colleagues (4) noted that the level of neurological involvement, severity of scoliosis, and recent history of significant medical problems were the greatest predictors of postoperative complication. The authors could not demonstrate that nutritional status, as measured by serum albumin level and lymphocyte count, was an independent risk factor for postoperative complication.

While we were unable to demonstrate the importance of low serum albumin or lymphocyte counts as a predictor of postoperative complication in our patient population, we do believe that improving the child's nutrition prior to surgery is important. However, there is little evidence to suggest that reaching a certain level of preoperative nutrition has a significant bearing on the postoperative outcome. Surgery for scoliosis need not be delayed or refused because of poor nutritional status, as any small benefit obtained by trying to improve nutritional status may be lost in the face of progression of curvature, especially if the curve is greater than 90 degrees. The surgeon should be prepared, however, for the need for aggressive postoperative nutritional support. I presently place a tunneled subclavian double-lumen venous catheter at the start of the spinal procedure, and intravenous hyperalimentation is commonly instituted by our gastroenterology and nutritional services early in the postoperative course.

B. Pulmonary Status

Chronic respiratory problems are common in children with cerebral palsy due to reactive airway disease secondary to frequent pneumonia, recurrent aspiration, gastroesophageal reflux, and swallowing disorders. Standard tests of pulmonary function are often difficult or impossible to administer in severely involved patients, making assessment of pulmonary status limited. Admission to the hospital 1 or 2 days prior to surgery for bronchopulmonary treatments or intravenous theophylline may be beneficial for patients with chronic reactive airway disease or bronchitis. The surgeon should be alert to the need for aggressive postoperative pulmonary toilet, with appropriate consultation with a pulmonologist or respiratory therapist as needed.

C. Latex Allergy

Latex allergy is an IgE- mediated hypersensitivity reaction thought to develop in response to repeated or chronic exposure to latex (natural rubber). Most of the patients reported have had multiple exposures to latex through previous surgery using latex rubber gloves or repeated catheterizations of the bladder. Latex allergy has been commonly reported in patients with myelomenigocele, but patients with cerebral palsy may be at risk for this life-threatening complications as well, especially if there is a history of placement of a ventriculoperitoneal shunt in infancy or a history of multiple previous operations (5). Reactions to latex may be severe, with an immediate onset of unexplained hypotension, bronchospasm, and oxygen desaturation that may lead to rapid cardiac arrest. A rash, urticaria, or flushing of the skin may occur but be obscured by surgical drapes in the operating room. The surgeon must therefore maintain a high index of suspicion for this complication. In order to prevent latex anaphylaxis, a careful allergic history must be obtained prior to surgery. If the history is suggestive of an allergy to latex, skin testing with a radioallergosorbent test (RAST) should be performed. The surgeon, anesthesiologist, and nursing staff need to be aware of the allergy, and appropriate precautions should be made to prevent patient contact with any latex-containing materials.

D. Shunt Evaluation

While the majority of patients with cerebral palsy do not have a previous history of shunted hydrocephalus, progressive ventricular dilatation secondary to intraventricular hemorrhage (IVH) in premature infants is the most common indication for placement of a ventriculoperitoneal shunt in the neonatal period. Shunt dysfunction has been extensively evaluated in myelomenigocele, demonstrating a decrease in the ultimate tensile strength and extensibility of shunt tubing with time. The majority of structural failures occur by fracture of the shunt within the cervical region, especially in cases where the shunt tube connector was placed in the thoracic or abdominal wall. Sneineh and colleagues (6) described two cases of intraoperative ventriculoperitoneal shunt fracture in the cervical region in children with cerebral palsy in whom a large surgical correction of scoliosis was performed, leading to progressive hydrocephalus and the need for shunt revision in the early postoperative period. A careful radiographic assessment of the structural integrity of the shunt should be made both pre- and postoperatively. If the cervical portion of the shunt is poorly visualized on the pre- or postoperative spinal radiographs, an anteroposterior cervical spine radiograph should be obtained to document shunt integrity in this region (Fig. 1). If the shunt is noted to be disrupted preoperatively, a baseline computed tomography (CT) scan of the head should be performed. Do not assume that a fractured shunt is a sign of arrested hydrocephalus, as these shunts can continue to function through a patent fibrous tract. If the postoperative radiograph documents disruption of the shunt or an increase in the distance between the ends of previously fractured tubing, an immediate CT scan of the head should be performed as a baseline with which to compare subsequent scans, should symptoms of hydrocephalus occur. This complication can be successfully managed by neurosurgical shunt revision.

E. Type of Instrumentation

Instrumentation systems for scoliosis have undergone a substantial evolution over the past several decades, including the use of Harrington instrumentation, the Luque method, Galveston technique for intrapelvic fixation, segmental hook-rod fixation systems, and unit rod instrumentation. A decrease in the rate of pseudarthrosis and instrumentation failure has paralleled the evolution of these newer systems and techniques. Unit rod instrumentation (Jantek, Inc., LaCanada, CA) is popular for correction of scoliosis and pelvic obliquity in patients with cerebral palsy and neuromuscular scoliosis, and the surgical technique has been described in detail (7). If unit rod instrumentation is unavailable to the surgeon, the concepts of a 1/4-inch stainless steel rod linked proximally, appropriately contoured to establish both coronal and sagittal plane alignment, placed down the body of the ilium within 2 cm of the sciatic notch and secured to the spine with segmental fixation, should be adhered to for optimal results.

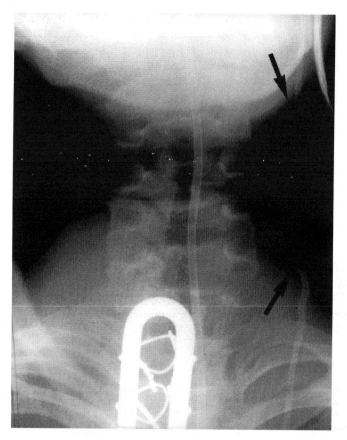

Figure 1 Anteroposterior cervical radiograph obtained immediately after posterior spinal fusion using unit rod instrumentation in a 12 year-old child with spastic quadriplegic pattern cerebral palsy and a history of shunted hydrocephalus. Substantial correction of a severe scoliosis from 80 degrees to 15 degrees was obtained, resulting in a fracture of a previously intact ventriculoperitoneal shunt in the cervical region (arrow). Hydrocephalus resulted, requiring shunt revision.

F. Fusion Levels

It is well recognized that junctional kyphosis is more frequent at the cephalad aspect of the spine when the fusion ends at or below the fourth thoracic vertebrae (8–10). One should consider extending the fusion and instrumentation to the first thoracic vertebrae to avoid this complication, although this can still occur in patients with preoperative kyphosis, osteopenia, and poor head control.

Whether to fuse to the pelvis in a child with cerebral palsy and scoliosis has been a topic of considerable debate. A fusion from T1 to the pelvis should be undertaken in all nonambulatory patients with quadriplegic pattern cerebral palsy with poor sitting balance, truncal decompensation, and fixed pelvic obliquity. A flexible pelvic obliquity left unfused in a quadriplegic child often progresses to a fixed obliquity as the patient matures. Although orthopedic literature has advocated not fusing to the pelvis in children who are ambulatory, many surgeons routinely fuse to the pelvis in ambulatory patients with neuromuscular scoliosis and pelvic obliquity using unit rod instrumentation without loss or deterioration of ambulatory ability. Preliminary data suggest that, on the contrary, ambulation may be improved due to better truncal balance in this select group of patients provided that there is restoration of sagittal balance. However, it is important to fully assess all other aspects of the patient's physical examination. Hip flexion contractures, for example, may subsequently require treatment to avoid a forward flexed gait.

G. Combined Anterior-Posterior Fusion

Anterior surgical release and fusion is indicated in cases of curve rigidity. There is not an absolute curve magnitude that determines the need for anterior release prior to posterior surgery, as even curves greater than 90 degrees may still maintain enough flexibility to allow for adequate correction by posterior surgery alone. The Miller test (7) is often used to determine curve flexibility preoperatively to assess the need for anterior release. When this is equivocal, bending films can be obtained. When anterior surgery is necessary, a standard retroperitoneal approach is used for lumbar curves, a 10th rib thoracoabdominal approach for thoracolumbar curves (or 12th rib extrapleural, retroperitoneal approach in cases in which it is imperative that the diaphragm not be taken down), or thoracotomy for thoracic curves (11). Video-assisted thoracoscopic surgery (VATS) may be limited by pulmonary scarring and adhesions from recurrent pneumonia in this patient population and is therefore not commonly used.

II. INTRAOPERATIVE COMPLICATIONS

A. Intraoperative Instrumentation Problems

When using the Galveston technique or unit rod instrumentation, the pelvic limbs of the rod(s) can perforate the pelvis anteriorly or posteriorly or enter the sciatic notch or acetabulum. Anterior penetration can cause injury to intrapelvic or abdominal viscera either acutely during surgery or postoperatively. Entrance of the limbs into the sciatic notch can cause injury to the sciatic nerve or superior gluteal artery. To help avoid these complications, adequate subperiosteal exposure of the outer wall of the pelvis is critical, and the location of the sciatic notch should be verified by finger palpation. The pelvic guide for the unit rod system is helpful in directing the drill hole into the area of bone approximately 2 cm above the sciatic notch, where the thickness of bone provides the strongest fixation and least chance of rod penetration (12,13). It should be kept in mind, however, that this guide is not rigid or fixed and does not guarantee placement of the drill tract down the ilium. Good spatial orientation, knowledge of anatomy and surgical exposure are the keys to directing this drill hole. A 1/4-inch drill bit on a power drill may be used, premarking the depth of the drill bit with a surgical marking pen to allow for drilling approximately 2 cm past the tip of the sciatic notch guide. In some cases, the guide does not sit favorably in relation to the iliac wing, and in these cases the tunnel can be drilled either freehand with the drill or, if the bone is soft, the tract can be created by hand using a pedicle probe. This can be done with the sciatic notch guide or finger in place within the notch to help direct the tract. The depth of the tract and its walls should be palpated carefully (a ball-tipped pedicle probe is used for this) to ensure that no breech has occurred.

The risk of anterior pelvic penetration when using the unit rod is especially high when there is significant lumbar lordosis present, due to the difficulty in getting the cephalad aspect of the rod anterior enough to direct the pelvic limbs down into the pelvic tracts. In cases where the lordosis is flexible, keeping the hips and knees maximally flexed on the spinal frame will help decrease the lordosis, and, if necessary, an unscrubbed assistant can direct upward pressure at the apex of the lordosis to help with seating of the pelvic limbs. In cases where the lordosis is more significant, one or both limbs can be cut off and placed into the pelvis separately and reconnected to the rod using 1/4-inch rod connectors (Fig. 2). If the lordosis is noted to be rigid, an anterior release should be performed before the posterior procedure. It may also be helpful to consider performing the spinal fusion procedure earlier, for lesser degrees of scoliosis, if a significant or progressive lordosis is noted. Careful attention to the patient's sagittal profile at each outpatient visit should therefore be emphasized.

Even with all of the above considerations, a pelvic breech may still occur. If a bony breech is palpated intraoperatively, after drilling the pelvic tracts, the surgeon has several options. If the breech is distal to the sciatic notch, the pelvic limb of the rod can be cut shorter on that side so that it does not reach the area of pelvic breech. If the breech is

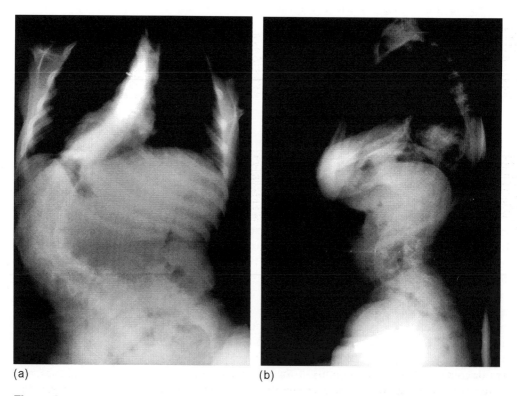

(a)   (b)

Figure 2 Preoperative and postoperative anteroposterior and lateral spine radiographs in an 11 year-old child with spastic quadriplegic pattern cerebral palsy and severe scoliosis and lumbar lordosis. (a) Preoperative sitting anteroposterior radiograph demonstrates a 115-degree scoliosis and marked pelvic obliquity. (b) Preoperative sitting lateral radiograph demonstrates exaggerated lumbar lordosis. (c) Postoperative sitting anteroposterior radiograph demonstrating substantial correction of the scoliosis and pelvic obliquity. Due to the marked lumbar lordosis, one of the limbs of the unit rod was cut-off and each limb was subsequently placed into the ilium separately to help avoid anterior perforation of the limb through the inner wall of the pelvis. The rod was subsequently reconnected using an end-to-end connector (large arrow) and a rod crosslink (small arrow) prior to performing the deformity correction. (d) Postoperative sitting lateral radiograph demonstrates restoration of sagittal balance.

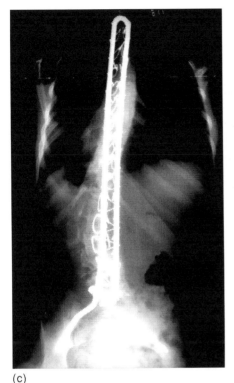
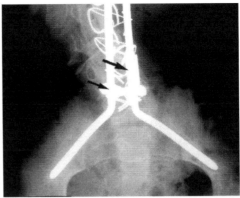

(c)

Figure 2 (*continued*)

proximal to the sciatic notch, cutting the limb at this level may not allow adequate pelvic fixation on that side. In this case the tract should be redirected, either with the drill or by hand, to establish a better trajectory within the bone. It is recommended in this situation to cut the rod and place the pelvic limb by hand to help assure that the limb follows the newly directed tract. The limb can then be reconnected to the rod using a rod connector as described above. If the procedure is being performed on a radiolucent table, fluoroscopic images of the pelvis can be made to confirm limb placement. In some cases the pelvic limb can be felt by direct external palpation anteriorly by an unscrubbed assistant. It is critical to perform adequate plain radiographs at the end of the procedure to evaluate specifically for this complication. A full-length anteroposterior spinal film as well as right and left iliac obliques of the pelvis can be performed while the patient is still under general anesthesia to confirm satisfactory rod placement. Significant rod penetration can be missed on an anteroposterior radiograph of the pelvis. If an anterior rod penetration is noted, the pelvic limb is revised immediately (Fig. 3).

Penetration of the rod through the outer wall of the ilium is usually not of much significance unless the tip of the rod is palpable under the skin. If palpable, skin breakdown or discomfort could result postoperatively. When this occurs, the surgeon has several choices depending on when it is discovered. If a breech of the outer wall is noted prior to placing the rod, the pelvic limb can be shortened accordingly or the tract redirected as described above. If it is noted postoperatively, it would be easier to approach the prominent rod directly over the area of prominence through a separate incision,

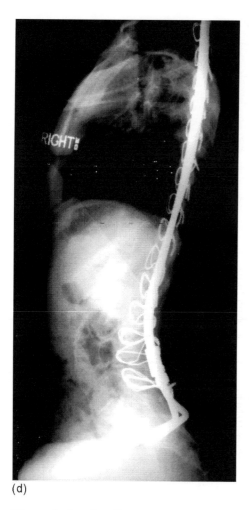

(d)

Figure 2 (*continued*)

shortening the rod using a metal burr (Midas Rex, Fort Worth, TX). This technique has also been described for an intra-articular penetration of a dysplastic hip joint (14).

In rare instances, the child's pelvis may be so dysplastic or thin that the ilium cannot be drilled to accommodate the 1/4-inch rod. In these circumstances, a 3/16-inch rod can be utilized, or the rod can be cut and fixed caudally using iliac or sacral screws.

B. Lamina Fracture or Wire Breakage

Once the pelvic limbs have been impacted into place, the surgeon gains great control over the pelvic obliquity. As the rod is secured to the spine during wire tightening, lamina fracture may occur due to the large corrective forces that occur during the time of rod placement. It is critical that constant pressure be maintained on the rod as the wires are being sequentially tightened from caudad to cephalad. Failure to do so can cause multiple lamina fractures due to cut-out of the wires ("unzippering"). Similarly, a failure of a wire

(a)

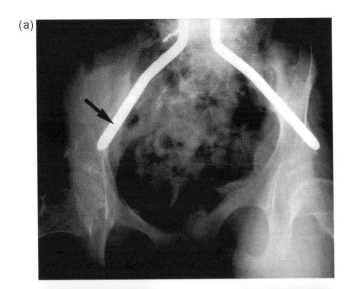

(b)

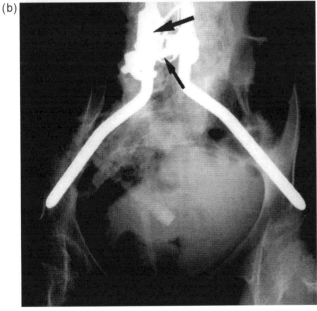

Figure 3 (a) Anteroposterior radiograph of the pelvis obtained immediately after posterior spine fusion using unit rod instrumentation. One of the pelvic limbs has perforated the inner wall of the pelvis (arrow), and was palpable anteriorly. The pelvic limb was immediately revised by loosening the lower sublaminar wires on that side, cutting the rod, redrilling the tract and replacing the limb by hand. (b) Anteroposterior radiograph demonstrating revision of the pelvic limb, with addition of an end-to-end connector (large arrow) and a rod crosslink (small arrow).

itself may occur from fatigue fracture if the wire is overtightened. Removal of a failed wire can cause neurological injury during removal and may require laminectomy. In these instances one would have to place either a pedicle screw or transverse process wire at the fractured level(s), depending on the number and location of the failed wires.

C. Neurological Injury

Neurological complications can occur during any spinal procedure. This risk may be higher when segmental spinal instrumentation using sublaminar wires is employed, although reports of neurological injury specifically in patients with cerebral palsy are sparse. This may be due in part to difficulties in identifying neurological sequelae in children with an underlying severe spastic quadriplegia. The principles recommended to decrease the risk of neurological injury during surgery for scoliosis in general (15) apply no less importantly to children with cerebral palsy, with some differences in how such complications may be managed when they occur.

In the severely involved cerebral palsy patient, the use of a "wake-up test" is not possible due to cognitive or physical impairment. Several recent studies, however, have established the feasibility of performing spinal cord monitoring in patients with neuromuscular scoliosis (16–18). Although the significance of spinal cord injury may be different in ambulatory patients versus nonambulatory patients, the nonambulatory patient with severe spastic quadriplegia may still benefit from protective sensation and, while usually incontinent, is still able to void spontaneously. Somatosensory and motor-evoked potential monitoring can be used for patients undergoing unit rod instrumentation, although in some cases monitoring has been aborted due to failure to obtain useful preoperative baseline signals.

Neurological injury during spinal fusion using segmental wiring has been attributed to multiple factors, including the passage of sublaminar wires, curve correction exceeding that of preoperative bending films, and surgeon inexperience (19). Attempting excessive correction on a rigid curve is best prevented by first performing anterior releases and, when necessary, closing-wedge osteotomies based at the apex of the convexity of the curve. Surgeons treating scoliosis in children with cerebral palsy should be experienced in the passage of sublaminar wires, which has been well described by others (20). Once the wire is passed, it should be pulled up tightly against the laminae by pulling the central loop caudad over the spinous process and the separated ends cephalad onto the laminae, while upward pressure is maintained. The wire ends are then bent outwards over the paraspinal musculature for additional support. This helps to decrease the chance of subsequent plunging of a wire within the canal as the remainder of the procedure is performed. For similar reasons, it is important to maintain an upward pull on the individual wires as they are tightened down onto the rod (Fig. 4).

Spinal cord injury secondary to stretch is uncommon when segmental wire fixation is utilized, as most of the corrective force is translational rather than distractive. In the patient with idiopathic scoliosis, spinal cord injury from corrective forces may be best treated by removal of instrumentation. In the severely involved nonambulatory spastic quadriplegic patient who has a postoperative neurological deficit, the risk of further spinal cord injury during removal of multiple level sublaminar wires and subsequent progression of the scoliosis may not justify removal of the instrumentation. In the ambulatory patient with cerebral palsy in whom the potential loss of ambulatory function by a neurological injury is profound, the course of treatment is best directed by the etiology of the injury. If an injury results from direct cord trauma, such as from the passage of a sublaminar wire, the wire can be removed safely only by laminectomy. It can be replaced by a transverse process wire or pedicle screw, if necessary, although in most cases a single wire is not critical to the integrity of the overall construct, except perhaps at T1. This is more likely to occur in the thoracic and thoracolumbar region because the epidural space is smaller and the spinal cord is more sensitive to direct contusion than is the nerve root. If injury occurs during the

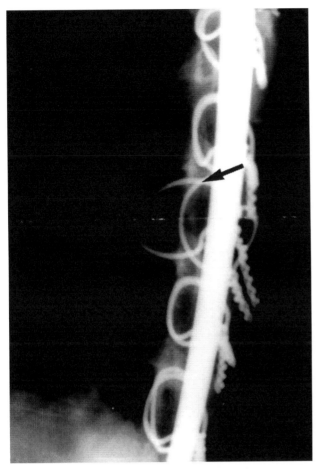

Figure 4 Lateral radiograph of the spine demonstrating a prominent wire loop within the spinal canal (arrow).

corrective portion of the procedure, it may be prudent to decrease some of the corrective force by bending the rod in situ rather than by removing the instrumentation in its entirety.

As in cases of nonneuromuscular scoliosis, monitoring of all intraoperative parameters, such as patient temperature, blood pressure, and hematocrit, is essential to allow maximal perfusion of the spinal cord. A precipitous drop in blood pressure can occur while the rod is being wired in place, as venous filling pressures in the vena cava are diminished by the acute spinal correction. The anesthesiologist needs to be prepared well in advance for this occurrence, maintaining the patient's pressure through the use of intravenous fluids and blood products, if necessary. An intraoperative loading dose of 30 mg/kg methylprednisolone, followed by a maintenance dose of 5.4 mg/kg every hour for 23 hours, is employed when acute spinal cord injury is recognized.

D. Excessive Blood Loss

Blood loss during spinal fusion in children with neuromuscular scoliosis can be excessive, in some cases exceeding more than two times the child's total blood volume. The surgeon and anesthesiologist must be prepared to handle major blood loss should it occur. Patients are usually routinely type and cross–matched for 6 units of packed red blood cells, and an adequate supply of fresh frozen plasma and platelets is routinely available. Cell-saver is utilized intraoperatively. Preoperative hemoglobin and hematocrit, prothrombin time, partial thromboplastin time, platelet count, and bleeding time is routinely measured. Platelet-mediated effects of seizure medications, especially valproic acid, may significantly increase blood loss as well, and thromboelastography, if available, should be considered preoperatively in these patients if a history of significant bleeding or bruising is elicited (21). Consultation with the patient's neurologist should be made to see if substitution of valproic acid by another antiepileptic medication can be made during the month prior to surgery. During the procedure, attention should be paid to maintaining normothermia, which has important implications for maximizing blood clotting capabilities. Patients with cerebral palsy often have abnormal thermoregulation, and a body temperature above 35°C should be maintained during the procedure through the use of adequate room temperature, heating blankets, and warming of intravenous fluids and blood products.

E. Cardiopulmonary Complications

Cardiopulmonary compromise is the most common cause for mortality after scoliosis surgery in cerebral palsy (8,22,23). Patients with a history of pulmonary problems are at especially high risk, and preoperative pulmonary status should be optimized. Consultation with the patient's other health care providers, or through a multidisciplinary medical team familiar with the gravity of the procedure and the medical complications that may occur postoperatively, is of paramount importance.

Intraoperative cardiopulmonary arrest may result from pulmonary compromise, hypovolemia, hypothermia, or air embolism. Pneumothorax or hemothorax, status asthmaticus, latex anaphylaxis, and disseminated intravascular coagulopathy (DIC) are complications that the surgeon and anesthesiologist must be prepared to handle should they occur.

III. POSTOPERATIVE COMPLICATIONS

A. Gastrointestinal Complications

Postoperative ileus is a frequent complication of spinal surgery and is common in children with cerebral palsy after a spinal fusion procedure. The preoperative spine films may suggest large amounts of stool in the lower colon and rectum, which can be further evaluated with plain radiographs of the abdomen. In children with a history of bowel difficulties, a preoperative bowel preparation may be helpful in preventing a prolonged postoperative ileus. In children with a history of feeding or swallowing difficulties, one should consider obtaining a preoperative swallowing evaluation (video flouroscopy and/or barium swallow) to look for possible silent aspiration. This may be especially important in the child who has poor head control or in the child who is to undergo surgery for a severe kyphoscoliosis who may have an underlying extension contracture of the neck musculature.

Postoperatively, the child is maintained on nasogastric suction, and oral intake is withheld until bowel sounds are auscultated. If a prolonged ileus occurs, nasogastric suction is continued and intravenous hyperalimentation is instituted. The surgeon must also maintain a high index of suspicion for mesenteric artery syndrome, particularly in the child who is malnourished. This complication may be managed successfully with nasogastric suction and intravenous hyperalimentation or jejunal feeding in most cases, although some patients may rarely require duodenojejunostomy or division of the ligament of Treitz. Acute pancreatitis has been observed in approximately 17% of patients with cerebral palsy undergoing posterior spinal fusion with instrumentation and may be secondary to intraoperative splanchnic hypoperfusion and activation of cytokines. Pancreatitis can lead to significant morbidity, and deaths from this complication have been reported. Serum amylase and lipase levels are routinely monitored, and a CT scan of the abdomen to look for a pancreatic pseudocyst requiring surgical drainage is necessary in cases where prolonged vomiting and feeding difficulties occur. As in mesenteric artery syndrome, nasogastric decompression and hyperalimentation or jejunal feeds are utilized in management. Gastroesophageal reflux or aspiration may also be exacerbated in some patients postoperatively. Appropriate medical management through the use of H2-receptor antagonists is usually successful in dealing with reflux. In some cases the child may refuse oral intake after surgery well after bowel function has returned. In these cases, consideration of nasogastric or gastrostomy tube placement should be made. The family may be somewhat reluctant to proceed with this ("he/she ate just fine *before* surgery..."), but the surgeon needs to stress the importance of proper nutrition for wound healing.

B. Genitourinary Complications

Urinary tract infections are not uncommon after spine surgery in cerebral palsy and should be treated with appropriate antibiotics when recognized. Urine output may decrease postoperatively due to the combined effects of hypovolemia and the syndrome of inappropriate antidiuretic hormone secretion (SIADH). The clinical hallmarks of SIADH include hyponatremia, hypo-osmolality, and an increase in urinary sodium secretion. Particular attention should be made to establish adequate fluid balance postoperatively, maintaining urine output at 0.5 mL/kg/h.

C. Pulmonary Complications

Early postoperative pulmonary complications may include atelectasis, bronchopneumonia, pleural effusion, and aspiration pneumonia. The patient is often left intubated for approximately 24 hours postoperatively and managed in the intensive care unit during this time to allow adequate control of respiratory parameters. After extubation, the patient is mobilized whenever possible to decrease postoperative atelectasis. Nonambulatory patients are moved out of bed to a reclining wheelchair several times each day. Aggressive postoperative pulmonary toilet is important and includes the use of chest physiotherapy and nebulizer treatments. Bronchopneumonia is treated by appropriate antibiotics after obtaining blood and sputum cultures. Aspiration pneumonia may occur as well, especially in cases where a preexisting swallowing disorder is present. Broad-spectrum antibiotics are utilized, and swallowing studies may be indicated. In some circumstances, bronchoscopy may be necessary to remove large mucous pugs, and large pleural effusions may require needle aspiration.

Deep venous thrombosis and pulmonary embolism are rare events after spine fusion in the child with cerebral palsy. I do not utilize prophylactic anticoagulants because of this rarity, but do pay particular attention to mobilization of the patient postoperatively. When a significant deep venous thrombosis is documented, however, anticoagulation therapy is indicated.

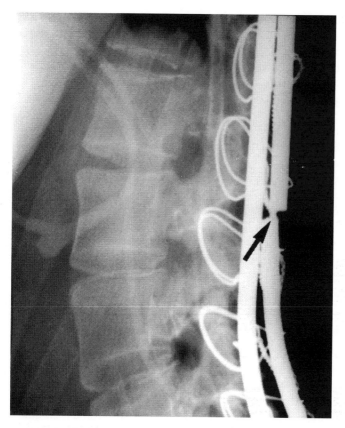

Figure 5 Lateral radiograph of the spine demonstrating breakage of a unit rod secondary to pseudarthrosis noted approximately two years after posterior spinal fusion in a 15 year-old male with cerebral palsy.

D. Infection

The incidence of postoperative wound infection after spinal fusion in children with cerebral palsy is higher than that seen in idiopathic scoliosis (23,24). The incidence of deep wound infection is higher in longer procedures, those with greater blood loss, and in those cases where prophylactic antibiotics are not utilized. As mentioned earlier, optimizing nutritional status may also be a significant factor in decreasing postoperative infection rates, particularly postoperative urinary tract infections.

Careful attention must be paid to performing a "water–tight" closure of the skin at surgery. Many of the patients are incontinent of urine and feces, and soiling, especially of the inferior third of the spinal incision, may occur postoperatively. Closure of the wound should not be delegated to an inexperienced member of the housestaff and should be closely supervised. Postoperatively, if the sterile dressing is left intact for several days, it must be checked frequently for soiling. Body temperatures must be monitored with each nursing shift. The incision must be checked frequently for signs of redness, swelling, or drainage, especially in the noncommunicative patient. Superficial infections may be managed with intravenous antibiotics, although a high index of suspicion for a deep infection must be maintained. If there is any doubt as to the depth of the infection or if

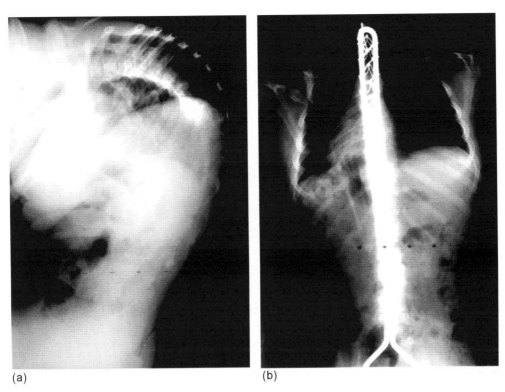

(a)   (b)

Figure 6 (a) Preoperative sitting lateral spine radiograph demonstrating a 100-degree kyphosing scoliosis in an 11 year-old child with spastic quadriplegic pattern cerebral palsy, osteopenia and poor head control. (b) Postoperative anteroposterior sitting spine radiograph demonstrates substantial correction of the scoliosis after spine fusion using unit rod instrumentation from T1 to the pelvis. The length of the rod appears adequate. (c) Postoperative lateral sitting spine radiograph demonstrates significant restoration of sagittal balance, however, there is proximal rod prominence secondary to proximal kyphosis and dissociation between the spine and the top of the rod. (d) Close-up of the proximal aspect of the rod. No further deformity occurred, and the prominent portion of the rod was removed after solid fusion was achieved.

fevers are associated with a palpable fluid collection, an aspiration of the wound may be considered using strict sterile technique, and any collected fluid should be sent for immediate Gram stain and culture. In cases where deep wound infection is confirmed, the patient is taken to the operating room for incision and drainage, opening the entire length of the incision down to the instrumentation and bone graft. Intraoperative tissue and fluid cultures for aerobic, anaerobic, and fungal organisms are again obtained, and all purulent and necrotic tissue is debrided. The wound is washed with sterile saline and antibiotic solution utilizing pressure irrigation. The instrumentation is not removed acutely, as doing so may be associated with a higher rate of pseudarthrosis. If the wound appears clean, it may be closed over suction drains. If the infection is extensive and the wound does not appear to be clean, it is packed with sterile gauze and covered, with repeated irrigation and debridement procedures performed every 1–2 days until the tissue appears healthy. Cultures are taken with each debridement, and if the wound appears clean and tissue cultures are negative, consideration is given to delayed primary wound closure. In some cases the wound is packed open and allowed to heal by secondary

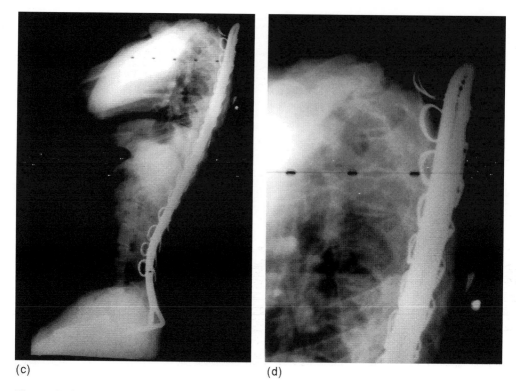

(c)   (d)

Figure 6 (*continued*)

intention. This may take up to 3 months to occur, although use of a vacuum-assisted closure device can help accelerate healing by approximately 2 months. Broad-spectrum antibiotics are initially utilized and then changed based on results of culture and antibiotic sensitivities. Parenteral antibiotics are continued until the infection appears to be under control, after which the patient is placed on oral antibiotics for the remainder of treatment.

If a chronic infection results, wound care is continued until a solid fusion is obtained. The instrumentation may then be removed. Late infection is similarly treated with removal of instrumentation after solid fusion has been obtained.

IV. LATE POSTOPERATIVE COMPLICATIONS

A. Pseudarthrosis

The use of segmental spinal instrumentation and pelvic fixation has greatly reduced the incidence of pseudarthrosis after spinal fusion in children with cerebral palsy. Meticulous attention to fusion technique is critical to success and cannot be overemphasized. To avoid excessive blood loss, the facet joints are extirpated and the transverse processes are decorticated following passage of the sublaminar wires (this sequence helps decrease overall blood loss and allows wire placement in a relatively bloodless field). Bone graft is then applied prior to rod placement. When fusing to the pelvis using unit rod instrumentation, posterior iliac crest autograft must be carefully harvested due to the need

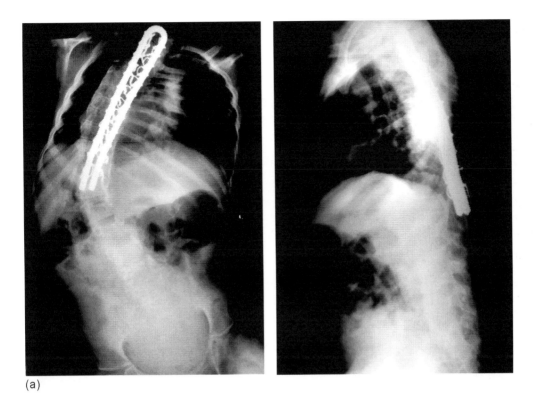

(a)

Figure 7 Thirteen year-old child with spastic quadriplegic pattern cerebral palsy who underwent a previous posterior spinal fusion at the age of 6 years from T1-T12, for an 80 degree scoliosis associated with a flexible pelvic obliquity. (a) Anteroposterior and lateral sitting spine films demonstrating progression of scoliotic deformity and fixed pelvic obliquity caudal to the previous fusion. (b) Anteroposterior and lateral sitting spine films obtained after revision surgery, consisting of anterior spinal release, wedge resection osteotomies and fusion, followed by same-day posterior fusion using unit rod instrumentation. Note the addition of two end-to-end rod connectors (large arrows) in addition to two crosslinks (small arrows).

for an intact ilium. A strategy to avoid the need for iliac crest autograft involves the use of corticocancellous allograft mixed with locally obtained spinal autograft and thrombin. This can be placed directly down onto the spine, so that the graft comes to lie underneath the rod. After placement of the rod, a large amount of additional corticocancellous allograft is then added.

Pseudarthrosis may present as back pain, instrumentation failure, or loss of correction (Fig. 5). Imaging studies, including plain radiographs, bone scan, or tomograms, may be helpful in establishing the diagnosis, but in some cases exploration of the fusion mass may be necessary.

When the diagnosis of pseudarthrosis is established, treatment is dictated by its clinical presentation. In the asymptomatic patient, observation may be warranted as long as no increase in deformity occurs. Symptomatic patients without instrumentation failure or increasing deformity can be managed by repeat bone grafting of the pseudarthrosis site. If a fracture of the rod has occurred at the site of pseudarthrosis, an end-to-end or parallel rod connector can be added to reconnect the rods after grafting. Any increase in deformity

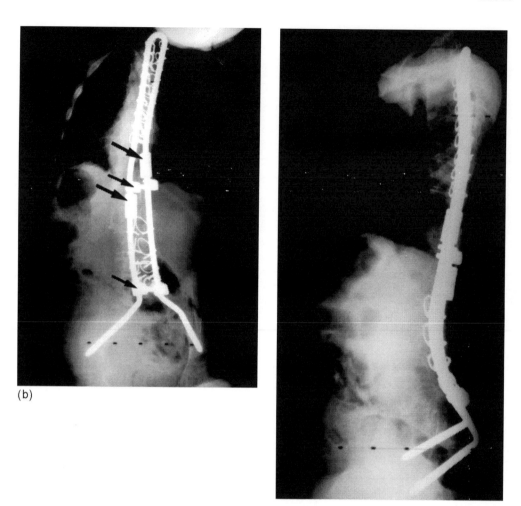

Figure 7 (*continued*)

will require surgical correction and may require addition of anterior osteotomies and fusion with or without instrumentation, posterior osteotomies, and revision or augmentation of posterior instrumentation. Compression across the pseudarthrosis aids in establishing fusion (25).

B. Instrumentation Failure or Prominence

Instrumentation failure in the form of rod breakage typically indicates the presence of a pseudarthrosis and should be managed as described above. Unit rod and Luque rod instrumentation failures have been more frequent with the use of a 3/16-inch rod rather than the 1/4-inch rod (8,9). Rod migration may occur in unlinked Luque rods. If this occurs with an increase in deformity, revision surgery would be indicated.

Prominence of a wire or of the top of the rod may be managed with removal of the prominent portion of the wire or rod. When using unit rod instrumentation, the cut rods will require the addition of crosslinks to prevent rod migration if the top portion of the rod is removed prior to achieving a solid fusion.

C. Extension of Deformity Cephalad or Caudad to the Fusion Level

Extension of deformity cephalad to the fusion is typically associated with failure to extend the fusion up to T1 or T2 (8,9,10), but may also be seen in patient's with preoperative kyphosis, osteopenia, or poor head control (Fig. 6). This is typically associated with prominence of the top of the rod(s). If a unit rod has been previously placed and the length was too short proximally, the top of the rod can be removed using a metal burr (Midas Rex, Fort Worth, TX) and the fusion can be extended with passage of sublaminar wires up to T1. Junctional kyphosis may require the addition of posterior osteotomies. The top portion of a unit rod or linked Luque rod can then be connected to the previous construct using side-to-side or parallel rod connectors.

Extension of deformity caudad to the fusion is typically associated with worsening of the scoliosis and pelvic obliquity. A previously flexible pelvic obliquity thought not to require fusion to the sacrum may become rigid as the child matures. This may present with a dislocated or significantly subluxated hip. In these cases, the pelvic obliquity should be corrected first, followed by hip reconstruction after the spinal fusion is solid. Pelvic obliquity and increasing scoliosis in these cases typically require extensive surgery, including anterior release and osteotomy, followed by posterior osteotomy, fusion, and revision of previously placed instrumentation (Fig. 7). The technique has been described in detail utilizing either Luque instrumentation (26) or unit rod instrumentation (25).

D. Crankshaft Phenomenon

Posterior spinal fusion performed in young, skeletally immature children may be associated with a phenomenon known as "crankshaft," a term used to describe a progressive three-dimensional loss of scoliosis correction due to continuation of anterior spinal growth associated with posterior spinal fusion (27). Crankshaft phenomenon has been associated with performing a posterior spinal fusion in patients with idiopathic scoliosis and an open triradiate cartilage before or during the onset of peak height (growth) velocity (28,29). Loss of spinal correction has been demonstrated in some young patients with cerebral palsy after posterior spinal fusion using Luque instrumentation (30). The crankshaft effect has not, however, been demonstrated in several recent large series of scoliosis in children with cerebral palsy treated with posterior spinal fusion using unit rod instrumentation, including those patients with the presence of an open triradiate cartilage (7,31,32). Based on these studies it seems likely that the addition of an anterior spinal fusion is not necessary to prevent crankshaft phenomenon in young patients with cerebral palsy when posterior spinal fusion using unit rod instrumentation is performed.

E. Residual Sagittal Plane Deformity

Attention to correction of sagittal plane spinal deformity is as important as the correction of the scoliosis in both ambulatory and nonambulatory patients with cerebral palsy. Utilization of a precontoured unit rod should allow for adequate restoration of sagittal balance in most instances. In the ambulatory patient, an anterior or posterior shift of the weight-bearing axis occurs when there is excessive lumbar kyphosis or lordosis, respectively. Failure to restore sagittal balance, especially when fusion is extended to the pelvis, can result in loss of ambulatory ability. In the sitting patient with cerebral palsy, a loss of lumbar lordosis causes a posterior shift of the weight-bearing axis from the posterior thighs to the ischial tuberosity and sacrum. This can result in ischial pressure ulcerations. Revision surgery to restore adequate sagittal balance may be required if deterioration of ambulatory function or decubitus ulcers occurs and may require anterior and posterior osteotomies with revision of instrumentation as described above.

REFERENCES

1. Drvaric DM, Roberts JM, Burke SW, King AG, Falterman K. Gastroesophageal evaluation in totally involved cerebral palsy patients. J Pediatr Orthop 1987; 7:187–190.
2. Jevsevar DS, Karlin LI. The relationship between preoperative nutritional status and complications after an operation for scoliosis in patients who have cerebral palsy. J Bone Joint Surg 1993; 75-A:880–884.
3. Mandelbaum BR, Tolo VT, McAfee PC, Burest P. Nutritional deficiency after staged anterior and posterior spinal reconstructive surgery. Clin Orthop 1988; 234:5–11.
4. Lipton GE, Miller F, Dabney KW, Altiok H, Bachrach SJ. Factors predicting postoperative complications following spinal fusions in children with cerebral palsy. J Pediatr Orthop 1999; 12:197–205.
5. Dormans JP, Templeton JJ, Edmonds C, Davidson RS, Drummond DS. Intraoperative anaphylaxis due to exposure to latex (natural rubber) in children. J Bone Joint Surg 1994; 76-A:1688–1691.
6. Sneineh KA, Lipton GE, Gabos PG, Miller F. Dysfunction of ventriculoperitoneal shunt after posterior spine fusion in children with cerebral palsy: an unusual complication. A report of two cases. J Bone Joint Surg 2003; 85-A:119–124.
7. Dias RC, Miller F, Dabney K, Lipton G, Temple T. Surgical correction of spinal deformity using a unit rod in children with cerebral palsy. J Pediatr Orthop 1996; 16:734–740.
8. Broom MJ, Banta JV, Renshaw TS. Spinal fusion augmented by Luque-rod instrumentation for neuromuscular scoliosis. J Bone Joint Surg 1989; 71-A:32–44.
9. Gersoff WK, Renshaw TS. The treatment of scoliosis in cerebral palsy by posterior spine fusion with Luque-rod segmental instrumentation. J Bone Joint Surg 1988; 70-A:41–44.
10. Stanitski CL, Micheli LJ, Hall JE, Rosenthal RK. Surgical correction of spinal deformity in cerebral palsy. Spine 1982; 7:563–569.
11. Watkins RG. Surgical Approaches to the Spine. New York: Springer-Verlag, 1983.
12. Bell DF, Moseley CF, Koreska J. Unit rod segmental spinal instrumentation in the management of patients with progressive neuromuscular spinal deformity. Spine 1989; 14:1301–1307.
13. Miller F, Moseley C, Koreska J. Pelvic anatomy relative to lumbosacral instrumentation. J Spinal Disord 1990; 3:169–173.
14. Givon U, Miller F. Shortening of a unit rod protruding into the hip joint: case report and description of a surgical technique. J Pediatr Orthop 1999; 12:74–76.
15. Mooney JF, Bernstein R, Hennrikus WL, MacEwen GD. Neurologic risk management in scoliosis surgery. J Pediatr Orthop 2002; 22:683–689.
16. Ecker ML, Dormans JP, Schwartz DM, Drummond DS, Bulman WA. Efficacy of spinal cord monitoring in scoliosis surgery in patients with cerebral palsy. J Spinal Disord 1996; 9:159–164.
17. Noordeen MHH, Lee J, Gibbons CER, Taylor BA, Bentley G. Spinal cord monitoring in operations for neuromuscular scoliosis. J Bone Joint Surg 1997; 79-B:53–57.
18. Padberg AM, Russo MH, Lenke LG, Bridwell KH, Komanetsky RM. Validity and reliability of spinal cord monitoring in neuromuscular spinal deformity surgery. J Spinal Disord 1996; 9:150–158.

19. Wilbur RG, Thompson GH, Shaffer JW, Brown RH, Nash CL. Postoperative neurologic deficits in segmental spinal instrumentation. A study using spinal cord monitoring. J Bone Joint Surg 1984; 66-A:1178–1187.

20. Zindrick MR, Knight GW, Bunch WH, Miller MC, Butler DM, Lorenz M, Behal R. Factors influencing the penetration of wires into the neural canal during segmental wiring. J Bone Joint Surg 1989; 71-A:742–750.

21. Chambers HG, Weinstein CH, Mubarak SJ, Wenger DR, Silva PD. The effect of valproic acid on blood loss in patients with cerebral palsy. J Pediatr Orthop 1999; 19:792–795.

22. Gau YL, Lonstein JE, Winter RB, Koop S, Denis F. Luque-Galveston procedure for correction and stabilization of neuromuscular scoliosis and pelvic obliquity: a review of 68 patients. J Spinal Disord 1991; 14:399–410.

23. Lonstein JE, Akbarnia BA. Operative treatment of spinal deformities in patients with cerebral palsy or mental retardation. J Bone Joint Surg 1983; 65-A:43–55.

24. Transfeldt EE, Lonstein SE, Winter RB, Bradford D, Moe J, Mayfield J. Wound infections in reconstructive spinal surgery. Orthop Trans 1985; 9:128–129.

25. Dias RC, Miller F, Dabney K, Lipton GE. Revision spine surgery in children with cerebral palsy. J Spinal Disord 1997; 10:132–144.

26. Ferguson RL, Allen BL Jr. The technique of scoliosis revision surgery utilizing L-rod instrumentation. J Pediatr Orthop 1983; 3:563–571.

27. Dubousset J, Herring JA, Shufflebarger H. The crankshaft phenomenon. J Pediatr Orthop 1989; 9:541–550.

28. Sanders JO, Herring JA, Browne RH. Posterior arthrodesis and instrumentation in the immature (Risser grade 0) spine in idiopathic scoliosis. J Bone Joint Surg 1995; 77:39–45.

29. Sanders JO, Little DG, Richards BS. Prediction of the crankshaft phenomenon by peak height velocity. Spine 1997; 22:1352–1357.

30. Sussman MD, Little D, Alley RM, McCoig JA. Posterior instrumentation and fusion of the thoracolumbar spine for treatment of neuromuscular scoliosis.

31. Bulman WA, Dormans JP, Ecker ML, Drummond DS. Posterior spinal fusion for scoliosis in patients with cerebral palsy: a comparison of Luque rod and unit rod instrumentation. J Pediatr Orthop 1996; 16:314–323.

32. Smucker JD, Miller F. Crankshaft effect after posterior spinal fusion and unit rod instrumentation in children with cerebral palsy. J Pediatr Orthop 2001; 21:108–112.

42
Complications Related to the Surgical Management of Patients with Myelomeningocele

Denise T. Ibrahim and John F. Sarwark
Northwestern University Feinberg School of Medicine and Children's Memorial Hospital, Chicago, Illinois, U.S.A.

I. INTRODUCTION

The surgical management of spinal deformities in children with myelomeningocele is a challenge for the surgeon due to the unique pathological features of the spinal deformity. Myelomeningocele patients experience an increased number of complications when compared to patients with idiopathic scoliosis. Occurence of complications such as deep wound infections, pseudarthrosis, skin ulcers, hardware failure, and urinary tract infection has been reported to range from 7.5% to as high as 61% of operative cases (1–3). Some of the features that separate these patients from others include dysraphic malformations of the posterior spinal elements, upper spinal cord anomalies leading to hydrocephalus, paralysis with asymmetry, and earlier onset of spinal deformities (4). These features must all be taken in consideration when treating spinal deformities in myelomeningocele patients. The overall complication rates in the past decade have decreased due to more stable implant constructs, multi-staged surgery in one anesthetic session, and multispecialty care.

The incidence of spinal deformity in myelomeningocele patients is approximately 69% and increases as the patient reaches adulthood. Piggott reported that 82.5% of patients will have scoliosis and 17.5% kyphosis by age 10 (5). Of thoracic-level myelodysplastic patients, nearly 100% will develop scoliosis, whereas when the neurological deficit occurs more caudally, the incidence of scoliosis decreases (6). The National Center for Health Statistics and U.S. Centers for Disease Control (CDC) reported a significant decrease in the overall rate of spina bifida in the past few years. The rate in 2000 was 20.85 per 100,000 live births as compared to 27.98 per 100,000 live births reported in 1995 (7). The decreased rate has not been fully explained. It can be postulated that public awareness of the importance of prenatal folic acid supplementation has contributed to the decline as has antenatal diagnosis of spinal cord defects with improved ultrasonography and pregnancy termination. The latter is not included in the CDC's statistical analysis.

The goals of surgical treatment of spine deformity myelomeningocele patients are to prevent progression of the spinal deformity, improve spinal stability and posture, improve respiratory function, and prevent or cure skin pressure ulcers (8). In addition, improved mobility, transfer ability, activities of daily living, urogenital care, and prevention of back pain are secondary gains (9). The key to preventing complications is understanding the special requirements of a patient with myelomeningocele with respect to timing of surgery, preoperative assessment of comorbidities, intraoperative precautions, and post-operative care. Taking into account published experiences from other surgeons should help the surgeon understand and prevent pitfalls. This chapter will review reported complications involving surgical treatment of scoliosis and kyphosis in myelomeningocele patients as well as discuss special issues that need to be addressed when considering spine surgery. The following information is divided into preoperative, intraoperative, and postoperative complications and avoidance.

II. PREOPERATIVE CONSIDERATIONS

Preoperative complications may occur if the patient has not had a full multidisiplinary team approach to his or her medical care and in assessing whether or not the patient is a candidate for surgery as well as the appropriate time for surgery.

A. Timing of Surgery

The progression of spinal deformity in myelomeningocele patients is greater at an earlier age than in nonmyelopathic patients. In the literature, progression rates have ranged from 2.5 to 6.2 degrees per year in myelomeningocele patients (10). It has been the experience of many surgeons that the earlier the surgery, the fewer the complications. Determining the appropriate age for surgery can be difficult; most corrective spinal deformity surgery is performed at an average of 12 years and 8 months (3). The selection for fusion is one of the most important preoperative planning choices. Dubousett et al. reported almost 100% progression of spinal curvature with isolated posterior fusion when performed before adolescence (11).

B. Fetal Surgery, Perinatal Surgery

The topic of appropriate timing of surgery would not be complete without discussing experimental fetal surgery of myelomeningocele. In utero closure of myelomeningocele has been recommended to prevent damage to the spinal cord secondary to amniotic fluid exposure through the spinal defect (12,13). It has been suggested that in utero treatment decreases the requirement of ventricular shunting for hydrocephalus, presumably because earlier closure provides a more normal spinal fluid circulatory pattern (14). Complications of in utero repair include induction of early labor, preterm delivery, infection, and death related to prematurity, as well as maternal morbidity, dermoid inclusion cysts, and spinal cord tethering (15). The risks and benefits of in utero surgery compared to surgery after birth are yet to be determined. In utero surgery is still in its investigational stages, and factors regarding appropriate gestational timing for the surgery versus no in utero surgery, as well as improvements in techniques to avoid the above-stated complications, are all subjects for future clinical investigation.

C. Tethered Cord Identification

When surgery of the spinal deformity is to be considered, the neurosurgery team should participate by evaluating the status of shunt functioning and the status of the spinal cord. A tethered cord may alter the timing of the surgery by requiring surgical untethering prior to spinal deformity correction. Pain, progressive spinal deformity, increasing spasticity, and decreasing motor function are indications for operative release of the tethered cord (13). Reigel et al. reported that the progression of scoliosis in lumbar and sacral levels plateaued or declined following the release of the tethered cord, but the release did not halt the progression of scoliosis in the thoracic level patients (16). They also believe that tethered cord release can decrease the incidence and magnitude of kyphosis (16). Having the appropriate information on spinal cord dynamics may help prevent perioperative traction complications on the tethered cord that otherwise should have been released prior to the corrective spinal curvature surgery. There is no clear evidence on whether traction of the tethered cord causes other neurological complications.

D. Shunt Malfunction

Approximately 90% of myelomeningocele patients have hydrocephalus requiring shunting (17). It is extremely important that the patient's shunt is functioning at full capacity to avoid malfunctions, including acute secondary hydrocephalus (18). Postoperative death has been reported due to an acute hydrocephalus from malfunctioning shunts (3).

E. Pulmonary Function

Altered pulmonary function of children with myelomeningocele is associated with complications at the time of surgery. Surgery is often performed to improve pulmonary function. Carstens et al. reported that 8 of 10 patients with preoperative restrictive pulmonary function improved their vital capacity and 6 patients had an increased forced expiratory volume after undergoing surgery, which included thoracotomies and diaphragm divisions (19). Banta and Park reported increases in peak flow postoperatively, thus improving their thoracic mechanics and enhancing greater endurance (20). Many surgeons, however, have reported an increased frequency of pulmonary complications due to the pulmonary dysfunction, comprising approximately 52–83% of total complications (21,22). Thorough preoperative pulmonary testing and evaluation will decrease the risk of this type of postoperative complication. Pulmonary complications include atelectasis, pleural effusion, delayed extubation, pneumonia, and acute respiratory distress syndrome (ARDS). Grossfeld et al. reported that a vital capacity of $< 40\%$ of the predicted value is a risk factor for a pulmonary complication (22).

F. Nutritional Assessment

The nutritional status of a myelomeningocele patient is included in the preoperative assessment of the patient. Maintenance of appropriate nutrition preoperatively and postoperatively decreases the risk of infection and promotes wound healing, thus lessening postoperative complications (23). Jevsevar and Karlin found that patients with preoperative albumin levels of $< 3.5\,g/dL$ and total lymphocyte count of $< 1500 \times 10^6/L$ had significantly higher infection rates, longer periods of postoperative mechanical ventilation, and longer periods of hospitalization (24).

G. Prophylactic Antibiotics, Urosepsis

The risk of infection is increased in children with myelomeningocele. The prevention of wound infections and sepsis may be anticipated preoperatively, intraoperatively, and postoperatively. The posterior skin region of the meningocele closure is scarred, poorly vascularized, and often insensate, posing an increased risk for skin flap problems and infection in the postoperative period (25). The high rate of recurrent urinary tract bacterial contamination places these patients at increased risk for infections. Perioperative antibiotics, including those directed at gram-negative organisms, is part of the preoperative routine to help avoid infections.

H. Latex Allergies

Myelomeningocele patients are now managed as having latex allergy. Eighteen to 40% of myelomeningocele patients develop latex sensitivity (26). Life-threatening anaphylaxis due to latex exposure has been of increasing concern. Myelomeningocele patients are exposed to latex derivatives early in life as a result of closure of the myelomeningocele and undergo continuous urinary catheterization, all contributing to their increased sensitivity (27). Prevention of complications comes from a careful history of reactions to balloons, catheters, gloves, and other latex products. If a history is suggestive of latex allergy, a radioallergosorbent (RAST) test is recommended (25).

I. Informed Consent

In addition to preparing the patients for surgery medically, the family is informed and educated as to the expected outcomes associated with spine surgery. Potential operative complications include impairment of current motor ability. Muller et al. (28) evaluated 14 myelomeningocele patients undergoing spinal surgery and found that 50% of the children developed increased flexion contractures, 13 had impaired motor ability, and 57% lost some ambulation capacity. Mazur et al. (9) also reported increased difficulty of ambulation following spinal correction and fusion. It is the surgeons' responsibility to communicate the risks and benefits clearly to the family.

III. INTRAOPERATIVE CONSIDERATIONS

Postoperative complications may be a result of an intraoperative adverse event. Proper preoperative planning concerning the technique and method of spinal deformity correction is paramount.

Stabilization of the spine, whether for scoliosis or kyphosis, has both short- and long-term goals. The earlier the correction is performed, the more manageable the curve. Lindseth stated that the correction goal in the coronal plane is usually limited to about 60 degrees in scoliosis and normal sagittal balance in kyphotic curves (4). Spinal deformities tend to be more rigid in younger patients with this problem than in idiopathic scoliosis patients. Myelomeningocele patients have higher complication rates of pseudarthrosis, loss of deformity correction, skin ulceration, and infection compared to other patients. A myelomeningocele patient's loss of posterior elements affects the adequacy of the instrumentation fixation, especially when pelvic obliquity correction is necessary. The approach to the deformity and instrumentation chosen will affect the incidence of pseudarthrosis, hardware failure, and loss of correction. The types of complications occurring in surgery for scoliosis and kyphosis are similar, but the rates may differ.

A. Pseudarthrosis

The rate of pseudarthrosis is reported to range from 14% to as high as 76% in scoliosis (3,29,30). When pseudarthrosis occurs, it often leads to loss of spinal fixation. Mazur et al. reported a 20% incidence of hardware failure, a 33% pseudarthrosis rate, and a 13% loss of normal lordosis with posterior Harrington rod alone, whereas combined Dwyer and posterior Harrington fusion decreased the loss of lordosis to 4%, the pseudarthrosis rate to 11%, and hardware failure to 9% (9). Osebold et al. lowered the pseudarthrosis rate by adding an anterior fusion (31). In general, it is currently accepted that an anterior and posterior fusion with instrumentation produces the best outcomes (30,32,33) in select cases (34). The necessity of an additional anterior approach with instrumentation remains controversial. Ward et al. (2) found that the addition of anterior instrumentation did not alter patient outcome, whereas, Geiger et al. (3) found that adding instrumentation anteriorly reduced their hardware-related complication. The inclusion of the pelvis in the fusion construct is also associated with a myriad of complications due to poor bone quality, ischial ulceration from altering sitting pressure points, the potential for loss of lordosis, and pseudarthrosis at this junction (35). Wild et al. reported that pelvic obliquity often spontaneously corrected when the scoliotic deformity was fused with inclusion of the sacrum (36).

B. Instrumentation Failure

Forms of instrumentation failure include rod breakage, hook disengagement, and pedicle screw migration. Loss of deformity correction has been associated with too short fusions with progressive compensatory curves and the performance of a stand-alone posterior or anterior fusion. The loss of correction may lead to breakage of instrumentation and increased pseudarthrosis rates. Mazur et al. reported that a fractured rod, cable, or hook displacement is often indicative of a pseudarthrosis (9). Pseudarthrosis can also cause loss of correction, affecting instrumentation failure rates. Banit et al. reported a sacral fixation complication of rod migration into the acetabulum with loss of iliac bolt fixation, requiring reoperation (8).

C. Allograft

Achieving a successful fusion of the corrected and instrumented spine commonly requires adjunctive bone graft extenders. Myelomeningocele patients may not have sufficient autogenous bone as a result of poor pelvic bone stock. Allograft is an acceptable graft material in this patient population. Sponseller et al. identified allograft, however, as being a possible significant risk factor for infection (37). The use of freeze-dried allograft in another study did not result in the occurrence of transmissible disease but was associated with a 5% superficial infection rate and no deep infections (38).

D. Infection

Infections in myelomeningocele patients undergoing spine surgery are not rare. Spinal infections may arise from urosepsis or be secondary to complications related to skin breakdown due to prominent hardware, poor skin quality, or insensate skin. Seromas often develop over the lumbo-sacral region and may become infected. The greater the exposure required for fusion and the more levels involved, the greater the incidence of postoperative infection. A straight-line posterior incision has a lower incidence of infection compared to a triradiate incision (25). Infections are more often polymicrobial and are often caused by gram-negative organisms as well as *Staphylococcus aureus* (37). It is imperative that meticulous preoperative evaluation of the skin and bladder be performed and preoperative antibiotics administered. Deep infections require aggressive surgical debridement and occasionally instrumentation removal. This may also contribute to the pseudarthrosis and loss of spinal correction. Osebold et al. reported an increased infection rate to 36% from 19% in patients whose dura was entered (31).

E. Decubitus Ulcers

Myelomeningocele patients have a constant threat of decubitus ulcers due to their more sedentary lifestyle and insensate skin. Prominent posterior instrumentation may produce ulceration of the skin, emphasizing the need for low-profile hardware. Also, fusion involving the lumbosacral junction may alter lordosis enough to increase the risk of sacral decubiti. Postoperative bracing may also contribute to skin pressure wounds. Hopf and Eysel reported that multisegmental anterior and posterior fusion procedures with segmental instrumentation allow for postoperative care without the need for external support (39).

F. Fractures

Bracing and casting may be required postoperatively. Immobilization may contribute to osteoporosis (25) in myelomeningocele patients. Long bone fractures have been reported to increase postoperatively. Osteopenic fractures may occur in the more severely involved and less mobile children. They are associated with prolonged immobilization. It is advised that lengthy periods of immobilization be avoided if possible (40). Early immobilization using a bivalved polypropylene body jacket minimizes osteoporosis, pressure sores, and social isolation (31).

G. Anesthesia

Anesthesiologists need to understand the complexity of medical problems that exist in myelomeningocele patients to provide safe anesthesia. Abnormalities in the control of ventilation are common in infants and children with myelomeningocele. At highest risk are those with lesions at L3 or above, severe brain stem abnormalities, abnormal pulmonary function tests, and airway patency disorders (34). A tidal volume of 5 mL/kg, appropriate arterial blood gases, and intact protective airway reflexes will help prevent premature extubation (34).

Inadequate intraoperative fluid management in the setting of increased blood loss may be underestimated resulting in postoperative tachycardia (3). Serial hematocrit levels will assist in transfusion requirements (34).

H. Complications Uniquely Associated with Kyphosis

In general, late or delayed surgical reconstruction has been associated with significant morbidity and mortality (18). Unrelenting kyphosis progression of approximately

8 degrees a year is seen in most patients with myelomeningocele with a tendency to develop this deformity, and therefore in these patients the preferred age of surgery is approximately 2–5 years (18). Preservation of growth is preferred in an attempt to preserve as much truncal height as possible (41). Intraoperative distal cord resection may be required with precautions not to ligate the cord/dural sac since it may alter the intraventricular pressure. This may occlude the central canal of the cord, which remains open in patients with hydrocephalus and may lead to acute hydrocephalus and death (31,42).

The amount of resection and spine shortening should be considered carefully. Spine shortening may lead to long-term respiratory complications (43). Perioperative respiratory distress syndrome resulting in death during kyphosis corrective surgery has been reported (44). The posterior transpedicular decancellation procedure with an instrumentation system extending to the lumbosacral junction as described by Nolden et al. has shown promising early results with decreased morbidity when compared to excisional techniques (41).

Anatomical variations of the aorta have been studied due to its perceived hazardous position in patients with kyphosis and myelomeningocele. Loder et al. reported their personal communications of complete obliteration of aortic blood flow after kyphectomy, which resulted in one death. Loder et al. (45) recommended a thorough preoperative evaluation of vascular anatomy in all patients with congenital kyphosis and myelomeningocele to access for abnormal aortic shortening with variability of branch anatomy, especially as it bridges the lumbar kyphosis. This was recommended in cases of extensive kyphosis resection, if a vascularized rib graft is considered, in the setting of previous abdominal surgery, or if major spinal distraction is anticipated (45).

Kyphosis correction has also been associated with apophyseolysis of the fourth and fifth lumbar disk space following a fusion from T8 to L4 for a 92 degree kyphosis (46). This complication required reoperation in which the fusion was later extended to the sacrum.

REFERENCES

1. Luque ER. Paralytic scoliosis in growing children. Clin. Orthop Relat Res 1982; 163: 202–209.
2. Ward WT, Wenger DR, Roach JW. Surgical correction of myelomeningocele scoliosis: a critical appraisal of various instrumentation systems. J Pediat Orthop 1989; 9:262–268.
3. Geiger F, Parsch D, Carstens C. Complications of scoliosis surgery in children with myelomeningocele. Eur Spine J 1999; 8:22–26.
4. Lindseth RE. Myelomeningocele spine. In: Weinstein SL, ed. The Pediatric Spine. 2nd. Philadelphia: Lippincott, 2001:845.
5. Piggott H. The natural history of scoliosis in myelodysplasia. J Bone Joint Surg 1980; 62B(1):54–58.
6. Mackel JL, Lindseth RE. Scoliosis in myelodysplasia. J Bone Joint Surg 1975; 57-A:1031.
7. National Vital Statistics System. Hyattsville, MD: NCHS, Centers for Disease Control, 2002.
8. Banit DM, Iwinski HJ, Talwalkar V, Johnson M. Posterior spinal fusion in paralytic scoliosis and myelomeningocele. J Pediatr Orthop 2001; 21:117–125.
9. Mazur J, Menelaus MB, Dickens DRV, Doig WG. Efficacy of surgical management for scoliosis in myelomeningocele: correction of deformity and alteration of functional status. J Pediatr Orthop 1986; 6:568–575.
10. Eysel P, Hopf C, Schwarz M, Voth D. Development of scoliosis in myelomeningocele. Neurosurg Rev 1993; 16(4):301–306.

11. Dubousett J, Herring JA, Shufflebarger H. The crankshaft phenomenon. J Pediatr Orthop 1989; 9:541–550.

12. Adzick NS, Sutton LN, Crombleholme TM, Flake AW. Successful fetal surgery for spina bifida. Lancet 1998; 352:1675–1676.

13. Tulipan NB, Bruner JP. Myelomeningocele repair in utero: a report of three cases. Pediatr Neurosurg 1998; 28:177–180.

14. Bruner JP, Tulipan NB, Paschall RL, Boehm FH, Walsh WF, Silva SR, Hernanz-Schulman M, Lowe LH, Reed GW. Fetal surgery for myelomeningocele and the incidence of shunt-dependent hydrocephalus. J Am Med Assoc 1999; 282:1819–1825.

15. Mazzola CA, Albright AL, Sutton LN, et al. Dermoid inclusion cysts and early spinal cord tethering after fetal surgery for myelomeningocele. N Eng J Med 2002; 347(4):256–259.

16. Reigel DH, Tschernoukha K, Bazmi B, Kortyria R, Rotenstein D. Change in spinal curvature following release of tethered spinal cord associated with spina bifida. Pediatr Neurosurg 1994; 20(1):30–42.

17. Beatty JH, Canale T, Banta JV, Lubicky JP. Current concepts review: orthopaedics aspects of myelomeningocele. J Bone Joint Surg 1990:626–630.

18. Sarwark JF. Kyphosis deformity in myelomeningocele. Orthop Clin Am 1999; 30(3): 451–455.

19. Carstens C, Paul K, Niethard FU, Pfeil J. Effect of scoliosis surgery on pulmonary function in patients with myelomeningocele. J Pediatr Orthop 1991; 11(4):459–464.

20. Banta JV, Park SM. Improvement in pulmonary function in patients having combined anterior and posterior spine fusion for myelomeningocele scoliosis. Spine 1983; 8(7):765–770.

21. Sarwahi V, Sarwark JF, Schafer MF, Backer C, Lee M, Aminian A, Grayhack J. Standards in anterior spine surgery in pediatric patients with neuromuscular scoliosis. J Pediatr Orthop 2001; 21:756–760.

22. Grossfeld S, Winter RB, Lonstein JE, Denis F, Leonard A, Johnson L. Complications of anterior spinal surgery in children. J Pediatr Orthop 1997; 17:89–95.

23. Mooney JF. Perioperative enteric nutritional supplementation in pediatric patients with neuromuscular scoliosis. J South Orthop Assoc 2000; 9(3):202–206, Fall.

24. Jevsevar DS, Karlin LI. The relationship between preoperative nutritional status and complications after an operation for scoliosis in patients who have cerebral palsy. J Bone Joint Surg Am 1993; 75:880–884.

25. Hensinger RN, Sidhu KS. Complication of spine surgery in children. Epps CH, Bowen JR, eds. Complications in Pediatric Orthopaedic Surgery. Philadelphia: JB Lippincott, 1995:91–124.

26. Banta JV, Bonanni C. Prebluda J. Latex anaphylaxis during spinal surgery in children with myelomeningocele. Dev Med Child Neurol 1993; 53:543–548.

27. Drennan JC. Current concepts in myelomeningocele. American Academy of Orthopaedic Surgeons Instructional Course Lecture 1999; 48:543–550.

28. Muller EB, Nordwall A, von Wendt L. Influence of surgical treatment of scoliosis in children with spina bifida on ambulation and motoric skills. Acta Paediatr 1992; 81(2):173–176.

29. Stella G, Ascani E, Cervellati S, Bettini N, Scarsi M, Vicini M, Magillo P, Carbone M. Surgical treatment of scoliosis associated with myelomeningocele. Eur J Pediatr Surg 1998; 8(suppl 1):22–25.

30. Banta JV. Combined anterior and posterior fusion for spinal deformity in myelomeningocele. Spine 1990; 15:946–952.

31. Osebold WR, Mayfield JK, Winter RB, Moe JH. Surgical treatment of the paralytic scoliosis associated with myelomeningocele. J Bone Joint Surg 1982; 64A(6):841–856.

32. Banta JV, Drummond DS, Ferguson RL. The treatment of neuromuscular scoliosis. American Academy of Orthopaedic Surgeons Instructional Course Lectures 1999; 48:551–562.

33. McMaster MJ. Anterior and posterior instrumentation and fusion of thoracolumbar scoliosis due to myelomeningocele. J Bone Joint Surg 1987; 69B:20–25.

34. Sarwark JF, Lubicky JP, Keyes M. Caring for the Child with Spina Bifida. Rosemont, IL: American Academy of Orthopaedic Surgeons, 2001: Chapter 43, 483.

35. Miladi LT, Ghanem IB, Draoui MM, Zeller RD, Dubousset JF. Iliosacral screw fixation for pelvic obliquity in neuromuscular scoliosis. A long-term study. Spine 1997; 22(15):1722–1729.

36. Wild A, Holger H, Kumar M, Krauspe R. Is sacral instrumentation mandatory to address pelvic obliquity in thoracolumbar scoliosis due to myelomeningocele? Spine 2001; 26(14):325–329.

37. Sponsellar PD, LaPorte DM, Hungerford MW, et al. Deep wound infections after neuromuscular scoliosis surgery: a multicenter study of risk factors and treatment outcomes. Spine 2000; 25(19):2461–2466.

38. Yazici M, Asher MA. Freeze-dried allograft for posterior fusion in patients with neuromuscular spinal deformities. Spine 1997; 22(13):1467–1471.

39. Hopf CG, Eysel P. One-stage versus two-stage spinal fusion in neuromuscular scoliosis. J Pediatr Orthop B 2000; 9(4):234–243.

40. Drummond DS, Moreau M, Cruess RL. Post-operative neuropathic fractures in patients with myelomeningocele. Dev Med Child Neurol Apr. 1981; 23(2):147–150.

41. Nolden MT, Sarwark JF, Vora A, Grayhack JJ. A kyphectomy with reduced perioperative morbidity for myelomeningocele kyphosis. Spine 2002; 27(16):1807–1813.

42. Winston K, Hall J, Johnson D, Micheli L. Acute elevation of intracranial pressure following transection of non-functional spinal cord. Clini Orthop Rel Res 1977; 128:41–44.

43. Lindseth RE, Stelzer L Jr. Vertebral excision for kyphosis in children with myelomeningocele. J Bone Joint Surg 1979; 61A:699–704.

44. Lintner SA, Lindseth RE. Kyphotic deformity in patients who have a myelomeningocele. J Bone Joint Surg 1994; 76-A(9):1301–1307.

45. Loder RT, Shapiro P, Towbin R, Aronson DD. Aortic anatomy in children with myelomeningocele and congenital lumbar kyphosis. J Pediatr Surg 1991; 11:31–35.

46. Bohm H, ElSaghir H. Apophyseolysis of the fourth lumbar vertebrae: an early postoperative complication following kyphectomy in myelomeningocele. Eur Spine J 2000; 9:586–587.

43

Postsurgical Sagittal and Coronal Plane Decompensation in Deformity Surgery

Kirkham B. Wood
St. Croix Orthopaedics, Stillwater, Minnesota, U.S.A.

In the spine with deformity, the vertebral column normally compensates above or below so as to maintain overall balance with the head positioned over the sacrum and pelvis. Decompensation, or spinal imbalance, is a complication after the surgical treatment of spinal deformities and represents a postsurgical loss of this ability to compensate. In the coronal plane, decompensation is most commonly associated with the surgical treatment of scoliosis, while decompensation in the sagittal plane may be seen with either scoliosis or kyphosis surgery. In general, postoperative decompression represents the iatrogenic failure to appreciate or fully understand normal alignment and compensatory mechanisms of the spine being treated.

This chapter will examine some of the causes of postsurgical decompensation in both the coronal and sagittal planes following deformity surgery in the adolescent.

I. SCOLIOSIS

A. Decompensation

Decompensation of spinal balance, wherein the postoperative C7 plumb line fails to fall in the midline of the sacrum or is made to lie further off balance, has become a significant issue in the past two decades with the introduction of powerful third-generation instrumentation systems, the first and most notable of which was that of Cotrel and Dubousset (1). Besides derotation, many other factors are associated with decompensation including incorrect choice of fusion levels (2–4), overcorrection of the thoracic curve (5–7), incorrect identification of curve patterns (5,8), progression of the lumbar curve after selective thoracic fusion (5,9), excessive lumbosacral fractional curve stiffness (10,11), and crankshafting or adding on.

Selecting proper fusion levels is critically important in maintaining coronal plane balance after surgery. Harrington originally emphasized the need to end the fusion distally at a vertebral level that was centered over the sacrum (12), so as to create a stable foundation. King et al. (13) later repeated this in his work, identifying this "stable" vertebra, centered over the midsacrum as the appropriate base to end the fusion. Other authors made similar recommendations: Moe (14,15) recommended ending the fusion at the neutrally rotated vertebra, while Goldstein (16) felt it should extend one level further. Either way, ending the fusion at a stable foundation was critical even early on.

While selecting the proper fusion end level was and remains important, early on it was also deemed important to assess the flexibility of the unoperated lumbar spine and its ability to "compensate" (or adjust itself so as to maintain overall spinal balance) once the cephalad thoracic curve was corrected. Side bending radiographs became important to distinguish a structural, less flexible (typically thoracic) primary curve from the more flexible lumbar compensatory curves. Misidentifying curve patterns was dramatically evident with these curves: they must be distinguished from a true double major curve with a truly structural lumbar curve, both of which required fusion.

When the rigid, double rod multihook systems were introduced in the 1980s, both greater curve correction and improved sagittal contour were seen compared with Harrington instrumentation (17). The King Type II or "false double major" curve became the classic curve pattern, requiring careful analysis wherein the rigid thoracic curve was balanced inferiorly by a similarly sized lumbar curve yet with varying flexibility—truly a compensatory curve. Issues with decompensation began to arise in greater numbers especially for those treating King Type II or false double major curves (Fig. 1). Thompson et al. (7), using computed tomography (CT) scans, studied adolescents who had undergone

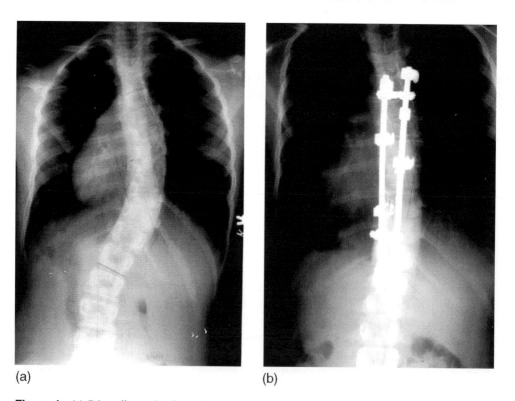

(a)   (b)

Figure 1   (a) PA radiograph of a right thoracic curve measuring 45 degrees with L3 as the stable vertebra. (b) Post-operative radiograph whereby instrumentation ended at T12. (c) Nine months post-operatively, there is imbalance of the trunk to the right with a recurrence of the Cobb angle measurement of the scoliosis. (d) By 18 months post-operatively the corrected curve now measures 56 degrees with severe decompensation to the right.

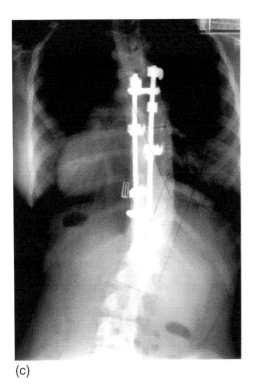

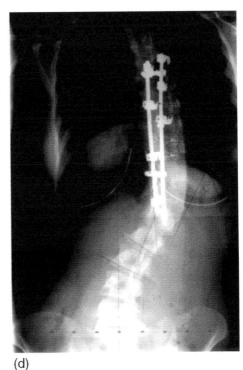

(c)   (d)

Figure 1 *(continued)*

posterior fusions with the new systems and noted that the derotation maneuver was capable of transmitting tremendous torque to the lumbar spine and that if that lower segment was unable to compensate, the result was decompensation. Extending the thoracic instrumentation distally and including the transitional segments between the curve areas, which would normally counterrotate to keep the spine balanced, was felt to be the source of the decompensation. Clinically, Richards et al. (18) reviewed their experience using the C-D derotation system and found that in Type II curves, those fused to or just below the stable vertebra were significantly out of balance to the left when compared with those fused short of the stable vertebra.

Eventually, as scoliosis surgeons have gained experience with these rigid segmental systems and C-D derotation maneuver came to be replaced with more translation, the incidence of postoperative coronal plane decompensation has decreased somewhat, but nonetheless remains a constant concern. Muschik et al. (19) compared postoperative spinal balance between two groups—one treated with a derotation maneuver and the other with translation and segmental correction—and found that those treated with a translation maneuver had much higher rates of postoperative balance than those treated with derotation, none of whom improved their balance (Fig. 2).

Another source of decompensation that has presented with the use of powerful modern instrumentation systems is that of overcorrection of the thoracic curve (5,7,20–23). Overcorrection of a thoracic curve above a relatively stiff lumbar curve can leave the spine badly decompensated to the left. Following correction of the primary curve, the lumbar spine must be able to compensate for whatever correction has been obtained in order to avoid unbalanced curves, or decompensation will result. In other words, the correction obtained within the thoracic spine must be tempered by the ability of the lumbar spine to self-correct as well (11,24).

Failing to understand a lumbar curve's natural history, i.e., its potential for worsening, can also lead to postoperative decompensation (21). Lenke et al. (5) evaluated their experience with C-D instrumentation and suggested that if the ratio of either the lumbar curve magnitude or the deviation of the apical lumbar vertebra compared to that of the apical thoracic spine was >1, then both curves should be fused; if <1, then careful selective posterior thoracic fusion and instrumentation is possible. Mason and Carango (25) similarly wrote that if the lumbar curve apex is more than 2 cm from the center sacral line, inclusion of the lumbar curve is necessary, otherwise the spine will be imbalanced to the left postoperatively.

Another aspect of the lumbar curve's ability to correct itself rests in the fractional lumbosacral hemicurve from L4 to the sacrum (10,11). Richards (11) reviewed 24 patients

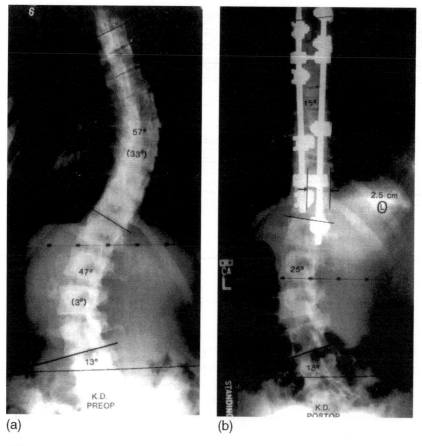

(a)   (b)

Figure 2 (a) PA radiograph of a 13 year old female with a King II Lenke 1C scoliosis. Note the 13 degree tilt of both L4 and L5 relative to the inter-crestal line. (b) Post-operative radiograph with correction of the high thoracic curvature to 15 degrees (side-bend correction to 33 degrees). The inability of the lumbar curve to compensate is in part due to the obliquity of L4 plus the over-correction of the thoracic curve. This has left the spine imbalanced to the left. (c) At 12 months postoperatively the decompensation has worsened with 38 degrees of left lumbar structural curvature.

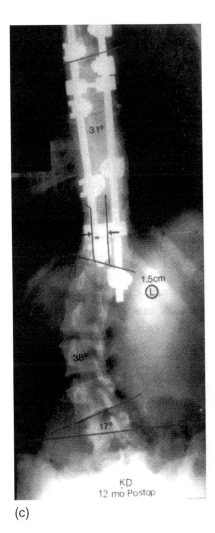

(c)

Figure 2 (*continued*)

with King II curves treated with selective thoracic fusion with either C-D or TSRH instrumentation, all with lumbar curves greater than 40°. The obliquity of L4 to the sacrum averaged 14° preoperatively and was essentially unchanged immediately postoperatively. Despite the lumbar curve's inherently greater flexibility, the thoracic curve correction was 61%, while the spontaneous lumbar correction was only 41%. The combination of a tilted L4 plus a large residual lumbar curve led to shifting of the trunk to the left in all cases. The lumbar curve's inability to correct could be found in this rigid inflexible lower lumbosacral hemicurve. In other words, even preoperative flexibility of the lumbar spine might not insure a balanced spine postoperatively.

Schwender (10) reviewed 50 similar patients with large lumbar curves and found that 80% were decompensated preoperatively to the left; postoperatively, this figure remained at 60% (Fig. 2). As was Richards' experience, all lumbosacral hemicurves remained unchanged by surgery. Their feelings were that because 90% of the individuals had some degree of sacral tilting, the spinal column must be assessed preoperatively, including right lumbar side bending films to check the capacity of the lumbosacral hemicurve to reverse itself with correction surgically. In the setting of a rigid, lumbosacral hemicurve, thoracic correction must again be carefully controlled so as to allow the remaining flexibility in the lumbar spine to maintain balance.

When decompensation does occur, two principal treatment options exist: (a) in the event that significant growth remains, orthotic containment can sometimes control and even correct the lumbar curve, bringing the spine into better balance; (b) if sufficient growth does not remain, the only real alternative is to extend the instrumentation and fusion down into the mid or lower lumbar spine, to a stable foundation, which unfortunately leaves fewer mobile segments below the fusion (26) (Fig. 3). Arlet et al. (27) described a novel approach in two patients who were postoperatively imbalanced to the left following selective thoracic fusion with a large lumbar curve. Removing one or more of the apical hooks allowed the spine to rebalance and level the shoulders and center the head more over the midline (Fig. 4).

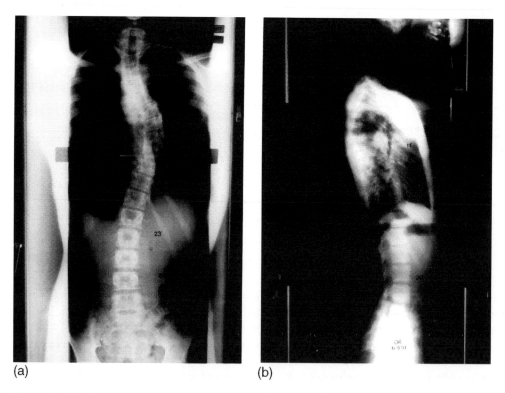

(a)   (b)

Figure 3 (a) PA and (b) lateral radiograph of a right thoracic curvature in a 16 year old boy. Note L1 would be considered the stable vertebra. (c) Postoperative PA radiograph detailing the instrumentation ending at T10 three levels short of the stable vertebra. (d) One year postoperatively there is a severe decompensation of the trunk to the right and recurrence of the coronal plane deformity. (e) PA and (f) lateral radiograph illustrating extension of the fusion down to L2 in order to regain coronal plane balance.

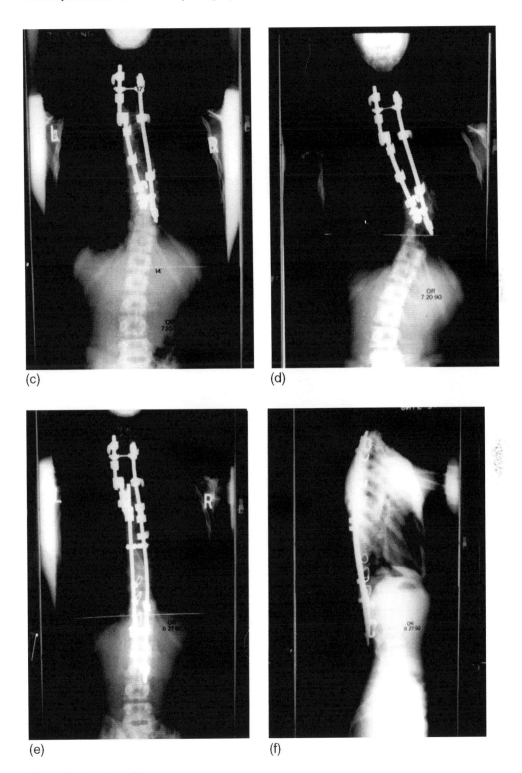

(c)

(d)

(e)

(f)

Figure 3 (*continued*)

B. Crankshaft

The crankshaft phenomenon—the long-term loss of the coronal plane Cobb angle curve correction—has been reported following posterior spinal fusion and instrumentation in the skeletally immature patient population (28–30). It has been described as continued

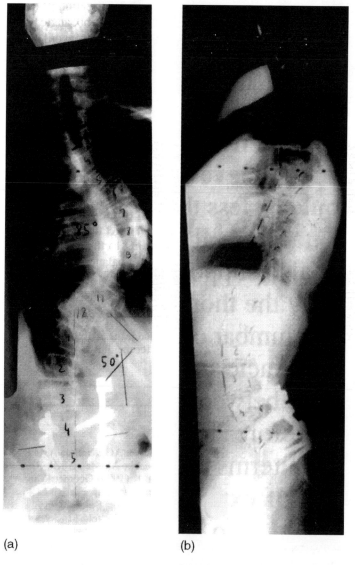

(a)   (b)

Figure 4   (a) PA and (b) lateral radiograph of a 13 year old female with a right thoracic curvature measuring 85 degrees. (c) Right side-bending radiograph reveals correction of the curve to 58 degrees. (d) Postoperative PA radiograph demonstrating correction of the curvature to 36 degrees with posterior instrumentation. (e) Postoperative photograph, however, demonstrates decompensation to the left and elevation of the right shoulder. (f) Removal of the apical pedicle hook on the right and two pedicle hooks on the left allows the curve to relax somewhat achieving overall coronal balance and leveling of the shoulders (g).

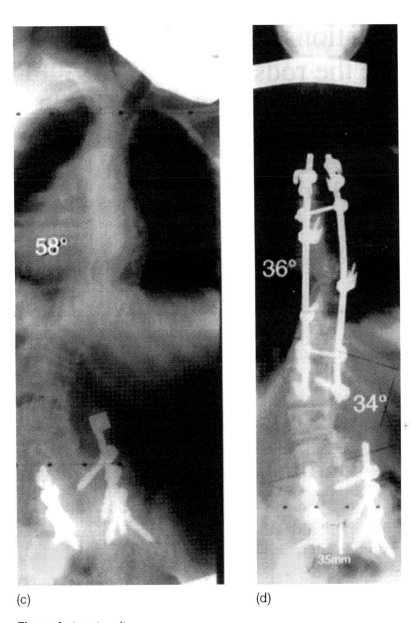

(c)   (d)

Figure 4 (*continued*)

anterior spinal growth in the presence of a solid posterior fusion. By nature, it thus has a higher prevalence in prepubertal (30), premenarchal, skeletally immature individuals especially those with open triradiate cartilage (31), or before their peak height velocity (31,32) (Fig. 5). Anterior surgery, with its attendant removal of the intervertebral disks and endplates, has been suggested by many to reduce the chances of postoperative crankshafting (33,30,33). Shufflebarger and Clark (33) recommended adding an anterior growth arrest to a posterior fusion for individuals Risser 0-1, Tanner 0-1, premenarchal, a Cobb angle greater than 60°, and Pedriolle rotation greater than 20°. Sanders et al. (31) also found

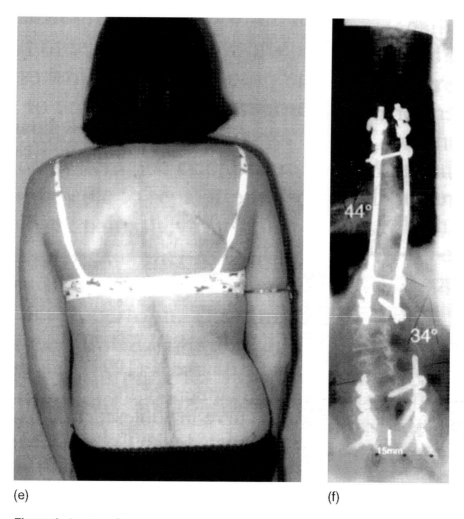

(e)   (f)

Figure 4 (*continued*)

a strong correlation between the patient's age (youth) and their open triradiate cartilage and postoperative crankshaft phenomenon, the average increase in Cobb measurement being 22°. Sanders et al. (32) further studied the risk of crankshaft phenomenon and correlated it with the peak height velocity in centimeters per year—a phenomenon that has been shown to correlate well with the period of rapid spinal growth and scoliotic curve progression (34,35) of the patient at the time of surgery. They found in their series, that all patients with closed triradiate cartilages were beyond their peak height velocity at the time of surgery and none crankshafted. Of those with open triradiate cartilages operated on before their peak height velocity, all crankshafted. Of those fused still with open cartilage, but after their peak height velocity, only two of 15 crankshafted ($p = 0.000009$).

Clinically there are differing opinions; Lee and Nachemson (36) followed 63 individuals operated on posteriorly alone with a Risser 0 and found an average progression over 5 years of only 3°. Only 7 (11%) progressed more than 10°, and thus "neither the patients nor the surgeons" felt this was of sufficient magnitude to warrant routine combined

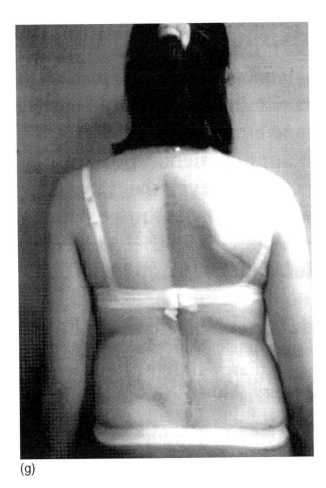

(g)

Figure 4 (*continued*)

anterior fusion. Some authors (37,38) have also questioned whether plain anterior-posterior radiography is really an accurate way of determining whether actual longitudinal growth—crankshafting—has taken place. By definition, the crankshaft phenomenon occurs in a fused spine. Whether adjacent, unfused segments may be also contributing to the phenomenon was studied by Delorme et al. (38) who measured three-dimensional radiographic reconstructions of 48 adolescents who had undergone posterior instrumentation and fusion. Although they did find the presence of a crankshaft phenomenon, i.e., significant increases in both spine length and Cobb angle, they also found equal numbers of individuals with increases in Cobb angles but no additional spine length, as well as others with increased spine growth but no Cobb angle changes. They concluded that Cobb angle changes as measured on plain radiography were not a reliable indicator of this complication. Even if anterior growth persists after a posterior fusion, Burton et al. (39) has suggested that the modern rigid multisegmental posterior instrumentation systems used today can prevent the crankshaft phenomenon in patients even as young as 10. They evaluated 18 patients, all Risser zero, 7 of whom had open triradiate cartilage, and none showed more than 2° loss of correction over a 39-month average follow-up.

C. Shoulder Imbalance

Postsurgical asymmetry of the shoulders is an unfortunate cosmetic effect of scoliosis surgery in both the adolescent as well as the adult. It is an example of a regional decompensation or imbalance following scoliosis surgery. Often cited causes include failure to recognize a structural left upper thoracic curvature (40–42), overcorrection of a right thoracic curvature (21,42), a preoperative shoulder imbalance left unaddressed (21,41), and a failing to recognize a tilted T1 vertebra tilted into the curve.

Double thoracic curves present the most vexing problem. Again, like the King II curves described earlier, the problem lies with the compensatory upper left thoracic curve's ability to compensate or balance the correction obtained with the more caudal midthoracic curve. Flexibility of the upper thoracic curve, however, is a little more difficult to appreciate on bending films due to the rigidity of the clavicle, shoulder girdle, and sternum.

Early uniplanar systems (e.g., Harrington) were not as liable to result in shoulder asymmetry. Frez et al. (43) treated 24 patients with segmental wiring and Harrington instrumentation. Seventy percent showed preoperative shoulder imbalances averaging 1.7 cm, yet all were reduced to within 1 cm at final follow-up. Lee et al. (41), in their review

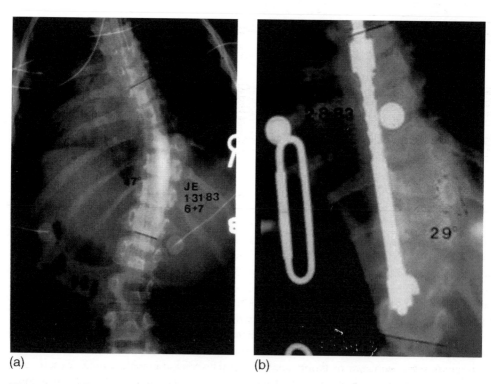

(a)   (b)

Figure 5   (a) PA radiograph of a 6–7 year old boy with congenital scoliosis measuring 47 degrees. (b) Postoperative PA radiograph demonstrating posterior spinal fusion and Harrington rod with correction of the curve to 29 degrees. (c) Four years postoperatively continued anterior growth has lead to crankshafting of the spine around the posterior instrumentation with the recurrence of the coronal curvature now measuring 56 degrees. (d) Six years postoperatively there is severe decompensation of the trunk to the left and crankshafting of the spine around the posterior instrumentation now measuring 74 degrees.

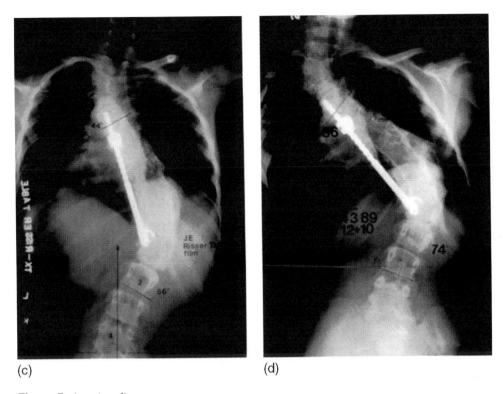

(c)   (d)

Figure 5 (*continued*)

of 294 patients treated with posterior instrumentation for thoracic scoliosis with upper curves greater than 20°, concluded that shoulder imbalance did not always correlate with the T1 tilt. Many patients had right shoulder elevation despite mild T1 tilt, and it was thus possible to limit the fusion to the lower curve. Their recommendation was that the more rigid the upper curve, the less correction of the lower curve that is needed, and, conversely, the more elevated the right shoulder, the more correction is needed in the lower curve so as to obtain balanced shoulders. Patients with large positive T1 tilts (i.e., T1 tilts into the concavity of the upper curve) are much more likely to have coronal imbalance and shoulder asymmetry issues unless the upper curve is included in the correction. Recently, Lenke et al. (40) suggested guidelines for the upper thoracic curve based on its Cobb angle and its degree of flexibility. Those structural curves over 30° and those who fail to correct on side bending to less than 20°, those with significant rotation, and those with positive T1 tilt should be included in the fusion. Suk et al. (42) reviewed their experience using pedicle screw segmental fixation and recommended fusing the proximal curve if greater than 25° and the left shoulder is level or elevated. If the left shoulder is lower inclusion is optional, unless it is more than 12 mm lower, in which case it should be left unfused. Overall, the consensus would seem to be that if the shoulders are level or the left shoulder is elevated at all preoperatively, the main thoracic curve correction should be reserved so as to maintain the balance. Conversely, the more the middle thoracic curve is corrected, the more likely the upper left curve will need to be corrected, and this will frequently entail extending the instrumentation proximally.

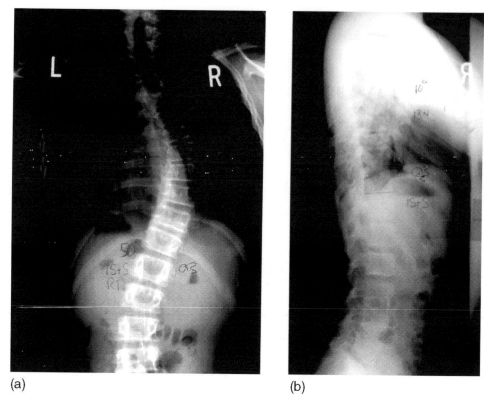

(a)   (b)

Figure 6 (a) PA and (b) lateral radiographs of a 15 year old boy with right thoracic scoliosis. (c) Right thoracic side-bend radiograph reveals correctability to 29 degrees. (d) Left lumbar curvature reveals an extremely flexible left lumbar curve. (e) Postoperative PA and (f) lateral radiographs. The right thoracic curvature has been corrected to 15 degrees which is resulted in moderate elevation of the left shoulder at one year postoperatively.

Anterior instrumentation is an attractive means of correcting scoliosis and, in many cases, saving distal fusion levels, but complete removal of the intervertebral disks plus correction using rigid rods and vertebral body screws is a very powerful means of spinal realignment. In the event of any preoperative left shoulder elevation, or an upper thoracic curve of any structural significance, the exuberance to correct the right thoracic curve must be carefully tempered so as to not leave the left shoulder excessively elevated postoperatively (Fig. 6).

Often, especially after a thoracotomy for anterior instrumentation, postoperative splinting from pain will imbalance the shoulders somewhat, giving the appearance of a decompensated shoulder girdle. Simply waiting 4–8 weeks for the postoperative pain and stiffness to subside will often allow the shoulders to spontaneously balance (44).

II. KYPHOSIS

Successful operative treatment of Scheuermann's kyphosis involves not only correction of the hyperkyphotic deformity, but a successful arthrodesis of the involved segments as well.

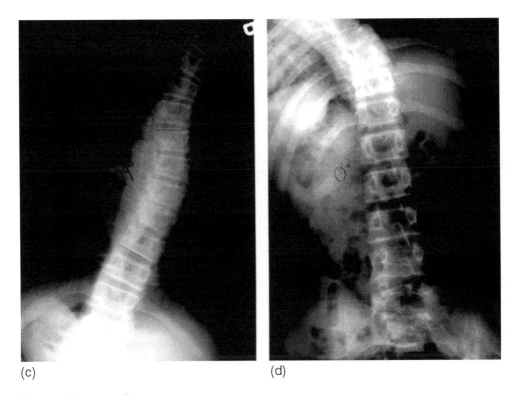

(c)   (d)

Figure 6 (*continued*)

Postoperative decompensation following the surgical treatment of Scheuermann's kyphosis typically manifests itself in the sagittal plane as either a proximal or distal junctional kyphosis. The two principal causes are either failing to include enough of the pathology in the fusion and instrumentation or overcorrection of the kyphotic deformity.

Originally, fusions to correct hyperkyphosis were performed posteriorly alone with Harrington compression instrumentation. However, follow-up often revealed not only implant failure and loss of correction, but also an unacceptably high rate of pseudarthrosis (45,46). Today, using rigid multilevel fixation hook/screw/rod systems, the mild-moderate curves can be treated posteriorly alone with a lower rate of pseudarthrosis and instrumentation complications. However, frequently both an anterior as well as a posterior fusion is performed, especially for those in whom the kyphosis is greater than 75°, when there is marked wedging of the apical vertebrae, or if the kyphosis cannot be corrected on a hyperextension lateral radiograph to less than 50° (20,46,47).

Although modern surgical techniques and rigid multisegmental posterior instrumentation can effect significant correction of most curves, largely because of its notable strength, some postoperative balance complications have been reported (48–52). Coscia et al. (48) reported a junctional hyperkyphosis in almost 70% of their patients treated with Luque sublaminar wiring and posterior fusion due in large part to this system's ability to affect great changes in the rigid spine. Their theory was also that in resecting the ligamentum flavum for the passage of the sublaminar wires, they had created additional local areas of sagittal plane instability and subsequent deformity developed. The thoracic spine is but

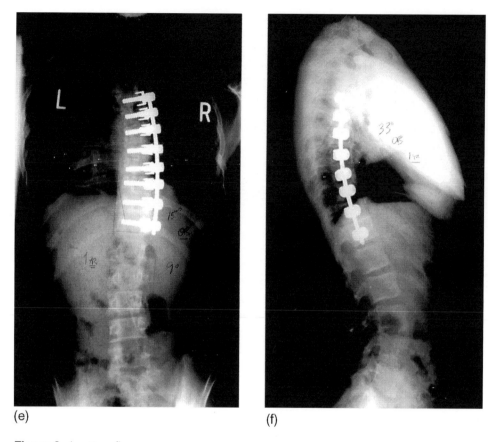

(e)   (f)

Figure 6 (*continued*)

one part of a rigid chest cage stabilized not only by the vertebral column and its ligaments, but by the connecting ribs and sternum anteriorly as well. Posterior instrumentation systems may exert a great deal of correcting force on a spinal segment, but the intact anterior structures (ribs, sternum, ALL) remain a kyphogenic force that will recreate angular deformities just beyond the instrumentation if too much correction is attempted.

Cotrel-Dubousset instrumentation, and similar rigid multisegmental hook and rod systems that followed, obviated the need for resection of the posterior ligaments at the limits of the fusion if the superior construct is a transverse process, infralaminar claw hook configuration. (Although, if supralaminar hooks are used in the superior foundation, some dissection of the intervertebral ligaments will be necessary and pose the risk of some kyphotic angulation.) Additionally, they pose a risk due to their inherent strength and rigidity. Numerous reports have presented cases of overcorrection of the kyphotic deformity leading to an acute postoperative kyphotic junctional deformity at the ends of the instrumentation (49,53). Based on these experiences, current recommendations would be as follows: because normal kyphosis in an adult can range from 20° to 50° (54,55) there would seem to be little need to correct any deformity to less than 40–50°. Hyperextension radiographs taken in the supine lateral position over a bolster preoperatively will provide some information as to the flexibility of the deformity and whether a combined surgical approach is necessary or not. Most authors currently recommend limiting the degree of correction to no more than 50% of the preoperative deformity (50,51,56).

Lowe (50,52) and others (51,53) have written that in order to avoid either proximal or distal junctional kyphotic deformities, the instrumentation should also typically extend to include the entire kyphotic deformity, normally from T2 down to and including the first lordotic segment of the lumbar spine, frequently L1–L2. This is notably different from scoliosis, where with modern techniques the instrumentation can often stop one or two segments short of the end Cobb vertebrae; in kyphosis correction, the whole Cobb deformity must be included.

In the event a proximal or distal kyphotic imbalance results, the only real treatment is extension of the instrumentation and fusion to include the pathological levels. No evidence exists to date to suggest that bracing plays any role in reversing this postoperative complication.

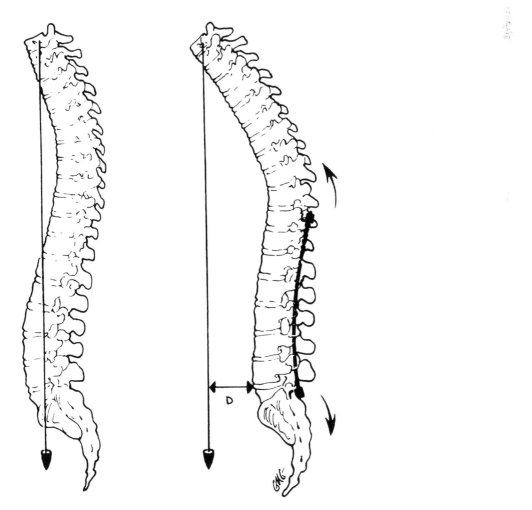

Figure 7 Diagram demonstrating the effects of distraction instrumentation within the lumbar spine on overall sagittal balance.

III. FLATBACK DEFORMITY

The first reports of flatback deformity as a phenomenon of postoperative sagittal plane imbalance were from the literature of Harrington instrumentation for the treatment of scoliosis (57). The principal offense was when the distraction instrumentation was extended down into the lower lumbar spine, typically L4 or L5. Harrington instrumentation corrected principally in the coronal plane, but it could not be adequately contoured to reflect the normal sagittal curvature, and as it worked in a distraction mode, this often resulted in the loss of the normal lumbar lordosis (Fig. 7). This then had the effect of pushing the patient's center of gravity forward of the pelvis (anterior decompensation) (Fig. 8). With upright activities over time, this would lead to painful fatigue of the lower back muscles, the need to flex the knees somewhat to maintain some sense of sagittal balance, and degeneration of the few remaining open segments down to the sacrum (57).

   Newer scoliosis instrumentation systems apply more of a three-dimensional corrective force to the deformed spine using multiple sites of hook, screw, or wire attachment correcting more with translation than distraction, and the operating surgeon is able to contour the rods to reflect the normal sagittal profile. Thus, postoperative sagittal plane imbalance—flatback syndrome—is much less common now than in the days of Harrington instrumentation. However, it can and does still exist, most often in the adult population. Yet even in the adolescent with scoliosis, if instrumentation is going to extend down in to

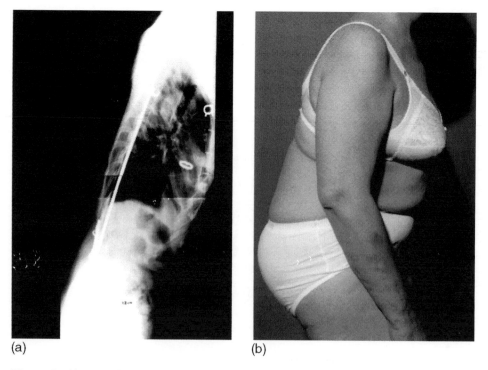

(a)   (b)

Figure 8 (a) Lateral radiograph and (b) clinical photograph demonstrating the effects of distraction instrumentation within the lumbar spine on overall sagittal balance.

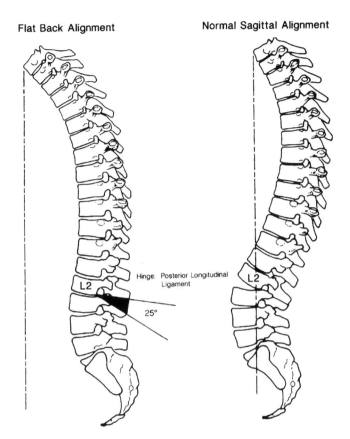

Flat Back Alignment   Normal Sagittal Alignment

Figure 9 A Smith Peterson posterior osteotomy hinging at the posterior longitudinal ligament.

Three Column Pedicle Subtraction Osteotomy

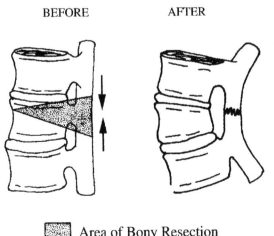

BEFORE   AFTER

Area of Bony Resection

Figure 10 A pedicle subtraction osteotomy hinges at the anterior longitudinal ligament.

the low lumbar spine, careful assessment of the preoperative sagittal profile must be made. Likewise, intraoperatively, proper contouring of the rods must reflect normal lordosis, not only to preserve the sagittal profile but to preserve and enhance the life of the few remaining intervertebral segments distal down to the sacrum.

Established flatback deformities are typically corrected in one of three ways: (a) posterior Smith-Peterson osteotomy with fusion and instrumentation; (b) anterior and posterior osteotomy, fusion, and instrumentation; and (c) posterior pedicle subtraction osteotomy. A Smith-Peterson posterior osteotomy (Fig. 9) can effect approximately 1° of sagittal plane correction for every millimeter of posterior fusion mass resected. This operation requires intact disk spaces anteriorly and hinges at the level of the posterior longitudinal ligament. In the setting of a solid fusion both anteriorly and posteriorly, two general options exist: (a) an anterior opening wedge osteotomy followed by a closing posterior osteotomy and instrumentation, or (b) a posterior pedicle subtraction osteotomy (Fig. 10) wherein a wedge resection of the posterior elements plus part of the vertebral body hinged at the anterior body wall is removed. This obviates the need for an additional anterior incision and exposure and can effect between 30 and 40° of correction per level. The blood loss, which can be extensive, tends to lessen somewhat with surgeon experience.

REFERENCES

1. Dubousset J, Graf H, Miladi L, Cotrel Y. Spinal and thoracic derotation with CD instrumentation. Orthop Trans 1986; 10:36.
2. Bridwell KH, McAllister JW, Betz RR, Huss G, Clancy M, Schoenecker PL. Coronal decompensation produced by Cotrel-Dubousset "derotation" maneuver for idiopathic right thoracic scoliosis. Spine 1991; 16:769–777.
3. Knapp DR, Price CT, Jones ET, Coonrad RW, Flynn JC. Choosing fusion levels in progressive thoracic idiopathic scoliosis. Spine 1992; 17:1159–1165.
4. Moore MR, Baynham GC, Brown CW. Analysis of factors related to truncal decompensation following Cotrel-Dubousset instrumentation. J Spinal Disord 1991; 4:188–192.
5. Lenke LG, Bridwell KH, Baldus C, Blanke K. Preventing decompensation in King type II curves treated with Cotrel-Dubousset instrumentation. Spine 1992; 17:S274–S281.
6. Sar C, Hamzaoglu A, Talu U, Kilicoglu O. Selection of fusion levels in surgical treatment of King type II curves. Orthop Trans 1995; 19:642.
7. Thompson JP, Transfeldt ET, Bradford DS. Decompensation after Cotrel-Dubousset instrumentation of idiopathic scoliosis. Spine 1990; 15:927–931.
8. King HA. Analysis and treatment of type 2 idiopathic scoliosis. Orthop Clin North Am 1994; 25:225–237.
9. Bridwell KH, Betz RR, Capelli AM, Huss G, Harvey C. Sagittal plane analysis in idiopathic scoliosis patients treated with Cotrel-Dubousset instrumentation. Spine 1990; 15:921–926.
10. Schwender JD, Denis F. Coronal plane imbalance in adolescent idiopathic scoliosis with left lumbar curves exceeding 40°: The role of the lumbosacral hemicurve. Spine 2000; 25:2358–2363.
11. Richards BS. Lumbar curve response in Type II idiopathic scoliosis after posterior instrumentation of the thoracic curve. Spine 1992; 17:S282–S286.
12. Harrington PR. Treatment of scoliosis, correction and internal fixation by spine instrumentation. J Bone Joint Surg (Am) 1962; 44:591–610.
13. King HA, Moe JH, Bradford DS, Winter RB. The selection of fusion levels in thoracic idiopathic scoliosis. J Bone Joint Surg (Am) 1983; 65:1302–1313.

14. Moe JH. A critical analysis of methods of fusion for scoliosis—an evaluation in two hundred and sixty-six patients. J Bone Joint Surg (Am) 1958; 40:529–554.

15. Moe JH. Methods and techniques of evaluating idiopathic scoliosis. In: Surgeons TAAoO, ed. Symposium on the Spine. St. Louis: CV Mosby, 1969:196–240.

16. Goldstein LA. The surgical treatment of idiopathic scoliosis. Clin Orthop 1973; 93:131–157.

17. Fitch RD, Turi M, Bowman BE. Comparison of Cotrel-Dubousset and Harrington rod instrumentation in idiopathic scoliosis. J Pediatr Orthop 1990; 10:44–47.

18. Richards BS, Birch JG, Herring JA, Johnston CE, Roach JW. Frontal plane and sagittal plane balance following Cotrel-Dubousset instrumentation for idiopathic scoliosis. Spine 1989; 14:733–737.

19. Muschik M, Schlenzka D, Robinson PN, Kupferschmidt C. Dorsal instrumentation for idipathic adolescent thoracic scoliosis: rod rotation versus translation. Eur Spine J 1999; 8:93–99.

20. Patwardhan AG, Rimkus A, Gavin TM, et al. Geometric analysis of coronal decompression in idiopathic scoliosis. Spine 1996; 21:1192–1200.

21. McCance SE, Denis F, Lonstein JE, Winter RB. Coronal and sagittal balance in surgically treated adolescent idiopathic scoliosis with the King II curve pattern. A review of 67 consecutive cases having selective thoracic arthrodesis. Spine 1998; 23:2063–2073.

22. Benli IT, Tuzuner M, Akalin S, Kis M, Aydin E, Tandogan R. Spinal imbalance and decompensation problems in patients treated wiht Cotrel-Dubousset instrumentation. Eur Spine J 1996; 5:380–386.

23. Kalen V, Conklin M. The behavior of the unfused lumbar curve following selective thoraic fusion for idiopathic scoliosis. Spine 1990; 15:271–274.

24. Kaneda K, Shono Y, Satoh S, Abumi K. Anterior correction of thoraic scoliosis with Kaneda anterior spinal system. Spine 1997; 22:1358–1368.

25. Mason DE, Carango P. Spinal decompensation in Cotrel-Dubousset instrumentation. Spine 1991; 16:S394–S403.

26. Lenke LG, Betz RR, Bridwell KH, Harms J, Clements DH, Thomas L. Spontaneous lumbar curves coronal correction after selective anterior or posterior thoracic fusion in adolescent idiopathic scoliosis. Spine 1999; 24:1663–1672.

27. Arlet V, Marchesi D, Papin P, Aebi M. Decompression following scoliosis surgery: treatment by decreasing the correction of the main thoracic curve or "letting the spine go." Eur Spine J 2000; 9:156–160.

28. Dubousset J, Herring JA, Shufflebarger HL. The crankshaft phenomenon. J Pediatr Orthop 1989; 9:541–550.

29. Stokes IAF, Shuma-Hartwick D, Moreland M. Spine and back shape changes in scoliosis. Acta Orthop Scand 1998; 59:128–133.

30. Roberto RF, Lonstein JE, Winter RB. Curve progression in Risser stage 0 or 1 patients after posterior spinal fusion for idiopathic scoliosis. J Pediatr Orthop 1997; 17:718–725.

31. Sanders JO, Herring JA, Browne RH. Posterior arthrosis and instrumentation in the immature (Riser-Grade-0) spine in idiopathic scoliosis. J Bone Joint Surg (Am) 1995; 77: 39–45.

32. Sanders JO, Little DG, Richard BS. Prediction of crankshaft phenomenon by peak height velocity. Spine 1997; 22:1352–1357.

33. Shufflebarger HL, Clark CE. Prevention of the crankshaft phenomenon. Spine 1991; 16: S409–S411.

34. Duval-Beaupere G. Pathogenic relationship between scoliosis and growth. In: Zorab PA, ed. Scoliosis and Growth. Edinburgh: Churchill Livingstone, 1971:58–64.

35. Burnwell RG. The relationship between scoliosis and growth. In: Zorab PA, ed. Scoliosis and growth. Edinburgh: Churchill Livingstone, 1971:131–150.

36. Lee CS, Nachemson AL. The crankshaft phenomenon after posterior Harrington fusion in skeletally immature patients with thoracic or thoracolumbar idiopathic scoliosis followed to maturity. Spine 1997; 22:58–67.

37. Papin P, Labelle H, Delorme S. Long term three-dimensional changes of the spine after posterior spinal instrumentation and fusion in adolescent idiopathic scoliosis. Eur Spine J 1998; 8:16–21.

38. Delorme S, Labelle H, Aubin CE. The crankshaft phenomenon. Is Cobb angle progression a good indicator in adolescent idiopathic scoliosis. Spine 2002; 27:E145–E151.

39. Burton DC, Asher MA, Min Lai S. Scoliosis correction maintenance in skeletally immature patients with idiopathic scoliosis. Is anterior fusion really necessary? Spine 2000; 25:61–68.

40. Lenke LG, Bridwell KH, O'Brien MF, Baldus C, Blanke K. Recognition and treatment of the proximal thoracic curve in adolescent idiopathic scoliosis treated with Cotrel-Dubousset instrumentation. Spine 1994; 14:1589–1597.

41. Lee CK, Denis F, Winter RB, Lonstein JE. Analysis of the upper thoracic curve in surgically treated idiopathic scoliosis. A new concept of the double thoracic curve pattern. Spine 1993; 12:1599–1608.

42. Suk S, Kim WJ, Lee CS, et al. Indications of proximal thoracic curve fusion in thoracic adolescent idiopathic scoliosis. Recognition and treatment of double curve pattern in adolescent idiopathic scoliosis treated with segmental instrumentation. Spine 2000; 25:2342–2349.

43. Frez R, Cheng J, Wong E. Longitudinal changes in trunkal balance after selective fusion of King II curves in adolescent idiopathic scoliosis. Spine 2000; 25:1352–1359.

44. Betz RR, Harms J, Clements DH, et al. Comparison of anterior and posterior instrumenation for correction of adolescent thoracic idiopathic scoliosis. Spine 1999; 24:225–239.

45. Bradford DS, Moe JH, Montalvo FJ, Winter RB. Scheuermann's kyphosis. Results of surgical treatment by posterior spine arthrodesis in twenty-two patients. J Bone Joint Surg (Am) 1975; 57:439–448.

46. Lowe TG. Scheuermann Disease. J Bone Joint Surg (Am) 1990; 72:940–945.

47. Kostuik JP. Anterior Kostuik-Harrington distraction systems for the treatment of kyphotic deformities. Spine 1990; 15:169–180.

48. Coscia MF, Bradford DS, Ogilvie JW. Scheuermann's kyphosis—results in 19 cases treated by spinal arthrodesis and L-rod instrumentation. Orthop Trans 1988; 12:1988.

49. Lettice J, Ogilvie JW, Transfeldt ET. Proximal junctional kyphosis following Cotrel-Dubousset instrumentation in adult scoliosis. Orthop Trans 1992; 16:162.

50. Lowe TG, Kasten MD. An analysis of sagittal curves and balance after Cotrel-Dubousset instrumentation for kyphosis secondary to Scheuermann's disease. Spine 1994; 19:1680–1685.

51. Tribus CB. Scheuermann's kyphosis in adolescents and adults: diagnosis and management. J Am Acad Orthop Surg 1998; 6:36–43.

52. Lowe TG. Scheuermann's disease. Orthop Clin North Am 1999; 30:475–487.

53. Papagelopoulos PJ, Klassen RA, Peterson HA, Dekutoski MB. Surgical treatment of Scheuermann's disease with segmental compression instrumentation. Clin Orthop Rel Res 2001; 386:139–149.

54. Schultz AB, Aston-Miller JA. Biomechanics of the human spine. In: Mow VC, Hayes WC, eds. Basic Orthopaedic Biomechanics. New York: Raven Press, 1991.

55. Bernhardt M, Bridwell KH. Segmental analysis of the sagittal plane alignment of the normal thoracic and lumbar spines and thoracolumbar junction. Spine 1989; 14:717–721.

56. Platero D, Luna JD, Pedraza V. Juvenile kyphosis: effects of different variables on conservative treatment outcome. Acta Orthop Belg 1997; 63:194–201.

57. Lagrone MD, Bradford DS, Moe JS, Lonstein JE, Winter RB, Ogilvie JW. Treatment of symptomatic flatback after spinal fusion. J Bone Joint Surg (Am) 1988; 70:569–580.

44

Complications in the Management of Neurofibromatosis in Children

Diane E. VonStein and Alvin H. Crawford
Cincinnati Children's Hospital Medical Center, Cincinnati, Ohio, U.S.A.

I. INTRODUCTION

Neurofibromatosis is a multisystem disease that primarily affects cell growth of neural tissue (1). The intent of this chapter is to identify the spinal complications most commonly associated with neurofibromatosis and present strategies for management.

Four distinctive forms of neurofibromatosis are recognized, although variant forms probably exist:

1. Neurofibromatosis-1 (NF-1), von Recklinghausen's disease, or peripheral neurofibromatosis is an autosomal dominant disorder. The entity is common and affects 1 in 4000 individuals. It is the most common single genetic disorder in humans. The gene locus of neurofibromatosis in humans has been identified and localized to the long arm of chromosome 17 (2–4).
2. Neurofibromatosis-2 (NF-2), or central neurofibromatosis, is also an autosomal dominant disorder, estimated to affect 1 in 50,000 individuals. Characteristically, there is a schwannoma of the eighth cranial nerve. Spinal complications have rarely been reported with NF-2.
3. Segmental neurofibromatosis is characterized by café au lait macules dispersed in bands on the skin. Complications are similar to those found in NF-1.
4. Mixed form neurofibromatosis.

Our discussion will be limited to NF-1.

Neurofibromatosis is the most common single gene disorder in humans. About 50% of all NF-1 cases are new mutations, occurring 100-fold more often than the usual mutation rate for a single locus (1,5). The manifestations of NF-1 may vary, but each individual that carries the gene eventually shows some clinical features of the disease. The Consensus Development Conference at the National Institutes of Health concluded in 1987 that the diagnosis of NF-1 could be assigned to a person with two or more of the following criteria (6):

1. More than six café au lait spots measuring at least 15 mm in adults and five café au lait spots of 5 mm in children

2. Two or more neurofibroma of any type or at least one plexiform neurofibroma
3. Freckling in the axilla or inguinal regions
4. Optic glioma
5. Two or more Lisch nodules (iris hamartomas)
6. A distinctive bony lesion (anatomic dysplasia or sphenoid wing distortion)
7. A first-degree relative with NF-1 by the above criteria

These criteria are useful even in young children (7). There seem to be two peaks of severe clinical problems for NF-1 patients: one from 5–10 years of age and the second from 36–50 years of age. At the second peak, 75% of the clinical problems are related to malignancy (8). The orthopedic complications usually present early and include spinal deformities of scoliosis and kyphoscoliosis. Other orthopedic complications include bony dysplasia with congenital bowing and pseudarthrosis of the tibia and the forearm (usually ulna), overgrowth phenomenon of the extremity, and soft tissue tumors.

Scoliosis is the most common skeletal manifestation of neurofibromatosis. The incidence of spinal deformities is reported to be between 10 and 60% (2,9–11). Spinal changes may occur throughout and are usually divided into soft tissue and bony pathology of the entire vertebral column. Some of the complications of treatment of spine problems reflect the treating physician's lack of understanding of the disease process and potential pitfalls with surgery. Other complications are inherent in the disease process itself. The goal is to prevent problems from occurring by understanding the unusual and unique characteristics of spine problems in NF-1. It is imperative that the patient understand the importance of careful follow-up observation because of the very real tendency for progression of spinal neuropathology that may continue throughout life.

II. CERVICAL SPINE

The cervical spine in NF-1 patients has not received enough attention in the literature (12,13). Cervical abnormalities occur more frequently when scoliosis or kyphoscoliosis is present in the thoracolumbar region, which distracts the examiner's attention to the more obvious deformity. Often the cervical lesion is asymptomatic. When symptomatic, pain is the most common presenting symptom (14).

The most common abnormality is a severe cervical kyphosis most often seen following decompressive laminectomy surgery, which itself is highly (Fig. 1) suggestive of the disorder (15). Ogilvie reported on the surgical treatment of cervical kyphosis by anterior fusion with iliac crest or fibular bone graft or both (14). He considered halo traction a useful prelude if the kyphosis is greater than 45 degrees. When progressive cervical kyphosis is the presenting deformity, preoperative halo traction of flexible deformities, followed by posterior fusion is the treatment of choice. If the deformity is rigid, then soft tissue release followed by traction is felt to be safer. If sufficient bone stock is present, internal fixation with rods, wires, screws, or hooks may be used. Sublaminar wire fixation may be difficult secondary to dural ectasia and osseous fragility. If there is osteolysis with poor bone stock of the vertebral body, anterior and posterior fusion is needed (14). Postoperative halo vest immobilization is recommended. Of Yong-Hing and coworkers' 56 patients with NF-1, 17 were found to have cervical abnormalities (13). Of these, seven were asymptomatic, whereas the rest had either limited motion or pain in the neck and four had neurological deficits, which probably could be attributed to cervical instability. Four of the 17 patients required fusion of the cervical spine. Curtis and associates described eight patients with

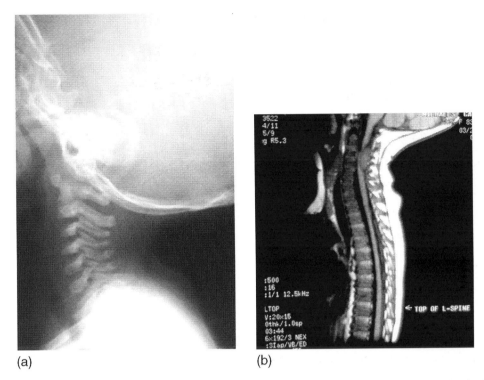

(a)   (b)

Figure 1 Spinal instability following laminectomy in a very young child who complained of neck pain and decreased range of motion. (a) Presenting lateral cervical spine radiograph with slightly decreased lordosis. (b) Magnetic resonance image illustrating extra dural neurofibroma at C3-C4 with spinal cord indentation. (c) Operative view of neurofibroma excision. (d) Lateral cervical spine radiographs 6 months following laminectomy and neurofibroma excision illustrating significant kyphosis of the entire cervical spine and a dystrophic appearance of the mid apical vertebra.

paraplegia and NF-1. Four cases were due to cervical spine instability or intraspinal pathology in the cervical spine (16).

Attention should also be paid to C1–C2. Isu and colleagues describe three patients with NF-1 who had C1–C2 dislocation with neurological deficit, and all improved after decompression and/or fusion (17). It is worthwhile to note that in none of these patients were any bony changes in the C1–C2 relation seen on flexion-extension. Therefore relying only on these views to detect instability is unwise. Most of the problems encountered occurred following excision of tumors, which involves resection of the laminae and posterior elements (Fig. 2). Postoperatively, the spine is unstable and tends to develop progressive kyphosis. Therefore, be aware of the NF-1 patient who presents with a scar in and about the neck and gives a history of having a mass removed in the past.

All patients with NF-1 who undergo surgery, require endotracheal anesthesia, require cranial traction, or present with neck tumors should have a cervical spine x-ray. If there is any suspicion of subluxation, computed tomography (CT) or flexion/extension extension magnetic resonance imaging (MRI) scans are appropriate studies. Other reasons for obtaining cervical spine x-rays in the NF-1 patient include torticollis and dysphagia (18). Always obtain skull x-rays prior to applying halo or Gardner–Wells pins.

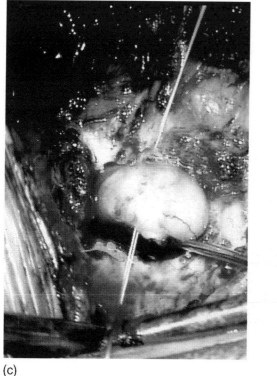

(c)

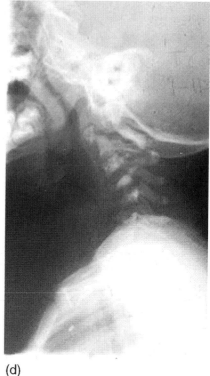

(d)

Figure 1 (*continued*).

III. THORACOLUMBAR DEFORMITIES

A. Nondystrophic Curves

Peculiar to NF-1 is the concept of dystrophic and nondystrophic spinal changes. Non-dystrophic scoliosis is the most common spinal deformity in NF-1 and the findings, treatment, and complications are similar to those of a normal idiopathic curve with the following exceptions (18–20): (a) NF patients present earlier than their idiopathic counter-part; (b) a somewhat worse prognosis can be anticipated for progression; and (c) there is a higher pseudarthrosis rate after spinal fusion (21). This may be due to a process termed modulation (see below) in which a nondystrophic curve takes on the characteristics of a dystrophic curve (21,22).

B. Treatment of Nondystrophic Curves

If the patient's curve is 20–25 degrees and has less than three of the dystrophic character-istics, treatment is observation (Fig. 3). Bracing is used when progression has been demon-strated or the patient presents with a curve greater than 25 degrees and is skeletally immature. Deformities exceeding 40 degrees need posterior spinal fusion with segmental instrumentation. Curves greater than 55–60 degrees are treated with anterior release with bone grafting, followed with instrumented posterior spinal fusion (21). This is necessary because the curve is usually more rigid than is a similar size curve in idiopathic scoliosis.

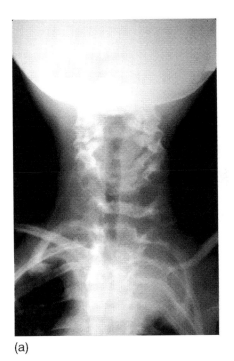
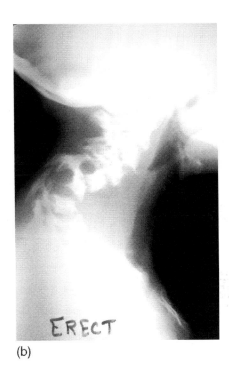

(a)   (b)

Figure 2 This child underwent multiple laminectomies for decompression of a large neurofibroma at the C5-C6 level. He subsequently presented with a severe kyphosis of the mid lower cervical spine. (a) Frontal view showing enlargement of the neuro foramina at the C7-T1 junction. (b) Lateral view illustrating severe kyphosis at the C6-C7 level following laminectomy. The loss of the posterior (tension) supporting structures has allowed each involved facet joint surface to slide and subluxate on its opposing surface producing increased compressive force on the anterior portion of the vertebral bodies. There has been an unhinging of the posterior articular facets, resulting in complete disengagement.

Many authors recommend postoperative orthotic immobilization, although others have treated these patients without postoperative immobilization, with good early results (19).

C. Dystrophic Curves

The concept of dystrophic curves is based on x-rays findings that can be detected as early as age 3 (10) (Fig. 3). The patient may present as a true scoliosis, with a normal kyphosis of less than 50 degrees, or frequently with a kyphoscoliosis, with severe kyphotic curves of more than 50 degrees.

A dystrophic curve is characterized by a short-segmented (usually involving 4, 5, or 6 vertebra) sharply angulated deformity, usually in the upper part of the thoracic spine (Fig. 4). There are nine radiographic characteristics of dystrophic spinal deformities (Table 1). These include scalloping of the vertebral bodies, sharpening of the vertebral margins, severe rotation of the apical vertebra, widening of the spinal canal or the intervertebral foramina, penciling of the ribs, spindling appearance of the transverse process, or a paravertebral mass (15,23). Apical vertebrae rotation can become so severe that it rotates out of the support axis such that the vertebrae are approximated against one another in a complex three-dimensional pattern (24) (Fig. 5). Plain x-rays may

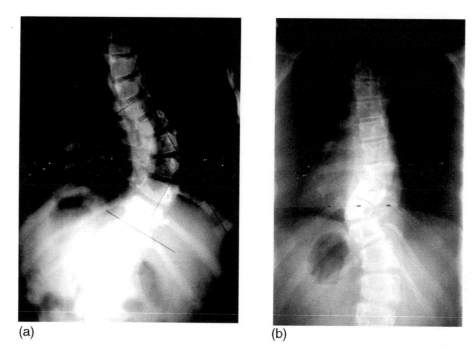

(a)   (b)

Figure 3 Two 13–year-old children with neurofibromatosis type I and scoliosis. One child has the nondystrophic type of scoliosis occasionally seen with neurofibromatosis, and the second has the characteristic dysplastic scoliosis felt to be associated with neurofibromatosis type I. (a) This 13-year-old child presented with multiple café-au-lait spots and referral from her pediatrician because of a positive Adams scoliosis bend test. This is a non-dysplastic idiopathic appearing curvature. She had a 45 degree curve and was recommended to have corrective surgery. (b) This 14-year-old child was known to have neurofibromatosis type I and a scoliosis deformity. She was being monitored for progression and subsequent to this radiograph was scheduled for surgery. This deformity typifies the characteristic, short segmented, sharply angulated, dysplastic spinal deformity of neurofibromatosis in a young child. In this patient there was a progression of the curvature of approximately 25 degrees over a 30-month period. (From Ref. 21.)

occasionally be interpreted as a congenital deformity. Rib penciling is present when the width of the rib is smaller than that of the narrowest portion of the second rib. Vertebral scalloping is present when the depth of scalloping is more than 3 mm in the thoracic spine or more than 4 mm in the lumbar spine. Although scalloping is found in all four planes, posterior scalloping is most consistent with the diagnosis of NF-1. The causes of these changes are in some cases intraspinal pathology such as tumors, meningoceles, or dural ectasia, but the changes may also occur with entirely normal intraspinal contents. In these cases, the dystrophic changes are explained by a primary bone dysplasia. Although all of these various features have been associated with dystrophic deformity, a universally accepted diagnostic criterion does not exist. It is important to detect those patients with a dystrophic curve because these curves are characterized by a rapid course of progression and higher rate of pseudoarthrosis following fusion.

Spinal deformity being followed as idiopathic may subsequently show dystrophic changes, a condition called modulation (21) (Fig. 6). Modulation refers to the ability of a spinal deformity to transform, by acquiring various dystrophic morphological features

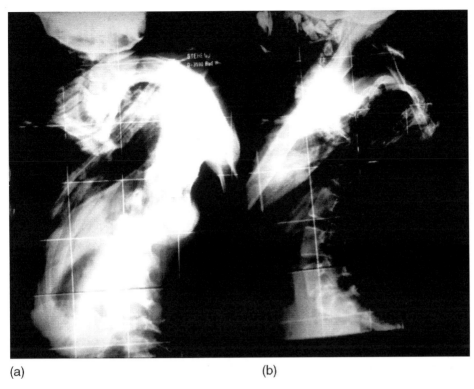

(a)   (b)

Figure 4 Radiograph of a 21-year-old scoliosis patient with severe rotation and angulation. (a) Coronal plane x-ray showing significant hairpin coronal plane curvatures, which is more than likely a manifestation of the child's significant kyphosis and rotatory deformity. (b) Sagittal plane x-ray showing the striking kyphosis. (Courtesy of Dr. Klaus Zielke, Badwildengen, West Germany.)

from non-dysplastic to dysplastic. A nondystrophic curve can become dystrophic, and a dystrophic curve can acquire further dystrophic changes. This is unique to spinal deformities in NF-1. These dystrophic changes may evolve slowly or aggressively. Progressively increasing dystrophic changes in a spinal deformity can, at a certain point, alter the behavior of the spinal curve and herald a course of rapid curve progression.

Table 1 Dystrophic Characteristics of NF-1 Spinal Deformities.

Dystrophic Features	%
Rib penciling	62
Vertebral rotation	51
Vertebral wedging	36
Posterior vertebral scalloping	31
Spindling of transverse processes	31
Anterior vertrebral scalloping	31
Widened interpediculate distance	29
Enlarged intervertebral foramina	25
Lateral vertebral scalloping	13

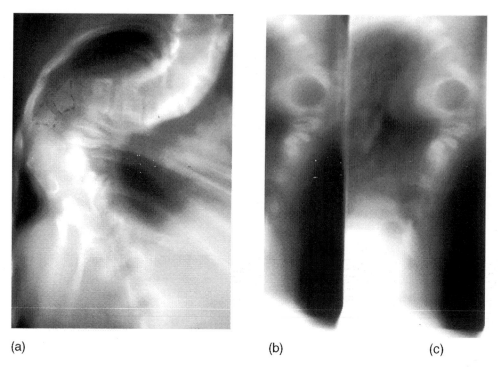

(a)   (b)   (c)

Figure 5 This 16-year-old child underwent polycycloidial tomography of what was considered to be a short segmented sharply angulated curvature. (a) The anterior view shows the upper limb of the curvature to be presenting horizontally. (b+c) The two lateral plain polytomography views illustrate the horizontal alignment of the curvature by virtue of the fact that one sees directly into the spinal canal. Even more impressive is the enlargement of the spinal canal, secondary to dural ectasia. One might note the inverse ratio of the widened canal and the anterior-posterior dimension of the verte-bral body reversed from its normal relationships. The A-P dimension of the body is usually up to twice the length of the canal.

With the large number of characteristics found in dystrophic curves, it would be ben-eficial to the patient and clinician to determine if one or more of these findings may be more predictive of those curves that are at greatest risk for progression. Funasaki's group, in 1994, found risk factors for substantial progression were early age of onset, a high Cobb angle at the first examination, an abnormal kyphosis, vertebral scalloping, severe rotation at the apex of the curve, location of the apex of the curve in the middle to caudal thoracic area, penciling of one rib or more on the concave side or on both sides of the curve, and penciling of four ribs or more (10). Based on 91 patients, a recent study made the following observations (25): (a) spinal deformity that develops before 7 years of age should be followed closely for evolving dystrophic features (modulation): (b) when a curve acquires either three penciled ribs or a combination of three dystrophic features, clinical progres-sion is almost a certainty.

D. Treatment of Dystrophic Curves

There is no justification to observe the dystrophic curve in NF-1 because it always pro-gresses (20,26). Studies have shown that curves treated with a Milwaukee brace progress

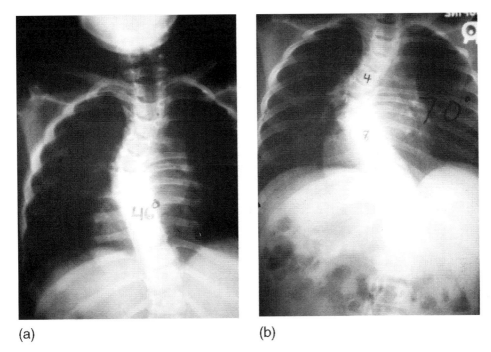

(a)   (b)

Figure 6 Progressive scoliosis in a very young child. The final deformity is short segmented, sharply angulated, and progressed 25 degrees over a $2\frac{1}{2}$-year period. (a) 46 degree thoracic curve at age 5 years 8 months. (b) 70 degree deformity at age 8 years 5 months illustrating more of the dysplastic characteristics. The curvature has modulated.

at a rate similar to those that are untreated (1). Early fusion is the best treatment. Fusion in the young individual stunts the growth of the truncal height only minimally because the curve is usually short with a poor growth potential in the involved vertebrae. The use of subcutaneous growing rods, in theory, would allow for further growth, although Mineiro and Weinstein questioned its value based on the small amount of growth achieved and number of procedures required (27). However only one of their patients had neurofibromatosis. More recent technological designs of universal instrumentation and localized fusion of anchor sites of "growing rods" may improve these results.

In spite of meticulous planning and treatment, major complications may occur with surgical treatment (31). Even in patients without neurological deficit, it is necessary to evaluate the contents of the spinal canal to minimize the possibility of neurological injury during correction. High-volume myelography or MRI can be used for identifying space occupying lesions.

A common recommendation is that curves between 20 and 40 degrees be fused posteriorly and instrumented from the neutral vertebra above to the neutral vertebra below (18,20,21). If the curve is more than 40 degrees or kyphosis is greater than 50 degrees, anterior surgery with discectomy and intervertebral fusion followed by posterior instrumentation and fusion is recommended. The current authors have used VATS to perform anterior release and fusion (Figure 7) (18).

Preoperative traction in severe curves with a flexible kyphosis is thought by Winter and coworkers to improve pulmonary function, improve minor neurological deficits, and diminish the curve before fusion (20) (Fig. 8). In 2002 Halmai and associates reported

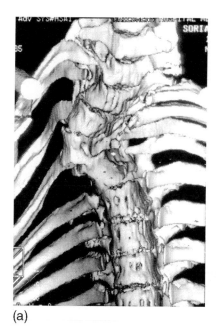

(a)

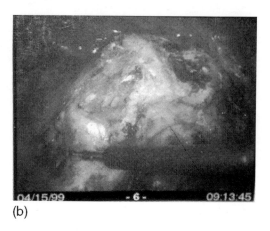

(b)

Figure 7   A 9-year-old child with dysplastic thoracic scoliosis who underwent anterior release and fusion by video-assisted thoracoscopic surgery. (a) Three-dimensional reconstructed CT illustrating significant rotation of the upper thoracic vertebra. (b) Thoracoscopic view of the anterior apical vertebra. The anterior longitudinal ligament has rotated completely posteriorly on the concave side and is attached to the concave rib heads. The vertebra appears to have spun around towards the convex side.

their protocol for treating dystrophic curves greater than 60 degrees using an average of 3 weeks of preoperative halo vest traction (28). They felt that the paraspinal ligaments and tissues in the intervertebral spaces would become less tight and more hydrated. This would assist in derotating the spine, which in turn would decrease the rate of intraoperative neurological complications. Careful neurological monitoring, especially motor strength, should be documented during periods of traction. The current authors recommend anterior release, N-J tube alimentation, and craniofemoral traction for rigid curves greater than 90 degrees. For curves greater than 100 degrees in any plane, anterior and posterior release is followed by tube alimentation and craniofemoral traction.

When posterior exposure is performed, careful decortication must be undertaken because erosion of the lamina is frequently seen due to dural ectasia. Dissection is often performed with electrocautery (Bovie dissection) because of the potential of plunging an elevator through a weakened lamina (29). Dural ectasia is an increase in the width of the thecal sac due to an increase in hydrostatic pressure that causes expansion, erosion, and ligamentous instability to the spinal canal and costovertebral complex. Meticulous fusion after decortication must be carried out using abundant bone graft over a broad area. Care should be taken to remove all soft tissue from interposition in the area of the bone graft (20,30). All the facet joints should be taken down, and autologous bone graft is preferred to bank bone. Instrumentation should be used when possible, but dystrophic vertebrae are not always good recipients for hooks because of osteoporosis and deformation of the posterior elements (26,32). Hook dislocation is therefore not infrequent. Pedicle screw anchors provides the best

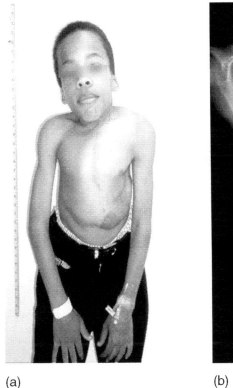
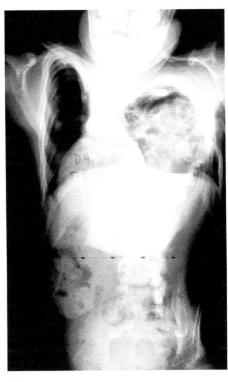

(a)   (b)

Figure 8 This 11-year-old child was referred with mild paraplegia after undergoing seven surgical procedures of the spine. The previous procedures were done with growing rods, which had been removed. (a) Frontal clinical view of the child showing significant café-au-lait spots as well as a plexiform neurofibroma over the left inferior-anterior rib cage. (b) PA of the thoracolumbar spine showing significant angular deformity in a hairpin turn of greater than 200 degrees. (c) A lateral clinical photograph of patient bending over illustrating the clinically significant kyphosis of the mid thoracic spine. In addition, there is a very large plexiform neurofibroma at the base of the kyphosis. (d) A standing lateral thoracolumbar sacral film illustrating the severe kyphosis in this child. Note at the mid-apical region there is an axial view of the spinal canal as one sees a cephalocaudal view. This confirms the fact that the severe rotation has caused the mid-portion of the spine to be horizontally positioned on this view.

foundation. In situ fusion and immobilization in a brace or cast is rarely necessary and represents a poor alternative.

If kyphoscoliosis is present (kyphosis > 50 degrees), anterior and posterior fusion should always be performed (18,20,21,33). When anterior fusion is performed, thorough intervertebral disk space exposure is extremely important. Fusion must be as long as possible, with the addition of strut-grafting. One should attempt to get the bone graft into the vertical weight–bearing axis of the torso (20). The recipient area should be well exposed (which is technically difficult due to severe apical rotation), and the strut graft that is inserted should be in contact with bone because graft material surrounded by neuro fibromatous soft tissue has a tendency to resorb. Multiple strut grafts should be used, and the fibula, being the strongest, should be placed most anteriorly. A rib graft

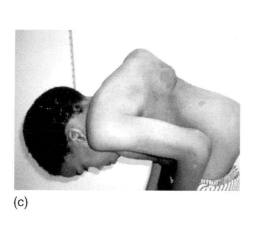

(c)

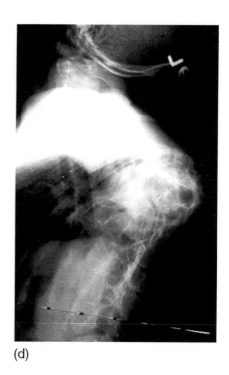

(d)

Figure 8 (*continued*)

swung on the vascular pedicle may also be helpful (24). The exposure is extremely difficult from the concave side, however, and often the apical vertebra may be subluxated or so severely rotated that it is not in alignment with the rest of the spine (34). Such malalignment makes it difficult to place anterior strut graft in the concavity of the kyphosis. Shufflebarger believes that the anterior procedure should be undertaken from the concave side with multiple strut grafts and that a convex discectomy would destabilize the spine (19). Others have not had a problem with the convex approach and continue to recommend it. Centers utilizing anterior and posterior release followed by craniofemoral traction for no less than 10 days have noted improved efficiency in obtaining correction of the kyphoscoliosis. Because of the ability to gain more correction with extensive release and traction, many surgeons are aggressive with anterior releases followed by posterior fusion.

In spite of rigid instrumentation, postoperative immobilization in NF-1 patients is always recommended in an effort to prevent pseudarthrosis (20). The external support should be maintained until a fusion mass with trabecular pattern is seen. Despite well-done surgery, pseudarthrosis with loss of correction is frequent, even in the hands of experienced spine surgeons. The reason for failure of the surgery is usually an inadequate anterior procedure. Crawford reported a 15% incidence of pseudarthrosis in 46 patients, and Sirois and coworkers reported a 31% incidence (18,35). Winter and associates had eight patients who underwent a planned two-stage anterior and posterior fusion (20). Of these, five healed, one died of respiratory complications and paraplegia, and two developed pseudarthrosis. The integrity of the fusion mass can be evaluated by bone scan, tomography, MRI, or second-look surgery about 6 months after the initial surgery. Sirois recommended planned 6-month reexploration and augmentation procedures in patients with an isolated posterior fusion (35).

Another complication during surgery may be bleeding. Soft tissue manifestations of NF-1 may complicate an otherwise well-planned surgery. Excessive plexiform venous channels are described around the vertebral bodies, making it difficult to access the vertebra (35). Soft tissue tumors from NF-1 may be highly vascular, so postoperative hematoma is not uncommon (20,35). Therefore, meticulous hemostasis must be carried out during surgery and hemovac drainage performed. Postoperative extradural hematoma causing paraplegia has been described (20,35).

Sirois reported complications that required additional surgery in 9 of 23 patients undergoing treatment of dystrophic curves (35). These included four reexplorations and augmentations 6 months postoperatively, two revisions for instrumentation dislocation, two extensions of the fusion mass for curve extension, and one multiple spinal osteotomy for increasing deformity despite a solid fusion mass for curve extension. In patients who are still growing, if anterior and posterior fusion is not done, there is an increased incidence of progression of the curve and the crankshaft phenomena. Additional reported and not infrequent complications include urinary tract infection, dural leak, and thrombophlebitis. After anterior surgery, pulmonary problems with pneumonia, atelectasis, and hemothorax may be seen. Ileus is observed especially during the period of time between staged anterior and posterior surgery, if the patient is kept in traction. The current authors strongly recommend N-J tube placement and hyperalimentation for all patients undergoing staged anterior posterior surgery.

IV. KYPHOSCOLIOSIS

Kyphoscoliosis is defined as a curve with 50 degrees or greater kyphosis. If kyphosis is present, appropriate dynamic x-rays, i.e., a hyperextension lateral over a bolster to evaluate the flexibility of the curve, should be performed. Paraplegia is not uncommon in patients with severe kyphosis. If a flexible kyphosis is causing paraplegia, the treatment should be halo-assisted traction (but with extreme caution), with close neurological or evoked potential monitoring during the course of the traction (18,36). An MRI of all patients with paraplegia to rule out rib protrusion into the spinal canal is mandatory (37–39).

If the kyphosis is flexible, the traction will correct some of the kyphosis and also reduce cord compression and possibly improve the neurological deficit (31) (Fig. 9). Following traction, anterior spinal cord decompression and fusion should be performed, followed by a posterior fusion. Deep hemovac drainage is necessary in all patients having anterior reconstructive surgery because of significant bleeding that may occur once the patient is normotensive. These patients should also be observed carefully afterward for the development of pseudarthrosis. Augmentation of the fusion mass should be performed at 6 months if pseudarthrosis is suspected because of loss of correction.

If the kyphosis is rigid, traction should not be used (36). Traction in these cases stretches the mobile spinal segments above and below the kyphosis, increasing the tension and point compression on the mid-apical spinal cord, which may cause further damage. Therefore, direct anterior release, disk excision, and intervertebral fusion followed by 7–10 days of traction and then posterior spine fusion is recommended. The vertebral bodies are occasionally extremely porotic and will tend to bleed freely from

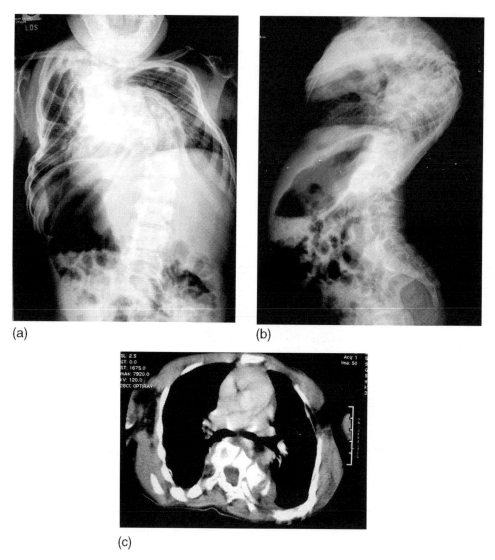

(a)   (b)

(c)

Figure 9 Pre- and postoperative x-rays of a 5-year-old child with severe dystrophic kyphoscoliosis. This child underwent bilateral open trapdoor procedures of the anterior cervicothoracic region, posterior soft tissue release, and cranio-femoral traction to achieve correction of her severe deformity. A posterior cervical–thoracic fusion using pediatric Isola growing rods was performed following 2 weeks of traction. (a) Frontal view illustrating the severe left cervical thoracic kyphoscoliosis. There was dural ectasia with widening of the thoracic canal and penetration of three ribs into the spinal canal. (b) Standing preoperative lateral cervical thoracolumbar sacral x-ray illustrating the severe kyphotic deformity in this child. (c) Axial MRI of thoracic spine at mid-apical region illustrating severity of deformity with three horizontal vertebra (lateral projection) and head of a rib in the spinal canal. (d) Postoperative posterior-anterior cervical thoracolumbar spine x-ray revealing the instrumentation construct, as well as the nasojejunal tube used to provide hyperalimentation for this child. (e) Standing lateral cervical/thoracolumbar x-ray illustrating the instrumentation construct. Note the stainless steel wire closures of the sternum following the trapdoor procedure, the nasojejunal tube for hyperalimentation, and a Medipore. The child was placed in a Minerva cast for additional immobilization.

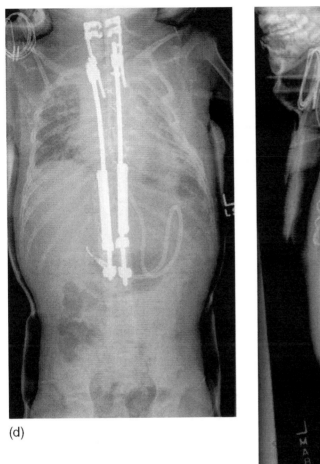

(d)

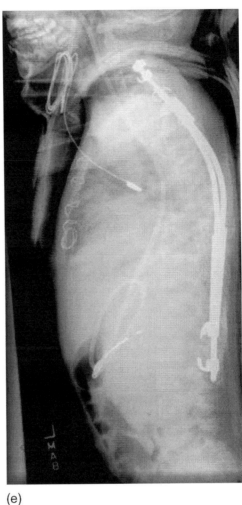

(e)

Figure 9 (*continued*)

the cancellous surfaces. The endplate is the strongest portion and should be protected with a meticulous anulus and discal release. Plenty of bone graft needs to be available.

Because of the association between paraplegia and kyphoscoliosis, there is a tendency to perform laminectomies to relieve pressure from the cord. Laminectomy only for cord compression in kyphoscoliosis is contraindicated, however (18,36). Occasionally, a neurological improvement may be seen after a posterior approach with incision of the dura because this may release pressure on the cord. Laminectomy does not completely decompress the spine because the compression is anterior and removal of bone posteriorly destabilizes the spine potentially increasing the kyphosis. Laminectomy alone also removes valuable bone stock required for a posterior spinal fusion. Occasionally paraplegia is related to protrusion of a rib into the spinal canal (Figure 10). This will usually be evident on CT or MRI. Removal of this protrusion should prevent neuropathy progression.

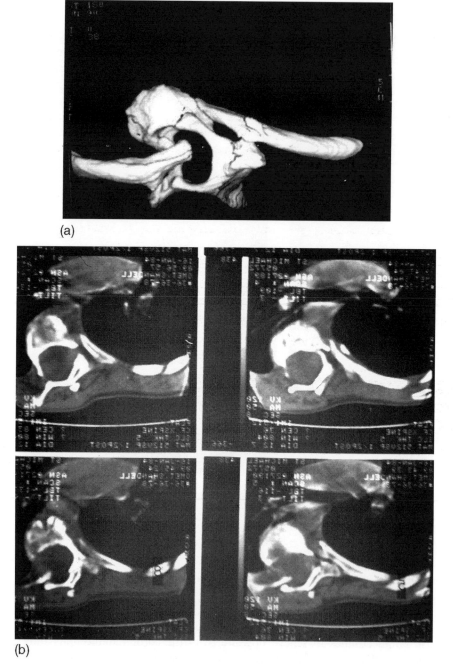

(a)

(b)

Figure 10 A three-dimensional reconstructed view of a mid-thoracic level as well as a CT, both illustrating significant spinal deformity, protrusion of the rib head into the vertebral canal, and widening of the canal secondary to dural ectasia. (a) The rib head has protruded into the very widened spinal canal, which has been expanded secondary to dural ectasia (Courtesy of Steve Tredwell Vancouver, BC). (b) Several axial CT images showing the erosive effects of dural ectasia. There is significant widening of the spinal canal and erosion of the lamina, transverse processes and pedicle on the right has permitted displacement of a rib into the canal.

V. PARAPLEGIA

Paraplegia is not an infrequent complication of spine deformities in NF-1 (16). The neurological compromise may be related to spinal deformity, instability of the costovertebral complex causing direct protrusion of a rib into the spinal cord, vertebral angulation, tumor, or dural ectasia. Paraplegia presenting in a younger age group is frequently caused by spinal deformity and in the older age group by tumor. Paraplegia after corrective surgery is often due to the compression exerted on the spinal cord by ischemia following hematoma are instruments occupying the intraspinal space. Rarely reported is the patient who presents with paraparesis due to rib displacement. This may have an insidious onset or may occur after a trauma (38). Bony dysplasia, intervertebral foraminal enlargement, and rotation of vertebral bodies all may contribute mechanically to allow the heads of the ribs to displace into the spinal canal. Increased kyphosis leads to excessive axial tension on the spinal cord and especially on the posterior dura, which compresses the spinal cord against the anterior vertebral body. Paraplegia is rare in a pure scoliotic curve; if present, a work-up for intraspinal pathology should be done. If paraplegia is present, MRI or CT myelogram is appropriate to find

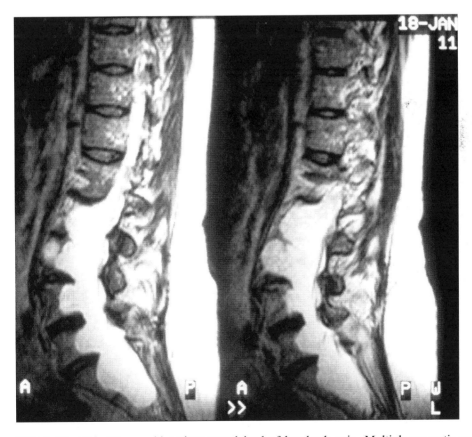

Figure 11 This 47-year-old patient complained of low-back pain. Multiple magnetic resonance images illustrate significant erosion of the lower lumbosacral spine from dural ectasia. (Courtesy of Dr. Courtney Brown, Denver, Colorado.)

the cause of paraplegia. With a severe deformity, interpretation of these images can be confusing, however, and often inconclusive.

Radicular symptoms have been reported, as well, due to vertebral arteriovenous fistulas (40). The most common form is a dural AV fistula sited in the sleeve of the thoracolumbar nerve root. Kahara reported recently of a posttraumatic AV fistula which caused radicular symptoms due to a mass effect of the dilated epidural venous space (40).

Prior to surgery the source of paraparesis, paraplegia or radiculopathy needs to be thoroughly investigated so that the surgeon is prepared to perform the necessary surgery and have the appropriate assistance available.

VI. SPONDYLOLISTHESIS

Spondylolisthesis in patients with NF-1 is rare (41–44). Spondylolisthesis is usually secondary to increased anteroposterior diameter of the spinal canal, with elongation and thinning of the pedicles, causing a pathological forward progression of the anterior

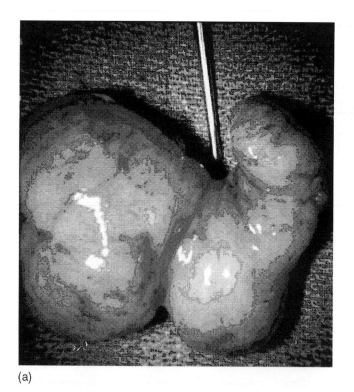

(a)

Figure 12 Example of a dumbbell tumor (neurofibroma) removed from the neural foramina at the time of surgery and a CT showing the neurofibroma in situ and an adjacent rib protruding into the spinal canal. (a) Dumbbell neurofibroma—the dumbbell appearance refers to the constriction of the neurofibroma that occurs where the lesion exits the neuraforamen. (b) The middle image of panel two shows the soft tissue shadow exiting the neural canal. The first image of panel three shows a rib to have protruded into the spinal canal. The child is asymptomatic.

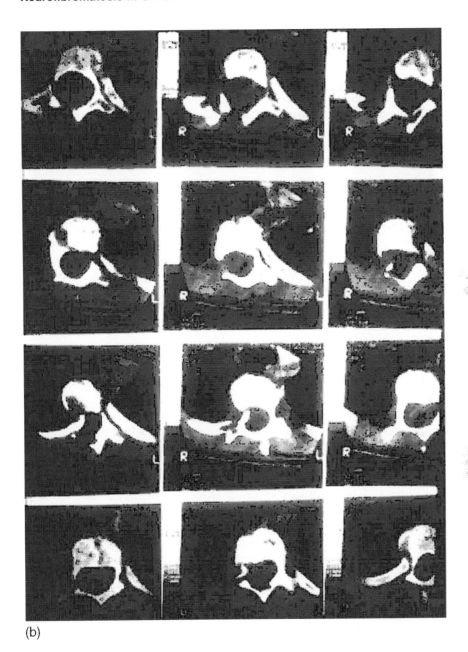

(b)

Figure 12 (*continued*)

elements of the spinal column. The causes of pathological instability are frequently dural ectasia, meningocele, and neurofibroma. Magnetic resonance imaging or CT/contrast scans are absolutely necessary for preoperative evaluation. The treatment in severe slips is anterior and posterior spinal fusion. Fusion is difficult to obtain because of the mechanical alignment of the lumbosacral region and poor bone formation. Often an L4-sacrum anterior and posterior fusion with lumbosacral instrumentation is recommended. Postoperative immobilization is also strongly recommended.

VII. SPINAL CANAL PATHOLOGY

A. Dural Ectasia and Intrathoracic Meningocele

A unique finding in NF-1 is dural ectasia. This is an expansion of the dural sac from an unknown etiology (45). Magnetic resonance imaging or high-volume CT myelography may distinguish dural ectasia from tumors. The expanding dura may cause erosion of the vertebral body and later, destabilization of the spine, with possible spontaneous dislocation (46–49) (Fig. 11). Dural ectasia may in some cases be so expansive to the spinal canal that the spinal cord is not injured, even if spine dislocation has developed. The treatment of dislocation is neurologically monitored traction, followed by fusion.

Meningocele is a protrusion of the spinal meninges through the intervertebral foramen or through an erosion of the vertebral body (49–55). It contains a subarachnoidal space filled with cerebrospinal fluid and causes a paravertebral cystic swelling. It is usually located in the thoracic spine. Meningocele and dural ectasia are a variation of the same phenomena, meningocele being more localized. Meningocele may often be an incidental finding on chest x-ray or symptoms such as pain or neurological compromise may be seen. If an intrathoracic meningocele expands, causing pressure on adjacent structures, it may cause coughing or dyspnea (55). If the symptomatic meningocele is massive, it should be approached, ligated and/or removed.

B. Dumbbell Lesion

A dumbbell lesion is a solitary neurofibroma that is constricted as it exits the neural foramen. The constriction gives the neurofibroma the appearance of a weightlifter's dumbbell (Fig. 12). With continued growth, erosion and widening of the intervertebral foramen occur. Erosion may, however, also be caused by meningocele, and MRI may be helpful to distinguish between the two. Spinal canal neurofibromas may be intradural or extradural and are most commonly seen in the cervical and thoracic level (56). It is recommended to fuse early in those patients who had a laminectomy for resection of a spinal canal tumor to prevent spinal column instability, usually kyphosis. Other tumors may come from the nerve sheath or from the nerve itself, presenting as interstitial hypertrophy, in which case the nerve is the tumor and the tumor is the nerve. The neurofibroma is usually benign, but it may cause complications by its local growth. The intraspinal portion of the tumor may cause cord compression and root failure. The peripheral tumor may create compression of blood vessels, nerves, lung, and pleura (56). Resection of the tumor originating from the nerve may result in a neurological loss. Patients need to be advised of this possible neurological deficit prior to surgery. Neurofibromas should be monitored for growth and pain symptoms possibly heralding malignant degeneration.

REFERENCES

1. Pulst SM. Prenatal diagnosis of the neurofibromatoses. Clin Perinatol 1990; 17(4):829–844.
2. Crawford A. Neurofibromatosis. In: SL Weinstein, ed. The Pediatric Spine: Principles and Practice. New York: Raven Press, 1994:619–649.
3. Goldberg NS, Collins FS. The hunt for the neurofibromatosis gene. Arch Dermatol 1991; 127(11):1705–1707.
4. Holt J. Neurofibromatosis in children. Am J Roentgenol 1978; 130:615.
5. Huson SM. Recent developments in the diagnosis and management of neurofibromatosis. Arch Dis Child 1989; 64(5):745–749.

6. National Institutes of Health Consensus Development Conference Statement: Neurofibromatosis. Neurofibromatosis 1988; 1:172.
7. Listernick R, Charrow J. Neurofibromatosis type 1 in childhood. J Pediatr 1990; 116(6): 845–853.
8. Riccardi VM, Kleiner B. Neurofibromatosis: a neoplastic birth defect with two age peaks of severe problems. Birth Defects Orig Artic Ser 1977; 13(3C):131–138.
9. Akbarnia BA, et al. Prevalence of scoliosis in neurofibromatosis. Spine 1992; 17(8 suppl): S244–248.
10. Funasaki H, Winter RB, Lonstein JB, Denis F. Pathophysiology of spinal deformities in neurofibromatosis. J Bone Joint Surg (Am) 1994; 76:692–700.
11. Rozaian S. The Incidence of scoliosis due to neurofibromatosis. acta orthop scand 1976; 147:534–539.
12. Heard GE, HJ, Naylor B. Cervical vertebral deformity in Von Recklinghausen's disease of the nervous system. J Bone Joint Surg Br 1962; 44:880.
13. Yong-Hing K, Kalamchi A, MacEwen GD. Cervical spine abnormalities in neurofibromatosis. J Bone Joint Surg Am 1979; 61(5):695–699.
14. Ogilvie JW. Neurofibromatosis. In: Bradford DS-Moe's Textbook of Scoliosis and Other Spinal Deformities. 3rd. Philadelphia: W. B. Saunders Co, 1995:338–347.
15. Holt J. The radiologic features of neurofibromatosis. Radiology 1948; 51:647.
16. Curtis BH, FR, Butterfield WL, Saunders FP. Neurofibromatosis with paraplegia. J Bone Joint Surg Am 1969; 51:843.
17. Isu T, et al. Atlantoaxial dislocation associated with neurofibromatosis. Report of three cases. J Neurosurg 1983; 58(3):451–453.
18. Crawford AH. Neurofibromatosis in children. Acta Orthop Scand Suppl 1986; 218:1–60.
19. Shufflebarger HL. Cotrel-Dubousset instrumentation in neurofibromatosis spinal problems. Clin Orthop 1989; 245:24–28.
20. Winter RB, et al. Spine deformity in neurofibromatosis. A review of one hundred and two patients. J Bone Joint Surg Am 1979; 61(5):677–694.
21. Crawford AH. Pitfalls of spinal deformities associated with neurofibromatosis in children. Clin Orthop 1989; 245:29–42.
22. Crawford AH. Neurofibromatosis in the pediatric patient. Orthop Clin North Am 1978; 9(1):11–23.
23. Hunt JC, Pugh DG. Skeletal lesion in neurofibromatosis. Radiology 1961; 76:1–19.
24. Winter RB, Lonstein JE, Anderson M. Neurofibromatosis hyperkyphosis: a review of 33 patients with kyphosis of 80 degrees or greater. J Spinal Disord 1988; 1(1):39–49.
25. Durrani AA, Crawford AH, Choudhury SN, Saifuddin A, Morley TR. Modulation of spinal deformities in patients with neurofibromatosis type 1. Spine 2000; 25(1):69–75.
26. Savini R, PP, Cervellati S, Gualdreini G. Surgical treatment of vertebral deformities in neurofibromatosis. Ital J Orthop Traumatol 1989; 15:13.
27. Minerio J, WS. Subcutaneous rodding for progressive spinal curvatures: early results. J Pediatr Orthop 2002; 22:290–295.
28. Halmai V, et al. Surgical treatment of spinal deformities associated with neurofibromatosis type 1. Report of 12 cases. J Neurosurg 2002; 97(3 suppl):310–316.
29. Kumar K, Crawford AH. Role of "Bovie" in spinal surgery: historical and analytical perspective. Spine 2002; 27(9):1000–1006.
30. Weiss RS. Von Recklinghausen's disease in the negro: curvature of the spine in Von Recklinghausen's disease. Arch Dermat Syph 1921; 3:144.
31. Jacobsen FS, CA, Crawford AH. Complications in neurofibromatosis. In: BJ, Epps CH, eds. Complications in Pediatric Orthopaedic Surgery. Philadelphia: Lippincott Company, 1995:649–683.
32. Konishi, K, et al. Hypophosphatemic osteomalacia in von Recklinghausen neurofibromatosis. Am J Med Sci 1991; 301(5):322–328.

33. Holt RT, Johnson JR. Cotrel-Dubousset instrumentation in neurofibromatosis spine curves.
     A preliminary report. Clin Orthop 1989; 245:19–23.
34. Hsu LC, Lee PC, Leong JC. Dystrophic spinal deformities in neurofibromatosis. Treatment by
     anterior and posterior fusion. J Bone Joint Surg Br 1984; 66(4):495–499.
35. Sirois JL, 3rd and J.C. Drennan, Dystrophic spinal deformity in neurofibromatosis. J Pediatr
     Orthop 1990; 10(4):522–526.
36. Lonstein JE, et al. Neurologic deficits secondary to spinal deformity. A review of the literature
     and report of 43 cases. Spine 1980; 5(4):331–355.
37. Flood BM, Butt WP, Dickson RA. Rib penetration of the intervertebral foraminae in neuro-
     fibromatosis. Spine 1986; 11(2):172–174.
38. Major MR, Huizenga BA. Spinal cord compression by displaced ribs in neurofibromatosis.
     A report of three cases. J Bone Joint Surg Am 1988; 70(7):1100–1102.
39. Khoshhal KI, Ellis RD. Paraparesis after posterior spinal fusion in neurofibromatosis second-
     ary to rib displacement: case report and literature review. J Pediatr Orthop 2000; 20(6):
     799–801.
40. Kahara V, et al. Vertebral epidural arteriovenous fistula and radicular pain in neurofibroma-
     tosis type I. Acta Neurochir (Wien) 2002; 144(5):493–496.
41. Crawford AH, Bagamery N. Osseous manifestations of neurofibromatosis in childhood.
     J Pediatric Orthop. 1986; 6:72.
42. Mandell GA. The pedicle in neurofibromatosis. AJR Am J Roentgenol 1978; 130(4):675–678.
43. Wong-Chung J, Gillespie R. Lumbosacral spondyloptosis with neurofibromatosis. Case report.
     Spine 1991; 16(8):986–988.
44. Winter RB, Edwards WC. Case report. Neurofibromatosis with lumbosacral spondylolisthesis.
     J Pediatr Orthop 1981; 1(1):91–96.
45. Klatte EC, Franken EA, Smith JA. The radiographic spectrum in neurofibromatosis. Semin
     Roentgenol 1976; 11(1):17–33.
46. Rockower S, McKay D, Nason S. Dislocation of the spine in neurofibromatosis. A report of
     two cases. J Bone Joint Surg Am 1982; 64(8):1240–1242.
47. Hvorslev V, Reiter S. A case of neurofibromatosis with severe osseous disease of the thoracic
     spine. Pediatr Radiol 1979; 8(4):251–253.
48. Stone JW, et al. Dural ectasia associated with spontaneous dislocation of the upper part of the
     thoracic spine in neurofibromatosis. A case report and review of the literature. J Bone Joint
     Surg Am 1987; 69(7):1079–1083.
49. Winter RB. Spontaneous dislocation of a vertebra in a patient who had neurofibromatosis.
     Report of a case with dural ectasia. J Bone Joint Surg Am 1991; 73(9):1402–1404.
50. Erkulvrawatr S, et al. Intrathoracic meningoceles and neurofibromatosis. Arch Neurol 1979;
     36(9):557–559.
51. Lipmann KAW. Intrathoracic meningocele, spinal deformity, and multiple neurofibromatosis.
     J Bone Joint Surg Am 1951; 33:87.
52. Nanson EM. Thoracic meningocele associated with neurofibromatosis. J Thorac Surg 1957;
     33:650.
53. Sengpiel GW, Ruzicka F, Lodmell EA. Lateral intrathoracic meningocele. Radiology 1948;
     50:515.
54. YaDeau RE, Clagett OT, Divertie MB. Intrathoracic meningocele. J Thorac Cardiovasc 1965;
     49:202.
55. Miles J, Pennybacker J, Sheldon P. Intrathoracic meningocele. Its development and association
     with neurofibromatosis. J Neurol Neurosurg Psychiatry 1969; 32(2):99–110.
56. Love DH, Dodge H. Dumbbell (hourglass) Neurofibromas affecting the spinal cord. Surg
     Gynecol Obstet 1952; 94:161.

45

Optimum Patient Selection

Richard P. Schlenk and Gordon R. Bell
Cleveland Clinic Foundation, Cleveland, Ohio, U.S.A.

I. INTRODUCTION

Determining which patients are most likely to achieve pain relief and functional improvement from spine surgery is a challenge even to the most experienced spine surgeon. The critical decision of whether and when to operate requires an understanding of the natural history of the condition, the likely outcome following surgery, and the factors that predict outcome. Predicting which patients are unlikely to benefit from surgery is important in order to prevent failed back syndrome and the development of chronic pain. The spine surgeon must identify those prognostic factors that will discriminate between patients who are likely to have favorable outcome following surgery and those who are not. This will enable patients and spine surgeons to have realistic expectations of the outcome following surgery.

The physical examination and radiographic assessment are the most objective measures available to the surgeon and form the basis of the surgical decision-making process. Although the preoperative physical examination and radiographic assessment can predict which patients are likely to do well after surgery, they are not the sole predictors of surgical outcome. Complications during surgery and inappropriate peri-operative management may certainly play a significant role in determining clinical outcome. Nevertheless, these factors do not explain why some operated patients, in whom technical goals of surgery are achieved, fail to achieve expected outcome.

Clinical results are determined by factors related not only to the physical illness, but also to emotional issues, social issues, lifestyle, and motivation for improvement. Proper attention should be paid to these other prognostic factors, which may play a significant role in outcomes. Non-organic clinical signs further help the clinician identify those patients who are unlikely to benefit from spine surgery (120). Worker's compensation and litigation factors also play a significant role in the outcome following spine surgery. Knowledge of how various psychological measures are utilized will assist the clinician in outcome prediction for patients with spinal disorders. Appropriate patient selection for spine surgery is therefore a dynamic process that requires consideration of all clinical, radiographic, social, and psychological factors in the decision-making process.

II. CLINICAL AND RADIOGRAPHIC PREDICTORS

In constructing a treatment strategy for pain related to spinal disorders it is essential that the source of pain be accurately identified. Identifying the etiology of radicular symptoms is more likely than identifying the cause of lower back pain. Accurate localization of the source of back pain may not be possible (84). Many anatomical structures, including the outer layers of the anulus fibrosus, facet joints, ligaments, muscles, and tendons, are potential sources for pain, and it is difficult to determine which spinal components might be pain generators (12). Without the ability to accurately localize which, if any, of these potential structures is responsible for back pain, it is difficult to know which structure or combination of structures should be treated. With nonspecific forms of conservative therapy, precise knowledge of the genesis of back pain may not be important. With surgical treatment, however, accurate localization of the pain is vital to the success of surgery. This fact underscores the unreliability of surgical procedures to cure low back pain, since failure lies as much in diagnosis as in treatment.

A. Lumbar Herniation

Objective clinical findings are an important parameter in the overall evaluation of a patient with a suspected herniated disk. The ability to prove that radicular pain is due to nerve root compression depends upon the demonstration of a neurological deficit or root tension sign and its confirmation by an objective imaging test (52,96). Relief of radicular pain can be treated successfully with surgery if it can be shown to have a compressive etiology (95). Spangfort performed a retrospective analysis of 2504 lumbar discectomies (102). He reported a direct correlation between physical, radiographic, and operative findings with clinical outcomes. The presence of a positive straight leg raising sign highly correlated with the degree of disk herniation. Patients who exclusively had back pain without radicular leg pain were reported to have a poorer outcome. Distinctly positive myelograms correctly predicted the presence of intraoperative pathology in 82% of patients. However, the single most important factor that predicted good outcome was the degree of disk herniation found at the time of operation. In other words, patients with a large herniation causing definite nerve root compression did much better following surgery than did patients having no herniation or a small herniation with minimal or no nerve root compression. Moreover, Spangfort also found that the outcomes after an exploration of a lumbar disk with negative findings were worse than the results of nonoperated conservative management. Hakelius (40) and Weber (123) confirmed that improper patient selection for lumbar disk surgery may be a major contributor to the development of chronic low back pain.

It is important to accurately and preoperatively predict which patients will have large protrusions causing definitive nerve compression that have a high likelihood of clinical improvement following surgery. Hirsch and Nachemson (52), in a study of 232 surgically proven disk herniations, demonstrated that the ability to correctly predict the presence of a herniated disk was 55% when diagnosis was based only upon the presence of an objective neurological finding. Accuracy increased slightly to 66% when the only clinical abnormality was a positive straight leg raising (SLR) sign. When an objective neurological abnormality was combined with a positive SLR sign, however, the ability to predict correctly the presence of a disk herniation increased to 86%. Finally, when both a positive neurological finding and a positive SLR sign were combined with a myelogram revealing a prolapse at a level consistent with the observed clinical findings, the chance of finding

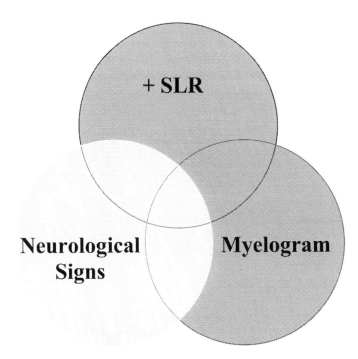

Figure 1 Venn diagram showing logic involved with surgical decision making for herniated lumbar disk. Surgery is likely to be palliative for pain when positive straight leg raising sign (+SLR), objective neurological signs, and a positive myelogram are all present.

a disk herniation at surgery was 95%. The importance of demonstrating an overlap of clinical and radiographic features of lumbar disk herniation is illustrated by a Venn diagram (Fig. 1).

Successful outcome following lumbar disk surgery has been reported to be between 49 and 97% (5,10,26,88). Patients who undergo lumbar discetomy for removal of a herniated lumbar disk have shown better short-term outcomes when compared with patients treated nonoperatively. However, the superiority of surgery over conservative treatment in the long term is not as clear. Weber randomized 126 patients with suspected lumbar disk herniation: half were operated on and the other half treated conservatively (123). At 1-year follow-up outcome was better in the operated group, but at 4 years and 10 years the difference between the two groups was not statistically different. However, a subgroup of patients "crossed over" from the conservative to the surgical group, and favorable outcomes of the conservative group may therefore have been overestimated. Other studies have demonstrated less favorable long-term outcome following surgery for lumbar disk herniation. Dvorak et al. performed a long-term retrospective study evaluating results 4–17 years after lumbar disk removal (27,60). Of the 371 patients reviewed, 70% reported occasional back pain, 23% significant back or leg pain, 44% residual sciatica, and 35% were under some kind of medical treatment. In addition, 14% were receiving disability and 17% had undergone a second back operation. Junge et al. followed patients 2 years after lumbar discectomy and observed good results in only 53%, moderate relief in 19%, and poor outcome in 28% (60).

The presence of nonorganic findings has been demonstrated to have a significant negative predictive value on patient outcome after lumbar disk surgery (59,105).

Neurological signs, sciatic tension signs, imaging studies, and absence of psychological factors have high predictive values for successful outcome when collectively considered. Based on strict selection criteria, Spengler et al. chose 84 patients for primary lumbar discectomy out of approximately 3600 patients (105). Utilizing an objective scoring system based upon a combination of physical signs, radiographic findings, and psychological measures, the presence of a lumbar disk herniation at the time of operation was successfully predicted in 81 of 84 patients. Junge et al. evaluated 381 patients who underwent lumbar discectomy and assessed multiple clinical, social, and psychological factors to determine which were predictive of outcome (59). Calculated predictors included physical mobility, duration of pain and disability, number of other pain locations, visual analog pain scale (VAS), disability pension, job level, depression, and diagnostic imaging. Utilizing these prognosticators, outcomes were correctly predicted in 79% of the patients with "bad" outcomes and 75% of patients with "good" outcomes. Patients with disabling radicular pain associated with nerve root tension signs had the best response to surgery, while those with primarily back pain had worse outcomes. Factors such as longstanding preoperative disability, multiple other painful regions in the body, and menial job level were also found to be associated with poor outcomes. The authors concluded that if predictive scores suggested a poor outcome, the indication for operation should be reevaluated via a multidisciplinary approach.

Prolonged duration of preoperative symptoms secondary to lumbar disk herniation has been reported to be a predictor of poor surgical outcome(54,87). Nygaard retrospectively reviewed 93 patients operated on for lumbar disk herniation (54,87). The duration of sciatic pain prior to surgery was significantly greater in the group with unsatisfactory outcome than in those with successful outcome. Patients with duration of sciatica of less than 6 months had significantly better outcomes compared with patients having symptoms of 6–12 months duration. Patients with symptoms more than 12 months duration had the poorest outcome. Kotilainen et al. reviewed 237 patients who underwent lumbar microdiscectomy and found that the mean duration of preoperative sciatica was 3.8 months in patients who finally returned to work compared to 6.3 months in those patients who did not return to work (69). Nygaard et al. also showed that protracted leg pain (lasting more than 8 months) correlated not only with unfavorable surgical outcome, but with failure to return to work (86). Length of preoperative sick leave has been reported to have direct effect on returning to work. Nygaard et al. found that those who returned to the same type of work postoperatively had a shorter duration of sick leave prior to surgery. Many factors including duration of conservative management, the patient's willingness to undergo surgery, and the insurance company's willingness to authorize surgery all play significant roles in the timing of surgical intervention. The reasons why prolonged preoperative symptoms are associated with less favorable outcomes remain unclear. Increased duration of symptoms may have important associations with neuronal injury, the acquisition of psychological factors associated with chronic pain syndromes, secondary gain issues, the development of narcotic addiction, and other factors known to be related with poor surgical outcome.

B. Lumbar Stenosis

Degenerative lumbar spinal stenosis is a frequent indication for spine surgery in the elderly. However, between 20 and 40% of patients who have surgery for spinal stenosis fail to benefit from surgery (1,58,62–65,99,111). As with lumbar disk herniation, the presence of back pain as the major preoperative symptom is a risk factor for poor outcome following surgery. Airaksinen et al. looked at preoperative factors on 438 patients who underwent decompressive surgery for lumbar stenosis (1). They demonstrated that clear myelographic stenosis and no history of prior surgical intervention were factors associated with a good surgical outcome. The presence of diminished canal cross-sectional area by computed tomography (CT) and magnetic resonance imaging (MRI) has been shown in some studies to have a definite relationship with symptoms of neurogenic claudication (17,41,126). Hamanishi et al. reported that a cross-sectional area less than $100\,mm^2$ at two or more intervertebral levels was highly associated with claudication symptoms (41). However, others have failed to demonstrate such a relationship (4,77). There is convincing evidence that two-level lumbar stenosis induces neurogenic claudication more frequently than single-level stenosis (17,89,126). Porter and Ward reviewed 49 patients clinically diagnosed with neurogenic claudication who underwent myelography and CT (89). Multilevel central canal stenosis or stenosis of both central and root canals was radiographically demonstrate in 46 of 49 patients. The authors hypothesized that the pathophysiology of neurogenic claudication is a result of two-level venous compression, with venous pooling of one or several nerve roots.

The risks and benefits of surgical decompression must be weighed against the natural history of lumbar stenosis. Johnsson et al. reported on 32 patients with lumbar stenosis who were conservatively managed for an average of 49 months (56,90). These patients had indications for decompression but refused surgery or were not cleared medically for an operation. At final follow-up, 41% of patients improved, 41% were unchanged, and 18% worsened. Walking capacity was improved in 37%, unchanged in 33%, and worse in 30%. Pain as measured by the VAS was unchanged in 70%. These results suggest that most patients either improve or remain unchanged and are unlikely to worsen if managed conservatively. Jonsson et al. compared surgical versus nonsurgical treatment for lumbar spinal stenosis (57,58). In a group of 44 patients treated surgically, clinical improvement was seen in 59% compared to 32% improvement in 19 patients treated conservatively. However, a greater percentage of patients were worse after surgery compared with nonoperative patients, 25% vs. 10%. Katz et al reviewed 88 patients undergoing laminectomy for lumbar stenosis and found poorer outcomes than had been previously reported (64). At one-year follow-up 11% of patients had poor outcome, while 43% had poor outcome at a minimum of 3-year follow-up. Severe pain was noted in 30% of patients, and 17% of patients required a second operation. Limited function was found in 35%, and an inability to walk 50 feet was present in 21%. There was a direct relationship between number of comorbidities and poorer outcome. The most common comorbidities associated with lumbar stenosis were osteoarthritis (32%), cardiac disease (22%), rheumatoid arthritis (10%), and chronic pulmonary disease (7%) (64). Their data demonstrated a cumulative effect of comorbidities, as no single comorbidity was significantly associated with a worse outcome. Katz et al. utilized a questionnaire in a long-term follow-up study of the 88 patients in the original cohort (63). At 7–10 years after surgery, 23% were deceased and 23% had undergone reoperation. Of the respondents, 33% had severe back pain and 53% were unable to walk two blocks. Patient perceptions of their own medical condition may have an effect on outcome after surgery for spinal stenosis. Katz et al. reported 199 patients with degenerative lumbar spinal stenosis and found that the most powerful predictor of greater walking capacity, milder symptoms, and greater satisfaction was the patient's perception of good or excellent health before surgery (66).

C. Degenerative Disk Disease

Low back pain (LBP) from presumed degenerative disk disease (DDD) remains an entity with historically low success rates from surgical intervention (25,37,38,72,125). Identifying a pain generator with patients with LBP is a difficult challenge (110). This is especially true in distinguishing patients with myofascial pain from those with symptomatic DDD. Myofascial pain tends to be associated with a sudden onset and improves with time. The onset of symptoms related to DDD is likely to be associated with an acute event, but symptoms tend to progress. Pain associated with DDD typically has a mechanical character. Patients frequently complain of sitting intolerance but have relief of symptoms when either reclined or lying.

DDD is a radiographic diagnosis best identified by the use of MRI. Early degenerative disk changes result in loss of hydration of the disk with resultant dark or isointense signal changes on T2-weighted images (81). As DDD progresses, endplate changes from an in-growth of vascularized fibrous tissue or from peridiscal marrow fatty degeneration may be evident on MRI (81–83). However, these changes on MRI do not necessarily correlate with LBP and are commonly present in the asymptomatic population. Boden et al. found that degenerative disks were present in 34% of asymptomatic patients 20–29 years old and in 93% of patients 60–80 years old (16). Correlating LBP with radiographic evidence of DDD remains elusive.

The use of discography as a provocative tool to assess the intervertebral disk as a potential pain generator is controversial. A concordant pain response requires the replication of the patient's pain upon injection of the degenerated disk, with a negative response at a normal level serving as a control. Holt performed lumbar discography on three levels in 30 asymptomatic patients. He reported that 37% of previously asymptomatic volunteers had positive discography (53). Although pain-related responses were noted, the criteria used for positive discography were solely determined by the presence of morphological abnormalities. Pain was demonstrated in 26% of discograms in asymptomatic subjects. Critics point out Holt's 24% incidence of misplacement of needle into the disk space using plain radiographs for guidance and argue that "correct" needle placement may have resulted in the anulus and not the disk nucleus being pressurized (100). Furthermore, the use of the contrast agent Hypaque in discography may have increased the incidence of false-positive responses. Hypaque, an irritant contrast material, when injected into ruptured disks may leak and come into direct contact with a nerve root, causing a false-positive pain response (100,122). If patients with herniated disks are removed from Holt's study, the false-positive rate is reduced to 4%. Walsh modified Holt's technique, utilizing a water-soluble agent injected under fluoroscopic guidance, in 7 patients who had low-back pain and in 10 asymptomatic volunteers (122). Injection at three levels was performed in both groups and all sessions were videotaped. They demonstrated a 0% false-positive rate for discography in asymptomatic subjects compared to 35% of symptomatic patients. Colhoun et al. retrospectively reviewed 195 patients 2 years after a technically successful lumbar fusion (21). They found that 89% of patients with provocative discography had significant and sustained benefit from fusion at the indicated level. Of 25 patients who had a discogram demonstrating morphological abnormality without provocation of pain, only 52% experienced good results after fusion. In contrast, others have demonstrated that discography has little value in predicting the outcome of spinal fusion (31). Schneiderman et al. found a high correlation between MRI and positive discography (97). Thirty-nine disks were evaluated by discography and compared with MRI findings. MRI was 99% accurate in predicting morphological normality or abnormality as determined by discography. However, others have not found such consistencies between MRI and discography. Discography has not been shown to be predictive of pain in patients with normal lumbar MRI.

The role of arthrodesis in the treatment of degenerative disorders of the lumbar spine remains a debated topic. Most patients with DDD can be successfully treated nonoperatively. Despite the ease of making a radiographic diagnosis of DDD, there are no findings that are pathognomonic for the diagnosis of clinically symptomatic DDD. Therefore, if the history, physical exam, and radiographic images are consistent with symptomatic DDD, surgery should only be considered after all conservative measures are exhausted. The goal of surgical fusion is to decrease the pain by limiting the movement over a dysfunctional motion segment. Herkowitz has recommended reserving single-level fusion for patients with pain and disability present for greater than one year, failure of aggressive nonoperative management over a 4-month period of time, MRI evidence of advanced DDD (preferable at a single level), and a negative psychiatric evaluation (47,98). Multilevel fusion for DDD is associated with greater risk of poor clinical outcome (9). Subach et al. performed a literature review for outcomes following fusion for DDD and reported a wide range of results: radiographic arthrodesis in 60–100%, satisfaction ratings 36–89%, and return to work 28–91% (108). Reported results after fusion for DDD largely consist of retrospective reviews with significant discrepancies in patient selection, operative technique, and patient outcomes. A lack of randomized, prospective trials that compare the natural history of DDD with surgical outcomes makes it difficult to draw definitive conclusions regarding optimal treatment.

D. Other Clinical Predictors

A number of other risk factors elicited in the medical history and physical exam can predict surgical outcomes. Patients at risk for poor surgical outcomes often have vague complaints, neurotic symptoms, dramatic pain descriptions, hostility, poor pain localization, and disparity between appearance and description of pain (114). The probability of good outcomes decreases with chronicity of pain, the number of previous spine surgeries for similar problems, and a history of multiple medical problems (20,75,112,117). Comorbid conditions are associated with advanced age and may significantly impact outcomes. Diabetes and cardiovascular disease have been shown to negatively influence results for surgical decompression of the lumbar spine (1). Obesity, as defined by weight greater than 50% over the ideal weight, is considered by many surgeons to be a risk factor for poor surgical outcomes (30). Patients who smoke have a higher incidence of poor results for both fusion and nonfusion spine surgeries (75).

III. NONORGANIC PREDICTORS

A. Addictive Disorders

The abuse of alcohol and narcotics has been shown to be associated with poor outcome after spine surgery (104). Chemical dependence, including alcoholism, is among the most common contributors to chronic pain syndromes (22,23). In addition, there is a high incidence of alcohol abuse in chronic back pain patients (6). Patients suffering from chronic pain are commonly given potent narcotic medications to relieve their symptoms. Unfortunately, when given over extended periods of time, this may result in psychological dependency and physical addiction. Drug craving provides an incentive for pain behavior, and the withdrawal of narcotics commonly produces hyperalgesia (61). Addiction is known to impair coping abilities, which, in turn, may significantly impact the postoperative physical rehabilitation process (23). Patients are often evasive about drug and alcohol use and may provide inaccurate information despite direct questioning. Preoperative interviews with the patient's family often provide clues, which may alert the surgeon to addictive disorders that might interfere with surgical outcome.

B. Preoperative Disability

Prolonged periods of preoperative disability may have adverse effects on outcome follow-ing spine surgery. It has been shown that individuals are more likely to return to work after surgery if they had been employed and were not receiving disability prior to surgery (101). Junge et al. found that prolonged preoperative disability was a statistically signifi-cant predictor of poor outcome following lumbar disk surgery (59). Trief et al. found that patients who were working up to the time of surgery were more likely to return to work at one year than those who were not (109). Airaksinen et al. found that only 31% of patients with spinal stenosis who were on sick leave prior to surgery returned to work following surgery (1). Preoperative work-leave and disability compensation issues are at times inseparable variables. However, keeping a patient working and out of the worker's compensation system prior to surgery may improve outcomes. Many factors other than the patient's symptoms may prevent this. The patient's eagerness to continue working, the clinician's attitude in regard to keeping a patient working, and the employer's willing-ness to be flexible with regard to type of work are factors that influence whether or not patients remain in the labor force up to the time of surgery. Not uncommonly, the clinician, patient, and employer may inadvertently account for needless and extended periods of preoperative disability.

C. Worker's Compensation and Pending Litigation

Industrial related low back injuries remain a significant medical problem in the United States. Approximately 85% of all persons have back pain at some time in their lives (14,15,33,103). LBP is a leading cause of worker's compensation claims. The incidence of LBP is highest during the ages of 25–60 years, and as a result work-related back injuries are of great economic concern. The Boeing Company study assessed the cost of 900 spine-related worker's compensation claims and evaluated multiple independent variables (1,14,15,103). Of interest, a highly statistical difference was found between appraisal ratings by employers of injured employees compared with those of uninjured workers (1,14). A disproportionate number of claimants, particularly those with high-cost back injuries, had the lowest appraisal rating by their employers. The authors concluded that psychosocial influences play a significant role in worker's compensation claims. Patients who are injured on the job may exhibit other issues including job dissatisfaction, lengthy time out of work, and anger directed toward the employer (10,29). In a follow-up Boeing Company study, job task dissatisfaction and distress defined by the Minnesota Multiphasic Personality Inventory (MMPI) were identified as significant risk factors for worker's compensation claims (13). This offers some explanation as to why the focus on purely physical and injury-related factors fails to explain work-related spine injuries. Clinically, these same nonphysical factors that significantly impact worker's compensation may also affect patients' responses to medical treatment.

Predicting which patients with worker's compensation will benefit from surgery and which patients have the motivation to return to work can be difficult. It is a general belief among healthcare providers that patients with worker's compensation claims are less motivated to return to work and therefore have less favorable outcomes following treatment. Symptoms of chronic pain in patients with pending litigation or compensation claims may be closely tied to financial gain. Some studies have demonstrated that patients receiving worker's compensation payments tend to have poorer outcome following spine surgery than those not receiving compensation (10,28,29,32,118). Dzioba and Doxey found that 43% of a group of patients receiving disability compensation had poor results following spine surgery (29). Turner and Leiding found significantly fewer good or excellent results in patients with pending compensation or litigation claims (114). They reported 47% good results for patients with compensation or litigation claims compared with 88% good outcome for patients without compensation or litigation. Some authors have asserted that patients with pending litigation during treatment are a greater risk for failure to improve and suggested that surgery should be withheld until litigation is resolved. Klekamp et al. found that 81% of patients without litigation or compensation had good results following lumbar surgery, while only 29% of patients who were actively involved in litigation and/or compensation had good outcomes (68). Worker's compensation patients with poor outcome following their initial surgery not surprisingly tend to have poor outcomes from subsequent operations. This was studied by Waddell et al., who retrospectively reviewed 103 industrial compensation patients who had one back operation and required reoperation (118). A second operation resulted in improvement in only 40–50% of cases, and 20% of the patients were reported to be worse. Although there was no control group, they concluded that compensation was a strong, relative contraindication to redo lumbar spine surgery.

Some critics claim that the poorer outcome in the worker's compensation population may be secondary to other issues. Some authors have not found a negative relationship between worker's compensation and outcome and have questioned the appropriateness of withholding treatment for these patients. Dworkin et al. examined the relationship between compensation and employment and reported on the short- and long-term outcome in a series of 454 chronic pain patients (28). When employment and compensation were evaluated as potential predictors of outcome, only preoperative employment status predicted short- and long-term outcome. Jamison et al. compared 110 chronic low back pain males who were divided into three groups: 44 receiving no compensation, 27 receiving time-limited worker's compensation, and 39 receiving unlimited Social Security disability benefits (55). All patients received nonsurgical treatment programs. They found that time-limited worker's compensation and non-compensation patients who were initially not working were more likely to return to work than disability patients receiving unlimited compensation. Whether these outcomes could be replicated in the surgical patient population remains uncertain. Although a significant body of evidence has identified litigation as a major risk factor for poor surgical outcome, it may not be appropriate to categorically deny surgery for patients with secondary gain issues. However, identification of secondary gain issues must alert the clinician to delve deeper into the patient's psychological profile and motivation prior to making a treatment decision.

D. Psychological Factors

Pain is a complex psychophysiological experience, and aspects of an individual's personality may alter the perception of pain and affect the patient's response to surgery.

Although physical factors are known to predict surgical outcome, much evidence indicates that psychological factors also significantly influence outcomes. Spine surgeons have become increasingly interested in the relationship between the psychosocial component of back pain syndromes and the response to conservative or operative therapy. These psychogenic contributors often become evident to the clinician when pain and disability seem out of proportion to what is usual. Recognition of "warning" signs may assist in identifying patients with significant psychological risk factors for poor outcome (120). Squirming and pacing about, sighing and groaning, bizarre gait or posture, minimal active voluntary spine motion, wincing and keeping eyes shut, tossing self about on examining table, jumping when touched, and staring or glaring at the examiner have been described as "red flags" to be recognized in the preoperative evaluation (114). Spengler et al. reported that psychosocial problems and personality disturbances adversely affected outcome following surgery (104). They noted that utilization of an objective preoperative evaluation that included preoperative psychological testing improved patient selection for lumbar discectomy.

Factors such as emotional stress and anxiety are psychological influences which may adversely affect outcome following spine surgery. Emotional distress has been found to be relevant to the genesis and treatment of many medical disorders (67,76,85) Anxiety can amplify physical symptoms as well as provide disincentives for recovery (22). Chronic tension, anger, and irritability can lead to physiological responses that generate pain (23). Trief et al. assessed patients before and after lumbar surgery, examining psychological predictors of lumbar surgery outcome (109). They found that premorbid anxiety predicted failure to return to work and failure to report functional improvement and pain relief. Greenough et al. demonstrated that preexisting anxiety significantly contributed to poor outcomes following anterior lumbar interbody fusion (36,38).

A strong association exists between chronic LBP and depression, although the nature of this relationship remains unclear. Krishnan et al. reported a 44% incidence of major depression, 11% minor depression, and 25% intermittent depression in the LBP patients studied (70). Many conservative spine surgeons feel that bone fide pain is magnified in the presence of depression and that initial treatment should, therefore, focus on treatment of the depression. On the other hand, major depressive disorders may be the cause of many somatic symptoms, including pain. Treatment specifically directed toward the affective disorder has been reported to improve painful symptoms (70,79). Five simple features elicited in the history give a clear indication of possible depression and should be sought whenever depression is suspected. These include anergia (lack of energy), anhedonia (inability to enjoy oneself), sleep disturbances, spontaneous weeping, and a general feeling of depression. Recognition of significant depressive elements may identify patients who are at higher risk for poor outcome and who are likely to respond to pharmacological treatment. However, it is important to recognize the duration of depressive symptoms. Patients who are chronically depressed are at risk for a poor response to surgical intervention aimed at improving pain. On the other hand, pain associated with recent-onset depression responds better to surgery (30). However, in many patients with depression this task may be difficult to determine.

A number of studies have attempted to combine clinical, radiographic, and non-organic risk factors in order to accurately predict surgical success. Hasenbring et al. examined risk factors associated with chronicity of pain in patients with lumbar disk herniation (43). Outcomes were accurately predicted in 86% of patients when combining physical factors with psychological and social testing. Herron and Pheasant (51) and Turner and Leiding (114) observed that patients with sensory and motor deficits without psychological impairment showed a better treatment outcome after lumbar discectomy than those with psychological factors. Patients with positive neurological and radiographic findings and no psychological impairment showed significantly better results following operative treatment than those with psychological abnormalities. Several studies have attempted to create an objective scoring system in which risk factors are weighted and recorded and then utilized in the treatment decision-making process (32,59,74,75,105). Spengler et al. reported on the use of a scorecard method and assigned a weight of 0–25 for predictor variables in four categories: neurological signs, sciatic-tension signs, personality factors (based on the score of the MMPI), and radiographic findings on lumbar myelography or computed tomography (105). They found that psychological factors accounted for 24% of the variance in clinical outcome and were much more predictive of outcome than any medical factors examined. Finneson and Cooper also utilized a scorecard method for predicting outcomes for patients undergoing lumbar disk surgery (32). Factors such as "sciatica is more severe than back pain," and "patients have realistic self-appraisal of future lifestyle" were assigned positive weight, whereas factors such as "gross obesity" and "secondary gain" were assigned negative weights. Patients who achieved good surgical outcome had higher ratings on the preoperative scorecard compared with those with poor outcome. Manniche et al. confirmed the predictive value of these methods and demonstrated that psychological factors strongly predicted long-term outcome following discectomy (74,75). Junge et al. created an evaluation system based on psychological, physical, and history of symptoms, which accurately predicted satisfactory surgical outcome in 74% of patients and poor outcomes in 89% (59).

IV. PSYCHOLOGICAL PROFILE MEASURES

Screening for presurgical emotional distress and depression may identify those patients at risk for poor outcome. Thoughtful assessment of patients being considered for spine surgery utilizing objective psychological measures may reduce the risk of unsuccessful spine surgery. It is important that psychosocial factors not only be considered but also measured, especially with bigger and more extensive spine surgery, when the patient's pain is protracted, or when the surgeon recognizes that the patient is under emotional distress (30).

A. MMPI

The Minnesota Multiphasic Personality Inventory profile (MMPI) is one of the most frequently administered psychological assessment tools for patients with low back pain. Considered the father of all psychological testing used to assess chronic pain patients, it was first published in 1943 and has been thoroughly researched as an objective personality assessment tool (44). MMPI is frequently used in the assessment of personality characteristics in back pain patients to distinguish between organic and functional back pain and to identify predisposing personality traits associated with poorer outcome (115,49,50,71,113,115). The MMPI has been utilized to classify personality and psychopathological characteristics of patients with chronic pain in which an emotional disturbance is a significant determinant of their pain experience. The MMPI has been subsequently revised to the MMPI-2 (45). The MMPI-2 is a broad-based, self-administered inventory consisting of 566 true-or-false questions yielding data on 10 clinical scales. Shorter versions of the MMPI have also demonstrated a high predictive value and seem suitable for screening patients with spinal disorders (93,94).

A frequent finding in patients with chronic back pain is the "conversion V" or somatization profile of the MMPI, defined as having elevations on the Hypochondriasis (Hs), Depression (D), and Hysteria (Hy) subscales. Sternbach characterized this subset of chronic pain patients as possessing a manipulative reaction pattern; these elevations on psychopathic deviance scales are closely associated with the intentional use of pain syndromes to obtain personal gratification (106). Other studies have confirmed this profile in patients as a predictor of poor outcome following spinal surgery (51,114,124). Hysteria and hypochondriasis scales assess similar characteristics, such as a tendency for excessive and multiple physical complaints. Both of these scales have been shown to predict poor surgical outcome in numerous studies (18,50,71,114). Turner and Leiding examined the MMPI to determine if it aided in the selection of lumbosacral fusion patients and found that patients with an abnormal MMPI tended to have poorer surgical outcome (114). Patients with the triad of elevation of hypochondriasis, hysteria, and depression had significantly fewer good or excellent results than those without conversion V disorders. Higher levels of depression alone, as measured by the MMPI, have also been associated with poor surgical outcome. Some studies have found the predictive value of the conversion V subscale is superior to clinical and radiographic factors in predicting surgical outcome (30,105).

A criticism of the MMPI is that it may reflect the status of the patient only at the time of testing. It is debatable whether personality traits, as measured by the MMPI, are static or dynamic and may therefore respond to external influences. Attempts have been made to determine which comes first: the pain or the personality disorder. Herron and Pheasant reviewed 69 patients who had completed both pre- and postoperative MMPI testing (51). They found that the MMPI profile was dynamic and not static. They reported that the identification of preoperative Hs and Hy scales were only modestly related to outcome. The same Hs and Hy scales measured in the postoperative period, however, were strongly related to outcome. The authors concluded that the MMPI is representative of the patient's current personality state and is not necessarily a measure of a permanent psychological state. Barnes found that patients successfully treated for chronic low back pain had a significant reduction in their MMPI profile levels to normal ranges (9). Hansen et al. reported a 20-year follow-up of MMPI profiles in patients with and without back pain (42). Elevations on conversion V scales were not present in subjects without LBP who later developed LBP. The results indicated that the onset of LBP may be followed by MMPI changes rather than preceded by them. The view that LBP is preceded by elevations in the MMPI profile is further refuted by Herron and Pheasant, who demonstrated that the MMPI Hy and Hs scores of LBP patients can be influenced by the success or failure of surgery (51).

Despite extensive use of the MMPI over the past several decades, there are serious concerns regarding the psychometric soundness of the MMPI and its clinical utility for the specific population of patients with back pain. Some authors state that it may not measure immutable personality traits but that it principally assesses mood states (109). Furthermore, mood states such as depression and anxiety are dynamic conditions likely to change in response to treatment. Other criticisms of the MMPI are that it is time consuming and has a low rate of satisfactory completion by patients (109). Perhaps the greatest criticism of MMPI is that, although it appears to identify profiles of patients likely to have poor outcome, it may not sufficiently help an individual patient. Therefore it may be inappropriate to reject a patient for spinal surgery based on the MMPI alone. The use of preoperative MMPI as a tool to identify individual patients at risk for poor surgical outcome remains controversial.

B. Waddell Signs

On the basis of the systematic observation of 350 patients with LBP, Waddell et al. described and standardized nonorganic physical signs in low back pain which are distinguishable from standard clinical signs (120). They identified nonorganic physical signs as a simple clinical screening tool for selecting patients who may require a more detailed assessment for potentially significant psychological factors preceding any treatment, particularly surgery. Identification of Waddell signs utilizes clinical judgment about the absence or presence of a sign in five categories: tenderness, simulation, regional disturbances, distraction, and overreaction to pain. Tenderness that is not localized to a particular skeletal or neuromuscular structure is nonorganic. Widespread nonanatomical skin tenderness or deep pain felt over a wide area constitutes a positive sign. Simulation tests give the impression that a particular examination is being carried out when in actuality it is not, for example, LBP upon vertical loading of the patient's skull or by passive rotation of the shoulders and pelvis in the same plane. These maneuvers should not produce LBP, and if back pain is produced, it constitutes a nonorganic finding. Distraction is the testing of a positive finding in a routine manner, then rechecking and confirming while the patient is not aware. Straight leg testing in the sitting position is the most useful distraction test. A discrepancy between the sitting and the supine SLR tests may signify nonorganic pathology. Regional disturbances are found over a widespread region and may be manifest as global weakness (partial cogwheel "giving away") or sensory loss that cannot be explained in an anatomical manner. Overreaction may be expressed by either verbal or nonverbal means. Facial expressions, tremor, and excessive sweating have been described. The presence of three out of five Waddell signs correlates with poor outcome following any form of treatment. Isolated positive signs are ignored. Patients with multiple Waddell signs have been shown to have more psychological distress (46). The presence of several Waddell signs are also associated with general affective disturbances, ineffective coping, and abnormal illness behaviors (119,121). It is generally believed that patients with multiple Waddell signs have more psychological distress, which correlates with failure of treatment, elevation of the Hy and Hs scores of the MMPI, and other psychological factors (78,120).

C. Pain Drawings

The pain drawing is used by many surgeons in the evaluation of spine-related pain symptoms. Drawings by low back pain patients depicting the severity, type, and location of their pain have been utilized as a brief screening technique for psychological involvement (90). The pain drawing has been described as a "poor man's MMPI." It consists of an outline drawing of the human body in which the patient is requested to map the distribution of pain. Pain is divided into four categorical descriptions: pins or needles, burning, stabbing, or deep ache. Pain drawn in multiple unrelated regions, in non-anatomical distributions, in bizarre patterns, or outside the confines of the body should alert the clinician to a potentially significant psychological component of the patient's symptoms (Fig. 2). Pain drawings may be numerically quantified by an overlay placed on the pain drawing itself. Chan et al. examined the reproducibility of the pain drawing test and reported a reliability of 73% and 78% using independent evaluators (19). They studied the correlation of pain

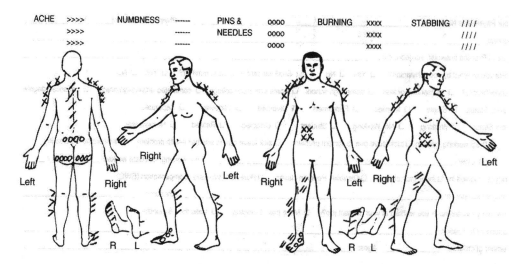

Figure 2 A pain drawing which demonstrates sensory complaints in multiple unrelated regions, in bizarre patterns, or outside the confines of the body may reflect a potentially significant psychological component of the patient's symptoms.

drawings with Waddell's signs and demonstrated that a large proportion of patients with high Waddell scores had nonorganic pain drawings. Ransford et al. developed a method of scoring the pain drawing and found a correlation between numeral pain drawing scores with MMPI Hs and Hy scores (90). However, there exists conflicting evidence demonstrating a direct correlation between pain drawings and MMPI scoring. Furthermore, the use of pain drawings to screen for psychological disorders appears to be associated with a high incidence of false-negative drawings. Von Baeyer et al. reviewed 212 patients with back pain and showed that more than half of the patients who demonstrated a significant psychological component of their pain, as assessed by MMPI criteria, had normal pain drawings (116).

D. SF-36

The SF-36 is a generic health outcome tool that evaluates the patient's perception of his or her health and physical well-being and was designed for use in clinical practice and research, health policy evaluations, and general population surveys (80,92,107). The SF-36 is a comprehensive short form with 36 questions and has been demonstrated to be an effective and valid measurement tool for patient satisfaction and quality-of-life improvement following surgery (2,3,7,8,34,35). The SF-36 measures three aspects of health: functional ability, well-being, and overall health. These are then quantified using eight health concepts: limitations in physical activities because of health problems; limitations in social activities because of physical or emotional problems; limitations in usual role activities because of physical health problems; bodily pain; general mental health (psychological distress and well-being); limitations in usual role activities because of emotional problems; vitality (energy and fatigue); and general health perceptions (Table 1) (80). For each variable, the scores are recorded and summarized to form a graphical health profile. The SF-36 has been shown to be a valid measurement tool for patients undergoing spine surgery (39) and is of prognostic value for lumbar spine surgery.

Table 1

Summary measures	Scales	Items
Physical health	Physical functioning (PF)	(PF1) Vigorous activities
		(PF2) Moderate activities
		(PF3) Lifting/carrying groceries
		(PF4) Climbing several flights
		(PF5) Climbing one flight
		(PF6) Bending or kneeling
		(PF7) Walking > 1 mile
		(PF8) Walking several blocks
		(PF9) Walking one block
		(PF10) Bathing or dressing
	Role physical (RP)	(RP1) Limited in kind of work and activities
		(RP2) Cut down in time in work and activities
		(RP3) Accomplished less than would like
		(RP4) Difficulty in performing work or activities
	Bodily pain (BP)	(BP1) Intensity of bodily pain
		(BP2) Extent pain interfered with normal work
	General health perception (GH)	(GH1) Is your health excellent, good, or fair
		(GH2) My health is excellent
		(GH3) I am as healthy as anyone I know
		(GH4) I seem to get sick a little easier than other people
		(GH5) I expect my health to get worse
Mental health	Vitality (VT)	(VT1) Feel full of pep
		(VT2) Have a lot of energy
		(VT3) Feel worn out
		(VT4) Feel tired
	Social functioning (SF)	(SF1) Frequency of health problems interfered with social activities
		(SF2) Extent of health problems interfered with normal social activities
	Role emotional (RE)	(RE1) Cut down the amount of times spent on work and other activities
		(RE2) Accomplished less than would like
		(RE3) Didn't do work or other activities as carefully as usual
	Mental health (MH)	(MH1) Been a nervous person
		(MH2) Felt downhearted and blue
		(MH3) Felt so down in the dumps nothing could cheer me up
		(MH4) Been a happy person
		(MH5) Felt calm and peaceful
	Reported change	(TRAN) Rating of health now compared with one year ago

Source: Ref. 80

It has been demonstrated that assessment of pain, social function, and mental health as measured by the SF-36 may be associated with an increased likelihood of a subsequent second procedure. Glassman et al. reviewed 235 patients treated by lumbar fusion who had a preoperative SF-36 (34). They compared the preoperative SF-36 of patients having a single operation with those requiring an additional procedure. Analysis of preoperative SF-36 responses revealed statistically significant higher scores in social function and pain for the 208 patients who underwent only a single fusion versus the 27 patients requiring a subsequent intervention. This study suggests that the SF-36 may have prognostic value for subsequent lumbar spinal surgery.

E. BDI

As discussed earlier, depression may adversely affect outcomes after spine surgery. Individuals with depression tend to focus on negative events, to have a low threshold for induced pain, and to report greater functional impairment. The Beck Depression Inventory (BDI) is a self-rating scale for measuring depression (11). The BDI consists of 21 questions with a cumulative scoring system that looks at manifestations of depression including sleep disturbance, weight change, irritability, sexual dysfunction, and anhedonia. It was developed as a means of identifying components of depression (24,48,55,59,60,73) and has been determined to have a high level of validity in differentiating between depressed and nondepressed people (91). The BDI has been demonstrated to be an important predictor of chronicity in patients with lumbar disk herniation (60,59,60). Recognition of patients with significant depressive elements may identify those who are at higher risk for poor outcome and to likely benefit from antidepressant agents.

V. CONCLUSIONS

Appropriate patient selection for spine surgery is a complex process. Most surgeons would anticipate a good outcome in a patient who possesses short duration of symptoms, is presently employed, has no pending compensation or litigation claims, has had no prior spine surgery, demonstrates anatomical neurological deficits, has correlative radiographic findings, and minimal psychological factors. Clinical, radiological, and psychological factors must all be collectively considered in the selection process for surgery to avoid poor outcomes and increase the likelihood of excellent surgical results.

REFERENCES

1. Airaksinen O, Herno A, Turunen V, Saari T, Suomlainen O. Surgical outcome of 438 patients treated surgically for lumbar spinal stenosis. Spine 1997; 22:2278–2282.
2. Albert TJ, Mesa JJ, Eng K, McIntosh TC, Balderston RA. Health outcome assessment before and after lumbar laminectomy for radiculopathy. Spine 1996; 21:960–962.
3. Albert TJ, Purtill J, Mesa J, McIntosh T, Balderston RA. Health outcome assessment before and after adult deformity surgery. A prospective study. Spine 1995; 20:2002–2004.
4. Amundsen T, Weber H, Lilleas F, Nordal HJ, Abdelnoor M, Magnaes B. Lumbar spinal stenosis. Clinical and radiologic features. Spine 1995; 20:1178–1186.
5. Andrews DW, Lavyne MH. Retrospective analysis of microsurgical and standard lumbardiscectomy. Spine 1990; 15:329–335.

6. Atkinson JH, Slater MA, Patterson TL, Grant I, Garfin SR. Prevalence, onset, and risk of psychiatric disorders in men with chronic low back pain: a controlled study. Pain 1991; 45:111–121.

7. Atlas SJ, Deyo RA, Keller RB, Chapin AM, Patrick DL, Long JM, Singer DE. The Maine Lumbar Spine Study, Part III. 1-year outcomes of surgical and nonsurgical management of lumbar spinal stenosis. Spine 1996; 21:1787–1794.

8. Atlas SJ, Keller RB, Robson D, Deyo RA, Singer DE. Surgical and nonsurgical management of lumbar spinal stenosis: four-year outcomes from the maine lumbar spine study. Spine 2000; 25:556–562.

9. Barnes B, Rodts GE, McLaughlin MR, Haid RW, Jr. Threaded cortical bone dowels for lumbar interbody fusion: over 1-year mean follow up in 28 patients. J Neurosurg 2001; 95:1–4.

10. Barrios C, Ahmed M, Arrotegui JI, Bjornsson A. Clinical factors predicting outcome after surgery for herniated lumbar disc: an epidemiological multivariate analysis. J Spinal Disord 1990; 3:205–209.

11. Beck A. Depression: Clinical, Experimental and Theoretical Aspects. New York: Harper & Row, 1967.

12. Bell G. Diagnosis of lumbar disk disease. Semin Spine Surg 1994; 6:186–195.

13. Bigos SJ, Battie MC, Spengler DM, Fisher LD, Fordyce WE, Hansson T, Nachemson AL, Zeh J. A longitudinal, prospective study of industrial back injury reporting. Clin Orthop 1992:21–34.

14. Bigos SJ, Spengler DM, Martin NA, Zeh J, Fisher L, Nachemson A. Back injuries in industry: a retrospective study. III. Employee-related factors. Spine 1986; 11:252–256.

15. Bigos SJ, Spengler DM, Martin NA, Zeh J, Fisher L, Nachemson A, Wang MH. Back injuries in industry: a retrospective study. II. Injury factors. Spine 1986; 11:246–251.

16. Boden SD, Davis DO, Dina TS, Patronas NJ, Wiesel SW. Abnormal magnetic-resonance scans of the lumbar spine in asymptomatic subjects. A prospective investigation. J Bone Joint Surg Am 1990; 72:403–408.

17. Bolender NF, Schonstrom NS, Spengler DM. Role of computed tomography and myelography in the diagnosis of central spinal stenosis. J Bone Joint Surg Am 1985; 67:240–246.

18. Cashion EL, Lynch WJ. Personality factors and results of lumbar disk surgery. Neurosurgery 1979; 4:141–145.

19. Chan CW, Goldman S, Ilstrup DM, Kunselman AR, O'Neill PI. The pain drawing and Waddell's nonorganic physical signs in chronic low-back pain. Spine 1993; 18:1717–1722.

20. Ciol MA, Deyo RA, Kreuter W, Bigos SJ. Characteristics in Medicare beneficiaries associated with reoperation after lumbar spine surgery. Spine 1994; 19:1329–1334.

21. Colhoun E, McCall IW, Williams L, Cassar PV. Provocation discography as a guide to planning operations on the spine. J Bone Joint Surg Br 1988; 70:267–271.

22. Covington EC. Psychiatric aspects of chronic back pain. Semin Spine Surg 1989; 1:35–42.

23. Covington EC. The psychiatry of chronic back disability. Semin Spine Surg 1994; 6: 269–281.

24. Crisson J, Keefe FJ, Wilkins RH, Cook WA, Muhlbaier LH. Self-report of depressive symptoms in low back pain patients. J Clin Psychol 1986; 42:425–430.

25. Dawson EG, Lotysch M, III, Urist MR. Intertransverse process lumbar arthrodesis with autogenous bone graft. Clin Orthop 1981; 154:90–96.

26. Deyo RA, Cherkin DC, Loeser JD, Bigos SJ, Ciol MA. Morbidity and mortality in association with operations on the lumbar spine. The influence of age, diagnosis, and procedure. J Bone Joint Surg Am 1992; 74:536–543.

27. Dvorak J, Gauchat MH, Valach L. The outcome of surgery for lumbar disk herniation. I. A 4–17 years' follow-up with emphasis on somatic aspects. Spine 1988; 13:1418–1422.

28. Dworkin RH, Handlin DS, Richlin DM, Brand L, Vannucci C. Unraveling the effects of compensation, litigation, and employment on treatment response in chronic pain. Pain 1985; 23:49–59.

29. Dzioba RB, Doxey NC. A prospective investigation into the orthopaedic and psychologic predictors of outcome of first lumbar surgery following industrial injury. Spine 1984; 9:614–623.

30. Epker J, Block AR. Presurgical psychological screening in back pain patients: a review. Clin J Pain 2001; 17:200–205.

31. Esses SI, Botsford DJ, Kostuik JP. The role of external spinal skeletal fixation in the assessment of low-back disorders. Spine 1989; 14:594–601.

32. Finneson BE, Cooper VR. A lumbar disk surgery predictive score card. A retrospective evaluation. Spine 1979; 4:141–144.

33. Frymoyer JW, Cats-Baril WL. An overview of the incidences and costs of low back pain. Orthop Clin North Am 1991; 22:263–271.

34. Glassman SD, Dimar JR, Johnson JR, Minkow R. Preoperative SF-36 responses as a predictor of reoperation following lumbar fusion. Orthopedics 1998; 21:1201–1203.

35. Glassman SD, Minkow RE, Dimar JR, Puno RM, Raque GH, Johnson JR. Effect of prior lumbar discectomy on outcome of lumbar fusion: a prospective analysis using the SF-36 measure. J Spinal Disord 1998; 11:383–388.

36. Greenough CG, Taylor LJ, Fraser RD. Anterior lumbar fusion. A comparison of noncompensation patients with compensation patients. Clin Orthop 1994:30–37.

37. Greenough CG, Taylor LJ, Fraser RD. Anterior lumbar fusion. A comparison of noncompensation patients with compensation patients. Clin Orthop 1994:30–37.

38. Greenough CG, Taylor LJ, Fraser RD. Anterior lumbar fusion: results, assessment techniques and prognostic factors. Eur Spine J 1994; 3:225–230.

39. Grevitt M, Khazim R, Webb J, Mulholland R, Shepperd J. The short form-36 health survey questionnaire in spine surgery. J Bone Joint Surg Br 1997; 79:48–52.

40. Hakelius A. Prognosis in sciatica. A clinical follow-up of surgical and non-surgical treatment. Acta Orthop Scand Suppl 1970; 129:1–76.

41. Hamanishi C, Matukura N, Fujita M, Tomihara M, Tanaka S. Cross-sectional area of the stenotic lumbar dural tube measured from the transverse views of magnetic resonance imaging. J Spinal Disord 1994; 7:388–393.

42. Hansen FR, Biering-Sorensen F, Schroll M. Minnesota Multiphasic Personality Inventory profiles in persons with or without low back pain. A 20-year follow-up study. Spine 1995; 20:2716–2720.

43. Hasenbring M, Marienfeld G, Kuhlendahl D, Soyka D. Risk factors of chronicity in lumbar disk patients. A prospective investigation of biologic, psychologic, and social predictors of therapy outcome. Spine 1994; 19:2759–2765.

44. Hathaway SR, Mckinley JC. Minnesota Multipahsic Personality Inventory Revised. Minneapolis, MN: University of Minnesota Press, :1943.

45. Hathaway SR MJ. MMPI-2, Minnesota Multipahsic Personality Inventory-2: Manual for Administration of Scoring. Minneapolis, MN: University of Minnesota Press, 1989.

46. Hayes B, Solyom CA, Wing PC, Berkowitz J. Use of psychometric measures and nonorganic signs testing in detecting nomogenic disorders in low back pain patients. Spine 1993; 18: 1254–1259.

47. Herkowitz HN, Sidhu KS. Lumbar spine fusion in the treatment of degenerative conditions: current indications and recommendations. J Am Acad Orthop Surg 1995; 3:123–135.

48. Herr KA, Mobily PR, Smith C. Depression and the experience of chronic back pain: a study of related variables and age differences. Clin J Pain 1993; 9:104–114.

49. Herron L, Turner J, Weiner P. Does the MMPI predict chemonucleolysis outcome?. Spine 1988; 13:84–88.

50. Herron L, Turner JA, Ersek M, Weiner P. Does the Millon Behavioral Health Inventory (MBHI) predict lumbar laminectomy outcome? A comparison with the Minnesota Multiphasic Personality Inventory (MMPI). J Spinal Disord 1992; 5:188–192.

51. Herron LD, Pheasant HC. Changes in MMPI profiles after low-back surgery. Spine 1982; 7:591–597.

52. Hirsch C, Nachemson A. The reliability of lumbar disk surgery. Clin Orthop 1963; 29: 189–195.

53. Holt EP, Jr. The question of lumbar discography. J Bone Joint Surg Am 1968; 50:720–726.

54. Hurme M, Alaranta H. Factors predicting the result of surgery for lumbar intervertebral disk herniation. Spine 1987; 12:933–938.

55. Jamison RN, Matt DA, Parris WC. Effects of time-limited vs unlimited compensation on pain behavior and treatment outcome in low back pain patients. J Psychosom Res 1988; 32: 277–283.

56. Johnsson KE, Rosen I, Uden A. The natural course of lumbar spinal stenosis. Clin Orthop 1992; 279:82–86.

57. Jonsson B, Annertz M, Sjoberg C, Stromqvist B. A prospective and consecutive study of surgically treated lumbar spinal stenosis. Part I: clinical features related to radiographic findings. Spine 1997; 22:2932–2937.

58. Jonsson B, Annertz M, Sjoberg C, Stromqvist B. A prospective and consecutive study of surgically treated lumbar spinal stenosis. Part II: five-year follow-up by an independent observer. Spine 1997; 22:2938–2944.

59. Junge A, Dvorak J, Ahrens S. Predictors of bad and good outcomes of lumbar disk surgery. A prospective clinical study with recommendations for screening to avoid bad outcomes. Spine 1995; 20:460–468.

60. Junge A, Frohlich M, Ahrens S, Hasenbring M, Sandler A, Grob D, Dvorak J. Predictors of bad and good outcome of lumbar spine surgery. A prospective clinical study with 2 years' follow up. Spine 1996; 21:1056–1064.

61. Kaplan H, Fields HL. Hyperalgesia during acute opioid abstinence: evidence for a nociceptive facilitating function of the rostral ventromedial medulla. J Neurosci 1991; 11:1433–1439.

62. Katz JN, Lipson SJ, Brick GW, Grobler LJ, Weinstein JN, Fossel AH, Lew RA, Liang MH. Clinical correlates of patient satisfaction after laminectomy for degenerative lumbar spinal stenosis. Spine 1995; 20:1155–1160.

63. Katz JN, Lipson SJ, Chang LC, Levine SA, Fossel AH, Liang MH. Seven- to 10-year outcome of decompressive surgery for degenerative lumbar spinal stenosis. Spine 1996; 21:92–98.

64. Katz JN, Lipson SJ, Larson MG, McInnes JM, Fossel AH, Liang MH. The outcome of decompressive laminectomy for degenerative lumbar stenosis. J Bone Joint Surg Am 1991; 73:809–816.

65. Katz JN, Lipson SJ, Lew RA, Grobler LJ, Weinstein JN, Brick GW, Fossel AH, Liang MH. Lumbar laminectomy alone or with instrumented or noninstrumented arthrodesis in degenerative lumbar spinal stenosis. Patient selection, costs, and surgical outcomes. Spine 1997; 22:1123–1131.

66. Katz JN, Stucki G, Lipson SJ, Fossel AH, Grobler LJ, Weinstein JN. Predictors of surgical outcome in degenerative lumbar spinal stenosis. Spine 1999; 24:2229–2233.

67. King KB. Psychologic and social aspects of cardiovascular disease. Ann Behav Med 1997; 19:264–270.

68. Klekamp J, McCarty E, Spengler DM. Results of elective lumbar discectomy for patients involved in the workers' compensation system. J Spinal Disord 1998; 11:277–282.

69. Kotilainen E, Valtonen S, Carlson CA. Microsurgical treatment of lumbar disk herniation: follow-up of 237 patients. Acta Neurochir (Wien) 1993; 120:143–149.

70. Krishnan KR, France RD, Pelton S, McCann UD, Davidson J, Urban BJ. Chronic pain and depression. I. Classification of depression in chronic low back pain patients. Pain 1985; 22:279–287.

71. Long CJ. The relationship between surgical outcome and MMPI profiles in chronic pain patients. J Clin Psychol 1981; 37:744–749.

72. Lorenz M, Zindrick M, Schwaegler P, Vrbos L, Collatz MA, Behal R, Cram R. A comparison of single-level fusions with and without hardware. Spine 1991; 16:S455–S458.

73. Lyles KW, Gold DT, Shipp KM, Pieper CF, Martinez S, Mulhausen PL. Association of osteoporotic vertebral compression fractures with impaired functional status. Am J Med 1993; 94:595–601.

74. Manniche C, Asmussen KH, Lauritsen B, Vinterberg H, Kreiner S, Jordan A. Low back pain rating scale: validation of a tool for assessment of low back pain. Pain 1994; 57:317–326.

75. Manniche C, Asmussen KH, Vinterberg H, Rose-Hansen EB, Kramhoft J, Jordan A. Analysis of preoperative prognostic factors in first-time surgery for lumbar disk herniation, including Finneson's and modified Spengler's score systems. Dan Med Bull 1994; 41:110–115.

76. Manuck SB, Henry JP, Anderson DE, Clarkson TB, Folkow B, Kaplan JR, Kaufmann PG, Lown B, Verrier RL. Biobehavioral mechanisms in coronary artery disease. Chronic stress. Circulation 1987; 76:I158–I163.

77. Mariconda M, Zanforlino G, Celestino GA, Brancaleone S, Fava R, Milano C. Factors influencing the outcome of degenerative lumbar spinal stenosis. J Spinal Disord 2000; 13:131–137.

78. Maruta T, GSCCIDKACR. Waddell's nonorganic signs and Minnesota Multiphasic Personality Inventory profiles in patients with chronic low back pain. Spine 1997; 1:72–75.

79. Maruta T, Vatterott MK, McHardy MJ. Pain management as an antidepressant: long-term resolution of pain-associated depression. Pain 1989; 36:335–337.

80. McHorney CA, Ware JE, Jr., Lu JF, Sherbourne CD. The MOS 36-item Short-Form Health Survey (SF-36): III. Tests of data quality, scaling assumptions, and reliability across diverse patient groups. Med Care 1994; 32:40–66.

81. Modic MT, Masaryk TJ, Ross JS, Carter JR. Imaging of degenerative disk disease. Radiology 1988; 168:177–186.

82. Modic MT, Ross JS. Magnetic resonance imaging in the evaluation of low back pain. Orthop Clin North Am 1991; 22:283–301.

83. Modic MT, Steinberg PM, Ross JS, Masaryk TJ, Carter JR. Degenerative disk disease: assessment of changes in vertebral body marrow with MR imaging. Radiology 1988; 166:193–199.

84. Mooney V. Where is the lumbar pain coming from?. Ann Med 1989; 21:373–379.

85. Nemeroff CB, Musselman DL, Evans DL. Depression and cardiac disease. Depress Anxiety 1998; 8(suppl 1):71–79.

86. Nygaard OP, Kloster R, Solberg T, Mellgren SI. Recovery of function in adjacent nerve roots after surgery for lumbar disk herniation: use of quantitative sensory testing in the exploration of different populations of nerve fibers. J Spinal Disord 2000; 13:427–431.

87. Nygaard OP, Romner B, Trumpy JH. Duration of symptoms as a predictor of outcome after lumbar disk surgery. Acta Neurochir (Wien) 1994; 128:53–56.

88. Pappas CT, Harrington T, Sonntag VK. Outcome analysis in 654 surgically treated lumbar disk herniations. Neurosurgery 1992; 30:862–866.

89. Porter RW, Ward D. Cauda equina dysfunction. The significance of two-level pathology. Spine 1992; 17:9–15.

90. Ransford A, Cairns D, Mooney V. The pain drawing as an aid to the psychological evaluation of patients with low-back pain. Spine 1976; 1:127–134.

91. Richter P, Werner J, Heerlein A, Kraus A, Sauer H. On the validity of the Beck Depression Inventory. A review. Psychopathology 1998; 31:160–168.

92. Riesenberg D, Glass RM. The Medical Outcomes Study. JAMA 1989; 262:943.

93. Riley JL, III, Robinson ME. Validity of MMPI-2 profiles in chronic back pain patients: differences in path models of coping and somatization. Clin J Pain 1998; 14:324–335.

94. Riley JL, III, Robinson ME, Geisser ME, Wittmer VT. Multivariate cluster analysis of the MMPI-2 in chronic low-back pain patients. Clin J Pain 1993; 9:248–252.

95. Rothman RH. Lumbar disk disease. In: Rothman, Simeone, eds. The Spine. Philadelphia: Saunders, 1982:508–645.

96. Rothman RH. A study of computer-assisted tomography. Spine 1984; 9:548.

97. Schneiderman G, Flannigan B, Kingston S, Thomas J, Dillin WH, Watkins RG. Magnetic resonance imaging in the diagnosis of disk degeneration: correlation with discography. Spine 1987; 12:276–281.

98. Sidhu KS, Herkowitz HN. Spinal instrumentation in the management of degenerative disorders of the lumbar spine. Clin Orthop 1997; 30:39–53.

99. Silvers HR, Lewis PJ, Asch HL. Decompressive lumbar laminectomy for spinal stenosis. J Neurosurg 1993; 78:695–701.

100. Simmons JW, Aprill CN, Dwyer AP, Brodsky AE. A reassessment of Holt's data on: "the question of lumbar discography." Clin Orthop 1988:120–124.

101. Sorensen LV, Mors O, Skovlund O. A prospective study of the importance of psychological and social factors for the outcome after surgery in patients with slipped lumbar disk operated upon for the first time. Acta Neurochir (Wien) 1987; 88:119–125.

102. Spangfort EV. The lumbar disk herniation. A computer-aided analysis of 2,054 operations. Acta Orthop Scand Suppl 1972; 142:1–95.

103. Spengler DM, Bigos SJ, Martin NA, Zeh J, Fisher L, Nachemson A. Back injuries in industry: a retrospective study. I. Overview and cost analysis. Spine 1986; 11:241–245.

104. Spengler DM, Freeman C, Westbrook R, Miller JW. Low-back pain following multiple lumbar spine procedures. Failure of initial selection?. Spine 1980; 5:356–360.

105. Spengler DM, Ouellette EA, Battie M, Zeh J. Elective discectomy for herniation of a lumbar disc. Additional experience with an objective method. J Bone Joint Surg Am 1990; 72: 230–237.

106. Sternbach RA. Pain Patients: Traits and Treatment. New York: Academic Press, 1974.

107. Stewart AL, Hays RD, Ware JE, Jr. The MOS short-form general health survey. Reliability and validity in a patient population. Med Care 1988; 26:724–735.

108. Subach BR, Haid RW, Rodts GE, Jr., McLaughlin MR. Do current outcomes data support the technique of lumbar interbody fusion? Clin Neurosurg 2001; 48:204–218.

109. Trief PM, Grant W, Fredrickson B. A prospective study of psychological predictors of lumbar surgery outcome. Spine 2000; 25:2616–2621.

110. Truumees E HH. Degenerative disk disease. In: Chapman's Othropaedic Surgery. Lippincott Williams & Wilkins. Philedelphia 2001:3775–3805.

111. Turner JA, Ersek M, Herron L, Deyo R. Surgery for lumbar spinal stenosis. Attempted meta-analysis of the literature. Spine 1992; 17:1–8.

112. Turner JA, Ersek M, Herron L, Haselkorn J, Kent D, Ciol MA, Deyo R. Patient outcomes after lumbar spinal fusions. JAMA 1992; 268:907–911.

113. Turner JA, Herron L, Weiner P. Utility of the MMPI Pain Assessment Index in predicting outcome after lumbar surgery. J Clin Psychol 1986; 42:764–769.

114. Turner RS, Leiding WC. Correlation of the MMPI with lumbosacral spine fusion results. Prospective study. Spine 1985; 10:932–936.

115. Uomoto JM, Turner JA, Herron LD. Use of the MMPI and MCMI in predicting outcome of lumbar laminectomy. J Clin Psychol 1988; 44:191–197.

116. Von Baeyer CL, Bergstrom KJ, Brodwin MG, Brodwin SK. Invalid use of pain drawings in psychological screening of back pain patients. Pain 1983; 16:103–107.

117. Waddell G. 1987 Volvo award in clinical sciences. A new clinical model for the treatment of low-back pain. Spine 1987; 12:632–644.

118. Waddell G, Kummel EG, Lotto WN, Graham JD, Hall H, McCulloch JA. Failed lumbar disk surgery and repeat surgery following industrial injuries. J Bone Joint Surg Am 1979; 61: 201–207.

119. Waddell G, Main CJ, Morris EW, Di Paola M, Gray IC. Chronic low-back pain, psychologic distress, and illness behavior. Spine 1984; 9:209–213.

120. Waddell G, McCulloch JA, Kummel E, Venner RM. Nonorganic physical signs in low-back pain. Spine 1980; 5:117–125.

121. Waddell G, Pilowsky I, Bond MR. Clinical assessment and interpretation of abnormal illness behaviour in low back pain. Pain 1989; 39:41–53.

122. Walsh TR, Weinstein JN, Spratt KF, Lehmann TR, Aprill C, Sayre H. Lumbar discography in normal subjects. A controlled, prospective study. J Bone Joint Surg Am 1990; 72: 1081–1088.

123. Weber H. Lumbar disk herniation. A controlled, prospective study with ten years of observation. Spine 1983; 8:131–140.
124. Wilfling FJ, Klonoff H, Kokan P. Psychological, demographic and orthopaedic factors associated with prediction of outcome of spinal fusion. Clin Orthop 1973; 90:153–160.
125. Wood GW, Boyd RJ, Carothers TA, Mansfield FL, Rechtine GR, Rozen MJ, Sutterlin CE, III. The effect of pedicle screw/plate fixation on lumbar/lumbosacral autogenous bone graft fusions in patients with degenerative disk disease. Spine 1995; 20:819–830.
126. Yukawa Y, Lenke LG, Tenhula J, Bridwell KH, Riew KD, Blanke K. A comprehensive study of patients with surgically treated lumbar spinal stenosis with neurogenic claudication. J Bone Joint Surg Am 2002; 84-A:1954–1959.

46

Complications Associated with House Staff Involvement in Patient Care

Louis G. Quartararo and Alexander R. Vaccaro
Thomas Jefferson University and the Rothman Institute, Philadelphia, Pennsylvania, U.S.A.

A university affiliation brings with it prestige, comradery, and the convenience of having house staff physicians to care for many of the simple, day-to-day patient care activities. Along with these positives comes the added responsibility of resident education. Residency training involves not only preparation for written examinations, but also training in surgical skills, patient interaction and interpersonal skills, and patient medical management. The "learning curve" for these activities has led many to believe that house staff participation is synonymous with increased complications, increased cost, and increased patient dissatisfaction.

I. THE "JULY PHENOMENON"

The July phenomenon is a theory that suggests that the yearly resident turnover is associated with increased hospital costs, increased mistakes, and higher complication rates. Several studies have tested this theory. Shulkin showed that there was no relationship between house officer experience and the occurrence of adverse events (42). Rich et al., in a study of over 21,000 patients, supported this contention, showing no relationship between house staff experience and hospital deaths, readmissions, or nursing home placement. They did, however, show that increased house staff experience is associated with a significant decline in length of stay and total hospital charges (33). When they revisited this problem several years later, Rich et al. performed a much larger study of over 240,000 patients and stratified the data between medical and surgical patients and teaching and nonteaching hospitals. They once again showed no relationship between the presence of house staff and mortality, operative complications, and nursing home discharge. The medical residents once again demonstrated the expected July phenomenon with declines in cost and increased length of stay as the academic year progressed. The surgical services, however, were ironically associated with an unexplained increase in length of stay and hospital charges throughout the year (34).

Other studies refute the July phenomenon more strongly. Buchwald et al. specifically examined cost as it relates to the academic year. They looked at matched cohorts of patients in July-August and April-May (beginning and end of the academic year). They found no differences in length of stay, total charges, or ancillary charges (6). Udvarhelyi et al. (48) also examined teaching hospital costs and found that, in spite of increased costs, teaching hospitals had shorter hospital stays and lower mean charges than nonteaching hospitals. They suggested that the increased costs of academic centers may be due not to a direct increase in resource utilization by inexperienced residents, but to the costs of teaching, including continuing medical education for nursing and medical staff, specialized patient care services, and the institution's specialized organizational structure (1,48).

Banco et al. (3) examined spine infection rate variations during the academic year. Over a 4-year period it was found that the month of January had the highest infection rate. No other monthly variations existed. No variations existed within the 4-month resident rotations or the 6-month fellowship rotations. It was concluded that since January did not coincide with the beginning of resident or fellow rotation that variation in spine infection rates had no association with the level of experience of the surgical house officers.

Other studies have examined the effects of changing intern and resident rotations through out the year. Rich et al. once again showed that changes in house staff rotation resulted in an increased length of stay and cost, but had no relation to mortality or readmission (35). Smith et al. showed that the end-of-the-month resident changes resulted only in increased length of stay (average of 1 day), but no increase in pharmacological charges, mortality, or morbidity (44). Another study measuring patient satisfaction showed that resident discontinuity resulted in decreased patient satisfaction with their care (14).

Therefore, the July phenomenon as it relates to house staff–induced morbidity is largely a myth. Most studies suggest no increase in patient risk, morbidity, or mortality in July. Some studies suggest increased costs in July are related to teaching services, while the majority do not. Patient satisfaction may suffer due to discontinuity in resident care at the conclusion of each rotation.

II. SLEEP DEPRIVATION

The length of the resident workweek has been the subject of much recent debate and has resulted in the ACGME's limitation of the resident workweek to 80 hours. The effect of sleep deprivation has been well documented. Military studies suggest that motor performance, particularly speed and accuracy, are affected by degree of sleep deprivation (21). Studies on resident performance have shown conflicting data. Some studies report negative effect on resident performance (10,30,40), while others do not. Jacques et al. demonstrated decreases in resident in-training test scores with sleep deprivation (18). Samkoff and Jacques showed that although sleep deprivation decreases performance on routine tasks and tasks requiring vigilance, there was no adverse effect on tests of dexterity, reaction time, and short-term recall (35). Reznick and Folse also found no significant difference in factual recall, concentration, and manual dexterity in sleep-deprived vs. non–sleep deprived individuals (32). This suggests an ability to compensate for sleep loss in challenging situations, but day-to-day tasks may suffer. Haynes et al. specifically examined surgical outcomes and the sleep deprivation status of the resident surgeon. They found in 6371 surgical cases no significant relationship between complication incidence and resident sleep deprivation (17).

Conversely, the solution to the problem may be, in itself, problematic. Laine et al. have shown that since New York State enacted limitations on resident work hours, there has been an increase in hospital complications and delays in test ordering by house staff (22). Other studies have shown reduced quality of care (30). The implementation of night float systems and cross-coverage systems has been shown to both increase "potentially preventable" adverse effects (29) and decrease patient satisfaction (14).

III. SURGICAL COMPLICATIONS ASSOCIATED WITH RESIDENTS

Many studies across several surgical disciplines directly address surgical complications related to residency training. The spine literature is scarce as it relates to these data. Banco et al., as mentioned above, found no relationship between the incidence of perioperative spine infection and the level of experience of house officers (3). Stranjalis (45) examined the differences between neurosurgical resident– and attending–performed cerebral aneurysm ablations. He showed a nonstatistically significant difference in these two groups, with lower Glasgow coma scales in the resident performed surgeries (45).

Other orthopedic studies suggest that there is no increased complication rate with resident teaching/training on patient care. Lavernia et al. (23) compared the outcome of total knee arthroplasty performed on a teaching service and nonteaching service at one hospital. They showed an increase in cost and operative time with residency training, but no increase in complication rate. A study on endoscopic carpal tunnel release demonstrated increasing complications with decreasing experience (not necessarily resident participation) and suggested cadaver practice of this technique before clinical application (24).

General surgeons have more extensively examined this phenomenon. Shaked et al. (39) showed no difference in resident gallbladder surgery performed under attending supervision versus attending performed surgeries. Similarly, Bickel et al. (4) showed no difference in complication rates or mortality, but did show an increase in conversion to open cholecystectomy with resident participation. Kazmers et al. (19) examined resident insertion of Greenfield filters, Praseedom et al. (31) looked at pancreatic surgery preformed by supervised residents, and Sussman et al. (47) examined appendectomies preformed by attendings versus residents with attending supervision. All three studies found no difference in complication rates when the house staff officers were adequately supervised.

Conversely, several studies have shown increased complication rates associated with resident involvement. Galandiuk and Ahmad showed a higher complication rate in colonoscopy preformed by residents when compared to surgeons and gastroenterologists (11). Massard et al. showed an increase in complications during pneumonectomies performed by interns (26). Khuri et al. (20) studied surgical outcomes of seven surgical departments in a Veterans Administration hospital, where medical training plays a major role. They found higher complication rates in six of the seven departments in this hospital versus a nonteaching hospital.

All three of the above studies did not quantify attending supervision. Most studies showing no difference in resident complication rates stipulate the condition of close attending supervision. Fallon et al. (9) specifically studied attending presence in the operating room and complication rates. They found that greater attending surgeon presence was significantly associated with lower mortality and complication rates. Haddad et al. showed the same correlation (16).

The ENT literature suggests that resident training/participation in certain types of procedures does result in higher complication rates. In particular, endoscopic sinus surgery and chronic ear surgery have shown higher rates of complications (15,50). Results of ENT studies examining thyroid surgery, parathyroid surgery, tracheotomy, sinus surgery, and rhytidectomy show no increase in complication rates with resident participation and close operative supervision (13,25,27,28,41,46,51). These studies suggest that more complicated procedures and procedures requiring endoscopic experience should have very close attending supervision to lower complication rates. The ophthalmology literature similarly suggests that the relatively simple procedures such as strabismus surgery and cataract extraction have no measurable difference between resident and attending complication rates, but that more technical procedures such as phacoemulsification and surgery requiring YAG lasers greatly benefit from close attending supervision (52,5,38,43,52).

Therefore, it can be concluded that close attending supervision of residents, particularly in complex procedures, results in the standard surgical complication rates associated with nonresident participation. Several studies suggest that newer technology such as telemedicine, computer simulations, and CT-guided instrumentation and procedures may result in better supervision and lower complication rates (7,37,53). The higher cost of academic centers may indeed not be due to inefficient resource utilization or the July phenomenon, as once thought. The often better clinical outcomes seen in most academic centers appear to justify the resource expenditure necessary to maintain these centers of excellence.

REFERENCES

1. Ayanian JZ, Weissman JS. Teaching hospitals and quality of care: a review of the literature. Milbank Q 2002; 80(3):569–593.
2. Badoza DA, Jure T, Aunino LA, Argento CJ. State-of-the-art phacoemulsification performed by residents in Buenos Aires, Argentina. J Cataract Refract Surg 2000; 26(6):794–795.
3. Banco SP, Vaccaro AR, Blam O, Eck JC, Cotler JM, Hilibrand AS, Albert TJ, Murphey S. Spine infections: variations in incidence during the academic year. Spine 2002; 27(9):962–966.
4. Bickel A, Rappaport A, Hazani E, Eitan A. Laparoscopic cholecystectomy for acute cholecystitis performed by residents in surgery: a risk factor for conversion to open laparotomy? J Laparoendosc Adv Surg Tech A 1998; 8(3):137–141.
5. Blomquist PH, Rugwani RM. Visual outcomes after vitreous loss during cataract surgery performed by residents. J Cataract Refract Surg 2002; 28(5):847–852.
6. Buchwald D, Komaroff AL, Cook EF, Epstein AM. Indirect costs for medical education. Is there a July phenomenon? Arch Intern Med 1989; 149(4):765–768.
7. Casiano RR, Numa WA Jr. Efficacy of computed tomographic image–guided endoscopic sinus surgery in residency training programs. Laryngoscope 200; 110(8):1277–82.
8. Coates KW, Kuehl TJ, Bachofen CG, Shull BL. Analysis of surgical complications and patient outcomes in a residency training program. Am J Obstet Gynecol 2001; 184(7):1380–1385.
9. Fallon WF Jr, Wears RL, Tepas JJ 3rd. Resident supervision in the operating room: does this impact on outcome? J Trauma 1993; 35(4):556–561.
10. Gaba DM, Howard SK. Fatigue among clinicians and the safety of patients. N Engl J Med 2002; 347:1249–1255.
11. Galandiuk S, Ahmad P. Impact of sedation and resident teaching on complications of colonoscopy. Dig Surg 1998; 15(1):60–63.
12. Garcia FA, Miller HB, Huggins GR, Gordon TA. Effect of academic affiliation and obstetric volume on clinical outcome and cost of childbirth. Obstet Gynecol 2001; 97(4):567–576.
13. Goldstein SI, Breda SD, Schneider KL. Surgical complications of bedside tracheotomy in an otolaryngology residency program. Laryngoscope 1987; 97(12):1407–1409.

14. Griffith CH 3rd, Wilson JF, Rich EC. Intern call structure and patient satisfaction. J Gen Intern Med 1997; 12(9):586.

15. Gross RD, Sheridan MF, Burgess LP. Endoscopic sinus surgery complications in residency. Laryngoscope 1997; 107(8):1080–1085.

16. Haddad M, Zelikovski A, Gutman H, Haddad E, Reiss R. Assessment of surgical residents' competence based on postoperative complications. Int Surg 1987; 72(4):230–232.

17. Haynes DF, Schwedler M, Dyslin DC, Rice JC, Kerstein MD. Are postoperative complications related to resident sleep deprivation? South Med J 1995; 88(3):283–289.

18. Jacques CH, Lynch JC, Samkoff JS. The effects of sleep loss on cognitive performance of resident physicians. J Fam Pract 1990; 30(6):632.

19. Kazmers A, Ramnauth S, Williams M. Intraoperative insertion of Greenfield filters: lessons learned in a personal series of 152 cases. Am Surg 2002; 68(10):877–882.

20. Khuri SF, Najjar SF, Daley J, Krasnicka B, Hossain M, Henderson WG, Aust JB, Bass B, Bishop MJ, Demakis J, DePalma R, Fabri PJ, Fink A, Gibbs J, Grover F, Hammermeister K, McDonald G, Neumayer L, Roswell RH, Spencer J, Turnage RH. VA National Surgical Quality Improvement Program. Comparison of surgical outcomes between teaching and nonteaching hospitals in the Department of Veterans Affairs. Ann Surg 2001; 234(3):370–383.

21. Kuo AA. Does sleep deprivation impair cognitive and motor performance as much as alcohol intoxication? West J Med 2001; 174:180.

22. Laine C, Goldman L, Soukup JR, Hayes JG. The impact of a regulation restricting medical house staff working hours on the quality of patient care. JAMA 1993; 269:403–404, 2987–2988.

23. Lavernia CJ, Sierra RJ, Hernandez RA. The cost of teaching total knee arthroplasty surgery to orthropaedic surgery residents. Clin Orthop 2000; 380:99–107.

24. Makowiec RL, Nagle DJ, Chow JCY. Outcome of first-time endoscopic carpal tunnel release in a teaching environment. Arthrosc Rel Surg 2002; 18(1).

25. Manolidis S, Takashima M, Kirby M, Scarlett M. Thyroid surgery: a comparison of outcomes between experts and surgeons in training. Otolaryngol Head Neck Surg 2001; 125(1):30–33.

26. Massard G, Roeslin N, Wihlm JM, Dumont P, Lion R, Witz JP, Morand G. The risks of surgical training. A study apropos of 348 pneumonectomies. J Chir (Paris) 1991; 128(3):116–119.

27. Mishra A, Agarwal G, Agarwal A, Mishra SK. Safety and efficacy of total thyroidectomy in hands of endocrine surgery trainees. Am J Surg 1999; 178(5):377–380.

28. Nguyen QA, Cua DJ, Ng M, Rice DH. Safety of endoscopic sinus surgery in a residency training program. Ear Nose Throat J 1999; 78(12):898–902, 904.

29. Peterson LA, Brennan TA, O'Neil AC, Cook EF, Lee TH. Does housestaff discontinuity of care increase the risk for preventable adverse events? Ann Intern Med 1995; 122(12):962–964.

30. Philibert I, Barach P. Resident's hours of work. BMJ 2002; 325:1184–1185.

31. Praseedom RK, Paisley A, Madhavan KK, Garden OJ, Carter DC, Paterson-Brown S. Supervised surgical trainees can perform pancreatic resections safely. J R Coll Surg Edinb 1999; 44(1):16–18.

32. Reznick RK, Folse JR. Effect of sleep deprivation on the performance of surgical residents. Am J Surg 1987; 154(5):520–525.

33. Rich EC, Gifford G, Luxenberg M, Dowd B. The relationship of house staff experience to the cost and quality of inpatient care. JAMA 1990; 263(7):994.

34. Rich EC, Hillson SD, Dowd B, Morris N. Specialty differences in the 'July phenomenon' for Twin Cities teaching hospitals. Med Care 1993; 31(1):73–83.

35. Rich EG, Gifford G, Dowd B. The effects of schedules intern rotation on the cost and quality of teaching hospital care. Eval Health Prof 1994; 17(3):259–272.

36. Samkoff JS, Jacques CH. A review of studies concerning effects of sleep deprivation and fatigue on residents' performance. Acad Med 1991; 66(11):687–693.

37. Sawyer MA, Lim RB, Wong SY, Cirangle PT, Birkmire-Peters D. Telementored laparoscopic cholecystectomy: a pilot study. Stud Health Technol Inform 2000; 70:302–308.

38. Schwartz SG, Holz ER, Mieler WF, Kuhl DP. Retained lens fragments in resident-performed cataract extractions. CLAO J 2002; 28(1):44–47.
39. Shaked A, Calderon I, Durst A. Safety of surgical procedures performed by residents. Arch Surg 1991; 126(5):559–560.
40. Shanafelt TD, Bradley KA, Wipf JE, Back AL. Burnout and self-reported patient care in an internal medicine residency program. Ann Intern Med 2002; 136(5):358–367, 391–393; 137(8):698–700.
41. Shindo ML, Sinha Uk, Rice DH. Safety of thyroidectomy in residency: a review of 186 consecutive cases. Laryngoscope 1995; 105(11):1173–1175.
42. Shulkin DJ. The July phenomenon revisited: are hospital complications associated with new house staff? Am J Med Qual 1995; 10(1):14–17.
43. Skolnick KA, Perlman JI, Long DM, Kernan JM. Neodymium:YAG laser posterior capsulotomies performed by residents at a Veterans Administration Hospital. J Cataract Refract Surg 2000; 26(4):597–601.
44. Smith JP, Mehta RH, Das SK, Tsai T, Karavite DJ, Russman PL, Bruckman D, Eagle KA. Effects of end-of-month admission on length of stay and quality of care among inpatients with myocardial infarction. Am J Med 2002; 113(4):288–293.
45. Stranjalis G. Ruptures cerebral aneurysm: influence of specialist and trainee-performed operations on outcome. Acta Neurochir (Wien) 1996; 138(9):1067–1069.
46. Sullivan CA, Masin J, Maniglia AJ, Stepnick DW. Complications of rhytidectomy in an otolaryngology training program. Laryngoscope 1999; 109(2 pt 1):198–203.
47. Sussman EJ, Kastanis JN, Feigin W, Rosen HM. Surgical outcome for resident and attending surgeons. Am J Surg 1982; 144(2):250–253.
48. Udvarhelyi IS, Rosborough T, Lofgren RP, Lurie N, Epstein AM. Teaching status and resource use for patients with acute myocardial infarction: a new look at the indirect costs of graduate medical education. Am J Public Health 1990; 80(9):1095–1100.
49. Let's keep residents out of community hospitals. Med Econ 1979; 56(3):80–83.
50. Vartiainen E. The results of chronic ear surgery in a training programme. Clin Otolaryngol 1998; 23(2):177–180.
51. Willeke F, Willeke M, Hinz U, Lorenz D, Nitschmann K, Grauer A, Senninger N, Klar E, Herfarth C. Effect of surgeon expertise on the outcome in primary hyperparathyroidism. Arch Surg 1998; 133(10):1066–1071.
52. Wisnicki HJ, Repka MX, Raab E, Hamad GG, Kirsch D, Nath A, Loupe DN. A comparison of the success rates of resident and attending strabismus surgery. J Pediatr Ophthalmol Strabismus 1993; 30(2):118–121.
53. Wolkomir MS, Beecher AC. "Virtual delivery": an interactive role play of abnormal labor Acad Med 1996; 71(5):550.

47

Legal Implications and Strategies for Managing Complications in Spinal Surgery

Joan M. Lewis
Superior Court Judge, San Diego, California, U.S.A.

Heather E. Hansen and John J. Gross
O'Brien & Ryan, LLP, Plymouth Meeting, Pennsylvania, U.S.A.

Steven R. Garfin
University of California, San Diego, California, U.S.A.

I. INTRODUCTION

Medical malpractice lawsuits are of great concern to physicians. As a result of these lawsuits, physicians face skyrocketing costs for medical malpractice insurance premiums and patients face shortages of qualified physicians, as more and more physicians decide it is financially impractical to practice in certain medical and/or geographical areas. Such problems are found to be especially rampant in large cities. Various states have dealt with medical malpractice claims differently. New York, Philadelphia, Washington, D.C., Chicago, and Miami for example, are at one end of the spectrum. They are the leading cities in the United States for jury verdicts against physicians (1). At the other end is California, which has passed laws limiting the noneconomical damages plaintiffs may be entitled to in such actions. Bills have been considered by the U.S. Congress to implement national limits for noneconomic and punitive damages awards to try to control regional legal/financial disparities.

II. OVERVIEW OF THE LEGAL PROCESS

This section presents a brief overview of physician involvement in civil litigation (i.e., medical malpractice). The civil litigation process in medical malpractice matters can be difficult for the practicing physician. It is both time-consuming and emotional for all involved.

In cases where an alleged wrong has occurred—anything from an unexpected scar to death—the injured party (plaintiff) may file a civil lawsuit against the party he or she feels is responsible (defendant). Depending on the nature of the alleged wrong, the plaintiff has a limited amount of time in which to file a lawsuit, i.e., statute of limitations. The statute of limitations varies from state to state. Depending on the jurisdiction, the plaintiff usually has 1–3 years from the date the injury is suffered or, in some cases, discovery of the injury, to file the lawsuit.

Once the complaint has been filed and served in the appropriate court, the attorneys for the defendant (doctor) respond, or answer, the complaint. Since this answer is early in the lawsuit, the response to the complaint may include objections to the complaint and may include allegations against plaintiff (counterclaims) or other defendants (cross claims). Thereafter, the parties to this civil action begin their arduous road to trial.

Once the answer is filed, the process of gathering information to be used at trial, or discovery, begins almost immediately. The two main ways parties conduct discovery is through interrogatories and depositions. Interrogatories are written questions presented to the opposing party, to which the opposing party responds under penalty of perjury. Depositions involve a witness (not necessarily a party to the action), where the witness gives sworn oral testimony in the form of responses to attorney's questions. The information obtained from the depositions and interrogatories lead to obtaining more information, which may be subject to further interrogatories, depositions, or subpoenas until the court-imposed discovery deadline date is reached.

Early in the discovery phase, the plaintiff will request basic information by way of interrogatory requests (written questions). Often the initial set of interrogatories request such information as name of insurance carrier, policy limits, prior lawsuits, and some personal information concerning the doctor's background, education and training. The initial questions call for information that may lead to the discovery of additionally relevant information.

The depositions of the parties occur further down the discovery road. Generally, the doctor's attorney will meet with the doctor prior to the deposition to review any necessary medical records or other relevant documents in preparation for the deposition. It is imperative that the doctor pay close attention to the predeposition instructions and follow the attorney's direction during the deposition. It has been the experience of many defense attorneys that professionals subject to a lawsuit have the mistaken belief they can relatively easily win the lawsuit, or have it dismissed, at the time of the deposition because of the "facts" presented. As a result, the deponent has an urge to give all information available, regardless of whether the questions call for such information. No matter what information is volunteered during the deposition process, it will not lead to the conclusion of the lawsuit. The only goal accomplished by volunteering information without attorney direction is to either lead to additional discovery or hinder the trial strategy of the physician's attorney.

Not long after the onset of the lawsuit or interrogatory and deposition time frame, both sides will enlist the help of a medical expert in the area of medicine subject to the lawsuit to render an opinion as to the appropriate standard of care. A number of other experts may also comment on the issue of causation and damages. "Damage experts" may include both medical professionals and professionals outside the medical arena, such as certified public accounts (CPA), vocational evaluators/counselors, and others.

If the matter cannot be resolved within a certain period of time (whether by settlement or dismissal), a trial will take place. At the trial the finder of fact (judge or jury) will hear testimony from the opposing expert(s), possibly prior and subsequent treating physicians, the parties, and other relevant witnesses. The finder (trier) of fact will often see enlargements of documents and illustrations, as well as pages from pertinent medical records. The parties will present their case clearly and passionately.

III. GROUNDS FOR PROFESSIONAL NEGLIGENCE/MEDICAL MALPRACTICE

In order to prevail in a medical malpractice action, the plaintiff must prove all of the following elements by a preponderance of the evidence: (a) defendant's duty to use such skill, prudence and diligence as other members of the profession possess and use, (b) conduct that breached that duty, (c) a (proximate) causal connection between defendant's negligence and the resulting injury, and (d) actual losses or damages resulted.

Medical specialists must possess and use the learning, care, and skill ordinarily possessed and exercised by practitioners of that specialty under similar circumstances. In fact, a doctor who has special training and experience in a particular field is subject to this standard, even if the doctor has not claimed to be a specialist. Additionally, a specialist who sends a nonspecialist to attend in his stead may be liable for any harm suffered by that patient. A doctor who is not a specialist is held to a standard of ordinary medical skill, knowledge or care, rather than the higher skill of a specialist (unless he or she holds himself or herself out as a specialist.)

A. Negligence in the Diagnosis and Treatment of a Patient

1. Duty to Possess and Use Professional Knowledge, Care, and Skill

A medical doctor is liable for injuries to a patient caused by failure to possess and exercise, in either diagnosis or treatment, the reasonable degree of skill, knowledge, and care that is ordinarily possessed and used by other medical doctors in similar circumstances. Suits often allege that one or more parties caused injury to another because of an act or omission. For example, in surgery, the negligence may be based on a number of aspects of the treatment, such as negligently deciding to perform the surgery, negligently performing the surgery, or failing to obtain informed consent before the surgery.

2. Duty to Consult a Specialist or Refer the Patient

A general practitioner who knows, or in the exercise of reasonable care should know, that special consultation is required, must consult a specialist or refer the patient to a specialist. Failure to do so constitutes malpractice unless the doctor conformed to the standard of a specialist.

3. Duty to Attend Diligently/Duty to Not Abandon Patient

A medical doctor has a duty to attend diligently, i.e., not to abandon the patient. An unwarranted lack of diligence in attending a patient my constitute malpractice.

A doctor is liable for injury resulting from abandonment, neglect, or other failure to attend to the patient throughout that patient's illness or disability, as long as medical attention is necessary.

A doctor may discharge the obligation to the patient by referring the patient to another health care provider or by giving the patient adequate notice and opportunity to find another health care provider.

4. Duty to Hospitalize

It is malpractice for a doctor to fail to hospitalize a patient under circumstances in which standard practice requires hospitalization. Additionally, it may be negligence to send a patient to a hospital that is not equipped to properly treat the patient's medical condition.

5. Duty to Inform

A physician is required to obtain informed consent from a patient before performing any nonemergency procedure. In the words of the famous Jurist Benjamin N. Cardozo (2), "every human of adult years and sound mind has a right to determine what shall be done with his own body." The doctrine of informed consent is designed to ensure that patients receive adequate information regarding the dangers and hazards anticipated, or possible, from the contemplated operation before the provider performs the procedure (3).

A doctor may be liable for a patient's injury that results from a course of treatment or procedure if (a) the doctor failed to make a reasonable disclosure to the patient of the choices of available treatment and the potential dangers inherent in each and (b) a prudent person in the patient's position who had been adequately informed of all significant perils would then not have consented to treatment (4). The doctor has a duty to disclose to the patient information regarding risks and complications of the procedure. While this must include what is likely to happen, as well as the possible adverse results and dangers of the operation, a physician is not required to disclose all known information (5).

The extent of information that must be communicated to the patient does not vary greatly nationally. In almost every jurisdiction the standard is patient oriented. This approach requires that the patient be given all material information that an average, reasonably prudent, person would need to determine whether to proceed with the procedure, remain in the present condition, or seek alternative treatments (6). It is important to note that physicians are not required to give their patients a "complete course in anatomy and to explain every risk, no matter how remote, before a consent [will] be valid" (7). Rather, a physician need only disclose matters that are "specifically germane to [the] surgical or operative treatment"(8). Surgeons must also inform their patients whether any alternative medical procedures exist (9).

Informed consent, in addition to being required before surgery, must be obtained before the patient is given anesthesia, receives radiation and/or chemotherapy, undergoes a blood transfusion, or a medication is given that is either experimental or being used in an experimental manner (10). Finally, and perhaps most relevant to spinal surgery, specific informed consent must be obtained before any surgical device is inserted.

Precisely what must be disclosed is not always clear. For example, as noted above, a surgeon must obtain the consent of the patient before inserting a surgical device. However, in Pennsylvania, for example, the surgeon need not inform the patient about the FDA classification of the device for consent to be "informed"(11). This was the holding of the state's supreme court in a case involving a claim of lack of informed consent where the implanted device was, at the time of implantation, classified by the Food and Drug Administration as Class III, which is the most heavily regulated category. The court found that the FDA classification of the device did not constitute a material fact, risk, complication, or alternative to a surgical procedure, thus informed consent was not required before its use (11). A physician's level of experience with a procedure is also not something that must be disclosed. In a Pennsylvania case, a physician, when asked, told the patient he performed the procedure in question on average once a month. In reality, the physician performed the procedure approximately nine times in the preceding 5 years. The Pennsylvania Superior Court noted that because the patient had asked about the physician's experience, it was clear that it was a relevant factor to the patient in deciding about the procedure thus going right to the purpose of informed consent (12). The state supreme court, however, reversed the decision, noting that the patient must be informed regarding the nature of the procedure itself, not the personal experience of the physician (12).

The Supreme Court of Hawaii reached a similar result where a patient, unhappy with her breast implants, sued her surgeon alleging, *inter alia*, that he had a duty to disclose the fact that he was certified as an otolaryngologist, facial surgeon, and cosmetic surgeon, not a plastic surgeon (13). Regarding actual experience, the Court of Appeals of Washington held a surgeon did not have a duty to inform a patient that he had only performed the laparoscopic procedure at issue on a pig (never a human) (14).

Some states have formed committees to determine precisely what must be disclosed. In Texas, the Texas Medical Disclosure Panel, made up of physicians and attorneys, establishes both the form and the degree of disclosure required (15). This system may have helped the defendant-physician who, before performing a lumbar laminectomy, informed the patient only that the surgery would be exploratory and a "piece of cake," as well as telling him he would be "up and walking around the next day." Obviously, the patient had not been informed of the risks that, unfortunately, occurred—loss of bladder and bowel control, increased leg and back pain, and sexual dysfunction (16).

Who must obtain the consent is probably the most straightforward of the informed consent-related questions. As a general rule, there is no independent duty for any nonphysician to obtain the informed consent of a patient (17). This is not true, however, in some cases. For example, where hospitals are involved in clinical investigations for the FDA, they are bound by federal regulations to obtain an informed consent from any patient undergoing experimental treatment. Thus, in such situations, the hospital assumes an independent duty that it would not ordinarily bear (18). Additionally, this is not to say that information a patient obtains from nonphysicians is not relevant to whether their consent was "informed." The Pennsylvania Superior Court held that information provided by a surgical nurse could be considered by the jury, along with that which was provided by the physician, noting that whether consent was valid is a function of the scope of the information received (19).

B. Battery—Unauthorized Surgery or Treatment

The requirement that informed consent be obtained is rooted in the fact that surgical or operative procedures amount to a battery if not consented to (20). In the law, a battery is considered a tort, or a civil wrong, one commits against another. It occurs when there is an unauthorized harmful, or offensive, contact with another's person or an object intimately connected thereto. Thus, in the eyes of the law, without proper authorization, a physician's procedure is equivalent to a thug's punch.

A doctor who performs an operation to which the patient has not consented, or that is substantially different from the treatment to which the patient consented, has committed a battery. Further, a doctor is liable for any injury or disability that results from the unauthorized treatment, even though it may have been skillfully performed. Since the failure of a physician to obtain informed consent amounts to a battery, the realm of negligence law is not entered (20).

Of note, a doctor can operate or treat without the patient's consent in an emergency or when immediate action is otherwise necessary and it is impracticable to obtain consent.

C. Liability for Inflicting Emotional Distress

Doctors, in the ways in which they interact with patients, can become liable for the torts of negligent, or intentional, infliction of emotional distress. In a California case the court agreed that doctors negligently and incorrectly told a patient that she had syphilis and that she needed to tell her new husband, which led to severe, unwarranted "emotional distress" for the plaintiff (21).

D. Fraud/Misrepresentation

A doctor may be liable to a patient for the intentional tort of fraud, in which case a longer statute of limitation may apply and punitive damages can be recovered.

E. Sexual Contact with, or Harassment of, a Patient

Sexual contact between a patient and a doctor may constitute malpractice or other potential torts. Under American Medical Association (AMA) guidelines, two broad types of physician misconduct are (a) misconduct arising from an inability to contain or control an emotional involvement with the patient, and (b) conscious exploitation of the doctor's status, knowledge, and the power to coerce or trick the patient into sexual conduct.

F. Causation

In a medical malpractice lawsuit, the plaintiff must establish by reasonable medical probability that the doctor's negligence was the legal cause of the patient's injuries. If this second element in a cause of action for medical negligence is not established, the plaintiff's case must fail.

G. Damages

The final element the plaintiff must establish in a medical malpractice claim is that the plaintiff suffered damages as a result of the doctor's negligence. Without establishing this element, the plaintiff's claim must fail. On occasion, a doctor may admit liability and have the trial proceed on the issue of damages alone.

IV. PROVING A MEDICAL MALPRACTICE CASE

Ordinarily, allegations of negligence must have the support of a medical expert. Without an expert, a plaintiff's case will fail as a matter of law. Depending on his or her expertise and why the plaintiff's attorney hired the medical expert, the expert testifies to establish the above elements—that there was a breach of the duty that caused damages to the plaintiff. The defense will obtain its own experts to testify as to the above. The two experts may end up criticizing each other before the litigation is through. The only time an expert is not required in a medical malpractice action is when the care and skill required in a particular circumstance is within the common knowledge of laypersons, such as leaving an object in a patient after surgery.

V. DEFENSES TO A MEDICAL MALPRACTICE CLAIM

A. No Relationship

An early resolution to a lawsuit can occur if it is established that there is a lack of a patient-physician relationship. If this can be established, there is no duty owed to the plaintiff. As a result, the plaintiff's case will fail as a matter of law.

B. Patient's Fault, or Contribution, to the Injury

A patient's failure to use ordinary care to prevent his or her own harm, including the failure to obtain treatment, may constitute contributory or comparative negligence. The defendant doctor has the burden of pleading, and proving, that the patient was contributorily/comparatively negligent and that the patient's negligence was a legal cause of the injury.

C. Statute of Limitations

A medical malpractice action for injury or death must be brought within the requisite time frame. The time frames in which to bring a lawsuit differ for adults versus minors and also differ from state to state. Generally, the statutory time frame for adult actions is 1–3 years after the date of injury, or 1–2 years after the discovery of that injury. For minors, the general rule is that the malpractice action be brought within 3 years from the date of the alleged wrongful act, or before the minor's eighteenth birthday, whichever provides the longer period. The statute of limitations is an important defense for doctors. It is imperative that the plaintiff consult with an attorney as to the state laws concerning the statute of limitations.

VI. DISCLOSURE

Problems concerning exactly what must be disclosed (provided) to patients are not confined to the area of informed consent. As an example, law in most states requires disclosure where a lethal weapon injury has occurred and when child abuse is suspected. Medical records must be provided when the patient, or an authorized representative, requests them.* More relevant to the focus of this chapter, however, are other areas where disclosure may or may not be required and/or authorized. These areas include situations where a medical error has occurred and litigation-related disclosures. Also, improper disclosure, actually leading to litigation, can be an issue.

VII. ALLEGED MEDICAL ERRORS

Medical errors can occur, some of which result in death. According to the Institute of Medicine (IOM), medical errors in hospitals kill between 44,000 and 98,000 patients annually (22). Although there is debate as to the accuracy of this estimate, the fact remains that, as with anything in life, errors are made in all areas of medicine, and not all of them result in death (23–25).[†] Even before this study was published, the Joint Commission on Accreditation of Health Care Organizations (JCAHO) was aware of the high number of medical errors occurring in the United States. In an effort to reduce the number of these errors, JCAHO in 1996 implemented the Sentinel Event Program. JCAHO defined a sentinel event as "an unexpected occurrence involving death or

---

*In Pennsylvania, these areas are governed by 18 Pa.C.S.A. 5106; 11 Pa.C.S.A. 2204; and 49 Pa.Code 16.61 (18); respectively.
[†]Some experts have suggested this study is flawed as it also included bad outcomes that may not have been due to mistakes.

serious physical or psychological injury, or the risk thereof" (26). Sentinel events include loss of limb or function, events resulting in unanticipated death or major permanent loss of function not related to the natural course of the patient's illness/underlying condition, suicide, infant abduction/discharge to wrong family, rape, hemolytic transfusion reaction involving administration of blood or blood products having major blood group incompatibilities, and surgery on wrong patient/body part. This program required hospitals to, on the occurrence of a sentinel event, conduct a root cause analysis, implement improvements to reduce risk, and monitor effects of improvements. It also encouraged hospitals to report events that result in death or serious injury, as well as corrective measures, to JCAHO.

Following the release of the 1999 IOM report, Dennis O'Leary, M.D., president of JCAHO, testified before a U.S. Senate subcommittee about the problems emanating from the nondisclosure of errors (27). Dr. O'Leary expressed the concern of JCAHO that fear of repercussion from disclosure of errors led to cover-ups and nondisclosure, resulting in increased patient harm/malpractice. According to O'Leary, "the blame and punishment orientation of our society drives errors underground" (27). Shortly thereafter, JCAHO modified its Sentinel Events Program. Most significantly, Rule 1.2.2 was implemented, requiring that "patients and, when appropriate, their families are informed about the outcomes of care, including unanticipated outcomes" (28). The intent of this new provision was that "the responsible licensed independent practitioner, or his or her designee, clearly explains the outcomes of any treatments or procedures to the patient and, when appropriate, the family, whenever those outcomes differ significantly from the anticipated outcomes" (28).

Under the JCAHO guidelines, individual organizations are allowed to set more specific parameters as long as they remain consistent with the JCAHO definitions. In Lexington, Kentucky, for example, one Veteran Affairs Medical Center does far more than is required. According to Steven Kraman, M.D., "it doesn't serve patients to hide from our mistakes" (29). As such, on the identification of a "serious error," the patient (or next of kin) is promptly notified by hospital administrators who admit the mistake, offer to further investigate the case, assist with the filing of claim forms, offer prompt compensation, and even encourage the injured to get a lawyer. While it is unclear whether their disclosure policy has decreased the frequency with which mistakes are made, it has reduced the amount the hospital has paid out in claims. The Lexington VA Center's average settlement is $83,000 less than the national VA average (29). This is believed to be the result of less hostility between the patient and/or family and the hospital. Some states have enacted laws requiring certain levels of disclosure. In Pennsylvania, hospitals are required to develop, implement, and comply with a Patient Safety Plan (30). This plan must provide for ease in, and nonretaliation for, medical staff reporting "serious events" or "incidents" which, under the law, they are required to report (31). This law also provides that patients be notified in writing within 7 days of the occurrence, or discovery, of a serious event (31).

The situation will usually dictate the proper person to relay the negative information to the patient or the family. Where surgery is involved, for example, the surgeon is usually the best choice to relay the complication or mistake. This may not be true, however, if the surgeon is distraught because of what has occurred, or is angered by other providers, or assistants, that "caused" the situation. It is advisable, in any case, to have another member of the medical staff present. The actual conversation should include a recitation of the facts of the incident, the effect it had or will have on the patient, what was or can be done, and an expression of regret. There should not be an admission of liability. According to the American Society of Healthcare Risk Management, "providing an explanation of what resulted from a test or treatment does not need to get into expression of fault or blame. Indeed, until all the facts are known about what occurred, what systems were implicated, etc., it may be inadvisable to do more than furnish an explanation regarding the unanticipated outcome" (32). It is important to remember that, during the course of any resultant litigation, the physician may be asked about any conversations he or she had with the patient or family. The physician should assume that the patient's attorney will explore any liability-oriented statements made during the discovery process and, more importantly, while the defendant sits alone in the witness chair at trial. Finally, the substance of any conversations that do take place should be documented in the patient's chart (see Sec. VIII).

Physicians can become involved in litigation even when they are not a party. Most frequently, the role of the physician will be limited to his or her experience as treater of an injured party. Most often this involves nothing more than providing the patient, or the patient's attorney, with a copy of the patient's chart. Should the physician be called to testify as to the treatment rendered, what he or she is permitted to discuss may be limited, not only by the terms of the Hippocratic Oath, but also by state law. Under Pennsylvania law, "no physician shall be allowed, in any civil matter, to disclose any information which he acquired in attending the patient in a professional capacity, and which was necessary to enable him to act in that capacity, which shall tend to blacken the character of the patient, without consent of said patient, except in civil matters brought by such patient, for damages on account of personal injuries" (33). Other constraints on the extent of testimony permitted exist under both the rules of evidence for the jurisdiction and the facts at hand.

Another way a physician can become involved in litigation via disclosure is to disclose too much. In such situations the physician can become the target of litigation. Pennsylvania courts have seen a number of such actions. Patients can sue a treating physician for defamation for conversations with defense counsel to the extent any disclosures made were unrelated to the action (34). They may also bring actions where the physician discloses to one spouse that the other has a sexually transmitted disease (35) or where the physician shows pictures of, and discloses information about, a patient at job activity (36).

As discussed in Sec. III.A, disclosing too little can also subject a physician to liability. It can also have an effect on the defenses allowed under the law. A clear example of this is where a patient brings a claim and the physician wishes to raise the expiration of the statute of limitations as a defense. Courts have prevented defendant physicians from doing so where, had the physician disclosed his or her error or the complication at the time, the patient could have brought the action within the statute. For example, the Supreme Court of Arizona reversed the dismissal of what appeared to be a claim filed outside the statute of limitations where the defendant dentist failed to disclose his error to the plaintiff, causing the plaintiff to be without reasonable notice to investigate whether negligence had occurred (37). A similar result was reached in Massachusetts, where the court found that where a physician has a duty to disclose, silence might amount to fraudulent concealment, which serves to toll the statute of limitations (38). An Arkansas court has placed an affirmative duty on the physician to disclose information where they have primary control over relevant information regarding an alleged wrong and plaintiff is unaware of the alleged wrong (39).

VIII. DOCUMENTATION

The manner in which the provider documents his or her treatment of the patient in the chart is of great significance, as mistakes or omissions can have medical, legal, and financial implications. A patient whose chart is not properly updated may receive duplicative, or otherwise wrong, medical care. The physician providing the duplicative, or otherwise wrong, care may find him or herself in legal trouble. From a legal aspect, documentation is essentially equivalent to the care itself (40). The records may be the only proof the physician has (or needs) in situations where an insurer questions that physician's billing (41). In fact, prosecutors may use chart entries to prove allegations of criminal activity, such as Medicare billing fraud (42).

JCAHO provides for the proper process of documentation in its guidelines (43). Some states have addressed the issue in statutes. In Pennsylvania, for example, state law specifically regulates the timing, corrections, and alterations to medical records (44). Noncompliance with the law can lead to the jury being made aware of the noncompliance and is grounds for license suspension (44). Many courts have commented on what should be included in a patient's chart. Most agree that it should be a concise, factual notation of the patient's progress, vital signs, and informational notes on the patient (45).

Liability has been imposed on physicians based on what was (or was not) in the patient's chart. In a Pennsylvania case the plaintiff's experts were permitted to testify that the defendant/attending physician failed to properly treat the patient based on failure to document certain procedures in the patient's chart (46). Specifically, the attending was alleged to have allowed a third year resident to deliver plaintiff's child without supervision. The experts were permitted to opine both that this had occurred and that the attending had been negligent based simply on the lack of notation in the chart that the attending was present (46). A Louisiana court reached a similar result where the family of the decedent patient brought an action based on alleged substandard monitoring of the patient as evidenced by the lack of notations in the chart (46). Operating under the maxim "not charted, not done," the court allowed plaintiff's experts to testify that the patient was not properly monitored based on the nurses' inability to specifically recall the patient and the lack of notation that monitoring had taken place (46). In a similar case, a court held that because no entries had been made in the chart, nothing had been done through the night for the patient, thus imposing liability was proper (47). Deciding whether the correct diagnosis was, or could have been, made often includes a review of the documentation by both physicians and nonphysicians (48).

IX. PROTECTION OF ASSETS*

The following provides limited discussion for general information only on this topic. The information should be considered with respect to specific needs and regional laws. Appropriate financial and legal advice should always be obtained.

Even the best and most careful physicians may find themselves in litigation. Once there, anything can happen. While it is unpleasant to have to consider, one should not underestimate the importance of shielding assets. The following sets forth the various ways

---

*This section was written by H. E. Hansen and J. J. Gross.

physicians can protect their assets. For most, insurance will be the most important (if not only) shield from personal liability they will need.

The first line of defense for physicians is the same as it is for the average home or car owner—insurance. Medical malpractice insurance, while expensive, is necessary. There are three main types of medical malpractice insurance: occurrence made, claims made, and tail. Occurrence made coverage provides insurance protection for a physician no matter when a lawsuit is filed, as long as that insurance company was the carrier at the time of the alleged event. Under a claims made policy, the insurer only has to provide coverage if it was the carrier both at the time of the event and the time the claim was filed. Tail insurance, on the other hand, covers claims that have occurred under a previous claims made policy. It is most commonly needed when a physician changes employment or insurance companies. While tail insurance is more expensive than the other types of insurance ($1\frac{1}{2}$–2 times a typical premium), it is a necessity for a physician. This cost is often incurred by the practice the physician is joining.

As with any insurance policy, physicians should review potential polices and consider such things as the limits, and the scope, of the coverage. They should also consider the consent/control over settlement rights the physician retains should litigation arise. Additionally, physicians may want to consult with colleagues and/or medical malpractice defense attorneys to gauge the reputation of the insurance company regarding such things as their policies on expenditures, including expert witnesses and their responsiveness to settlement requests/negotiations.

Other types of insurance are available to physicians. One is an umbrella liability policy, which provides excess personal injury protection. In short, it covers the "over" of liability insurance. It also covers such things as false claims and intentional acts. Another type of insurance is a litigation expense policy. Only offshore insurance companies issue these. They cover attorneys' fees and costs, but have no cash value and will not pay creditors. There is also a settlement option included in this—the physician can normally choose to use the money to settle the case rather than as fees for their attorneys. Besides the security of the coverage, the biggest advantage to this type of policy is that a large portion of the "unearned premiums" is refunded. However, the refund of these premiums can have tax implications, such as showing as income or leading to the loss of deductions. One benefit is that the amount paid in premiums comes off of the physician's ledger, which may be useful should a debtor/creditor situation arise.

The second line of defense physicians might consider is transferring assets. Any transfer made, however, must not run afoul of the Uniform Fraudulent Transfer Act (UFTA). As its name implies, the UFTA prohibits fraudulent conveyances. Most commonly, these are conveyances performed without any, or sufficient, consideration, usually to shield assets from a creditor. Some common fraudulent conveyances are gifts over which the transferor retains control, transfers made during insolvency, and transfers made with the intent of keeping assets from creditors. Courts will allow circumstantial evidence in these cases, and if the court deems the conveyance fraudulent, the transfer will be set aside and the transferee will be forced to forward the assets to the creditor. Transfers to a trust set up after a claim has been made are almost always deemed fraudulent and lacking consideration. Even transfers to offshore trusts may not protect the assets from creditors.

Another type of transfer is gift giving to a spouse. If done correctly, this strategy can reduce federal and state taxes. However, as with trusts, the transfer must occur before the creditor issue arises. It is also important to remember that if the spouse dies, the protection continues only if the proper estate planning has occurred (i.e., planning that prevents the property from coming back to the transferee on the death of the spouse). Additionally, this can result in tax issues, as an increased tax cost can result from the failure to utilize the tax credits available to both spouses. Another potential problem with spousal transfers is, obviously, the effect of divorce. A court is unlikely to return assets to a transferring spouse when the transfer was for the purpose of avoiding creditors.

Transfers are also sometimes accomplished via an asset return arrangement where one transfers assets to another with a "secret understanding" that the assets will be returned once the creditor issue has passed. This strategy is not advisable for many reasons. First, if the matter goes to court, one of two things can happen: the arrangement will be disclosed, resulting in the court undoing the transaction and making the assets available to the creditor, or the arrangement is not disclosed, the transferee denies it under oath and opens himself up to a perjury charge. Another problem is that this type of transfer is essentially a gift and thus will be taxed as one. Additionally, the transferred assets become available to the creditors of the transferee. Of course, the most fundamental problem with this strategy is that one is literally giving one's assets away.

As noted above, another popular method is transferring assets into a trust. Trusts can be broken down into two general categories: revocable and irrevocable. Revocable trusts are those that allow one to retain control over the disposition and use of the assets. This type of trust is useful in reducing probate costs on the death of the individual, but is not as useful in asset protection, as most courts allow claimants and creditors to get to the assets in a revocable trust. An irrevocable trust, on the other hand, is one in which control over the assets is relinquished, although some indirect control is permitted.

Trusts set up in, and under, the laws of a foreign nation, or offshore trusts, are sometimes used to protect assets. Before doing this, however, one should consider not only the laws and stability of the foreign government, but also the recently increased scrutiny by the Internal Revenue Service IRS of such transactions. Using these types of trusts to avoid civil liability can result in criminal liability for such things as tax evasion and conspiracy. Finally, courts are often not receptive to arguments that one has truly relinquished their control in the assets they place in offshore trusts and thus may not uphold the expected protection.

The third line of defense physicians might consider is called transformation of assets. Transformations involve the conversion of assets from unprotected forms (cash, etc.) to property protected by the law. For example, one could purchase personal residences, annuities, and life insurance policies or transfer the assets into a business such as a limited partnership or nonmanaging limited liability company in a state that limits creditors' remedies to charging these entities. Numerous legal and financial considerations must be carefully evaluated before undertaking any aggressive form of asset-protection procedures.

For physicians practicing with a group, there are separate liability issues to be considered. The actions of others in your group, especially nonphysicians or physicians with no ownership interests in the practice, can subject the physician to liability. Nonmedical liability can exist as well, where, for example, a practice fails and creditors go to its constituents for their money. For the most part, protection from types of claims described in this paragraph exists in the physician's choice of entity form. There are a few entity choices for physicians. It is important to note that no corporate form can shield one from his or her own individual actions or acts.

Simply incorporating is the most common form of physician practices. Many states have a special type of corporation available only to professionals (physicians, attorneys, accountants, architects, and engineers). In Pennsylvania this type of entity is called a professional corporation, or PC. The corporate form has its share of problems, but does provide comprehensive protection for the owners or shareholders. Additionally, the IRS now allows small corporations to make a subchapter S election, eliminating the double taxation problem that plagued corporations for years.* The other main choices for physician practices are the limited liability entities—partnerships and companies, or LLPs and LLCs. Like corporations, these entities shield its constituents from certain important types of liability. As far as physician practices are concerned, they are not very different from the S corporations. They offer substantially the same protection and use the same flow-through tax model. However, there are important differences as well, which is why, as with any important business decision, the physician may need to consult both an accountant and an attorney.

REFERENCES

1. National Association of Insurance Commissioners, 1998.
2. Schloendorff v. The Society of New York Hosp. 105 N.E. 92 (1914)(NY Ct. of App.).
3. Gray v. Grunnagle, 223 A.2d 663, 670 (1966).
4. Rogers v. Lu, 485 A.2d 54, 56 (1984). See also Festa v. Greenberg, 511 A.2d 1371, 1373 (1986), allocatur denied, 527 A.2d 541 (1987).
5. Cooper v. Roberts, 286 A.2d 647, 650 n.3 (1971); Gouse v. Cassel, 615 A.2d 331, 334 (1992); Nogowski v. Alemo-Hammad, 691 A.2d 950, 957 (1997); Rowinsky v. Sperling, 681 A.2d 785, 788 (1996), allocatur denied, 690 A.2d 237 (1997); Hoffman v. Brandywine Hosp., 661 A.2d 397, 401 (1995).
6. Southard v. Temple, 781 A.2d 101 (2001); 40 P.S. 1303.504; Texas Medical Liability and Insurance Improvement Act, Tex.Rev.Civ. Stat.Ann. art. 4590i, subchapter F, sec. 6.01–6.07.
7. Nogowski, 691 A.2d at 957 (quoting Jeffries v. McCague, 363 A.2d 1167, 1171 (1976)).
8. Kaskie v. Wright, 589 A.2d 213, 217 (1991).
9. Gouse, 615 A.2d at 333–34.
10. 40 P.S. 1303.504.
11. Southard, 781 A.2d at 101.
12. Duttry v. Patterson, 741 A.2d 199 (1999).
13. Ditto v. McCurdy, 947 P.2d 952 (1997).
14. Whiteside v. Lukson, 947 P.2d 1263 (1997).
15. Tex. Rev. Civ. Stat. Ann. art. 4590i, subchapter F, sec. 6.04(b).
16. Walsh v. Kubiak, 661 A.2d 416 (1995).
17. Watkins v. HUP, 737 A.2d 263 (1999); Southard, 781 A.2d at 101.
18. Friter v. Iolab Corporation, 607 A.2d 1111 (1992).
19. Foflygen v. Kislin, 723 A.2d 705 (1999).
20. Montgomery v. Bazaz-Sehgal, M.D. 798 A.2d 742 (2002).
21. Molien v. Kaiser Found. Hosps., 616 P.2d 813 (1980).
22. "To Err is Human: Building a Safer Health System." Institute of Medicine. December 1999.
23. Brennan, TA. The Institute of Medicine report on medical errors – could it do harm? *N Engl J Med* 342:1123–1125. 2000.

---

*Corporations are separate entities and, as such, must pay taxes. The shareholders of corporations must pay taxes on their gains from the corporation. With small corporations, this often resulted in shareholders personally paying tax twice, thus the "double taxation problem." The subchapter S election allows tax to "pass through" to the shareholders as with partnerships to its members.

24. McDonald CJ, Weiner M, Hui SL. "Deaths Due to Medical Errors Are Exaggerated in Institute Of Medicine Report." JAMA. 284:93–95. July 5, 2000.

25. Leape LL. Institute of Medicine medical error figures are not exaggerated. JAMA 2000; 284:95–97.

26. Joint Commission on Accreditation of Health Care Organizations, R.I. 1.2 (effective July, 2001).

27. Dennis O'Leary, M.D., testimony before the United States Senate Committee on Appropriations Subcommittee on Labor, Health and Human Services, Education, and Related Agencies, February 22, 2000.

28. Joint Commission on Accreditation of Health Care Organizations, R.I. 1.2.2.

29. John McKenzie, An honest hospital: hospital cuts malpractice damage by admitting errors to patients. ABCNEWS.COM. June 28, 2001.

30. 40 P.S. 1303.306–307.

31. 40 P.S. 1303.308.

32. American Society of Healthcare Risk Management. Perspectives on Disclosure. April 2001.

33. 42 Pa. C.S.A. 5929.

34. Moses v. McWilliams, 549 A.2d 950 (1988).

35. Haddad v. Gopal, 787 A.2d 975 (2001).

36. McKay v. Geadah, 50 Pa. D. & C.3d 435 (1988).

37. Walk v. Ring, 44 P.3d 990 (2002).

38. Gonzalez v. U.S., 284 F.3d 281 (2002).

39. Roberts v. Francis, 128 F.3d 647 (1997).

40. Frank J. Cavico, Nancy M. Cavico, The Nursing Profession in the 1990's: Negligence and Malpractice Liability. 43 Clev. St. L. Rev. 557 (1995).

41. John B. Reiss, PhD, Esq. [see generally, "Coding, Documenting, and Billing Physician Services: A Growing Target for Government Enforcement Agencies?" The Health Lawyer. 9 NO.4 Health Law. 9 (1997)].

42. State v. Romero, 574 So.2d 330 (1990).

43. Joint Commission on Accreditation of Health Care Organizations regulations.

44. 40 P.S. 1303.511.

45. Smith v. State (La.), 517 So.2d 1072 (1987).

46. Gates v. Harris, 29 Phila. Co. Rptr. 94 (1995).

47. Harrington v. Rush-Presbyterian, 569 N.E.2d 15 (1990).

48. Smith v. Rossman, 23 Phila. Co. Rptr. 87 (1985).

Index